Infections:

*Recognition,
Understanding,
Treatment*

Infections:

Recognition, Understanding, Treatment

EDITED BY

J.-C. Pechère

J. Acar
M. Armengaud
B. Grenier
R. Moellering Jr.
M. Sande
F. Waldvogel
S. Zinner

With The Special Assistance of
C. Cherubin

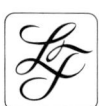

Lea & Febiger   *1984*   *Philadelphia*

Lea & Febiger
600 Washington Square
Philadelphia, PA 19106-4198
U.S.A.
(215) 922-1330

Library of Congress Cataloging in Publication Data

Pechère, J.C. (Jean-Claude)
  Infections: Recognition, Understanding, Treatment

  Bibliography: p.
  Includes index.
  1. Communicable diseases. I. Title. [DNLM:
1. Communicable diseases—Diagnosis. 2. Communicable diseases—Therapy.
WC 100 I4027]
RC111.P43   1983   616.9   83-9855
ISBN 0-8121-0900-7

Les Infections. Copyright © 1984 by Edisem.
Infections: Recognition, Understanding, Treatment. Copyright © 1984 by Lea & Febiger.
Copyright under the International Copyright Union. All Rights Reserved. This book is protected by copyright. No part of it may be reproduced in any manner or by any means without written permission of the Publisher.

PRINTED IN THE UNITED STATES OF AMERICA

Print Number: 5 4 3 2 1

Preface

In Alice's Wonderland, a School of Bakery Science was established. Prestigious teachers taught basic phytology, comparative phytobiology, and, for obvious practical reasons, an advanced course on the respective properties of angiosperms and apetalous dicotyledons within the class of Phanerogamae, as well as geography (Where does wheat grow?), the physics of solids (elucidating at long last the mysteries of leavening agents), and, of course, the behavioral sciences and statistics. What became of the young bakery science graduates after a 3-year course of studies? They set up shop and baked bad bread.

In their choice and presentation of the subject matter, the authors of this book have made a special effort to stay close to the patient. Instead of the usual nosologic and academic format, they have attempted to proceed along the different steps that a physician follows in practice. As an example, let us take acute hematogenous osteomyelitis. The patient generally has a fever, as well as swelling and tenderness over an osteoarticular structure. When these presenting signs are found, one must first determine clinically whether the lesion appears to be of infectious origin and whether bone, joint, or some more superficial involvement is present. An effort is made to confirm the bone involvement by means of radiologic examinations and scintiscans while different specimens are taken, to try to identify the causative organism. It is then possible to plan treatment based on the organism that has been discovered and its susceptibility to antibiotics. If we now consult the chapter on osteoarticular infections (see Chapter 28), we see that this practical sequence is followed.

To underscore this "true-to-life" approach and to facilitate the learning process by the reader, the text is provided with many educational objectives, for example, "Decide when a chest roentgenogram is necessary in patients with fever and cough." This objective includes several implicit or explicit elements: (1) a practical situation, that is, consultation of a physician by a patient for fever and cough; (2) the principal problem that underlies this situation, such as the possible identification of pneumonia; (3) the solution to the problem, for instance, preparation of a chest roentgenogram in certain cases. The objective nearly always begins with a verb, so the principal action required is clear; in this case, the verb is "decide," which tells us that a chest roentgenogram should not be ordered for all patients with fever and cough. In addition, at least insofar as is possible, the successive objectives are linked together, to reflect the different steps of the diagnosis and treatment. Thus, for septicemia and bacteremia, the path is as follows (Objectives 13–1 through 13–6): establish the indication and prepare adequate blood cultures; rapidly consider the organism or organisms most likely responsible for the infection; look for signs of shock; begin immediate treatment; interpret the results of the blood cultures; and modify the treatment if necessary following the study of the causative organism in the laboratory. Simply by reading the objectives, one can obtain a picture of the general scope of a question.

The chapters also include boxes that provide additional information, whether microbiologic (What is a Rickettsia?), epidemiologic (such as in infectious mononucleosis), clinical (as in the mucocutaneous lymph node syndrome), or practical (the Schick test). This presentation was adopted to avoid breaking the continuity of the main text.

Even the best of books can never, by itself, enable us to bake good bread, much less to practice good medicine. We hope at least to be useful to physicians and their patients.

Québec   J.C. Pechère, M.D.

Contributors

Jacques F. Acar, M.D.
Professor of Medical Microbiology,
Université Pierre et Marie Curie;
Chief, Microbiology and Infectious Diseases
  Department,
Hôpital St-Joseph and Hôpital Broussais,
Paris, France

Maxime Armengaud, M.D.
Professor of Infectious and Tropical Diseases,
Faculty of Medicine,
University P. Sabatier;
Head of the Infectious and Tropical Disease
  Service,
Hôpital Purpan
Toulouse, France

Michel G. Bergeron, M.D.
Professor of Medicine and Microbiology,
Université Laval;
Chief, Infectious Disease Service,
Le Centre Hospitalier de L'Université Laval,
Québec, Canada

Phillippe Bernard, M.D.
Associate Professor, Department of Ear, Nose,
  and Throat,
University of Ottawa;
Head, Department of Otolaryngology,
Children's Hospital of Eastern Ontario (Ottawa);
Member of the Staff,
The Hospital for Sick Children, Toronto
  (Otolaryngology),
Ottawa, Canada

Denise Blum, M.D.
Pediatric Intensive Care Unit,
Hôpital Saint-Pierre,
Brussels, Belgium

Henry F. Chambers, M.D.
Clinical Instructor, Medical Service,
San Francisco General Hospital,
San Francisco, California

Charles Cherubin, M.D.
Clinical Professor of Medicine,
Hahneman College of Medicine;
Director of Medicine
Bayley Seton Hospital
Staten Island, New York

Yvon Cormier, M.D.
Lecturer, Department of Medicine,
Université Laval;
Pulmonary Specialist, Center for Pneumology,
Le Centre Hospitalier de L'Université Laval,
Québec, Canada

André Dachy, Ph.D.
Professor of Pediatrics,
Université Libre de Brussels;
Head of Pediatrics Department,
Hôpital Saint-Pierre,
Bruxelles, Belgium

Patrick Demol, Ph.D.
Associate Professor,
Université Libre de Brussels;
Resident,
Hôpital Saint-Pierre,
Brussels, Belgium

Pierre Déry, M.D.
Professor of Pediatrics,
Université Laval;
Department of Pediatric,
Le Centre Hospitalier de Université Laval,
Québec, Canada

Marc Desmeules, M.D.
Associate Professor, Department of Medicine,
Université Laval;
Director, Center for Pneumology,
Le Centre Hospitalier de Université Laval,
Québec, Canada

Jacques Drucker, M.D.
Pediatrics Assistant,
Centre Hospitalier Regional de Tours,
Centre de Pediatrie Gatien de Clocheville,
Tours, France

François Fékété, M.D.
Faculty of Medicine,
Microbiology Laboratory,
Université Laval,
Québec, Canada

Pearce Gardner, M.D.
Director of Infectious Diseases Training Program,
Program Director of Internal Medicine Training Program,
University of Chicago, Division of the Biological Sciences and the Pritzker School of Medicine;
Physician,
University of Chicago Hospitals and Clinics,
Chicago, Illinois

Alasdair M. Geddes, M.D.
Professor of Infectious Diseases,
University of Birmingham;
Consultant Physician,
East Birmingham Hospital,
Birmingham, England

Fred W. Goldstein, M.D.
Assistant of Microbiology and Infectious Disease,
Department of Microbiology,
Hôpital St-Joseph,
Paris, France

Pierre C. Gosselin
Lecturer, Department of Obstetrics and Gynecology,
Faculty of Medicine,
Université Laval;
Member, Department of Gynecology,
Hôtel-Dieu de Québec,
Québec, Canada

Bernard Grenier, M.D.
Professor of Infectious Diseases,
Faculty of Medicine,
Université François Rabelais Tours;
Chief, Medical Department,
Centre de Pédiâtrie Gatien de Clocheville,
Tours, France

Jean-Marie Hubrechts, M.D.
Clinical Biology Specialist,
Head of Department, Bacteriology and Serology,
Centre Hospitalier J. Bracops,
Brussels, Belgium

Jean Joly, M.D.
Faculty of Medicine,
Microbiology Laboratory,
Université Laval,
Québec, Canada

Jean H. Jonas
Professor, Department of Microbiology and Immunology,
Université de Montréal;
Director, Department of Microbiology and Immunology,
Hôpital Ste-Justine,
Montréal, Canada

André Kahn, M.D.
Associate Professor of Pediatrics,
Université Libre de Brussels;
Pediatric Intensive Care Unit,
Hôpital Saint-Pierre,
Brussels, Belgium

Jacques LaForge, M.D.
Lecturer, Department of Medicine,
Université Laval;
Center for Pneumology,
Le Centre Hospitalier de L'Université Laval,
Québec, Canada

Michel Laverdiere, M.D.
Associate Professor of Clinical Medicine, and Microbiologist,
Department of Microbiology,
Université de Montréal,
Montréal, Canada

Daniel Lederer, M.D.
Assistant Professor, Section of Medicine,
Brown University;
Director, Pulmonary Division,
The Miriam Hospital,
Providence, Rhode Island

Raymond Lessard, M.D.
Associate Professor of Medicine,
Université Laval;
Department of Dermatology,
Hôtel-Dieu de Québec,
Quebéc, Canada

Bernard Mansheim, M.D.
Clinical Assistant Professor of Medicine and Infectious Diseases,
University of Florida College of Medicine;
Consultant Epidemiologist,
Alachua General Hospital,
Gainesville, Florida

John McGowan, M.D.
Professor of Pathology and Laboratory Medicine,
Professor of Medicine (Infectious Diseases),
Emory University School of Medicine;
Director, Clinical Microbiology,
Grady Memorial Hospital,
Atlanta, Georgia

Contributors

Rollande Michaud
Clinical Professor of Medicine,
Université Laval;
Clinician, Department of Ophthalmology,
Le Centre Hospitalier de L'Université Laval,
Québec, Canada

Robert C. Moellering, Jr.,
Shields Warren-Mallinckrodt Professor of
 Clinical Research,
Harvard Medical School;
Physician-in-Chief, Department of Medicine,
New England Deaconess Hospital,
Boston, Massachusetts

Yves Morin, M.D.
Professor, Department of Medicine,
Université Laval;
Department of Cardiology,
Hôtel-Dieu de Québec,
Québec, Canada

Gilles J. Murray, M.D.
Professor of Medicine and Microbiology,
Université Laval;
Microbiologist and Consultant in Infectious
 Diseases,
Hôpital du Saint-Sacrement,
Québec, Canada

M. Para, M.D.
Assistant Professor of Medicine,
Assistant Professor of Medical Microbiology,
The Ohio State University;
Division of Infectious Diseases,
University Hospital,
Columbus, Ohio

Jean-Claude Pechère, M.D.
Head, Microbiology Department
Hôtel-Dieu de Québec
Québec, Canada

Michael Rein, M.D.
Associate Professor of Medicine,
Division of Infectious Diseases,
University of Virginia School of Medicine,
Charlottesville, Virginia

Michel Rey, M.D.
Professor of Infectious and Tropical Diseases,
Chief, Infectious Diseases Unit,
Le Centre Hospitalier Universitaire Hôtel-Dieu
Paris, France

Jean Robert, M.D.
Clinical Professor of Medicine,
Department of Microbiology,
Université de Montréal;
Microbiologist,
Chief, Department of Community Health,
Montréal, Canada

Jean-Claude Rolland, M.D.
Professor of Pediatrics,
Université François Rabelais Tours;
Chief, Pediatrics Service,
Centre de Pédiâtrie Gatien de Clocheville,
Tours, France

Alain Rousseau, M.D.
Professor and Chairman of Ophthalmology,
Université Laval;
Chairman, Department of Ophthalmology,
Le Centre Hospitalier de L'Université Laval,
Québec, Canada

Merle A. Sande, M.D.
Professor and Vice-Chairman, Department of
 Medicine,
University of California;
Chief, Medical Service,
San Francisco General Hospital,
San Francisco, California

Phillippe Solal-Céligny, M.D.
Pulmonary Fellow, Centre de Pneumologie,
Le Centre Hospitalier de L'Université Laval,
Québec, Canada

Jean-Louis Vildé, M.D.
Lecturer,
University Paris 7;
Hospital Staff Physician, Infectious Disease
 Service,
Hôpital Claude Bernard,
Paris, France

Jean Vincelette, M.D.
Assistant Professor of Clinical Medicine,
Université de Montréal;
Microbiologist and Infectious Disease
 Consultant,
Hôpital Saint-Luc,
Montréal, Canada

Francis Waldvogel, M.D.
Professor of Medicine,
Université de Genève;
Chief, Infectious Diseases Division and Clinical
 Bacteriology Laboratory,
Physician-in-Chief,
Clinique medicale therapeutique, Hopital
 cantonal universitaire,
Geneva, Switzerland

Stephen H. Zinner, M.D.
Professor of Medicine,
Brown University;
Head, Division of Infectious Diseases,
Roger Williams General Hospital,
Providence, Rhode Island

Contents

CHAPTER		
1	Wound Infections . . . *J.C. Pechère, F. Fékété*	1
2	Rhinitis, Sinusitis, Otitis, and Laryngitis . . . *P. Déry, P. Bernard, J.C. Pechère*	21
3	Sore Throat and Fever . . . *P. Déry, J.C. Pechère, J. Joncas, P. Bernard*	37
4	Oral Infections . . . *B.J. Mansheim*	61
5	Influenza Syndrome . . . *G. Murray*	71
6	Acute Pneumonias in Adults . . . *J.C. Pechère, J. Joly*	77
7	Acute Pneumonias in Infants . . . *J.C. Rolland*	103
8	Pulmonary Tuberculosis . . . *M. Desmeules, Y. Cormier, J. Laforge, J.C. Pechère, P. Solal-Céligny*	113
9	Pulmonary Mycosis . . . *D.H. Lederer, A.A. Medeiros*	125
10	Pleural Effusion . . . *F.A. Waldvogel*	145
11	How to Approach a Fever . . . *M. Armengaud*	153
12	Fever in the Drug User . . . *C. Cherubin*	163
13	Bacteremia and Septicemia . . . *J.C. Pechère, M. Laverdiere*	171
14	Infective Endocarditis . . . *H.F. Chambers, M.A. Sande*	189
15	Pericarditis and Myocarditis . . . *Y. Morin*	205
16	Typhoid Fever . . . *A.M. Geddes*	215
17	Acute Infectious Diarrhea . . . *B. Grenier*	221
18	Intestinal Helminthic Infections . . . *J. Vincelette*	237
19	Abdominal Infections . . . *M.G. Bergeron*	249
20	Liver Infections . . . *F.A. Waldvogel*	267
21	Urinary Tract Infections . . . *J.F. Acar, F. Goldstein*	281

CHAPTER		
22	Genital Infections . . . G. Murray, J.M. Hubbrecht, P.C. Gosselin, J. Robert, J.C. Pechère	303
23	Syphilis . . . M.F. Rein	335
24	Infection and Pregnancy . . . B. Grenier	349
25	Infectious Adenopathy . . . J.L. Vildé	369
26	Primary Skin Infections . . . R. Lessard	385
27	Infections with Rashes . . . A. Dachy, A. Kahn, D. Blum, P. Demol, J.C. Pechère	403
28	Bone and Joint Infections . . . F.A. Waldvogel	431
29	Encephalitis and Parameningeal Infections . . . M.F. Para, P. Gardner	451
30	Acute Infectious Meningitis . . . M. Armengaud, C. Cherubin	465
31	Infections Affecting the Peripheral Nervous System . . . J. Drucker	489
32	Eye Infections . . . R. Michaud, A. Rousseau	501
33	Infections in the Immunocompromised Host . . . S.H. Zinner	529
34	Nosocomial Infections . . . J. McGowan Jr., J.A. Acar	551
35	Travel to Tropical Countries . . . M. Rey	561
36	Principles of Antimicrobial Treatment . . . R.C. Moellering, Jr.	575
	Index	589

CHAPTER 1

Wound Infections

J.C. Pechère and F. Fékété

> Objective 1–1. Describe the balance between host and microbe on the surface of the skin using a small skin wound superinfected with *Staphylococcus aureus* as an example.

Let us assume that a young boy has cut himself with a knife and has forgotten about it only to discover, several days later, that the cut has become infected. The infection is obvious from the pus that oozes from the wound and from the classic signs of inflammation: redness, swelling, pain, and heat.

If the physician were to Gram stain this pus on a slide and examine it microscopically, gram-positive cocci, grouped in clusters resembling bunches of grapes, would be visible. These microbes would probably be staphylococci (Fig. 1–1). Leukocytes would also be present, but for the most part, they would be altered, incomplete, or in dissolution: they specifically constitute pus. The microscopic examination would, therefore, identify the opponents normally present on the "battlefield" of an infection: the invader, in this case, the staphylococcus, and the mobile defenses of the host, the leukocytes.

MICROBE OR "INVADER"

Obviously, the first step in solving the problem of an infection is to secure positive identification of the invading microbe. This may be accomplished by inoculating the pus on agar or in broth. Because the staphylococcus is not a demanding organism, a single nutrient agar suffices in this case. The clinician should streak the pus on the surface of the agar and let it incubate at 37° C for 18 to 24 hours. Rounded, shiny colonies, 1 to 2 mm in size, with a yellowish tint that may range from beige to golden, appear. At this point, the bacteriologic identification is practically certain; however, it is still necessary to perform several other tests in order to be absolutely positive of the organism's identity.

To rule out the possibility of a micrococcus, an organism that resembles staphylococci morphologically and that can sometimes produce yellowish colonies, an aerobic fermentation of glucose should be used. Because this medium is positive only for staphylococci, it helps to confirm the diagnosis. Several other characteristics of the isolate should also be evident, such as the presence of coagulase, the occasional presence of a hemolysin, and, in particular, the fermentation of mannitol.

Only when all these tests have been completed can the organism responsible for the infection be positively identified. In this particular instance, the invading organism is *Staphylococcus aureus*. The method of introduction to the wound could have been the

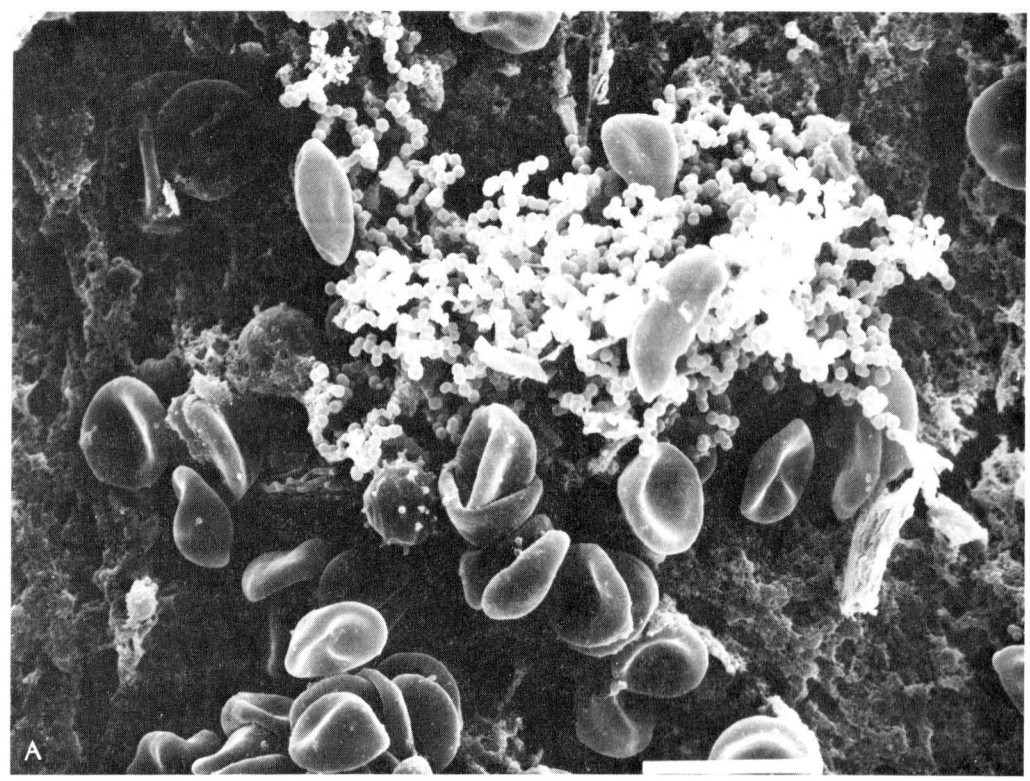

Fig. 1–1. *A*, Staphylococci in an infected vascular prosthesis.

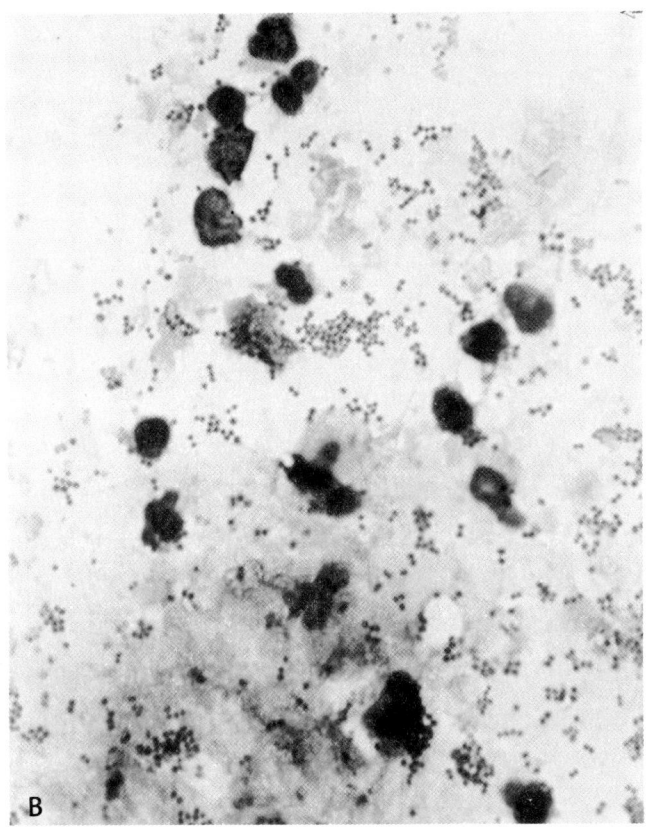

Fig. 1–1. *B*, Pus from an abscess due to *Staphylococcus aureus*.

knife, but it is much more likely that the microbe was actually present on the child's skin before the injury occurred.

Staphylococcus aureus is, in fact, an ordinary inhabitant of the body and is normally found on the skin of healthy individuals (Table 1–1). In addition to the skin's surface, it exists in body cavities and in the intestines, as part of the saprophytic flora, the density and the composition of which varies according to the area under consideration and, to a certain degree, from one individual to another. On the skin, these organisms colonize the stratum corneum and the hair follicles. A distinction should be made between the superficial flora, which is easily eliminated by washing, and the deep flora, which penetrates the hair follicles from which it can re-expand and reconstitute the surface flora. One to ten million bacteria ordinarily reside on one square centimeter of skin, but this number is increased tenfold in warm, wet areas such as the axillary folds. *Staphylococcus aureus* is a quasi permanent resident of the anterior nares and may also be part of the perineum in 10 to 40% of normal individuals. From these sites, the bacterium can disseminate elsewhere on the skin.

The physiologic role of this skin flora in man is poorly understood. It causes difficulties of interpretation when the organism is cultured from a specimen. Is it an innocuous saprophyte or the pathogen responsible for the illness? In the case of the child's knife wound, the organism was found in large numbers, in pure culture, without other representatives of the normal skin flora. In addition, the child's symptoms were compatible with a staphylococcal infection; therefore, the diagnosis was acceptable.

Pathogenicity of Staphylococcus Aureus. Adherence of bacteria to the host's cells is an essential step in the development of an infection. Other chapters discuss the way in which certain fibrillar proteins, the pili, permit the adherence of *Escherichia coli* to the mucosa of the small intestine (Objective 17–2) or to epithelial cells of the urinary tree (see Objective 21–3), as well as the adherence of *Neisseria gonorrhoeae* to the cells lining the urethra (see Chap. 22).

In some cases, the bacteria are surrounded by a mass of polysaccharide fibrils or glycocalyx, which permit microcolonies of organisms to adhere to the various host cell surfaces. Examples are enteric bacteria and pseudomonas. Glycans and dextrans secreted by some streptococci seem to contribute to the adherence of the bacteria to the endocardial surface, causing endocarditis, or to the dental surface, causing caries. Lipoteichoic acid and certain so-called M proteins (see Chap. 3) play an analogous role in the pathophysiology of streptococcal group A pharyngitis. In the case of *Staphylococcus aureus*, adherence is probably necessary, but the exact mechanism remains unknown. It has been suggested that the teichoic acid situated on the bacterial surface mediates the process.

When several microbial species reside in a given area, as in the skin, a sort of competition exists among the species. The phenomenon of interference has been observed in numerous instances, and *Staphylococcus aureus* has been particularly involved. The possible mechanisms of this bacterial interference remain theoretic: nutritional competition, re-

Table 1–1. Normal Cutaneous Flora: Usual Species

Species	Remarks
Staphylococcus epidermidis	Nearly always present; sometimes pathogenic (foreign body), may cause folliculitis (Objective 26–4)
Propionibacterium acnes	Gram-positive bacillus, anaerobic; slightly pathogenic; often contaminates blood cultures
Diphtheroids	Gram-positive bacillus, aerobic; slightly pathogenic
Staphylococcus aureus	Important potential pathogen; major cause of skin infections
Candida (not *C. albicans*)	Especially *C. parasilopsis*; slightly pathogenic
Malassezia furfur	Lipophilic yeasts; cause of tinea versicolor (Objective 26–4)

lease of toxic metabolites, or direct competition for sites of adherence. Nevertheless, the equilibrium may be broken by an external event such as the ingestion of an antibiotic, which suppresses the sensitive species, or as in the case of the boy in this chapter, a wound, an injury that favors the multiplication of bacteria better adapted to this new situation.

Once the bacteria cross the cutaneous or mucosal barrier, the process of infection begins. *Staphylococcus aureus* appears to be particularly well equipped for this task because it is the most frequently implicated pathogen in skin infections, superficial abscesses, and infection of hemodialysis cannulas and shunts. Table 1–2 lists the various substances secreted or those parts of the bacterial cell wall that seem linked to the pathogenicity of *S. aureus*. These toxins, enzymes, and various molecules taken one by one do not explain the virulence of the entire organism, but they each contribute to it. To illustrate the role of these factors, a comparison with *Staphylococcus epidermidis* can be helpful. *S. aureus* and *S. epidermidis* belong to the same genus, but have different characteristics (Table 1–3). *S. epidermidis* is less well armed and less pathogenic than *S. aureus*.

PATIENT

The host, or patient, possesses several lines of defense against the invading microbes. The skin and mucosa form a barrier that has an important protective role. In our example of the boy's wound, the cutaneous barrier was broken by the knife blade. Practically speaking, staphylococci cannot cross intact skin; they must take advantage of a break or wound, or, in the case of the mucosa, a preceding viral infection (Table 1–4).

Some microorganisms, however, can succeed in penetrating skin even without a visible lesion. Examples are *Francisella tularensis*, the agent of tularemia, and the cercariae of *Schistosoma haematobium*, the agent of bilharziasis.

Once the skin barrier has been crossed, the second major line of primary defense comes into play: phagocytosis by tissue macrophages, polymorphonuclear neutrophils, and monocytes. Phagocytosis ordinarily comprises a series of steps—opsonization, chemotaxis, attachment, and ingestion—followed by the death and digestion of the microbe.

Table 1–2. Factors Linked to the Pathogenicity of *Staphylococcus aureus*

Factors	Mode of Action and Commentary
Enzymes	
Coagulase	Coagulates plasma of many animals; inhibits leukocytosis(?)
Hyaluronidase	Splits hyaluronic acid, a substance found in connective tissue, and the eye, skin, bones, and synovial fluid; favors the spread of the staphylococci(?)
Phosphatase	Degrades phosphate bonds, such as in nucleotides
Proteases	Heterogeneous group of enzymes that are capable of hydrolyzing certain proteins (gelatin, fibrin)
Lipase	Liberates fatty acids that could degrade coenzyme A; the formation of furuncles has been linked to the secretion of lipase
Catalase	Inhibits intraleukocytic bacterial activity
Toxins	
Alpha hemolysin	Causes necrosis of a number of cells; lethal in rabbits when given intravenously
Beta hemolysin	Action is similar to that of alpha hemolysin
Leukocidin	Kills human polymorphonuclear leukocytes and macrophages by acting on their membranes
Enterotoxins	Causes food poisoning
Exfoliative toxin	Splits the granular layer of the epithelium
Superficial molecular fractions	
Protein A	Reacts with the F_c fraction host IgG; the aggregate that results fixes complement
Capsular antigens	Some isolates are encapsulated, thus are less susceptible to phagocytosis
Peptidoglycan	A pyrogen; reduces leukocytic chemotaxis

Table 1–3. Distinctive Characteristics of *Staphylococcus aureus* and *Staphylococcus epidermidis*

Bacteriologic characteristics not implicated in virulence	*Staphylococcus aureus*	*Staphylococcus epidermidis*
Yellow pigment	Usual	No
Fermentation of mannitol anaerobically	Definite	No
Requirement for biotin for growth	—	Definite
Characteristics implicated in virulence		
Coagulase	Usual	Exceptional
Alpha-toxin	Usual	No
Leukocidin	Usual	No
Nuclease	Usual	No
Protein A	Usual	No
Infections in man	Frequent infections causing furuncles, abscesses, sinusitis, superficial mastoiditis, parotitis, pneumonias, prostatitis, renal abscesses, orchidoepididymitis, perinephric abscesses and cellulitis, pelvic abscesses, septicemia, and endocarditis	Rare infections of prostheses (cardiac valves, bone, or ventricular shunts), endocarditis, infrequent urinary infections

Table 1–4. Predisposing Causes for Staphylococcal Infections

Breaks in the skin: accidental and surgical wounds, burns, dermatoses
Foreign bodies: dust and dirt in a wound, sutures, catheters, prostheses
Preceding viral infection: particularly influenza and measles
Preceding use of antibiotics ineffective against staphylococci
Leukocyte defects: quantitative (leukopenia) or qualitative (chronic granulomatous disease)
Humoral immune deficiencies
Various other conditions: diabetes, arteriosclerosis with tissue ischemia, alcoholism, renal insufficiency

In the case of the staphylococcus, opsonization is accomplished by means of IgG antibody or, in nonimmune sera, by the intermediary of the complement. Antibody or C3b complement fraction is deposited on the surface of the cell, which is thus rendered recognizable to the phagocytes.

The phagocytes are drawn by chemotaxis toward the focus of infection by the intermediary of activated complement fractions (C5a fraction in particular) and by the various substances secreted by the staphylococcus. Then the opsonized bacteria attach themselves to the phagocyte's membrane, which forms pseudopods that ingest the staphylococci. These bacteria are rapidly killed and digested in the phagocytic vacuoles, following a complex process that includes both oxygen-dependent and oxygen-free steps.

There are several other immune defense mechanisms whose role appears less clear. Antibodies against bacterial cell constituents and toxins have been identified, as well as a cellular immune response in patients infected with *Staphylococcus aureus*.

The invading staphylococcus thwarts the host defenses. Its leukocidins and toxins inhibit the chemotaxis of neutrophils and monocytes. Some encapsulated isolates escape opsonization with complement and can only be phagocytosed by means of specific antibody directed against the capsule. Opsonization is also inhibited to a certain degree by protein A because chemotaxis may be reduced by the peptidoglycan portion of the cell wall. In addition, the ability of some staphylococci to destroy complement can have serious consequences for the host.

The final issue of this sort of battle depends heavily on the condition of the host. If the patient is in good health, most infections will be resisted and will remain local and minor. Local therapy, simple cleaning, disinfection, and drainage are sufficient under these conditions. When the patient's defenses are compromised or when circumstances favor the infection (Table 1–4), however, there is a risk that the infection will spread, as in cellulitis, lymphangitis, and adenitis, or even become generalized and lead to septicemia. If this occurs, it then becomes necessary to prescribe antibiotic therapy to obtain a prompt cure (see Objective 1–4).

Objective 1–2. Prevent wound infections.

The purpose of wound infection prophylaxis is to limit the risk of local infection (cellulitis, abscess, and gangrene), regional infection (lymphangitis, adenitis, and suppurative thrombophlebitis), or systemic infection (septicemia) and to prevent tetanus. (Mammal bites and rabies prevention are special cases and are discussed in Objective 1–3.)

FACTORS CONTRIBUTING TO WOUND INFECTION

Bacterial contamination is the most important contributing factor in wound infection. Although ideally, a surgical wound is aseptic and carries a minimal risk of infection, a massively contaminated accidental wound has an excellent chance of becoming infected. The bacteria may be exogenous, that is, coming from soil, dust, or dirty objects, or endogenous, meaning from the individual himself because the skin, colon, vagina, and mouth contain many bacteria that can be the source of contamination. Thus, the site of a wound directly influences the risk of infection; wounds close to or involving densely colonized structures carry a higher risk of infection.

The nature of the wound is also important; wide, irregular wounds and those accompanied by crushing injury are more dangerous than limited wounds with clean edges. A deep, nearly inapparent, innocuous-looking puncture wound may be the source of tetanus or other clostridial infection. Burns are often clean initially, but without their cutaneous protection, the burned areas are vulnerable to environmental contamination. Ischemia from local compression, edema, or vascular injuries can inhibit the defense and healing processes by limiting the local arrival of fibrin, antibodies, platelets, polymorphonuclear leukocytes, macrophages, lymphocytes, and fibroblasts (to mention only the principal factors). Necrotic or nearly necrotic tissues, clots, and hematomas are perfect culture media for microbial growth. Therefore, delays in therapeutic intervention considerably increase the danger of infection, particularly if treatment is delayed beyond 4 to 6 hours. In addition, the presence of foreign bodies promotes bacterial proliferation. For example, although 10^7 to 10^8 staphylococci must be injected under the healthy skin of a rabbit to produce an abscess, a much smaller number (10^2 to 10^3) cause pus formation in the immediate vicinity of a suture. Therefore, it is essential that the objects and debris often present in a wound be meticulously removed.

The general condition of the patient may increase the risk of infection. Hypoxemia, hypovolemia, malnutrition, shock, and immunosuppression all increase this risk.

PREVENTION OF WOUND INFECTIONS

Because a variety of factors contribute to wound infection, one may prevent such infection in a number of ways.

Local therapy is the mainstay of prevention. Healthy tissue is the best antiseptic and skin the best bandage. Therefore, all devitalized tissues should be debrided. Clots, organic debris, and foreign bodies of all sorts should be eliminated by a thorough cleansing and by irrigation with sterile physiologic saline solution. Careful hemostasis should be performed if needed. Local circulation should be restored as much as possible by decompression and vascular reconstruction. A wound with a high risk of infection should not be sutured, to avoid creating anaerobic conditions and introducing foreign bodies and to facilitate the drainage of future secretions. In small third-degree burns of less than 20% of the body surface, the risk of later contamination can be reduced by early excision followed by immediate skin grafting. Once local therapy is complete, the injured parts can be left alone.

Applying local antiseptics to inhibit bacterial growth is of lesser importance; however, solutions containing iodine quaternary ammonium or sodium hypochlorite may be used for this purpose.

General preventive measures include restoration of the patient's blood volume and the fluid and electrolyte balance, treatment of shock, and correction of malnutrition.

Use of prophylactic antibiotics remains controversial. Such use is justified only when definitely indicated, as in the following examples:

1. Massive contamination has or may have taken place subsequent to penetration of the colon or after a perineal wound. In some cases, an actual infection is already established, and the prescription is more therapeutic than prophylactic.
2. The wound is extensive and irregular, and debridement has not been complete because it was necessary to preserve essential structures such as tendons.
3. Local ischemia exists or the potential for clostridial infection (gas gangrene) is present, such as after severe crush injuries to muscles or following arterial wounds.
4. A joint space or the meninges have been opened.
5. The patient has an open fracture.
6. Surgical debridement has been delayed or cannot be performed.

When indicated, it is best to prescribe antibiotics as quickly as possible. In most cases, a cephalosporin is selected because it is active against many staphylococci, streptococci, Enterobacteriaceae, and clostridia, these being the most likely infecting organisms. For an adult of average weight, one may administer cephalothin, 2 g intravenously, just before or during debridement, then 1 g 4 and 8 hours later, or cefazolin, 1 to 2 g each 6 to 8 hours for 3 doses. Aside from cases of overt infection, it is not necessary to continue further medication. When specific risks are identified, one may administer more specific antimicrobial agents. Thus, if following contamination by intestinal contents, one fears infection by anaerobes, *Bacteroides fragilis* in particular, and Enterobacteriaceae, one should choose agents specific against these organisms. Cefoxitin, or the combination of metronidazole or clindamycin and an aminoglycoside, are administered in 3 doses as described for cefazolin. In burns, moderate doses of penicillin G can be prescribed for the first few days when the patient appears vulnerable, to prevent *Streptococcus pyogenes* infections, especially the classic scarlet fever of burn patients. Penicillin G may also be used when a clostridial infection is considered likely. Apart from these indications, the practitioner should remember that, in the majority of wounds he is called upon to treat, antibiotic prophylaxis is unnecessary.

Tetanus. That this frightful disease exists in an economically developed society where effective means of prevention are available is unacceptable. The disease is caused by a toxin secreted by *Clostridium tetani*, a gram-positive bacillus frequently found in the intestines of herbivores as well as in the soil. The bacterium produces spores that permit it to survive for several months or years under hostile conditions. Wounds contaminated with soil may contain the bacillus or its spores. It is a strict anaerobe; the spores cannot germinate nor can the bacteria multiply in healthy, normally oxygenated tissues. In contrast, in an ischemic, necrotic wound, filled with clots or various debris or infected by pyogenic organisms, the oxidation-reduction potential is sufficiently reduced to permit the microbe to proliferate. Therefore, the cleansing and debridement of wounds previously mentioned is the first form of prevention. *C.*

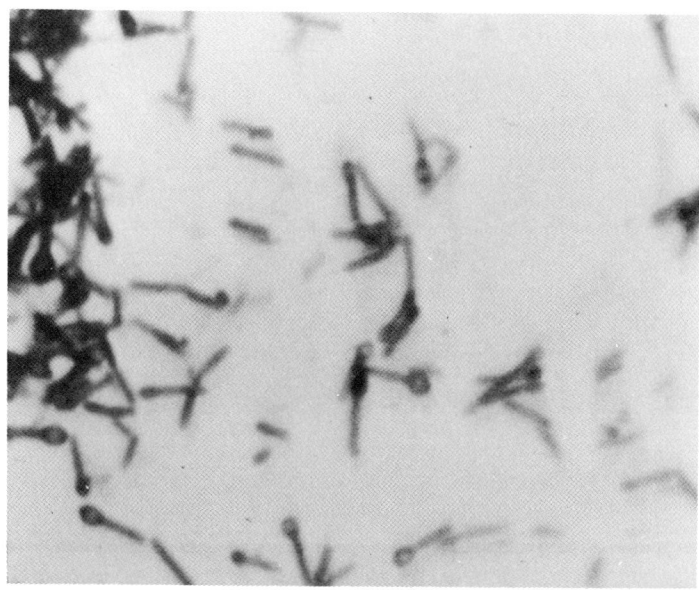

Fig. 1–2. *Clostridium tetani* is a spore-forming organism. The spores are located on the end of the bacterium, which then resembles a pin. The spore enables the bacterium to survive under unfavorable conditions for months or even years.

tetani can invade adjacent tissues, but this is not the mechanism of its pathogenicity. Once in the growth phase, the bacterium secretes a powerful toxin, tetanospasmin, lethal in a dose of one millionth mg/kg animal. This powerful neurotoxin follows the neural pathways and is, no doubt, also carried by the circulation to the central nervous system where it exerts its effects and precipitates the disease. The toxin particularly accumulates in the spinal cord where it inhibits impulses of the internuncial neurons (Fig. 1–2), causing impressive and painful muscle spasms (Fig. 1–3).

Antibodies (antitoxins) are available to counter the toxin; however, they have no effect once the toxin has been fixed by the nervous tissue. Therefore, protection against tetanus requires that antitoxins be present when the toxin is produced. Under these conditions, 0.01 U antibodies per ml serum generally protects the injured patient. In practice, only two ways ensure protection: immunization before the accident or serotherapy afterwards.

Immunization of the population is by far the better method. Tetanus toxin treated with heat and formalin loses its toxicity while retaining its antigenicity and thus becomes an anatoxin or toxoid. When injected into a nonimmune subject, it stimulates the development of antitoxin. Today, we use purified,

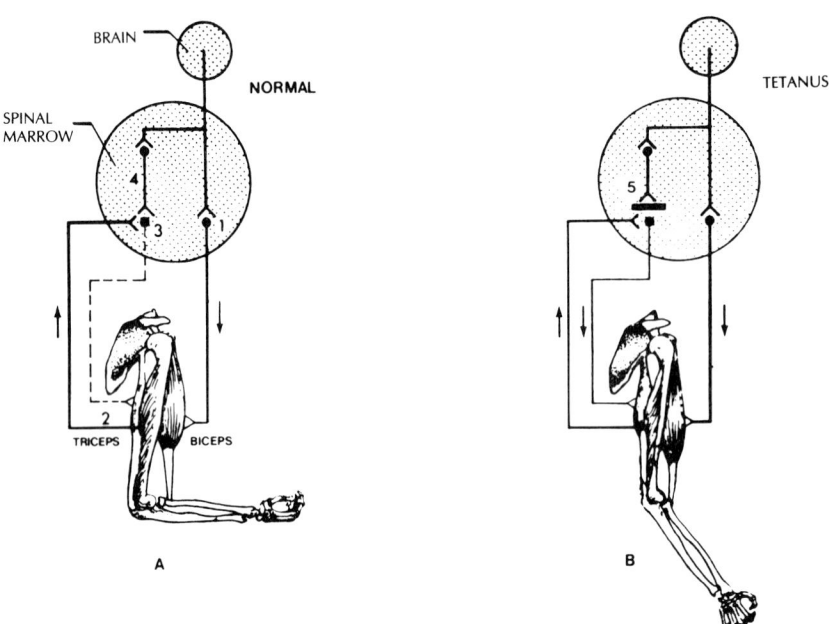

Fig. 1–3. In a normal individual, when an impulse from the brain causes the biceps to contract (1) a stretch-sensitive receptor orders the triceps to oppose the stretching, but this opposition is inhibited by impulses from the inhibitory nerve (4). In tetanus, the inhibitory impulses to the triceps motoneuron are blocked (5); both muscles contract and cause a spasm. (From Van Heyningen, W.E.: Tetanus. Sci. Am., *218*:69, 1968.)

Table 1–5. A Comparison of Primary Tetanus Immunization Series in Two Countries*

United States	France
First dose	First dose
Second dose: 4–6 weeks after the first	Second dose: 1–3 months after the first
Third dose: 6–12 months after the second	Third dose: 1–3 months after the second
Booster injection every 10 years	Booster infection 1 year after the third. Then, a booster injection every 10 years
Intramuscular injection	Subcutaneous injection

*The physician should always provide a written vaccination certificate.

absorbed preparations that are usually well tolerated. These preparations can be combined with other vaccines, diphtheria vaccine in particular. Several inoculation schedules are available (Table 1–5). The protection given is remarkable; fewer than 4 failures per 100 million. Neonatal tetanus can be prevented by immunizing the mother in the first 6 months of pregnancy.

Unfortunately, many individuals are as yet unvaccinated. When such an individual requires protection, it is necessary to use passive immunization, which is more costly and less well tolerated than the preferred active immunization just described. Homologous antitoxin (human) is preferred over heterologous antitoxin (horse), despite the higher cost, because it evokes practically no allergic response and provides longer protection (its half-life is approximately 25 days).

The practical aspects of tetanus prevention include the following:

1. Decision as to whether the wound is tetanus-prone. Examples are large wounds that have been neglected or are seen late, wounds associated with multiple fractures, crush injuries, bullet wounds; deep puncture wounds, wounds containing foreign bodies or devitalized tissues, already infected wounds, wounds contaminated with dirt or feces, wounds resulting from induced abortion, and neglected umbilical wounds in newborns.
2. Local treatment of the wound as previously described.
3. Ensuring that the patient has adequate immunologic protection against tetanus (Table 1–6).
4. If the wound is considered tetanus-prone, prescription of penicillin, 1 or 2 million U orally or intramuscularly for a few days; in allergic patients, oral tetracycline, 2 g/day.

Objective 1–3. Respond appropriately to mammal bites.

Physicians often see patients who have been bitten by a mammal, usually a dog. The mouth is one of the most highly contaminated areas of any animal. Each ml saliva contains over 10 million bacteria of a varied flora, mostly anaerobic. Therefore, animal bites are frequently complicated by infection, usually leading to a local cellulitis caused by a variety of microbes (Table 1–7). The most dangerous complications are rabies and tetanus.

PREVENTING INFECTION OF ANIMAL BITES

Preventive measures begin with local therapy as described in Objective 1–2. In view of the high bacterial density of saliva (in this connection, human bites seem particularly likely to become infected), the question of prophylactic antibiotic treatment naturally arises. If the wound is deep or multiple, antibiotics are usually prescribed. Penicillin G or V is often chosen because most bacteria

---

RECOGNIZING TETANUS AT THE OUTSET: TRISMUS

Even though effective prophylaxis is available, more than a million cases of tetanus are reported annually worldwide. In developed countries, the disease is seen, though less and less, in older persons who have not been vaccinated or who neglected their booster injections. Drug addicts constitute a new and increasing population. In underdeveloped areas, neonatal forms are predominant. To improve the grave prognosis of this disease (as high as 30 to 50% mortality rate), one must diagnose tetanus from its first sign, trismus. This sign is in essence a painful contraction of the masseter muscle aggravated by all efforts to overcome it (Fig. 1–4). In over 90% of cases, the wound through which the bacillus was introduced, for example, deep punctures, heroin injection sites, various lacerations, or chronic ulcers, is found, and the patient's history reveals an incubation period of 1 to 2 weeks. Typically, the patient has not been properly immunized. If he asserts that he has been actively immunized, his serum antitoxin level can be assayed, and if that level is greater than 0.01 U/ml, the diagnosis should be reconsidered.

The differential diagnosis broadly includes temporomandibular arthritis, which can be confused with tetanus when it occurs concurrently with serum sickness following the injection of antitetanus serum. Trismus accompanying tonsillar abscess, dental abscesses, various ear, nose, and throat infections, tetany, encephalitis, or meningitis can be recognized by its setting. Rabies begins with difficulty in swallowing rather than with true trismus, whereas poisoning due to tranquilizers can be diagnosed by the patient's history and by blood levels. If tetanus is suspected, 500 to 10,000 U human immunoglobulin and a first dose of toxoid should be injected immediately. The administration of 1 to 2 million U penicillin G to eliminate any remaining tetanus bacilli is often recommended but is of questionable value. Moreover, a specialized center should be contacted. Some severe cases may require early tracheostomy.

Full-blown tetanus is easy to recognize by its prolonged, generalized contractions, which are exacerbated by the slightest stimulus. At any time, the patient may become unable to breathe, and a tracheostomy is thereby justified. The principal causes of death are respiratory insufficiency and cardiac arrhythmia. In contrast, localized tetanus, characterized by minor muscular contractions in the area close to the portal of entry, has a subacute course and is most often diagnosed late and with much difficulty in patients who are incompletely immunized. The demonstration of *Clostridium tetani* in a wound does not itself confirm a diagnosis of tetanus.

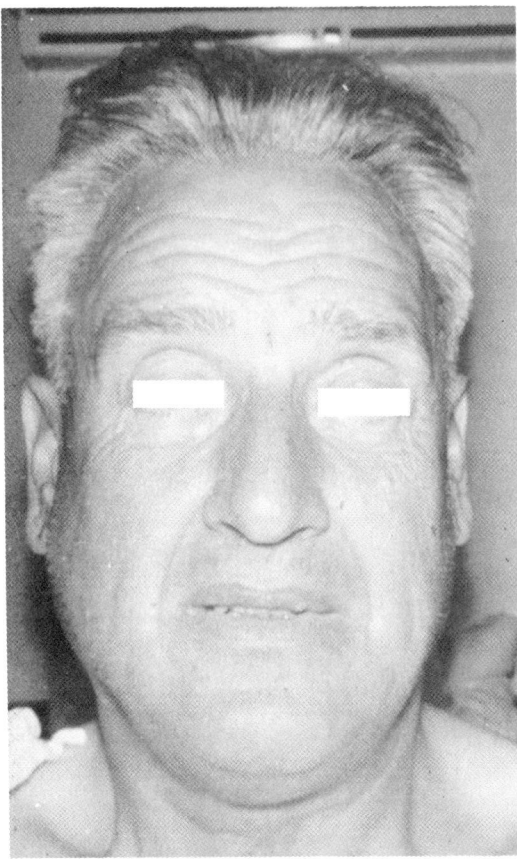

Fig. 1–4. In tetanus, spastic muscles of the head and neck, retracted lip commissures, elevated alae nasi and eyebrows, and accentuated wrinkles of the forehead give the patient a smiling and surprised look.

likely to develop in the wound are sensitive to penicillin (Table 1–7). Although no controlled study has established that prophylactic antibiotic therapy is beneficial in *Pasteurella multocida* infection from dog and cat bites or in rat-bite fever, the infecting organisms are sensitive to penicillin.

Tetanus prophylaxis should always be instituted (Objective 1–2) after a mammal bite.

Rabies must be prevented. Rabies, a disease on the increase in several countries, exists mainly in wild animals, is transmitted to humans through infected saliva, and is almost inescapably fatal once symptoms have appeared. Effective individual prophylaxis is available, but it must be decided upon rapidly and judiciously. Such treatment should be considered for any individual who has been the victim of a mammal bite; the decision to institute rabies prophylaxis should be determined by the following information:

1. The geographic region. Rabies is either endemic or epidemic among the mammalian fauna of most countries of the world. Some islands have been protected effectively and are free of the disease. These include Borneo, Hong Kong, Japan, the United Kingdom, Iceland, Australia, New Zealand, New Caledonia, several islands of the Caribbean, and, for reasons that are less clear, Scandinavia; in these countries, prophylaxis against rabies is not required. Some areas remain free of the disease while other adjacent areas are endemic; for example New York City as opposed to New York State.
2. The animal species. The principal vector varies with the particular region: stray dogs in Africa, Asia, Latin America, and the Mediterranean countries; the fox in Europe; foxes, skunks, dogs, bats, and sometimes cats and cattle in North America; the mongoose in Puerto Rico; the jackal in India; and the wolf in Iran. It is unusual for rabies to be contracted and transmitted by small rodents, rabbits, or hares, or by animals that have been previously vaccinated.
3. The circumstances surrounding the bite. The probability of rabies is greater when the animal attacked without provocation; some affected animals, such as the cat, are abnormally quiet ("dumb" rabies).
4. The wound itself. Severe wounds of the face, neck, hands, feet, or genitals are considered at high risk. A wound may become infected if licked by the animal or with its contaminated saliva, even without an actual bite.

If, on considering these points, rabies is still plausible, the physician should proceed as indicated in Table 1–8. Rabies antiserum provides rapid, but short-lasting, protection

Table 1–6. Practical Tetanus Immunization Program in a Patient With a Wound

		Clean (Not "Tetanus-prone") Wounds	"Tetanus-prone" Wounds
Completed primary vaccination			
Time since last booster injection	<1 year	No immunization	No immunization
	1–5 years	No immunization	Toxoid booster
	5–10 years	No immunization	Toxoid booster
	>10 years	Toxoid booster	Toxoid booster and homologous serum* (250–500 units IM in another site)
Unvaccinated (or vaccination incomplete or uncertain)		Single dose of toxoid	Single dose of toxoid and homologous serum* (250–500 units IM in another site)
		Completion of the vaccination later if necessary	Completion of the vaccination later if necessary

*If homologous serum is not available, use horse serum (1500–3000 units) in 3 successive injections to avoid anaphylactic shock, except if the patient is known or proves to be allergic. If that is the case, serotherapy should not be used.

RABIES

The incubation period for rabies in humans ranges from 10 to 240 days, with an average of about 2 months. The disease begins with nonspecific prodromes: fever, nausea, anorexia, headache, and sore throat. The patient becomes anxious and irritable; he may complain of increased salivation. Often, the first sign that worries him is the appearance of "abnormal sensations" at the site of the bite, such as burning, tickling, or pain, even though the wound may be healed by then. From 2 to 4 days later, the excitement stage begins. Anxiety and agitation increase. Random paralysis or muscle weakness is manifested by strabismus, diplopia, dilatation or contraction of the pupils, urinary retention, and hoarseness. Hydrophobia becomes so severe that the mere sight of liquids produces spasmodic contractions of the glossopharyngeal muscles. Later, paralysis progresses, and disorders of consciousness appear; up to this point, the patient, unfortunately, will have remained lucid. If untreated, the course of the disease is almost invariably fatal.

(half-life of approximately 3 weeks); specific immunoglobulin of human origin (20 IU/kg) is preferred to that of equine origin (40 IU/kg), which is less well tolerated. If possible, half the dose is injected around the wound, and the rest is given intramuscularly; the syringe should be changed.

Several vaccines are available. The older, poorly tolerated vaccines are now obsolete. The vaccine prepared in human diploid cell culture (HDCV) is now considered the best, particularly from the standpoint of tolerance. According to the recommendations of the Center for Disease Control of the United States Public Health Service (CDC), 5 intramuscular doses of 1 ml must be given (for example, into the deltoid muscles), the first as soon as possible and the others 3, 7, 14, and 29 days later. The World Health Organization (WHO) recommends a sixth dose at 90 days. Protective antibodies, which can be assayed, appear in 7 to 10 days and persist for at least a year. If HDCV is not obtainable, duck embryo vaccine (DEV) can be used although it stimulates lower antibody levels. The series includes 23 doses of 1 ml each, administered subcutaneously in changing sites on the abdomen, waist, and back. The first 21 injections are given consecutively (1 daily for 21 days or 2 daily for 7 days and then 1 per day for 7 days); the other 2 doses should be administered as booster injections 10 and 20 days after the twenty-first dose.

Finally, persons with a high risk of exposure to rabies, such as veterinarians and forest rangers, should be vaccinated before any ex-

Table 1–7. Infections Transmitted by Mammal Bites

Infection	Microorganisms	Mammal Incriminated	Incubation	Principal Clinical Manifestations
Miscellaneous local infections	Staphylococcus aureus, streptococcus (group A, viridans, anaerobic), Bacteroides melaninogenicus, and Fusobacterium and Spirochaeta species	All, human bites particularly dangerous	A few hours to a few days	Cellulitis, sometimes septicemia
Pasteurellosis	Pasteurella multocida	Cat and dog especially, but many others	A few days	Cellulitis, sometimes septicemia (in cirrhotics)
Rabies	Rabies virus	Many, especially foxes, dogs, cats, cattle, bats, skunks, mongoose, jackals	About 2 months (10–240 days)	Encephalitis
Rat-bite fever				
Haverhill fever	Streptobacillus moniliformis	Rat, mouse, weasel	2–10 days	High fever, morbiliform or petechial rash and polyarthritis
Sodoku	Spirillum minor	Rat, squirrels	>10 days	Relapsing fever and macular rash
Tetanus	Clostridium tetani	All	7–10 days	Trismus and contractions

Table 1–8. Measures to Take When Rabies is Suspected

Biting animal
Wandering dog or cat, wild animal: insist on its capture. Destroy the animal immediately, but save the head and forward it to the nearest diagnostic center for a direct immunofluorescence examination of the brain.
Pets and domestic animals presenting clinical signs of rabies: same as above.
Apparently healthy pets: confine and keep under observation for 14 days. If the animal remains normal for 5 days, rabies contamination is unlikely; in 14 days, the diagnosis can be excluded. If the animal becomes sick, destroy it and examine the brain.

Wound care
Wash generously with soap and water. When all the soap has been removed, apply a 0.1% solution of quaternary ammonium. Do not suture.

Immunization
If the wounded patient has had a harmless contact with the animal, no treatment is necessary.
If the patient was bitten or if a cutaneous or mucosal wound was contaminated with saliva, organic fluids, or tissue, determine whether the animal is one of the following and treat accordingly:
1. Rabid, presumably rabid, or not captured: use antirabies immunoglobulins, locally and intramuscularly in addition to vaccination (see text). Discontinue vaccination if the postmortem examination of the animal is negative for rabies.
2. Apparently healthy: keep animal under observation. At the first sign of rabies in the animal, use antirabies immunoglobulin, locally and intramuscularly, in addition to vaccination (see text). If no rabies in animal during observation, treatment is not necessary.

posure (HDCV: 3 doses of 1 ml on days 0, 7, 21, and 28, sometimes with a booster injection if the antibody titer is not sufficiently elevated; DEV: 4 doses of 1 ml on days 0, 7, and 14 and 5 to 6 months after the third dose).

> **Objective 1–4.** Identify the cause of superficial cellulitis in order to start appropriate treatment.

Any cutaneous wound can be complicated by cellulitis, which is an infection of the subcutaneous tissues. Certain forms of cellulitis, mentioned in the discussion following Objective 1–5, invade the deep tissues. These deep infections generally involve anaerobic bacteria or a mixed aerobic-anaerobic flora. They can be life-threatening and often require wide surgical excision. On the other hand, superficial cellulitis, to which the present discussion is limited, is much less serious. With proper treatment, every chance of uncomplicated recovery exists.

The nature of the initial lesion varies. It

can be an insect bite, a chicken pox vesicle, a thorn, a small, inapparent scratch, or an open wound. In a few days, local pain, redness, and swelling intensify rapidly. The degree of extension and its rate of progression are important indicators of the severity of the lesion and must be evaluated. Lymphangitis, satellite adenopathy, thrombophlebitis in the vicinity, or even a combination of high fever, chills, and indications of toxicity that indicate septicemia are grave signs. The character of the periphery of the cellulitis should be noted; it may be sharply demarcated and edematous in erysipelas, for example. Vesicles should be looked for locally, and the lesion should be palpated with a finger to detect crepitation, an alarming finding indicating gas gangrene from anaerobic organisms (see Objective 1–5).

Foremost among the likely infectious agents are *Streptococcus pyogenes* and *Staphylococcus aureus*. An abrupt onset of the first signs, sometimes only a few hours after the initial lesion, points to a streptococcal infection, whereas staphylococcal cellulitis usually begins as a furuncle. Actually, a precise origin is difficult to establish clinically because the list of causes includes many other organisms, such as *Haemophilus influenzae*, especially in young children and in cases of periorbital cellulitis, Enterobacteriaceae such as *Escherichia coli* and *Proteus* species, *Pseudomonas* species, *Streptococcus pneumoniae*, or even *Candida albicans*, particularly in the immunosuppressed. A deep cellulitis may appear superficial at first. A wound inflicted while swimming may become infected by gram-negative organisms such as *Aeromonas hydrophila*, found in fresh water, or *Vibrio parahaemolyticus*, found in salt water.

A definitive diagnosis is established by bacteriologic culture of blood and appropriate local specimens. Appropriate samples may be obtained by collecting a small quantity of serous fluid at the portal of entry, if there is one, or by needle puncture (if necessary, one should inject a small amount of sterile physiologic saline and then withdraw it promptly), as well as by a small cutaneous biopsy (punch biopsy). The sample is taken from the most inflamed area, and immediate Gram staining and microscopic examination are always performed. In view of the organisms likely to be present, blood agar and chocolate agar, for *Haemophilus influenzae*, in particular, should be inoculated. Samples from a deep cellulitis should be cultured under anaerobic conditions, such as thioglycolate broth.

SPECIFIC DISORDERS

Some special types of cellulitis warrant more detailed discussion.

Erysipelas. This disorder is caused by group A streptococcus. Because the suppurative element is minor, it is difficult to isolate and to culture the organisms responsible for the infection. Erysipelas spreads by the lymphatic system and occurs mainly in children and in the aged. Lymphedema and the nephrotic syndrome are sometimes noted as predisposing causes in the periumbilical, neonatal form, which is rare today. The portal of entry is often a tiny wound. The onset is surprisingly rapid. The clinical picture includes high fever, chills, and an inflammatory patch whose borders progress rapidly in a centrifugal fashion. When it involves the face, erysipelas takes on a typical appearance, with a butterfly pattern over the patient's cheeks and nose (Plate 1A). The inflammatory signs are predominant at the periphery, and the raised indurated border can be palpated. The edges are sharply demarcated, with small vesicles at the surface. When the disorder develops outside the facial area, the patch of erysipelas loses some of its characteristics; in these cases, the sharp, raised edge can be lacking. In persons suffering from lymphatic obstruction, after a mastectomy, for example, erysipelas recurs and often becomes milder from one attack to the next. Like other forms of cellulitis caused by group A streptococcus, erysipelas may be complicated by glomerulonephritis 2 to 3 weeks after the initial infection (Table 3–3).

Periorbital Cellulitis. This disorder primarily affects children. The list of predispos-

Table 1–9. Periorbital and Orbital Cellulitis: Differential Diagnosis

	Lid Swelling	Proptosis	Ophthalmoplegia	Impaired Vision	Prostration, Papilledema
Orbital cellulitis	+	+	+	+	0
Periorbital cellulitis	+	0	0	0	0
Subperiostal abscess	0	Lateral displacement	0	0	0
Cavernous sinus thrombosis	+	+	+	+	+

+, Present; 0, absent.
(Modified from Barkin, R.M., Todd, J.K., and Amer, J.: Periorbital cellulitis in children. Pediatrics, 62:390, 1978. Copyright American Academy of Pediatrics.)

ing causes includes local wounds, underlying sinusitis, otitis, or even dental abscesses; however, more than half the cases occur without apparent reason. The bacteria involved are *Haemophilus influenzae*, observed particular in children under 5 years of age, *Staphylococcus aureus*, and less frequently, *Streptococcus pyogenes* or *Streptococcus pneumoniae*. Anaerobes, such as *Peptostreptococcus* and *Fusobacterium* species, can also be found, particularly extending from sinusitis in adults. Clinically, periorbital cellulitis must be differentiated from various other orbital infections and from cavernous sinus thrombosis (Table 1–9), primarily to determine whether the patient's eye is threatened. This distinction is not always easy to make, especially in the presence of extensive edema, but if any doubt exists, an ophthalmologist should be called upon to perform a decompression operation without undue delay.

Malignant Staphylococcal Infection (Facial). This infection develops as a complication of a furuncle of the upper lip or of the angle of the nose, usually as a result of being unduly squeezed. Fortunately, this infection is rare today. The lesion is painful, sometimes cyanotic, and cool due to local thrombophlebitis. This infection is serious because septicemia is nearly always present and it may lead to cavernous sinus thrombosis (Table 1–9).

Pasteurella multocida Cellulitis. This form of cellulitis is caused by a small gram-negative coccobacillus, *P. multocida*, that inhabits the gums and oropharynx of many animals; more than two-thirds of all cats and half of all dogs are affected. Humans are generally contaminated from a bite or a scratch. The cellulitis (Plate 1B) is of abrupt onset, but regresses slowly, even with appropriate treatment. An abscess frequently forms. When the bite is deep, tenosynovitis, osteomyelitis, or arthritis may be present (Plate 1C). *P. multocida*, like *Streptococcus pneumoniae*, has a capsule that may interfere with phagocytosis by the host's cells; this factor accounts for the risk of systemic infection in certain compromised hosts. For example, in cirrhotic patients, *P. multocida* septicemia and superinfection of ascitic fluid ("spontaneous peritonitis") have been observed after a bite or a scratch. Septicemia and meningitis may also be noted in the elderly.

Anthrax. Caused by *Bacillus anthracis*, anthrax has become rare in developed countries. Cutaneous infection generally occurs as a result of industrial handling of contaminated animal products, such as goat hair or skin, wool, or bones. Because the bacterium is spore-forming, these products remain dangerous for months or years. Generally, the contaminated animal products originate from Asia or Africa, where anthrax is still endemic. Infection also results from contact with infected animals, nowadays chiefly swine, horses, cattle, and wild animals, or from accidental autoinoculation with the vaccine. Therefore, anthrax is primarily an occupational disease among leather workers and ranchers. A vesicle or a crop of vesicles filled with a reddish fluid appears in a few days. These lesions rupture and ulcerate, forming a dark eschar surrounded by extensive edema

(Plate 2A). The lesions are pruritic but painless. The sites of predilection include the head, neck, forearms, and hands. General health remains good, except in the 20% of patients who develop septicemia.

***Erysipelothrix* Infections.** These infections are caused by a gram-positive bacillus, *Erysipelothrix rhusiopathiae*. The infection usually begins in the hand, one or more days after a small wound has been inflicted during the course of handling salt water fish, crustaceans, poultry, or various other meats. Along with the lesions, which are a violet color, a known occupational exposure among butchers, cooks, and fishermen, constitutes one of the most reliable clinical clues to a diagnosis of erysipelothrix. As with erysipelas, erysipelothrix infection progresses centrifugally, with most signs occurring at the periphery of the lesion and the border sharply defined (Plate 2B). Neither fever nor systemic signs are present, however. Even if left untreated, the disease heals within 2 or 3 weeks, although rare complications, such as arthritis in an adjacent structure, septicemia, and endocarditis, have been described.

TREATMENT

The presumptive treatment of cellulitis is based on the clinical findings and the microscopic examination of Gram-stained local secretions. If a streptococcal infection is probable, penicillin G is chosen (500,000 to 1,000,000 U intravenously), followed by similar doses of procaine penicillin G, every 8 to 12 hours intramuscularly. For a patient allergic to penicillin or for a minor form of the disorder, the alternative is erythromycin (adult dose: 500 mg orally every 6 or 8 hours). If a staphylococcal infection is suspected, as in the majority of cases, or if the origin of the cellulitis is undetermined, the treatment must include an antistaphyloccocal agent, usually a penicillinase-resistant penicillin, such as nafcillin or oxacillin, 1 to 1.5 g intravenously every 4 hours in serious cases, or dicloxacillin, 1 g orally every 6 to 8 hours for a less severe form of the disorder. These penicillins are also active against streptococci.

In an immunosuppressed patient, establishing the cause of the cellulitis is especially important because of the gravity of the infection and the greater number of possible causes. If no clues are present, an attempt must be made to cover the whole range of infective agents by using a cephalosporin or a combination of an antistaphylococcal penicillin and an aminoglycoside.

Erysipelothrix rhusiopathiae is susceptible to penicillin, and an intramuscular injection of 1,200,000 U benzathine penicillin may be sufficient to treat a local infection. Alternatives are oral penicillin, 250 mg 4 times daily for 7 days, or erythromycin.

Orbital cellulitis due to *Haemophilus influenzae*, in which the threat of losing an eye exists, calls for a reliable antibiotic. The appearance of strains of *H. influenzae* resistant to ampicillin (5 to 30% in North America) has raised doubts concerning the regular use of this antibiotic in this instance. Chloramphenicol (50 mg/kg/day) or a third-generation cephalosporin such as cefotaxime (Table 13–7) may be preferred initially, with the option of returning to ampicillin if the organism is found to be susceptible to it. The recommended dosage for ampicillin is 200 to 300 mg/kg/day intravenously. Surgical orbital decompression is sometimes necessary.

Pasteurella multocida cellulitis is treated with penicillin (procaine penicillin, 600,000 U intramuscularly every 12 hours; ampicillin 500 mg orally every 6 hours). Tetracycline, 500 mg orally every 6 hours, is an alternative in individuals allergic to penicillin, or when resistance to penicillin is detected by antibiotic sensitivity tests. Treatment should be continued for 2 to 4 weeks to prevent recurrences.

Cutaneous anthrax can be treated by one of the following regimens: penicillin V, 500 mg orally, 4 times daily for 7 days; procaine penicillin, 600,000 U intramuscularly, twice daily for 5 days; sulfadiazine, 3 g orally and then 1 g every 4 hours for 7 days; or tetracycline 500 mg orally every 4 to 6 hours for 7 days.

> **Objective 1–5. Recognize deep cellulitis as rapidly as possible and take appropriate action.**

Deep cellulitis can be extremely serious, and its development can be incredibly rapid. It is life-threatening, and an immediate, energetic treatment is the only hope for a cure.

In the presence of cellulitis, the following signs should alert the physician to the possible development of a deep, severe infection: (1) the patient has a rapidly worsening, toxic appearance with tachycardia, hypotension, and mental changes; (2) the cellulitis spreads from hour to hour; (3) palpation of the lesion locally gives the impression of crepitation because of the formation of gas in the tissues, which must not be confused with air that may have been introduced into the tissues by an injury, by surgical intervention, or following a pneumothorax; and (4) a fetid odor is observable.

SPECIFIC DISORDERS

Several entities can be distinguished on the basis of clinical and bacteriologic criteria.

Clostridial Myonecrosis. This disorder, with an incidence of 3 to 8 cases annually per million population in Canada, is a complication of certain limb injuries, such as a fracture of the femur after an accident, often on a motorcycle, or following a wound. The disorder is also observed postoperatively particularly after amputation of a lower limb for vascular insufficiency in a diabetic, following a biliary operation with exploration of the bile duct, or after a surgical opening of the large intestine. Some cases are secondary to an intramuscular injection, and one may even see "spontaneous" gas gangrene in immunosuppressed individuals. In all such patients, *Clostridium perfringens*, or more rarely other clostridia, such as *C. septicum*, *C. novyi*, or *C. sordellii*, takes advantage of the conditions of anaerobiosis and the presence of crushed or necrosed tissues to multiply. The infection is manifested initially by increasing local pain 1 or 2 days after the injury has occurred. In addition, a dark, foul-smelling serous discharge, edema, and darkening of the tissues are present. These local signs are rapidly followed by systemic signs of toxicity and fever. When it is not masked by edema, significant local crepitation is present.

The diagnosis is easy, but it should be confirmed without delay by Gram staining of secretions, to reveal numerous, fat, "box-car"-like, gram-positive rods (Fig. 1–5) and few polymorphonuclear leukocytes. A plain roentgenogram of the limb shows small gas bubbles, which, in the case of myonecrosis, have a fern-like pattern. This situation calls for immediate action, with a high dose of penicillin G and radical surgical excision of the necrosed tissues; amputation may even be necessary. In facilities where equipment is available, hyperbaric oxygen therapy may be administered without delaying the other measures, but without assurance that it will improve the prognosis.

Gangrenous Cellulitis. Caused by anaerobic organisms, this type of cellulitis is produced by clostridia and a variety of nonsporogenic anaerobes, such as different bacteroides, peptostreptococci, and peptococci. Sometimes, these infections are associated with Enterobacteriaceae, staphylococci, or other streptococci. In contrast to clostridial myonecrosis, the underlying fascia and muscle are not invaded; this infection is more frequent, less spectacular, and less serious. Its incubation period is longer, local pain is absent or minor, edema is limited, and systemic toxicity is less serious. The infection is characterized, however, by extensive gas formation in the tissues with evident crepitation. The treatment is similar to that of clostridial myonecrosis.

Myositis. In myositis due to anaerobic streptococci, such as peptostreptococci, sometimes associated with *Streptococcus pyogenes* or *Staphylococcus aureus*, the clinical picture is less dramatic than in clostridial myonecrosis. The infection develops 3 to 4 days after the causative wound, that is, more slowly. Pain develops later, and the progres-

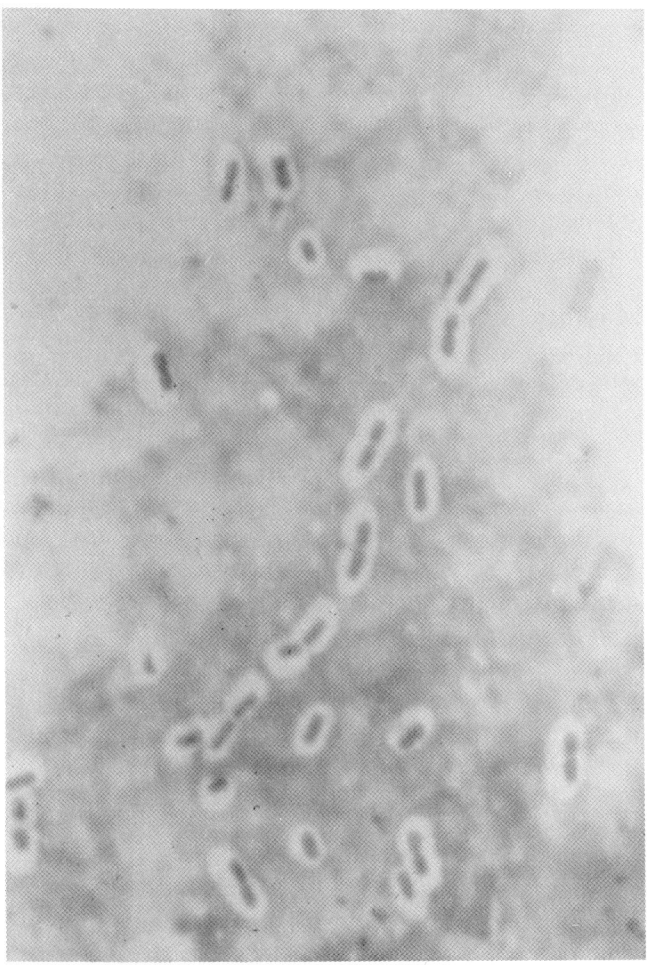

Fig. 1–5. Microscopic appearance of secretions during the course of *Clostridium perfringens* gas gangrene in a diabetic patient. Several gram-positive bacilli are in an active state of division. The bacilli are surrounded by a nonstaining capsule. The absence of polymorphonuclear cells indicates that host defense mechanisms are overwhelmed.

sion of gas in the tissues is more limited, although an intense cutaneous erythema appears at the surface. The secretions, which are more frankly purulent than in clostridial myonecrosis, contain gram-positive cocci and large numbers of polymorphonuclear leukocytes. A more uncommon and clinically similar group A streptococcus myositis has also been identified. The treatment is based essentially on penicillin G in high doses and on wide surgical drainage.

Necrotizing Fasciitis. This disorder is caused by group A streptococcus, occasionally accompanied by the bacteria mentioned in Table 19–7. It is secondary to a limb injury, but certain cases occur without a visible portal of entry. An erythema with edema develops in 2 to 3 days, becomes covered with a few bullae containing a yellowish or brownish fluid, and then undergoes central necrosis. The lesion is sharply demarcated at the periphery. The overall picture resembles a third-degree burn. Gram staining of the secretions reveals a mixed flora or chains of gram-positive cocci. The infection progresses along the fascial planes and may result in an impressive necrosis, septicemia, metastatic abscesses, and death unless appropriate treatment is given. Treatment consists of radical surgical debridement down to the healthy tissue and antibiotic therapy as suggested in Table 19–7. The mortality rate for treated patients is about 15%. A regional variant of necrotizing fasciitis is Fournier's gangrene, which affects the scrotum and perineum, and can sometimes extend to the penis and the abdominal wall.

Synergistic Necrotizing Cellulitis. This disorder is a variant of necrotizing fasciitis and involves the skin, subcutaneous tissues, fascia, and underlying muscles. This entity is also caused by a mixed infection, by anaerobes, such as streptococci and bacteroides, and aerobic-anaerobic organisms, often gram-negative. Age, obesity, diabetes, and cardiac or renal disease are predisposing factors. The infection is even more serious than necrotizing fasciitis, with a severe toxic appearance, positive blood cultures in more than half the patients, and a high risk of mortality. No gas appears in the tissues in three cases out of four, and the foul-smelling secretions ("dishwater pus") contain a mixed flora revealed by Gram staining. Radical surgical excision, sometimes amputation, and broad-spectrum antibiotic therapy effective against both *Bacteroides fragilis* and Enterobacteriaceae, for example, cefoxitin, or an aminoglycoside in addition to clindamycin, should be given without delay.

SUGGESTED READINGS

Anonymous: Human diploid cell rabies vaccine. Med. Lett. Drug Ther., 22:93, 1980.

Committee on Trauma, American College of Surgeons: Early Care of the Injured Patient. 2nd Ed. Philadelphia, W.B. Saunders, 1976.

Corey, L., and Hattwick, M.A.W.: Treatment of persons exposed to rabies. JAMA, 232:272, 1975.

Defore, W.W., Jr., et al.: Necrotizing fasciitis, a persistent surgical problem. J. Am. Coll. Emerg. Physicians, 6:62, 1977.

Finegold, S.M.: Anaerobic Bacteria in Human Disease. New York, Academic Press, 1977.

Francis, D.P., Holmes, M.A., and Brandon, G.: Pasteurella multocida: infections after domestic animal bites and scratches. JAMA, 232:42, 1975.

Gerding, D.N., Khan, M.Y., Ewing, J.E., and Hall, W.H.: Pasteurella multocida peritonitis in hepatic cirrhosis with ascites. Gastroenterology, 70:413, 1976.

Ginsberg, M.B.: Cellulitis: analysis of 101 cases and review of the literature. South. Med. J., 74:530, 1981.

Giuliano, A., Lewis, F., Jr., Hadley, K., and Blaisdell, F.W.: Bacteriology of necrotizing fasciitis. Am. J. Surg., 134:52, 1977.

Goldstein, E.J.C., et al.: Bacteriology of human and animal bite wounds. J. Clin. Microbiol., 8:667, 1978.

Hitchcock, C.R., Demello, F.J., and Haglin, J.J.: Gangrene infection: new approaches to an old disease. Surg. Clin. North Am., 55:1403, 1975.

Kaplan, M.H., and Tenenbaum, M.J.: Staphylococcus aureus: cellular biology and clinical application. Am. J. Med., 72:248, 1982.

Kizer, K.W.: Epidemiologic and clinical aspects of animal bites injuries. J. Am. Coll. Emerg. Physicians, 8:134, 1979.

Ledingham, I.M., and Tehrani, M.A.: Diagnosis, clinical course and treatment of acute dermal gangrene. Br. J. Surg., 62:364, 1975.

Middleton, D.B., and Ferrante, J.A.: Periorbital and facial cellulitis. Ann. Family Pract., 21:98, 1980.

National Advisory Committee on Immunization: Statement on rabies prophylaxis. Canada Dis. Weekly Rep., 6:125, 1980.

Parker, M.T.: Postoperative clostridial infections in Britain. Br. Med. J., 3:671, 1969.

Recommendations of the Immunization Practices Advisory Committee: Rabies prevention. Morbid. Mortal. Weekly Rep., 29:265, 1980.

Sabath, L.D.: Mechanisms of resistance to beta-lactam antibiotics in strains of *Staphylococcus aureus*. Ann. Intern. Med., 97:339, 1982.

Saphir, D.A., and Carter, G.R.: Gingival flora of the dog with special reference to bacteria associated with bites. J. Clin. Microbiol., 3:344, 1977.

Stevens, D.L., Higbee, J.W., Oberhofer, T.R., and Everett, E.D.: Antibiotic susceptibilities of human isolates of Pasteurella multocida. Antimicrob. Agents Chemother., 16:322, 1979.

Stone, H.H., and Martin, J.D., Jr.: Synergistic necrotizing cellulitis. Ann. Surg., 175:702, 1972.

Verhoef, J., and Verbrugh, H.A.: Host determinants in staphylococcal disease. Annu. Rev. Med., 32:107, 1981.

CHAPTER 2

Rhinitis, Sinusitis, Otitis, and Laryngitis

P. Déry, P.A.M. Bernard, and J.C. Pechère

> **Objective 2-1.** Differentiate simple coryza from upper respiratory tract infections requiring medical attention.

Respiratory infections comprise a large portion of the physician's practice. These infections have considerable social and economic impact in Western countries because they are involved in more than half the deaths caused by disease. Respiratory infections are also responsible for an incalculable amount of job absenteeism and for enormous medical and pharmaceutical expenses.

Simple coryza may be differentiated from infections that require medical attention on the basis of clinical symptoms such as rhinorrhea, fever, headache, sore throat, earache, cough, and respiratory difficulties.

The microbiology laboratory is occasionally useful in diagnosing certain suspicious and purulent respiratory infections.

RHINORRHEA

Rhinorrhea as a Sign of Coryza. Rhinorrhea is the earliest, the most frequent, and the most important sign of upper airway infection. It is usually due to a coryza or common cold, which is man's most frequent infection; 80% of the population suffer from at least one episode a year. The following description is familiar: the patient's nose becomes congested and then secretes a watery discharge, which may yellow or thicken in a few days because of bacterial superinfection. Coughing, sneezing, headache, and tearing are often associated symptoms. Colds are contagious and other cases occur in a patient's circle of contacts more often than not.

In about a quarter of patients, the infection is due to a rhinovirus from the Picornaviridae family (Tables 2–1 and 2–2). The hundred different types of these rhinoviruses can be distinguished from each other by neutralization tests. Each type induces a specific immunity of short duration (about 2 years), which, however, does not protect against heterologous types, except during the first few weeks after an infection. This immunity has a higher correlation with the titer of IgA in nasal secretions than with IgG serum levels.

Other viruses that produce cold symptoms are, for example, coronavirus, parainfluenza

Table 2–1. Principal Viruses Implicated in Respiratory Infections in Man

Genus	Nucleic Acid	Form	Symmetry	Size (mm)	Species or Types	Serologic Specifity
Adenovirus	DNA	Spherical	Icosahedral	70–80	Types 1–31	Group or type
Orthomyxovirus	RNA	Spherical or filamentous	Helicoidal	80–110	Influenza A,B,C	Type or strain
Paramyxovirus	RNA	Spherical or filamentous	Helicoidal Icosahedral	100–200	Parainfluenza 1–4	Type
					Respiratory syncytial	Species
					Rubella	Species
Picornavirus	RNA	Spherical	Icosahedral	20–30	Rhinovirus, 100 types	Type
					Coxsackievirus A–124	Type
					Coxsackievirus A–16	Type
					Echovirus 1–32	Type
Coronavirus	RNA	Spherical	Helicoidal	80–120	Types 3	Group or type
Reovirus	RNA	Spherical	Icosahedral	50–80	Types 3	Group or type
Herpesvirus	DNA	Spherical	Icosahedral	150	Herpes simplex, type 1	Species and type
					Cytomegalovirus	Species
					Epstein-Barr	Species
					Varicella-zoster	Species

Table 2–2. Viral Infections of the Respiratory Tract

Site of Infection	Virus Usual	Less Common
Rhinitis and pharyngitis	Rhinovirus	Adenovirus 1–7,14,21
	Coronavirus	Coxsackievirus A 21,24,B2–5
	Parainfluenza 1–3	Echovirus
	Respiratory syncytial	Parainfluenza 4
	Herpes simplex type 1	Epstein-Barr virus
Laryngitis	Parainfluenza 1–3	Rhinovirus
	Influenza AA	Adenovirus
	Respiratory syncytial	Rubeola
Bronchiolitis	Respiratory syncytial	Influenza A
	Parainfluenza 1,3	
Pneumonia	Respiratory syncytial	Adenovirus 3,4,7
	Parainfluenza 1,3	Rubeola, varicella
	Influenza A	Cytomegalovirus

(Modified from Fenner, F., and White, D.O.: Medical Virology. 2nd Ed. New York, Academic Press, 1976.)

viruses 1 and 3, respiratory syncytial virus, adenovirus, and coxsackie virus. The multiplicity of agents renders natural or vaccine-induced immunity almost useless. Thus, precise virologic diagnosis is hardly useful in current practice, and no effective specific therapy exists.

Antibiotics are not indicated even when the patient is febrile. Many controlled prospective studies have shown that therapy with penicillin, tetracycline, or a macrolide neither influences the course of the disease nor diminishes the frequency of bacterial superinfection either in young children, or when fever is present.

Isolation is generally ineffective, except possibly in the case of young infants or the newborn, who should be kept away from people with colds.

Persistent or Bloody Rhinorrhea. Rhinorrhea due to coryza rapidly resolves and is rarely the reason for medical consultation. On the other hand, when it persists or is bloody, it does deserve special attention.

Frequent episodes of watery rhinorrhea in a patient suggest an allergic rhinitis. Periodic recurrence outside the usual season for colds and without the usual epidemiologic context, along with a personal or familial allergic diathesis and the presence of eosinophils in the nasal secretions, all support this hypothesis.

A thick, purulent, greenish discharge, which lasts more than 10 to 15 days, should lead one to suspect a pneumococcal infection. This diagnosis can be confirmed by direct examination of the pus or by isolation of the organism on a culture medium. A complete investigation should include a search for a foreign body in the nose and an examination of the sinuses. A short course of penicillin therapy can be beneficial.

If the rhinorrhea is slightly bloody or is accompanied by superficial scaling and crusting around the nostrils, it indicates a possibility of Group A streptococcal infection (impetigo), which is usually seen in this form in children under 4 years of age. Culture confirms the diagnosis. Penicillin therapy is indicated (see Objective 3–4).

Rarely, a serosanguineous discharge in an infant is a sign of diphtheria, in which case an intranasal membrane can be seen by speculum examination. Diagnosis and treatment are discussed under Objectives 3–5, 3–6, and 3–7.

The presence of serosanguineous discharge in a neonate might suggest a diagnosis of congenital syphilis, which is now, fortunately, uncommon (see Objective 23–1).

OTHER CLINICAL SYMPTOMS

Fever. With coryza, the temperature remains normal or is only slightly elevated. When the fever is high, persistent, or more important, reappears after a period of convalescence, the physician should suspect a complication, such as otitis, sinusitis, or pneumonia, caused by either a viral agent or a bacterial superinfection. In children under 4 years of age, however, the combination of coryza and elevated temperature is common, and the fever may reach 39° C (102° F) or more without complications.

Rhinorrhea and fever can also be signs of one of the various contagious exanthems of childhood. Therefore, possible contacts should be tracked down, and the beginnings of a rash should be looked for, especially in school-age children.

One could devote an entire chapter to the subject of fever without rhinorrhea. Upper respiratory infections are a frequent cause of unexplained fever of short duration and should be searched for in febrile patients, especially in children. Often, patients lack suggestive symptoms, but clinical examination may reveal otitis, stomatitis, dental abscess, or pharyngitis. A pharyngeal culture may reveal a streptococcal infection, and a roentgenogram may show sinus involvement.

Cough. Cough is usually a sign that the lower respiratory tract is involved; however, it may sometimes be the presenting complaint of a patient with an upper airway infection. Children with rhinorrhea, for example, may cough at night because the nasal discharge flows backwards into their throats while they are lying down.

Sore Throat. For the first 24 to 48 hours after the onset of a coryza, the patient may complain of pain in the throat. This discomfort is a sign of irritation of the posterior choanae (nares) leading to the nasopharynx. Such a patient is afebrile, and examination of the throat reveals little of value. On the other hand, if pharyngeal pain is the dominant symptom, if fever is present, and if pharyngitis is observed in the physical examination, then the physician must investigate the possibility of a streptococcal infection (see Objectives 3–1 to 3–4). Polyadenopathy in association with splenomegaly should suggest the diagnosis of infectious mononucleosis (see Objective 3–8). General systemic involvement, a toxic appearance, an odor of mustiness on the breath, and pharyngeal membranes should indicate the possibility of diphtheria, especially in an appropriate epidemiologic context (see Objectives 3–5 to 3–7).

Earache. Pain in the ear, often following a coryza, can prompt the patient to consult a physician and suggests acute otitis media. In young children who cannot express themselves, a parent may suspect an ear infection because of the infant's irritability. The diagnosis is established by examination of the eardrum (see Objective 2-4).

Headache. A patient without a history of migraine or other localized headaches who has a severe headache in conjunction with rhinorrhea does not usually have simple coryza. In particular, if the pain is localized, either frontally, maxillarily, temporally, or occipitally, one should rule out a sinusitis (see Objective 2-2). This local pain is often accompanied by a frequent, purulent nasal discharge or a flow of pus down the back of the pharynx, seen when this airway is examined.

Respiratory Difficulty. The nasal discharge associated with a coryza is accompanied by a certain degree of respiratory difficulty due to the accumulation of nasal secretions. True dyspnea rarely occurs, except in the young infant.

If dyspnea is present, one must look either for involvement of the lower respiratory tract, as in pneumonia, bronchitis, or asthma, or an obstruction of the upper airways. The presence of inspiratory dyspnea suggests that the difficulty is situated within the extrathoracic air passages. When the onset of the dyspnea is abrupt, one must rule out the possibility of foreign body ingestion, spasmodic laryngitis, or epiglottitis. An inspiratory dyspnea of gradual onset suggests laryngotracheobronchitis or a retropharyngeal abscess. Both spasmodic (stridulous) laryngitis and laryngotracheobronchitis (also known as croup) are usually preceded by a seemingly ordinary rhinorrhea (see Objective 2-6).

USE OF THE MICROBIOLOGY LABORATORY

With the exception of epidemiologic studies, upper respiratory infections rarely necessitate laboratory investigations because most virologic testing is expensive and misleading. Laboratory examinations may, however, be useful or possibly indispensable in the following cases; (1) purulent drainage of

Table 2-3. Organisms Found in the Nose and Oropharynx

	Nose	Oropharynx
Staphylococcus aureus	+ +	+
Staphylococcus epidermidis	+ +	+
Streptococcus pneumoniae	+	+
Streptococci, alpha-hemolytic	+	+ +
Streptococci, group A	*	*
Streptococci, group B	*	+
Corynebacteria, aerobic	+ +	+ +
Haemophilus influenzae	+ +	+ +
Haemophilus parainfluenzae	*	+
Branhamella catarrhalis	+ +	+ +
Enteric bacteria	*	*
Peptococci	*	+ +
Veillonella	*	+ +
Spirilla, anaerobic	*	+ +
Bacteroides fragilis	*	+
Bacteroides, other species	*	+
Actinomyces	*	+
Candida	*	+
Herpesvirus	+	+
Respiratory viruses	*	*

*Fewer than 10% are carriers
+ 10-50% are carriers
+ + More than 50% are carriers

recent origin from a sinus or from an ear; (2) suspicion of diphtheria or group A streptococcal pharyngitis; and (3) diagnosis of infectious mononucleosis or influenza.

Interpretation of the cultures is not always easy because the ear canal, the nose, and the upper part of the respiratory tract are normally colonized by numerous bacterial species (Table 2-3). The isolation of an organism by culture increases in diagnostic significance under the following conditions:

1. The site from which the organism was cultured is normally sterile, such as the middle ear or a sinus.
2. The specimen has not passed through a highly contaminated area. Thus, culture of organisms recovered from pus in the external auditory canal yields less-reliable information.
3. The organism is not a normal inhabitant of the respiratory tract. *Bordetella pertussis* found in the throat is much more

significant than pneumococci found in the same area.
4. The organism is found in pure culture. Growth of a pure culture of pneumococci from pus obtained by a transmeatal sinus puncture is stronger evidence that this organism is the causative agent of a sinusitis than is growth of a mixed culture containing the same organism.
5. The sample is obtained before any antibiotic therapy is begun. Even a few hours of therapy can change the ecology of the respiratory tract and can lead to an over-representation of gram-negative bacilli in the upper airways.
6. The sample is taken from the exact site of the infection; for example, pus from the middle ear and not pus crusting in the outer ear canal.
7. The organism can be isolated at the onset of symptoms.

> **Objective 2–2. Diagnose acute sinusitis by its clinical, radiologic, and microbiologic findings.**

Sinusitis is an inflammation of the mucosa of one or several of the air-filled cavities of the cranium. This inflammation can be precipitated by cold, by the penetration of water, such as during swimming, by an allergy, or by a viral infection. Normally, the sinuses remain sterile because of the action of the ciliary epithelium and because of local immunity. Once the mucosa is inflamed, however, bacterial superinfection may develop.

CLINICAL SIGNS OF SINUSITIS

Clinically, local pain is the principal presenting complaint: it is orbitofrontal for ethmoid and frontal sinusitis, and subzygomatic for maxillary sinusitis. The pain of sphenoid sinusitis is not as well localized. Usually pressure causes pain on the forehead, the cheek bones, or in the vicinity of the emergence of the supraorbital or the suborbital nerves in frontal or maxillary sinusitis, respectively.

Purulent nasal discharge is common, most often draining through the anterior nares, but sometimes posteriorly, when a sheet of pus is seen draining down into the pharynx. During the physical examination, the physician should look for the origin of the discharge with the aid of a nasal speculum (anterior rhinoscopy) and then a pharyngeal mirror (posterior rhinoscopy). In general, the pus exudes from the middle meatus, on one or both sides. This examination is also used to check the condition of the nasal mucosa, which is often red and tender. Fever is inconstant. Polymorphonuclear leukocytosis is common in this condition.

Radiologic examination generally involves four views: the frontal film, for outlining the frontal sinuses and the anterior portion of the ethmoid bones; the oblique nasal films such as the Waters view for delineating the maxillary and frontal sinuses, albeit with some distortion, and the Caldwell view for the frontal and ethmoid sinuses; the lateral film, chiefly for viewing the sphenoid and maxillary sinuses together; and the base of the skull (Hirtz) or submental-vertex views, which are better for observing the ethmoid sinuses. In addition, panoramic dental films are used to show the relation of the maxillary sinuses to the roots of the molars as well as the condition of the latter.

Unilateral opacification and a visible fluid level form the radiologic diagnosis of sinusitis (Fig. 2–1). If the opacification is bilateral, the diagnosis becomes more difficult. Asymmetric opacification, with little in the way of clinical signs, does not strongly indicate a true bacterial sinusitis; this picture could also be due to simple catarrhal (inflammatory) or vasomotor (allergic) sinusitis, a mucosal polyp, or an intrasinus cyst.

To diagnose an ethmoid sinusitis, it is better to rely on the disappearance or the thickening of the ethmoidal partitions rather than on the appearance of opacification, except if this feature is clearly unilateral and correlates well with the clinical signs.

MICROBIOLOGIC DIAGNOSIS OF SINUSITIS

Microbiologically, the identification of a causative organism can be difficult because

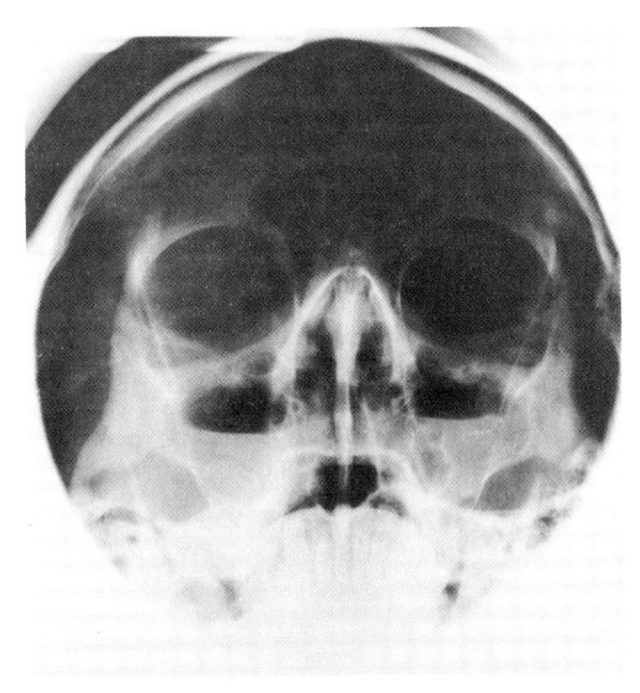

Fig. 2–1. Bilateral maxillary sinusitis with fluid levels.

abundant saprophytic flora colonize the nasal cavity. Sampling at this site is generally of no value unless the suppurative drainage is profuse. Pus collected directly from the sinus by aspiration after disinfection of the nasal mucosa gives more reliable information. Samples can be collected by transmeatal puncture of the maxillary sinus or by direct puncture of the frontal sinus. The pus thus obtained should be examined immediately by Gram staining and microscopy; it generally exhibits a pure culture or one clearly predominant organism. Direct puncture is only used when the sinusitis appears especially severe, for example when a direct intracranial extension of the infection is feared. This procedure is also useful after a failure of empiric antibiotic therapy, therapy that is begun as soon as the diagnosis has been made.

The organisms responsible are *Haemophilus influenzae* or *Streptococcus pneumoniae* in half the cases. The rest include anaerobes, often a mixed flora, *Staphylococcus aureus*, *Streptococcus pyogenes* (group A), *Branhamella catarrhalis*, enteric bacteria, and *Pseudomonas* species. Viruses account for about 15% of cases.

> **Objective 2–3.** Outline appropriate treatment for simple sinusitis, relapsing sinusitis, and severe sinusitis.

Acute sinusitis is painful and can lead to several serious complications. This possibility prompts the physician to treat the patient immediately on the supposition that the responsible organism is either a *Haemophilus* species or a pneumococcus, unless microsopic examination of the pus suggests another cause. Experience has shown that by the time the identity and sensitivities of the causative organism are reported, the patient who was treated quickly is usually much improved.

COMMON ACUTE SINUSITIS

Acute sinusitis is most often a uni- or bilateral maxillary sinusitis, or, more rarely, a frontal sinusitis. Antibiotics are chosen based on the type of bacteria most likely to be re-

> **PLASMID-MEDIATED RESISTANCE OF HAEMOPHILUS INFLUENZAE**
>
> The resistance of *Haemophilus influenzae* to the penicillins is dependent on the presence of a plasmid. A plasmid is a fragment of DNA distinct from the chromosome and situated either in the cytoplasm or incorporated into the chromosome. At the time the bacterium divides, the plasmid, having replicated independently from the chromosome, is found in the daughter cells. It can also pass from one bacterium to another by conjugation or by transport by a bacteriophage (transduction). In this way, plasmids spread new genetic information, sometimes in epidemic fashion. Many examples of the transmission of genetic information are seen in the chapters that follow: biochemical properties, production of antigens and toxins, as in diphtheria, scarlet fever, and *Escherichia coli* endotoxin, and resistance to antibiotics. Antibiotic resistance is usually due to plasmid-directed enzymes that destroy or inactivate the antibiotics. Thus, the resistance of *Haemophilus influenzae* to ampicillin is usually due to a plasmid-mediated beta-lactamase, which is capable of hydrolyzing penicillin G, ampicillin, amoxicillin, carbenicillin and certain cephalosporins. In this particular instance, resistance is sometimes missed by ordinary disc sensitivity tests, and it is necessary to look specifically for the beta-lactamase by special techniques such as nitrocefin discs; however, it is frequently detected empirically, when therapy fails. The frequency of this resistance varies from 5 to 30%, depending on the area surveyed.

sponsible (see Objective 2–2). Oral amoxicillin or ampicillin is often prescribed: 50 mg/kg/day for children, 1.5 to 3 g/day for adults. When a penicillinase-producing staphylococcus is suspected, these agents are useless and are replaced by an antistaphylococcal penicillin, such as oral dicloxicillin or parenteral oxacillin. When penicillin allergy is suspected, the trimethoprim-sulfamethoxazole combination is effective, in a dose of 2 tablets (80 mg trimethoprim and 400 mg sulfamethoxazole) morning and evening, especially against *Haemophilus* species and pneumococci; this combination is also useful against a beta-lactamase-producing *Haemophilus* species.

Antibiotic treatment is continued for 10 days, and a decongestant is usually added, as follows:

By mouth: Pseudoephedrine, preferably pure, because combined products have the disadvantage of producing drowsiness, which is potentially dangerous in an active adult. Combined products are only preferred for children. Doses vary according to the particular preparation.

Locally: Applied for short periods, local decongestants, such as nose drops or spray, can bring an overall relief of symptoms, but it is necessary to warn the patient against the danger of habituation. Only 3 or 4 applications are advisable per day.

Further, one should recommend clearing the nose frequently by blowing it *softly* and applying petrolatum to the outside of the nares to prevent irritation.

Underlying causes should also be investigated, especially those that can be corrected. Sinusitis may follow swimming or diving. In the winter, the combination of dry, warm air inside the house and cold air outside contribute to the development of sinusitis. Several local factors that decrease the ventilation and drainage of the sinuses also contribute; examples are a deviated nasal septum, edema of the mucosa due to vasomotor or allergic rhinitis (a common condition), or polyposis, which is in itself a long-term result of allergic rhinitis. Less often, one finds general factors that weaken the defense mechanisms, such as a systemic illness, recent viral infection, immunosuppressive therapy, or hypogammaglobulinemia. Mucoviscidosis is often complicated by infections of the sinuses and by the presence of polyps on the abnormal mucosa. In the adult, dental infections are a frequent source of maxillary sinusitis.

By the end of 10 days of treatment, the symptoms should be gone, and the roentgenograms should be normal. If infection persists, a specialist should be consulted.

RELAPSING SINUSITIS

A first recurrence of sinusitis is treated as previously described. If this illness is the patient's second or third relapse, the search for the underlying condition should be carried further. The interval between exacerbations is often characterized by a reduced but tenacious pain.

The roentgenograms may show a sinus that remains opacified. In this case, a specialist should be consulted to decide on the appropriate course of action: puncture, lavage, correction of the underlying causes, or surgical drainage. In the meantime, nasal washing by bulb syringe with a warm solution of sodium chloride (1 tsp/L hot water) morning and evening and the administration of oral decongestants, are recommended.

SEVERE SINUSITIS

Severe sinusitis is mainly a condition of infants and children. Adult cases arise as a complication of anterior nasal polyposis or trauma. The ethmoidal or frontal sinuses are the usual sites. Clinically, few "nasal" signs occur, but the patient may have extreme local pain, palpebral edema with immobilization of the globe, prostration, or an elevated temperature with shaking chills (an invitation to take a blood culture). On fundal examination, venous dilation may indicate intracranial venous thrombosis (see Table 1–9); on the least suspicion, a lumbar puncture is indicated.

Admission of the patient to the hospital is mandatory. Parenteral therapy should be instituted as soon as cultures are taken. Unless otherwise indicated by microscopic examination of the pus, antibiotic therapy must be directed against *Haemophilus influenzae*, pneumococci, and *Staphylococcus aureus*. Where *S. aureus* infection is likely, an antistaphylococcal-penicillin of the oxacillin type is generally given (8 to 12 g for an adult). When bacteriologic clues are lacking, the use of a third-generation cephalosporin such as cefotaxime or ceftazidime is recommended; remember that, on the whole, these products have less antistaphylococcal activity than oxacillin. After several hours of treatment, surgical drainage should be considered.

> **Objective 2–4. Diagnose acute otitis media clinically.**

Acute otitis media is an inflammation of the middle ear characterized by the presence of local exudate or pus. It is the second most common infection in children after coryza: 10 to 15% are affected by it each year, half of whom are under 3 years of age. Young children are particularly susceptible partly because their lack of immunologic experience, but also because of the anatomic orientation of the eustachian tube, which represents the usual portal of entry for acute infections of the middle ear. In the young child or infant, this tube lies in a nearly horizontal position; hence it has no dependent drainage. In addition, the orifice is still small and is surrounded by an abundance of lymphoid tissue. Repeated nasopharyngeal infections at this age lead to swelling of the mucosa and hypertrophy of the adenoids, which quickly obstruct the eustachian tube; an exudate then accumulates in the middle ear. This exudate is rendered purulent by the infiltration of polymorphonuclear cells. The intracavitary pressure then increases; the tympanic membrane bulges out and may rupture. The pus can also penetrate the air-filled cavities of the petrous bone and can produce an osteitis. Mastoiditis is now rare, however, as are meningitis and brain abscesses, because of the use of antibiotics.

PATHOGENESIS OF OTITIS

Otitis is rarely a primary infection. Generally, it is a complication of a nasopharyngeal viral infection or, more rarely, an allergic response to an allergen. Bottle feeding while a child is lying down is another contributing factor in young infants, who are often fed in this manner. Finally, in many cases, a serous effusion persists in the middle ear after treatment; this effusion is often the source of a repeated otitis at the time of a subsequent upper respiratory tract infection.

Even though the stage is usually set by a viral infection, the majority of cases of otitis media result from bacterial superinfection, as has been clearly shown by systematic transtympanic aspirations. Positive results vary, but they may exceed two-thirds of the cases. In other patients, the fluid aspirated appears sterile or, more rarely, contains a virus, such as respiratory syncytial, influenza A, coxsackie virus, parainfluenza, adenovirus, or *Mycoplasma pneumoniae*.

The bacteria responsible for the greatest

number of cases of otitis media (more than 90% in some studies) belong to only three species: *Streptococcus pneumoniae* predominates, and *Haemophilus influenzae* follows closely, chiefly in children under 5 years of age; *Streptococcus pyogenes*, a frequent cause before the introduction of antibiotics, has become rare. *Branhamella catarrhalis* is a recently recognized cause of acute otitis. Other bacteria are clearly less common, except in the intubated newborn, in whom staphylococci and enteric bacteria are frequent causes. *Staphylococcus aureus* is also often the cause of relapses, especially when the tympanic membrane has been perforated. In chronic otitis, *Pseudomonas* species are frequently implicated.

CLINICAL SIGNS OF OTITIS

Recognizing an otitis clinically is often difficult. In an infant, the warning signs, which are fever, refusal to eat, diarrhea, abdominal pains, vomiting, and irritability, scarcely suggest a disease of the ear. Even if the child is old enough to speak, or if the patient is an adult, hearing loss and earache are neither constant nor characteristic. Ear drainage, though indeed characteristic, is not common today. Practically speaking, the diagnosis of otitis media is made by demonstrating fluid in the middle ear, which is sometimes a difficult task, for it requires accurate examination of the eardrum.

In order to view the eardrum of a young child, the child is laid down with his arms held to his sides. With one hand, the physician holds the infant's head while pulling the pinna of the ear gently upwards and backwards with the thumb and index finger in order to straighten out the external canal. If the infant is under 6 months of age, it is necessary to do the opposite, that is, to pull down on the earlobe. With the other hand, the physician gently pushes an otoscope forward into the ear, taking care not to push in any wax. If it is impossible to view the eardrum conveniently because of obstruction, the external ear must be cleaned by suction or with the aid of a curette.

Otitis is easily confirmed when a spontaneous perforation of the eardrum releases a purulent discharge that, if recent, can be examined by Gram staining and microscopy. Generally, gram-positive cocci such as streptococci or pneumococci or small pleomorphic gram-negative bacilli such as *Haemophilus* species can be seen.

A red, bulging eardrum and an absent light reflex make the diagnosis of otitis nearly certain. It is rare for an otitis to be hidden behind a flat membrane that retains its light reflex, whether the tympanic membrane is red or not. "Red eardrums" are sometimes due simply to crying or to fever, without any specific local ear inflammation.

A retracted eardrum indicates a negative pressure within the middle ear and precludes an acute otitis.

Bullous myringitis is a special case characterized by a red eardrum spotted by one or several blisters. It is often associated with a mycoplasmal infection, although this is probably not the exclusive cause.

Actually, interpretation of a red eardrum is difficult, especially in a child who has already had several episodes of otitis or in the young infant. When in doubt, the use of a pneumatic otoscope, which is unfortunately sometimes a painful procedure, allows the physician to determine whether the eardrum is mobile, the possibility of otitis is remote. Detection of diminished mobility of the eardrum depends on the experience of the examiner. Recourse can be made to an objective method such as tympanometry. Sound waves are directed at the membrane and the quantity reflected by the eardrum is then measured. The more mobile the eardrum, the more sound is absorbed. The mobility of the eardrum is affected by the presence of liquid in the middle ear. The practical value of this objective technique for the diagnosis of otitis media remains to be shown, however, especially in the infant. When the diagnosis is still in doubt, simply observe the child for 48 hours; a therapeutic decision at this point is probably easier to make.

> **Objective 2–5. Treat acute otitis media appropriately.**

Once the diagnosis of acute otitis media is certain, antibiotic therapy is required. If it is well chosen, it will reduce the risk of relapse, decrease the duration of symptoms, and diminish the occurrence of complications.

CHOICE OF AN ANTIBIOTIC

The choice of antibiotic depends upon the following considerations:

Otitis in the first few weeks of the life of a hospitalized newborn usually accompanies a more serious illness. The bacterial origin is unpredictable; it varies from staphylococci to gram-negative bacilli. Consequently, a culture taken by transtympanic puncture or paracentesis is necessary to establish the identity and sensitivities of the causative organism. Most of the time, an intravenous antistaphylococcal penicillin and an aminoglycoside are indicated.

After the neonatal period, the first choice of therapeutic agents is a penicillin. When it is likely that *Haemophilus influenzae* is responsible, amoxicillin, whose intestinal absorption and penetration into the middle ear exceeds that of ampicillin, should be given (50 mg/kg/day). Amoxicillin is particularly appropriate in children under 5 years of age with a rhinorrhea lasting more than 2 weeks or with otitis accompanied by purulent conjunctivitis, or when a *Haemophilus* species has actually been isolated from the culture of nasopharyngeal secretions. Clinical studies have not demonstrated the superiority of amoxicillin or ampicillin to penicillin when the etiologic agent has not been identified, however. A difference appears only if otitis due to *Haemophilus influenzae* is considered separately. Nevertheless, the increasing importance of this organism as a cause of otitis, even in adults, has made amoxicillin or ampicillin the agent of choice no matter what the patient's age.

The appearance of *Haemophilus influenzae* resistant to ampicillin modifies this scheme (see Objective 2–3). In most situations the number of resistant colonies is small enough that initial therapy does not need to be changed from that previously recommended, that is amoxicillin. When initial treatment has failed, however, a change in therapy should be considered. Actual evidence of beta-lactamase production by *H. influenzae* in the nasopharyngeal sections of the middle ear necessitates the use of another antimicrobial agent. Chloramphenicol (50 mg/kg/day) would be appropriate and is usually effective, but it is not indicated because, unfortunately, it may cause aplastic anemia (1 in 25,000 to 40,000 patients treated). The combination of trimethoprim and sulfamethoxazole (trimethoprim, 6 mg/kg/day and sulfamethoxazole, 30 mg/kg/day) can also be recommended. Cross-resistance between ampicillin and trimethoprim-sulfamethoxazole has thus far appeared rarely in *H. influenzae*. An oral cephalosporin, cefaclor (40 to 60 mg/kg/day), is probably another alternative to chloramphenicol, but its cost prevents it from replacing amoxicillin as the drug of initial choice.

In children allergic to penicillin, erythromycin is the treatment of choice (50 mg/kg/day); a sulfonamide such as sulfisoxazole (120 mg/kg/day) is added to it in cases of otitis due to *Haemophilus influenzae*. This combination of erythromycin and a sulfonamide has been a pediatric favorite in the United States for a long time. The trimethoprim-sulfamethoxazole combination or cefaclor are alternatives.

In bullous myringitis, owing to its likely association with a mycoplasma, erythromycin (30 mg/kg/day in the adult) is a logical choice.

Treatment of 10 days' duration has always been considered sufficient; however, this belief is now in question. Indeed, after 10 days of antibiotic therapy, the middle ear can, in nearly 50% of cases, still contain fluid that is positive on culture. It may be that, in the future, standard therapy will be 10 days of amoxicillin followed by a sulfonamide until the serous otitis disappears. The use of decongestants or antihistamines does not reduce the incidence of residual serous otitis and may even increase it.

MYRINGOTOMY

Myringotomy was an important procedure before the days of antibiotics, but is rarely indicated today. On the whole, it neither improves the course of otitis in the short run nor reduces complications in the long run. The frequency of prolonged or relapsing otitis in antibiotic-treated patients is not altered by myringotomy.

Several elective indications for this procedure still remain, however. It is necessary if the patient has intolerable pain or an eardrum so distended that spontaneous perforation seems imminent. Culture of the pus is needed mainly after a failure of antimicrobial therapy, in an immunodeficient patient, or during the neonatal period. When the physician merely needs to obtain a sample for a culture, simple puncture under microscopic control is usually preferable to myringotomy.

> Objective 2–6. Evaluate the risk of airway obstruction in laryngitis and treat appropriately. Recognize the cases of laryngitis that require specific treatment.

Laryngeal infections are common. The predominant cause is viral, and most cases resolve without treatment. These infections can, however, be threatening when they produce respiratory obstruction. Therefore, it is important that the physician know how to identify those clinical situations in which obstruction is a major risk, to treat the patient appropriately and in time. Furthermore, he must know when to suspect an early diphtheria or a retropharyngeal abscess—rare contingencies, but ones requiring specific responses that cannot be delayed.

The various different laryngeal infections do not have the same risk of laryngeal obstruction. In distinguishing one infection from another, the evidence is essentially clinical. It is based principally on the age of the patient and on the rapidity of the onset of the symptoms and dyspnea.

LARYNGITIS IN THE ADULT

In the adult, laryngitis is manifested most often by a hoarse or barely audible voice; respiratory difficulty may occur. Rhinorrhea or a slight fever may complete the picture. Laryngitis is usually of viral origin, and no particular treatment is necessary once the history and physical exam have ruled out other causes, such as trauma, neoplasm, or allergy.

It should be pointed out, however, that cases of acute epiglottitis due to *Haemophilus influenzae*, diphtherial laryngitis, and retropharyngeal abscess are possibilities in adults and present problems similar to those in children.

Laryngeal tuberculosis generally appears in a clinical picture already strongly suggestive of pulmonary tuberculosis in a severely ill patient. The diagnosis relies on the laryngoscopic appearance of small, yellowish tubercles and the microbiologic examination of direct specimens by smear or culture.

LARYNGITIS IN THE CHILD

The risk of respiratory difficulty in a child with laryngitis requires a much more elaborate approach. Customarily, a child with laryngitis has hoarseness of the voice, frequently accompanied by a cough. The voice may be completely silenced. The physician should pay strict attention to the possible development of dyspnea, which results from a narrowing of the airway.

Laryngeal obstruction expresses itself mainly as difficulty in taking a breath. Inspiration is prolonged, eventually becoming noisy (stridor) and is accompanied by respiratory indrawing, that is, pulling inward of the supra-and infraclavicular spaces, the intercostal spaces, and sometimes even the epigastric space, with inspiration. In contrast, expiration proceeds rapidly and without difficulty, at least when the obstruction is not too severe. Cyanosis is a sign of the utmost gravity.

The physician should try to determine, through the patient's history, whether the dyspnea is of recent appearance, that is, within the past several hours, or whether it has developed progressively. Although the list of possibilities is extensive, a recent appearance suggests, above all, an epiglottitis or a spasmodic laryngitis, whereas a progressive onset should bring to mind a viral laryngotracheobronchitis or "croup."

Dyspnea of Progressive Onset. The symptoms start one or several days before the child is brought to a physician. If the child is under 3 years old, if a rhinopharyngitis preceded the laryngitis and if the fever is moderate, this illness is probably a subglottal infection or a laryngotracheobronchitis, which, when severe, is commonly called "croup." Respiration is audible with inspiratory stridor and a hoarse, barking cough. Viral isolation from pharyngeal secretion is at its highest in this respiratory infection, with a definite predilection for parainfluenza viruses (see Table 2–4). Remember, however, that viral studies can, in practice, be omitted because they do not influence therapy.

Before the diagnosis can be definitively established, several rare possibilities must be excluded. The physical examination, for example, may uncover a retropharyngeal abscess by revealing a fluctuant mass in the posterior pharyngeal wall. Hospitalization in a specialized care unit is needed in this case so that the abscess may promptly be drained by surgical means. Because anaerobes from the oropharyngeal flora are usually involved, penicillin G is generally recommended as antimicrobial therapy.

Diphthereal laryngitis must be considered when the specific epidemiologic or clinical evidence mentioned in Objective 3–5 is present. This infection is serious because the special risks presented by diphtheria toxin are added to the dangers of respiratory obstruction. The approach to this type of patient is given in Objectives 3–6 and 3–7.

TREATMENT OF VIRAL LARYNGOTRACHEOBRONCHITIS ("CROUP"). The child with laryngotracheobronchitis requires close observation with as little disturbance as possible. A mist tent can be used to maintain a humidified atmosphere for the child; this helps to liquify and to mobilize the secretions that contribute to the obstruction. The experience in some centers indicates that the use of racemic epinephrine can reduce the frequency of intubations and tracheostomy. A solution of 2.25% is diluted 1 to 8 in sterile water and is given with intermittent positive pressure (15 cm H_2O) by facial mask. Each treatment should run from 10 to 15 minutes.

In the majority of patients, with or without epinephrine, neither intubation nor tracheostomy is necessary. Even when endotracheal intubation is necessary, it does not produce as good a result as in epiglottitis. In fact, endotracheal tubes seem to maintain the subglottal inflammation, which delays extubation and may make tracheostomy necessary. The use of corticosteroids is controversial. One approach is to use them for a short period (such as methylprednisone 4 mg/kg every 4 hours for 3 doses) in severely affected patients or when the condition is worsening despite the use of other therapeutic techniques, such as a humidified atmosphere.

In laryngotracheobronchitis, antibiotics are not indicated because this infection is viral. A rare but extremely severe form of this disease is called necrotizing laryngotracheobronchitis. It is characterized by the appearance on the mucosa of a thick, purulent exudate. Even though this form probably has a viral origin, bacterial superinfection of the altered mucosa is likely to occur rapidly. In

Table 2–4. Organisms Identified in 132 Children Hospitalized for Laryngotracheobronchitis

	Frequency (%)
Parainfluenza virus	42
Respiratory syncytial virus	6
Influenza virus	6
Rhinovirus	6
Adenovirus	3
Echovirus	2
Mycoplasma pneumoniae	1
Sterile samples	34

(Data from Dowsham, M.A.P.S., McQuillan, J., and Gardner, P.S.: Diagnosis and clinical significance of parainfluenza virus infections in children. Arch. Dis. Child., *49*:8, 1974.)

this case, antibiotic therapy, selected according to the culture results, is useful.

Inspiratory Dyspnea of Rapid Onset. In this instance, the physician must distinguish among several possible diagnoses: dyspnea due to a foreign body, acute epiglottitis, or spasmodic laryngitis.

FOREIGN BODY INGESTION. The sudden appearance, over a few minutes, of inspiratory dyspnea in a child who has been eating or playing with small objects should quickly orient the physician toward the diagnosis of foreign body ingestion. The child is afebrile, and removal of the object clears the obstruction.

ACUTE EPIGLOTTITIS. This dreaded life-threatening infection is a true medical emergency. The cause is almost exclusively *Haemophilus influenzae* type B (streptococci have also been known to produce it rarely), which can be isolated from the blood or from pharyngeal culture in more than 90% of these patients.

The illness starts abruptly in a 2- to 6-year-old, previously healthy child. Within a few hours, the mother notices dysphagia and dysphonia. A striking picture of respiratory insufficiency then develops: the child sits upright, the mouth open and drooling. Fever often exceeds 39° C (103° F). Palpable cervical adenopathy is present.

The risk of provoking respiratory arrest is so great that it is generally preferable not to examine the patient's throat too closely. Even though oral examination may reveal a cherry-red, swollen epiglottis rising over the base of the tongue, the procedure endangers the patient, and, furthermore, is unnecessary because the epiglottitis can be easily and safely visualized by a lateral roentgenogram of the neck. The shadow of the epiglottis is enlarged and rounded, looking like a thumb when normally it resembles the tip of the little finger (Fig. 2–2). Incidentally, this film is useful in the differential diagnosis: both laryngotracheobronchitis and spasmodic laryngitis show visible glottal narrowing; the bulging of a retropharyngeal abscess is easily noted; and sometimes, a radiopaque foreign body is seen.

If the clinical or radiologic diagnosis of epiglottitis is suggested, the child can be taken to an operating room or similar facility to confirm the diagnosis. Visualization of the swollen, cherry-red epiglottis leads to the placement, under anesthesia, of a nasotracheal tube. Blood and local cultures are taken, and ampicillin therapy (200 mg/kg/day IV) is instituted immediately.

The patient is then transferred to an intensive care unit and is kept in a humidified atmosphere. Once the effect of the anesthetic wears off, administration of tubocurarine is generally not necessary because the child, relieved of the obstruction, seems to accept the tube well. If this is not the case, diazepam, given intravenously at a dose of 0.2 mg/kg, is sufficient. Extubation is attempted in an operating room 36 to 48 hours later, and antibiotic therapy is continued for 10 days.

When no significant respiratory distress is seen, some authors recommend commencing antibiotic therapy and keeping the patient under close observation. We believe this approach is risky, even with experienced personnel because antibiotic treatment does not, in general, completely prevent subsequent respiratory deterioration, which may sometimes be difficult to control. Intubation, a simple procedure, removes the risk.

As discussed, the diagnosis of epiglottitis directly implies a *Haemophilus influenzae* infection. In spite of the existence of ampicillin-resistant strains, we believe it reasonable to continue to use ampicillin as the drug of first choice. Here, in contrast to meningitis, the infection itself is not likely to be an immediate cause of death; airway obstruction is the real danger. Our attitude would be different, however, when evidence suggests dissemination of the organism to other areas of the body, as in pneumonia or meningitis, when the case occurs in a part of the world where the incidence of ampicillin-resistant *H. influenzae* is high, or when a resistant strain has been isolated on culture. In these patients, chloramphenicol becomes the drug of choice. The new cephalosporins, cefotaxime and moxalactam, because of their high activity against

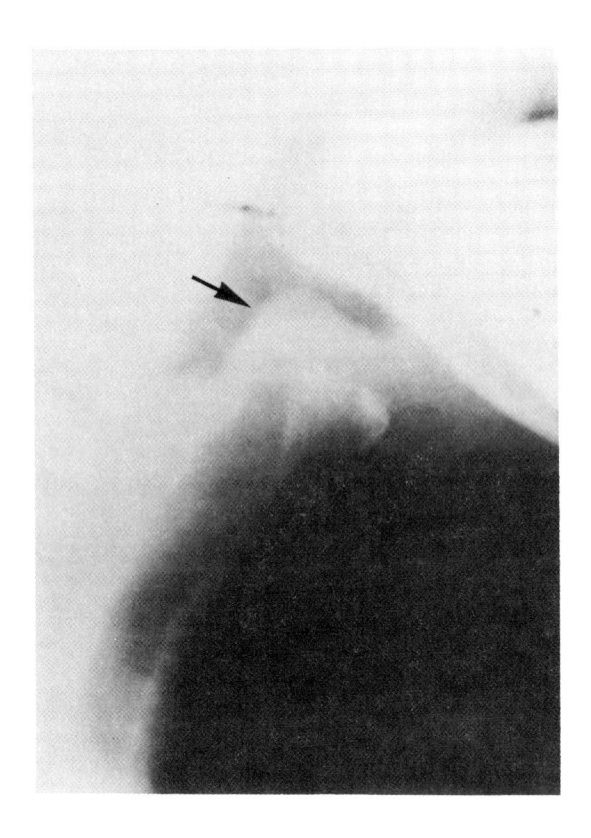

Fig. 2–2. Epiglottitis. Arrow indicates the enlarged epiglottis.

H. influenzae, their resistance to beta-lactamases, and their good tolerance, may, in the future, become the agents of choice in the treatment of epiglottitis, pending the results of the sensitivity tests.

SPASMODIC LARYNGITIS. Spasmodic laryngitis is a curious illness; impressive, but more benign than epiglottitis. Its origin is poorly understood. Although parents may notice a mild rhinorrhea in their child during the day, the illness seems to appear suddenly, usually during the night. The child, usually 2 to 4 years of age, is awakened by an abrupt onset of respiratory distress, without fever. Again, it is advisable not to examine the throat too closely; a roentgenogram of the neck is recommended instead. A highly humidified atmosphere, such as a home bathroom or a mist tent, greatly improves the child's condition. The use of racemic epinephrine often results in spectacular relaxation of the anxious child; however, its effect only lasts 2 hours. A single dose may give rise to a false sense of security, and the child may be sent home only to have the dyspnea reappear later with the same intensity. In fact, close observation is necessary. The obstruction can, on occasion, be sufficiently severe to warrant intubation or tracheostomy, especially in the young. Given the contradictory results obtained with corticosteroids, we feel that a trial is justified only in order to avoid intubation in these children (dexamethasone, 0.3 mg/kg at 2-hour intervals for 2 doses). Antibiotics are not indicated.

SUGGESTED READINGS

Berman, S.A., Blakany, T.J., and Simmons, M.A.: Otitis media in infants less than 12 weeks of age: differing bacteriology among in-patients and out-patients. J. Pediatr., 93:453, 1978.

Berman, S.A., Balkany, T.J., and Simmons, M.A.: Otitis media in the neonatal intensive care unit. Pediatrics, 62:198, 1978.

Evans, F.O., et al.: Sinusitis of the maxillary antrum. N. Engl. J. Med., 293:735, 1975.

Fearon, B.W., and Bell, R.D.: Acute epiglottitis: a potential killer. Can. Med. Assoc. J., 112:760, 1975.

Gellady, A.M., Shulman, S.T., and Ayoud, E.M.: Periorbital and orbital cellulitis in children. Pediatrics, 61:272, 1978.

Giebink, G.S., et al.: The microbiology of serous and mucoid otitis media. Pediatrics, 63:915, 1979.

Hamory, B.H., et al.: Etiology and antimicrobial therapy of acute maxillary sinusitis. J. Infect. Dis., 139:197, 1979.

Hays, G.C., and Mullard, J.E.: Can nasal bacterial flora be predicted from clinical findings? Pediatrics, 49:596, 1972.

Leipzig, B., et al.: Prospective randomized study to determine the efficacy of steroids in treatment of croup. J. Pediatr., 94:194, 1979.

Lexomboon, U., et al.: Evaluation of orally administered antibiotics for treatment of upper respiratory infections in Thai children. J. Pediatr., 78:772, 1971.

Nelson, J.D., Ginsburg, C.M., Clahsen, J.C., and Jackson, L.H.: Treatment of acute otitis media of infancy with cefaclor. Am. J. Dis. Child., 132:992, 1978.

Pelton, S.I., Teele, D.W., Shurin, P.A., and Kelin, J.O.: Disparate cultures of middle ear fluids: results from children with bilateral otitis media. Am. J. Dis. Child., 134:951, 1980.

Schwartz, R., Rodriguez, W.J., Khan, W.N., and Ross, S.: Acute purulent otitis media in children older than 5 years. Incidence of Haemophilus as a causative organism. JAMA, 238:1032, 1977.

Shurin, P.A., Pelton, S.I., Donner, A., and Klein, J.O.: Persistence of middle-ear effusion after acute otitis media in children, N. Engl. J. Med., 300:1121, 1979.

Shurin, P.A., Pelton, S.I., and Finkelstein, J.: Tympanometry in the diagnosis of middle-ear effusion. N. Engl. J. Med., 296:412, 1977.

Wald, E.R., et al.: Acute maxillary sinusitis in children. N. Engl. J. Med., 304:749, 1981.

Wortzman, D., and Holgate, R.C.: Special radiological techniques in maxillary sinus disease. Otolaryngol. Clin. North Am., 9:117, 1976.

CHAPTER 3

Sore Throat and Fever

P. Déry, J.C. Pechère, J. Joncas, and P. Bernard

Objective 3–1. Determine which patient with pharyngitis requires a throat culture for streptococci.

Pharyngitis and tonsillitis affect many people each year and have a considerable socioeconomic impact. These disorders are the most common reason for consulting a physician. Unfortunately, however, they are also among the worst treated of all illnesses, primarily because of the overprescription of antibiotics.

Before treating pharyngitis with antibiotic therapy, the physician should attempt to determine whether the condition requires this treatment. In making the decision, the following five factors should be considered:

1. More than eight times out of ten, the pharyngitis is of viral origin and requires no antimicrobial treatment. Therefore, it is gross abuse to treat all pharyngitis with antibiotics. Patients that require antibiotic therapy, such as those with infections due to group A streptococci, must be identified, however.
2. It is nearly impossible to establish the diagnosis of streptococcal pharyngitis by clinical means alone.
3. Identification of the streptococcus by means of a throat swab and culture is the best way to confirm the diagnosis.
4. The major goal of antibiotic therapy for streptococcal pharyngitis is to prevent acute rheumatic fever, but it is not proved that antibiotics provide relief to the patient or modify the illness.
5. Antibiotics effectively prevent rheumatic fever even if treatment is put off for several days—specifically, the time required to obtain the results of a throat culture.

It is well established that group A streptococci are responsible for many cases of pharyngitis. Every throat swab yields, in culture, numerous different bacteria; only a change in flora incriminates a particular organism. Group A streptococcus is the bacteria most frequently isolated in patients with pharyngitis. By comparison, *Staphylococcus aureus*, *Pneumococcus* species, and *Haemophilus influenzae* appear with equal frequency in all patients, whether or not they have pharyngitis. Table 3–1 describes other bacterial causes of pharyngitis and tonsillitis.

A viral origin is much more common, however. Although practically absent in asymptomatic individuals, viruses are found in 20 to 30% of patients with pharyngitis and tonsillitis. Additional evidence suggests that

Table 3-1. Causes of Pharyngitis and Tonsillitis

Organisms	Main Clinical Characteristics	How to Confirm the Diagnosis
Bacteria		
Streptococcus pyogenes	Reddened pharynx, with or without whitish exudate; sometimes scarlet fever	Throat culture (medium: sheep blood agar) (Objective 3-2)
Mycoplasma pneumonia	Reddened pharynx, without exudate or membrane formation; sometimes interstitial pneumonia, bullous myringitis (Objective 6-6)	Serologic study (Objective 6-6)
Neisseria gonorrhoeae	Reddened pharynx; sexual history; sometimes urethritis, proctitis, cervicitis	Throat culture (medium: Thayer-Martin) (Objective 22-3)
Corynebacterium diphtheriae	False membrane, toxic appearance, large satellite adenopathies (Objective 3-6)	Throat culture (medium: tellurite agar) (Objective 3-7)
Combination of anaerobic bacteria (Vincent's angina)	Pharyngeal ulcerations and edema, toxic appearance	Gram stain of pharyngeal secretion shows fusobacteria and spirochetes
Virus		
Epstein-Barr	Reddened pharynx, with or without exudate or false membrane; extrapharyngeal signs of infectious mononucleosis	Atypical lymphocytes, heterophile and EBV antibodies (Objective 3-9)
Coxsackie A	Herpangina; small vesicles in the palate, pillars, tonsils, and posterior pharyngeal wall, but not in the anterior portion of the mouth	Isolation of virus and serologic study
Herpes simplex type I (sometimes type II)	Gingivostomatitis; vesicular or ulcerated lesions mainly affect the anterior portion of the mouth (gums, etc.), but can be found in the posterior pharyngeal wall	Isolation of virus from the lesions; Tzanck smear from ulcer (intranuclear inclusion bodies and giant cells); serologic study
Adenoviruses and others	Reddened pharynx with or without exudate; often rhinitis, conjunctivitis, and bronchitis	Generally not done
Fungi		
Candida albicans	Reddened pharynx with whitish exudate	Gram stain of pharyngeal secretion and culture (medium: Sabouraud)
Unknown		
Kawasaki disease	Reddened pharynx, strawberry tongue, and clinical criteria (Chap. 27)	No specific tests available

more than 80% of pharyngitis is of viral origin: included are adenoviruses, herpesviruses such as herpes simplex, Epstein-Barr, and cytomegalovirus, echoviruses, myxo- and paramyxoviruses, rhinoviruses, and coronaviruses.

UNCERTAINTY OF THE CLINICAL DIAGNOSIS OF PHARYNGITIS

Distinguishing between viral and streptococcal pharyngitis by physical examination is difficult except in the following clinical situations:

1. When the patient has scarlet fever, which indicates a streptococcal origin (Objective 27-7).
2. When the pharyngitis is vesicular, which suggests a viral origin. This disease is called herpangina and is caused by several types of coxsackievirus A (Fig. 3-1).

Otherwise, the clinical diagnosis is subject to numerous errors. The so-called "typical" patient with streptococcal pharyngitis has an acute illness with a painful throat, an intense

Sore Throat and Fever

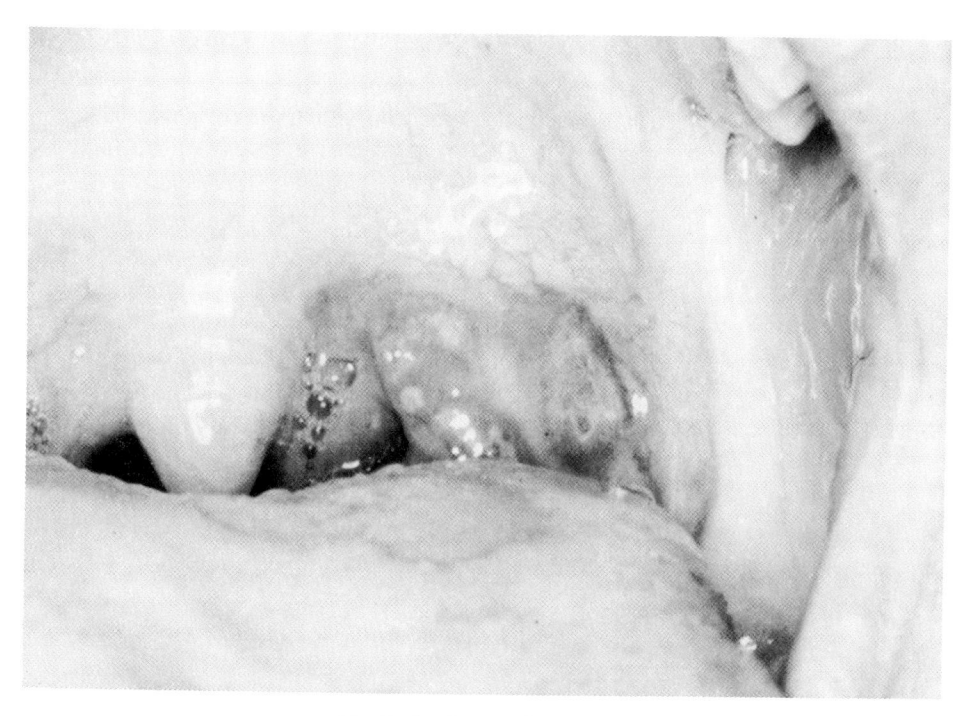

Fig. 3–1. Herpangina vesicles.

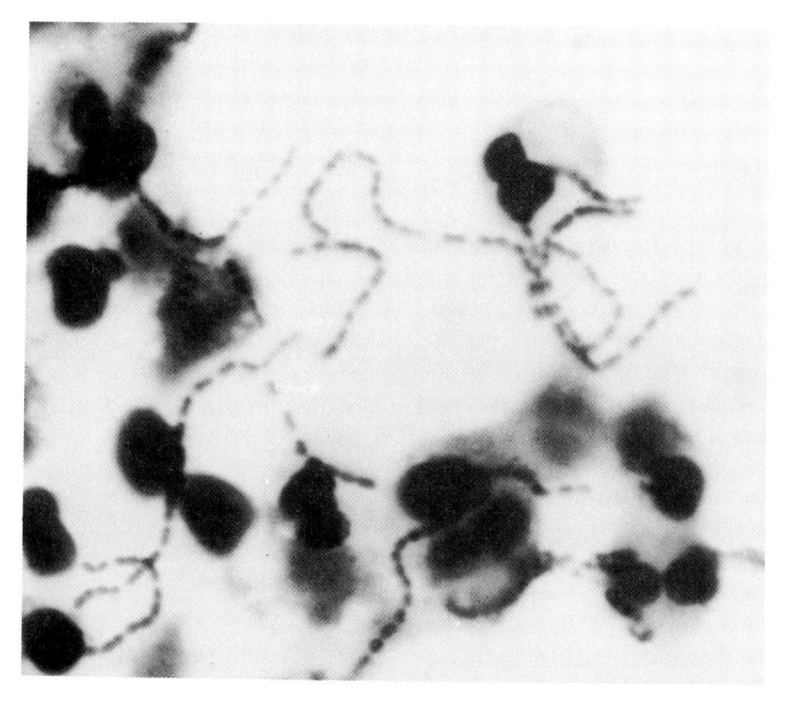

Fig. 3–2. Chains of *Streptococcus pyogenes* (group A) in a smear of pus.

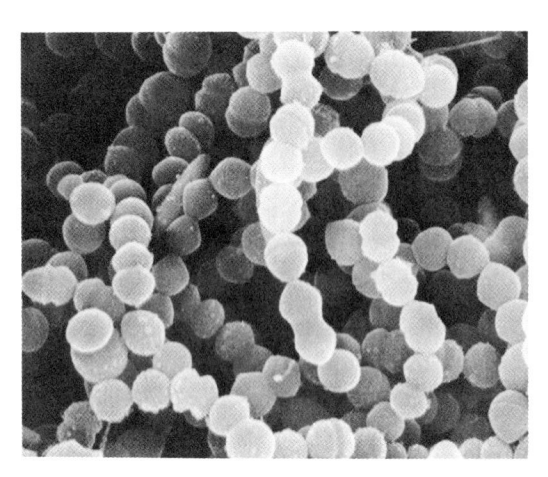

Fig. 3–3. *Streptococcus pyogenes* as seen under a scanning electron microscope. Note that cell divisions are always in the same plane; this phenomenon explains the chain-like configuration after several generations. (1 cm = 1 micron). (Courtesy of R. Guindoin.)

sensation of malaise, nausea, and an elevated fever. Throat examination reveals a striking, intense erythema, the tonsils and the uvula are swollen, petechiae are scattered on the soft palate; a whitish exudate, easily detachable with a tongue blade, usually covers the tonsils, and painful adenopathy fills the anterior cervical spaces. Unfortunately, several studies have shown that one cannot rely upon this clinical picture, partly because fewer than two-thirds of cases of streptococcal pharyngitis produce these findings, and partly because viral pharyngitis can present an identical picture. Overall, the physician who bases prescription of antibiotic therapy solely on the clinical appearance treats far too many cases of viral pharyngitis and, at the same time, leaves some patients with true streptococcal pharyngitis untreated.

INDICATIONS FOR THROAT CULTURE

Throat culture clearly is required to establish a diagnosis; however, it would be undesirable to take a throat culture from every patient. Therefore, some guidelines must be followed to ensure that most cases of streptococcal pharyngitis are sampled without sampling every sore throat.

Certainly, throat cultures are mandatory in all patients with the classic clinical picture, as previously described, especially because the frequency of rheumatic fever (RF) is higher (2 to 3%) following a severe pharyngitis with a purulent exudate than when the symptoms are less severe (less than 1%). Otherwise, the indications for throat culture depend on the age of the patient.

Children under 4 years of age form a group with a high incidence of upper respiratory infections, but their risk of RF is small. Group A streptococcal infections are uncommon in this age group. When they do occur, they take on the appearance of a purulent rhinitis, often with a blood-tinged discharge, and with scabs and weeping lesions around the nose (impetigo); they may even appear as fever of undetermined origin without pharyngitis. Therefore, one can justifiably limit the search for streptococci to patients with classic, severe pharyngitis, suspicious rhinorrheas, and fevers of unknown origin.

Between 4 years of age and adolescence, throat cultures are taken more frequently. They are indicated in all patients in whom the fear of RF appears justified, as follows: (1) fever above 38° C (100.4° F)—the risk is small when pharyngitis occurs without fever; (2) lower socioeconomic milieu; and especially (3) a history of RF in the individual or in his family.

In the adult, the danger of RF is minimal. Indications for throat culture are limited to patients with "typical" pharyngitis and to those with a history of RF.

Sore Throat and Fever

GROUP A STREPTOCOCCI OR *STREPTOCOCCUS PYOGENES*

Streptococci are characterized by their morphologic features, such as gram-positive cocci in chains (Figs. 3–2 and 3–3). These organisms have an anaerobic metabolism, but tolerate atmospheric oxygen. The medium of choice for their isolation is sheep blood agar because it contains the nutrients necessary for their growth and permits detection of their hemolytic properties. Complete or beta hemolysis produces a clear zone, as seen surrounding streptococci in pharyngitis; incomplete or alpha hemolysis leaves a greenish zone, as seen with pneumococci and alpha-hemolytic streptococci; hemolysis may also be absent.

Although hemolysis is the first means of identification, it is, unfortunately, not sufficient. Full classification of the streptococci depends principally on immunologic criteria, Deep within the cell wall is a polysaccharide, or C antigen, which can be extracted in the laboratory. When this antigen is injected into rabbits, the antisera obtained distinguish among 20 serologic groups, lettered A through H and K through P (Table 3–2).

Streptococcus pyogenes comprises group A. This organism is remarkable mainly for its delayed, nonsuppurative sequelae (Table 3–3). Its C antigen, composed of rhamnose and N-acetyl glucosamine, may be implicated in the etiology of acute rheumatic fever, as suggested by two observations. First, N-acetyl glucosamine and certain glycoproteins of the heart valves in man fix the same specific antibody. Next, persistently elevated levels of antipolysaccharide C antibody are detected in rheumatic carditis, whereas in the usual course of a *Streptococcus pyogenes* infection they are barely detectable.

In addition to the C antigen, *Streptococcus pyogenes* has several surface antigens, one of which, the M protein (Table 3–4), has over 50 immunologic varieties. These surface antigens permit group A to be subdivided, by means of slide agglutination tests, into as many types as there are monospecific sera. M protein seems to play a role in pathogenicity, as suggested by the following observations:

1. Streptococci do not adhere to pharyngeal cells when the M protein is absent or masked by specific antibody (IgA antibodies are found in the parotid saliva). Therefore, the spicules of M protein must attach themselves to specific epithelial receptor sites, the first requirement for pathogenicity.
2. Streptococci deprived of M protein, or covered with anti-M antibody, are easily phagocytosed by polymorphonuclear cells. In the absence of antibody, complete streptococci are resistant to phagocytosis.
3. In man, a *Streptococcus pyogenes* infection gives rise to an apparently protective anti-M antibody. Thus, although no group immunity is present, a specific immunity for each M type exists.
4. Acute poststreptococcal glomerulonephritis is associated with certain M types of group A streptococci, especially type 12, but also types 1, 4, and 18 following a pharyngitis and types 2, 31, 49, 52, 57, and 60 after a cutaneous infection. Table 3–5 illustrates the relationship between the M types and the possible sequelae.

T protein is a third antigen. Like M protein, T protein is superficial. Although anti-T sera are occasionally used for epidemiologic purposes, T protein does not seem to play a specific role in virulence.

Group A streptococci also secrete a large number of substances. The principal ones are described in Table 3–6.

Table 3–2. Major Pathogenic Streptococci in Man

Name	Group	Hemolysis	Disease in Man
S. pyogenes	A	β	Pharyngitis, rheumatic fever, glomerulonephritis, scarlet fever, erysipelas, septicemia
S. agalactiae	B	β	Neonatal infections, septicemia
S. faecalis	D	None, α or β	Urinary infections, endocarditis
S. mutans	Nongroupable	α	Endocarditis, dental caries
S. pneumoniae	Nongroupable	α	Pneumonia, otitis, meningitis

Objective 3–2. Select the proper method for taking a throat culture for group A streptococci.

TECHNIQUE FOR THROAT CULTURE

The patient should be seated, or supported if an infant, head hyperextended, mouth open widely, with the tongue drawn down and the pharynx well exposed. The tonsillar areas should be touched firmly with a sterile swab. Swabbing the posterior wall of the pharynx is optional because it provokes a gag reflex and nausea without increasing the likelihood of positive culture. Contact of the swab with the tongue and buccal mucosa should be carefully avoided.

LABORATORY PROCEDURES

Direct microscopic examination of the exudate usually gives little information.

Table 3–3. Clinical and Epidemiologic Characteristics of the Sequelae of Group A Streptococcal Infection

	Scarlet fever	Erysipelas	Glomerulo-nephritis	Rheumatic fever	Erythema nodosum	Chorea
Usual age	4–8	all ages	2–12	4–25	Child, adult	Child
Site of initial infection						
Skin	rare	yes	yes	no (except)	no	no
Throat	yes	rare	yes	yes	yes	yes
Other mucosa	yes	rare	no	rare	no	no
Delay between initial infection and sequelae	1–2 days	1–4 days	1–3 weeks	2–4 weeks	1–2 weeks	1–6 weeks
Presence of streptococci in distant lesions	0 exceptional with associated septicemia	yes	no	no	no	no
Blood culture positive	rare	occasionally	no	no	no	no
Familial predisposition	yes	no	no	yes	no	yes
Possibility of relapse	rare	yes	rare	yes	slight to none	rare

Table 3–4. Group A Streptococci: The Two Key Antigens

Polysaccharide C
 Basis of grouping streptococci
 All group A streptococci having the same polysaccharide C
 Polysaccharide C not giving rise in man to formation of antibody
 No group immunity
Protein M
 Basis for typing group A streptococci
 More than 50 different M proteins recognized (that is, more than 50 types of group A streptococci)
 Relationship between virulence and presence of M protein
 M antigen leading to the formation of protective antibody
 Type-specific immunity

The sample can be seeded directly onto blood agar, or if the swab can reach the laboratory within 2 to 3 hours, it is sufficient simply to place it in a sterile tube. For longer delays, blood agar in a tube may be used. If the sample is to be sent by mail, acceptable results can be obtained by rapid drying, for example, by placing the sample in a tube with a desiccating agent, such as aluminum hydroxide gel, or by absorbing the moisture with a piece of sterile filter paper.

The culture medium of choice is fresh moist agar containing 5 to 10% sheep blood. When the swab has been desiccated for transport, it is first passed for several hours in broth; if not, the plate may be streaked directly by quadrants in order to obtain isolated colonies.

The throat contains many bacterial species, but group A streptococci stand out on blood agar because of their beta hemolysis. Ordinarily, only colonies surrounded by a halo of complete hemolysis are identified further, but because streptolysin O, in contrast with streptolysin S, is inactivated by atmospheric oxygen, and because certain strains secrete only streptolysin O, hemolysis is sometimes

Table 3–5. Relationship Between Types of Group A Streptococci and Possible Sequelae

Clinical Entity	Types of Streptococci
Scarlet fever	All types, provided they are parasitized by a bacteriophage that induces the formation of erythrogenic toxin
Rheumatic fever	All types
Acute glomerulonephritis	If initial infection is pharyngeal, 12.1, 4
	If initial infection is cutaneous, 49.2, 31
Erysipelas	At least 14 different types
Erythema nodosum	No data available

Table 3-6. Some Enzymes and Toxins Secreted by Group A Streptococci

Material Secreted	Antigenic Response in Man	Properties
Erythrogenic toxin	Yes, antitoxin protective	Responsible for some symptoms of scarlatina such as rash, vomiting, early nephritis
Streptolysin O	Yes, antistreptolysins	Destroys red cells
Streptolysin S	No	Destroys red cells
Streptokinases A and B	Yes, antistreptokinases	Lyse fibrin; transform plasminogen to plasmin
Deoxyribonucleases A, B, C, D	Yes	Depolymerize DNA
Nicotinamide-adenine dinucleotidase	Yes	Splits coenzyme A
Proteinase	Yes	Degrades protein

more accurately detected under anaerobic conditions, such as in an atmosphere of 10% CO_2 and 90% N_2 (incidentally, this atmosphere also favors the growth of streptococci). If this procedure fails, a low O_2 tension can be created by stabbing the agar with the inoculating loop and thus permitting the colonies to grow within the agar.

A nonhemolytic group A streptococcal epidemic with several cases of RF has been reported.[1] The frequency of such a phenomenon remains uncertain. It is probably exceptional, but it could lead to an error that would not be detected by the usual microbiologic procedures; without beta hemolysin, group A streptococci are much like a rattlesnake without its rattle.

At least 5%, and occasionally up to 70%, of beta-hemolytic streptococci belong to groups other than A, such as B, C, or G, and do not possess the slightest risk of producing RF. It is usually preferable to identify the isolate positively rather than to treat unnecessarily all those patients who are carrying non-group A streptococci. Note that in school-age children the prevalence of non-group A hemolytic streptococci in the throat seems to be increased; prevalence also varies geographically.

The reference method for grouping, which involves precipitation of a heat-liberated extract of the isolate with specific antisera, is a long and tedious procedure. Several simpler methods are available, as follows:

1. Sensitivity to bacitracin, by disc diffusion on an agar plate. About 85% of group A streptococci are inhibited by bacitracin, whereas 85% of the non-group A streptococci are not. This method is certainly the easiest to perform and is the most commonly used, although it has a much larger potential for error than the precipitation method.
2. Immunofluorescence. This method is rapid and gives a 94% correlation with the reference method. Its use is limited by a lack of reliable commercial antisera.
3. Slide agglutination tests. One such test, in which the C (or group) antigen is exposed by removing the outer antigenic proteins with trypsin, could perhaps combine both speed and accuracy. Another slide test is even simpler to use and involves a coagglutination technique.

> **Objective 3-3. Interpret the results of throat culture and specify their limitations.**

Whatever the method used to interpret throat culture results, grouping is necessary to complete identification. Establishing antibiotic sensitivities is not required in this case because sensitivity to penicillin may be assumed initially. In all, the microbiologic workup of a throat culture takes about 2 days. Such a delay before determining proper therapy is acceptable because it poses no increased risk to the patient. A negative result is not absolute; each step from throat swab to identification contains inherent sources of potential error. Because therapy is based on the results of this procedure, the best possible technique should be used to limit the frequency of these errors.

FINAL DIAGNOSIS

Even when the organism is detected in the throat, the diagnosis of pharyngitis or tonsillitis due to group A streptococci is not automatic. Indeed, some people are simply carriers, without any clinical or biologic evidence of infection. The percentage of carriers in a population varies, with a predilection for young children, especially at the end of winter and the beginning of spring. Furthermore, epidemics of pharyngitis are preceded by an increase in the number of carriers in the population; the incidence sometimes reaches 60%.

The discovery of group A streptococci in the pharynx is compatible with three possibilities: (1) streptococcal pharyngitis; (2) nonstreptococcal pharyngitis in a carrier; and (3) a carrier state without pharyngitis.

In an attempt to achieve greater diagnostic precision, the quantity or concentration of streptococci in the throat has been investigated, but unfortunately, without finding a satisfactory correlation. In any case, the usual sampling techniques do not permit a useful quantitation of the number of colonies; only a semiquantitative description of heavy, medium, or slight growth is possible.

The serologic approach is equally disappointing. Theoretically, a streptococcal infection should be distinguishable immunologically from a carrier state. In an infection, an elevation of specific antibodies should be expected, but not in the carrier state. Indeed, antistreptolysin O and anti-DNase B can be quantitated by the laboratory, but this quantitation does not help clinically for the following reasons:

1. The antibody levels measured in the laboratory do not always show a significant rise. In a study in Minnesota, 57% of children with group A streptococcal pharyngitis failed to show a significant rise in antibody titer; 16% had an elevation of antistreptolysin alone; 8% had a rise of anti-DNase B alone; and only 19% showed an increase in the titers of both. Numerous individuals have elevated levels of antibodies at the beginning of their pharyngitis as a result of previous infections. In more than 80% of these individuals, the antibody titer remains stable throughout the course of their illness.
2. In order to judge changes in antibody levels, it is necessary to take 2 samples 10 or even 15 days apart. Although treatment decisions can wait a few days for culture results, such decisions cannot be put off this long.

In conclusion, in clinical practice it is impossible to distinguish between streptococcal pharyngitis and nonstreptococcal pharyngitis in a carrier. The possibility of overtreatment must be accepted, and all patients with pharyngotonsillitis in which group A streptococci are demonstrated should be treated. Specific antibody titers can be omitted.

> **Objective 3–4. Plan the treatment of a streptococcal pharyngotonsillitis.**

Penicillin is the usual therapy for streptococcal pharyngitis. Contrary to widespread opinion, this antibiotic, though active against streptococci, does not modify the clinical course of the disease. The duration of fever, dysphagia, and cervical adenitis may be shortened, but only by 24 to 48 hours. Acute glomerulonephritis seems not to be prevented by treatment, even if antibiotics are administered when the first symptoms appear. Penicillin, given in the usual oral doses, suppresses the pharyngeal streptococci in only 80% of cases. Treatment is possibly of value in preventing the suppurative sequelae, such as sinusitis, mastoiditis, otitis media, and suppurative cervical adenitis, complications usually found in children under 4 years of age.

The main reason for treatment, however,

is for the prophylaxis of RF, a disease that is disastrous for the individual affected and financially ruinous for society as a whole. The monetary cost of a single episode of RF has been estimated to be equivalent to 5000 office visits.

The risk of RF after a streptococcal pharyngitis of any type is about 0.5 to 3%. Fortunately, the frequency seems to have declined in developed countries, although the reason for the decline is not known. On the other hand, RF remains a major public health problem in underdeveloped nations. Rheumatic fever appears 2 to 4 weeks after the onset of a pharyngitis. Penicillin can usually prevent RF, but the drug must be given no later than 9 days after the onset of the pharyngeal infection.

Penicillin is most often given orally (penicillin V) at a dose of 50,000 U/kg/day for children or 125 mg (200,000 U) 4 times a day in adults. The duration of therapy must be sufficient to eliminate the streptococci from the throat; a 10-day course is necessary. When the compliance of the patient is uncertain, a single intramuscular injection of benzathine penicillin (1.2 million U) is preferred. In case of penicillin allergy, erythromycin is the agent of choice, at a dose of 30 to 50 mg/kg/day for children and 1 g/day in adults for 10 days. Some strains of group A streptococci are resistant to erythromycin, however, notably in Japan and in Europe. Tetracycline should not be used.

The following procedure, which we have adopted in our practice for several years now, is convenient. A throat swab is taken, and a prescription is given to the patient, who is instructed to have it filled only when a telephone call has confirmed that the culture results were positive. This approach may be readily employed by a physician who practices in a hospital or at a reasonable distance from a microbiology laboratory.

The physician whose practice is located far from these facilities should be equipped with a small incubator and a supply of blood agar plates, to treat those patients whose throat cultures may grow beta-hemolytic streptococci. That some patients are unnecessarily treated must be accepted in these circumstances; however, this approach does diminish antibiotic overuse in the treatment of upper respiratory infections. In addition, once the organism is isolated, it can be sent to a reference laboratory for grouping.

In underdeveloped countries or in lower socioeconomic areas, the conditions of medical practice and the high risk of RF have led some medical groups, without taking cultures, to prescribe penicillin to all patients who have pharyngitis at least within the critical ages.

The attitude toward carriers is unsettled. In the absence of a well-defined risk, such as a familial RF diathesis or an epidemic situation, attempts to suppress the carrier state seem to be of little practical value. For this reason, routine throat cultures of asymptomatic contacts of patients with streptococcal pharyngitis are not done, except in a family in which RF has occurred.

> **Objective 3–5. Explain why diphtheria must be treated before microbiologic confirmation.**

In contrast to streptococcal pharyngitis, diphtheria requires immediate therapeutic action based solely on faith in the clinical signs. If left untreated, the disease has a high mortality rate. The effectiveness of therapy depends on its promptness, and a laboratory is not able to produce any useful information for several days.

In man, *Corynebacterium diphtheriae* multiplies preferentially in the nasopharynx, and less often on the larynx, conjunctivae, or skin. Once established, the infection does not disseminate; it produces satellite adenopathy, but not bacteremia. The club-shaped bacteria multiply in the superficial layers of the colonized epithelium. The toxin they produce necrotizes the neighboring tissues; this necrosis favors local extension of the infection and elicits an inflammatory reaction characterized by the secretion of a thick exudate—

the false membrane. When toxin production is sufficient, diphtheria takes the form of a severe systemic illness. The mortality rate reaches 16% in children under 5 years, 5.8% in 5- to 10-year-old children, and 5% in patients over age 20.

> **Objective 3–6. Define the indications for emergency antidiphtheria therapy.**

Although diphtheria is still rampant worldwide, immunization and improving socioeconomic conditions have reduced its annual incidence to about 1 per million in industrialized countries. The disease is, however, 20 or 30 times more frequent in poorer areas of the world.

Diphtheria appears sporadically or in small epidemics that develop because physicians are no longer able to recognize the disease. It is spread by infected individuals during the periods of incubation or convalescence, and more important, by asymptomatic carriers. Transmission is by nasopharyngeal secretions such as coughing and sneezing, or more rarely, by contact with personal effects. Epidemics occur all year round, with a slight predilection for autumn and winter.

DIAGNOSIS OF DIPHTHERIA

The medical approach depends on the epidemiologic context. Once one or several recent cases have been recognized within a specific area, all cases of pharyngitis should initially be considered suspect. Throat cultures for *Corynebacterium diphtheriae* should be taken systematically, and treatment for diphtheria should be started on the slightest suspicion.

Outside an epidemic context, the physician should rely on the clinical appearance and must be alerted by unusual symptoms in the course of a pharyngitis. The patient's general state of health is often altered; these patients have great fatigue, pallor, and a toxic appearance, but, at the same time, a fever that generally does not exceed 38.5° C (101.3° F). Signs of toxicity, such as epistaxis, prostration, and disordered consciousness, may even be in the forefront in what is called malignant diphtheria. Unusually abundant adenopathy, which distorts the upper part of the neck, a serous or sanguineous nasal discharge, or a

---

DIPHTHERIA TOXIN

The seriousness of diphtheria is due principally to the potent exotoxin produced by certain strains of *Corynebacterium diphtheriae,* once also known as Klebs-Loeffler bacillus. These gram-positive, aerobic, non-sporeforming rods are typically dumbbell- or club-shaped and contain metachromatic granules. Because of their mode of multiplication, they form themselves into small groups with the bacteria lying at acute angles to one another ("Chinese letters"). *C. diphtheriae* can grow rapidly on deficient substances, such as Loeffler medium, which is based on coagulated serum, or an inhibitory media-like tellurite agar, which permits some degree of separation from the other pharyngeal flora.

The organism would have little pathogenicity were it not infected by a temperate bacteriophage that carries the "tox" gene; nonlysogenized isolates lack this gene. The "tox" gene furnishes the genetic information necessary for the synthesis of the notorious toxin, a simple polypeptide of around 62,000 daltons. Hydrolysis of a disulfide bond activates the toxin molecule by exposing 2 complementary fragments, A and B. Fragment A represents the true toxic portion. It blocks the translocation of amino acids from the transfer RNA to the ribosomes by combining with nicotinamide-adenine dinucleotide and forming a complex that inhibits transferase II. This process halts the incorporation of amino acids into polypeptide chains, shuts off protein synthesis, and quickly leads to cell death.

When injected into a guinea pig (traditionally used in laboratory studies of diphtheria), diphtheria toxin kills the animal in 1 to 3 days. At necropsy, necrosis is found around the site of injection, congestion and hemorrhage are seen in the adrenals, and multiple foci of cellular damage occur in the myocardium, liver, and kidneys. In man, the toxin attacks most organs during the course of the illness, with some predilection for nervous tissue, in which it produces demyelination, and for the heart. These lesions usually take several days to become clinically evident. When the intoxication is not too severe, the lesions are reversible; paralysis, for example, may regress completely.

The toxin's antigenic properties are used in the production of a vaccine; toxicity is removed by treating the toxin with heat and formalin. The resulting toxoid confers immunity. Protection diminishes in 10 years, however, and booster injections are recommended for persons at high risk.

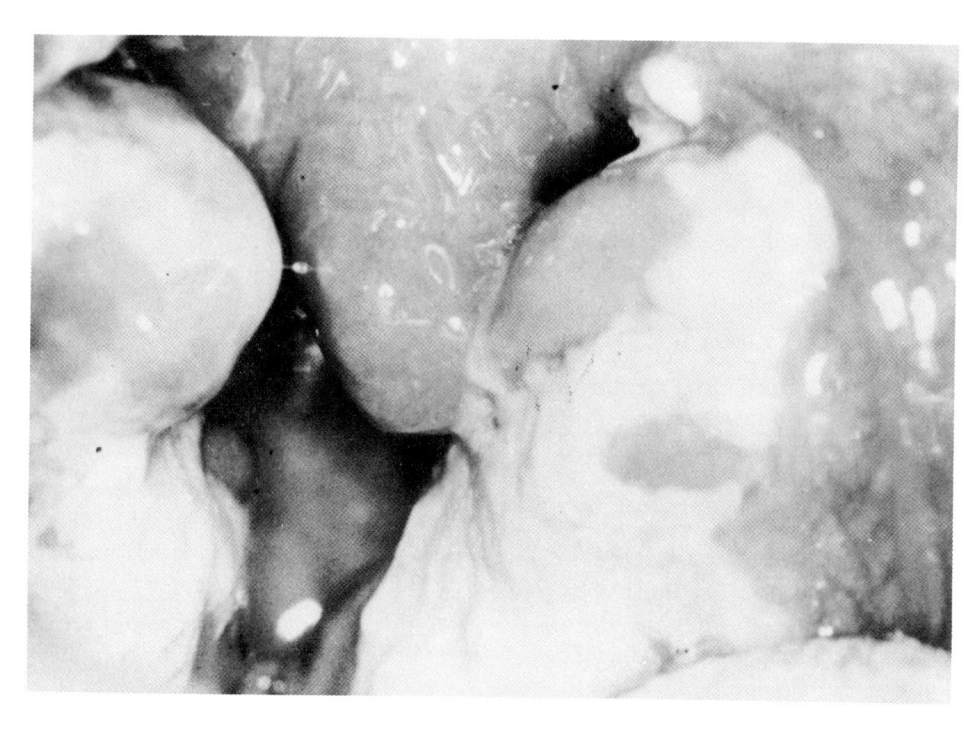

Fig. 3–4. Diphtheritic pharyngitis. Note the important edema. (Courtesy of the Departments of Pediatrics and Microbiology, CHUL, Québec, Canada.)

moldy odor on the breath should attract the physician's attention. Although dysphagia is only moderate, the intensity and extent of the pharyngeal lesions are surprising. A grayish false membrane, which stretches out beyond the tonsillar bed, lies on edematous, sometimes hemorrhagic, tissue from which it cannot be easily disassociated or detached (Fig. 3–4). Invasion of the larynx or even the trachea is possible, accompanied by a "barking" cough and voice loss. Paralysis of the palate, a serious prognostic sign, can sometimes be recognized by the nasal voice and reflux of ingested fluids through the nose. Another disquieting sign, cardiac arrhythmia such as atrioventricular dissociation, may suggest the diagnosis in a child. The presence or absence of a history of immunization against diphtheria is only relative evidence because the disease can occur in immunized individuals, although in attenuated form.

On the whole, recognizing diphtheria is difficult for someone who has never seen it, and confusion is all too possible. *Streptococcal pharyngitis* can form false membranes and may produce toxicity. Keep in mind also that the combination of streptococcal pharyngitis and diphtheria has been described.

Infectious mononucleosis is the usual cause of a pharyngeal false membrane in an adolescent or a young adult. Theoretically, in this instance, the patient should appear less toxic; the false membrane should not extend to the soft palate; adenopathy should not be restricted to the neck, but should occur in various other areas; and splenomegaly should often be found. In practice, however, some doubt is possible. The complete blood count (CBC) and rapid slide test for infectious mononucleosis (Monotest) may be done quickly and are useful here. The CBC is equally helpful in recognizing the cause of a necrotizing pharyngitis, which occasionally is seen in the course of leukemia or agranulocytosis with a clinical picture that could sometimes be mistaken for diphtheria. When the false membrane is hidden by edema, tonsillar abscess should be ruled out by careful pharyngeal examination.

Localized diphtheritic infections without pharyngitis, such as laryngitis or rhinitis in the infant, conjunctivitis, or even cutaneous ulcerations, make the differential diagnosis even more difficult. In these exceptional cases, the most reliable clinical indications are the epidemiologic context, the formation of local false membranes on the lesions, and the signs of general toxicity.

> **Objective 3–7. Respond appropriately when diphtheria is suspected.**

THROAT CULTURE

Although treatment is generally undertaken on a clinical basis, a throat culture is indispensable for confirming the diagnosis. An extensive and costly epidemiologic investigation is undertaken only once the disease has been microbiologically ascertained. To obtain material for culture, one should gently lift the false membrane; then, one should rub a swab along and behind the membrane's edge. An immediate microscopic examination can sometimes be useful. Gram-positive rods with the appropriate morphologic features, granulations, and groupings suggest *Corynebacterium diphtheriae*. Unfortunately, the normal throat flora contains related species, appropriately called diphtheroids, which may be a source of confusion. Immunofluoresence tests can provide an early warning, but they do not eliminate the need for culture and for conventional microbiologic identification.

The swab must be quickly dispatched to the laboratory with a label specifically stating that diphtheria is suspected, so that the proper media will be used for culture. Loeffler medium, which is three parts heated beef serum to one part nutrient broth, or the newer, more commonly used tellurite agar is preferred because either medium inhibits the growth of common throat flora, such as streptococcus and neisseria. A blood agar plate is inoculated to detect the group A streptococci sometimes associated with diphtheria. Within a few hours, *C. diphtheriae* appears on tellurite agar as small, black colonies; the color is due to the reduction of tellurite to tellurium. The next step in the identification process is the demonstration of toxin production. For this purpose, an agar gel precipitation test, the Elek test (Fig. 3–5) is generally used; it produces results within 24 hours.

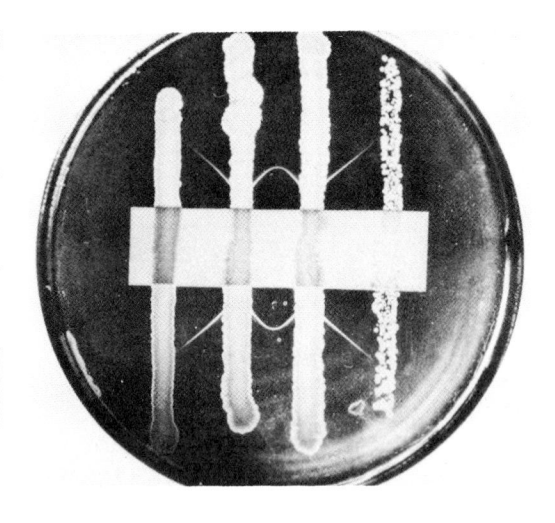

Fig. 3–5. Elek test. The perpendicular stripes are seeded from right to left, with a control nontoxigenic isolate, a control toxigenic isolate, and two suspected isolates. For the toxin-producing isolates, two identical arcs of precipitation are observed (stripes 2 and 3).

SPECIFIC THERAPY

Specific therapy is undertaken as soon as the culture has been taken and without waiting for the results. This therapy is primarily aimed at neutralizing diphtheria toxin.

Serotherapy is the principal method of treatment, but it works only while the toxin is extracellular. Consequently, it is necessary to administer treatment before the toxin fixes irreversibly to the cells. An old experiment[3] clearly demonstrated that the prognosis worsens when therapy is delayed: the mortality rate was 0, 4, 11, 16, or 18%, according to whether the antitoxin was administered on the first, second, third, fourth, or fifth day of the illness, respectively. After the fifth day, serotherapy probably does not curb the course of the disease.

Because diphtheria antitoxin is of equine origin, it can produce hypersensitivity reactions, such as anaphylactic shock immediately or serum sickness in several days. The patient should be asked whether he has received horse serum previously and whether he is allergic. Hypersensitivity to the serum must be tested in every patient who is going to receive it, by administering an intradermal injection of 0.1 ml of a 1:1000 dilution of diphtheria antitoxin. The test is considered positive if an urticarial reaction greater than 10 mm appears within 20 minutes. The conjunctival test used to be given simultaneously, but the nonspecific irritations produced made it difficult to interpret. When allergy to horse serum is evident, desensitization should be attempted by a series of injections every 20 minutes in increasing doses. First, 0.1 ml of a 5% solution is injected subcutaneously. Then, the quantity is increased progressively until 0.5 ml pure serum is given at one time.

For cases of average intensity, 20,000 to 40,000 U antitoxin are indicated: 40,000 to 80,000 U are given in severe cases, and extremely high doses (up to 120,000 U) have been administered to patients with malignant diphtheria. If more than 40,000 U are administered, at least half the dose should be given intravenously to obtain adequate circulating concentrations as quickly as possible; in this case, the serum should be diluted by a ratio of 1 part serum to 20 parts physiologic saline solution and infused over an hour.

Antibiotic therapy should be prescribed to eliminate the source of toxin production, to limit the risk of spread, and, in certain cases, to eliminate associated pharyngeal infections, group A streptococci, in particular. Erythromycin, at a dose of 25 to 50 mg/kg/day, orally if possible, for 15 days seems to be the most effective agent at the present time. Penicillin, although active in vitro, may not be the drug of choice because it appears less likely to eliminate the carrier state.

Bed rest under close observation for several weeks is essential because myocarditis and sudden death can occur at any time. Furthermore, paralysis of the soft palate or the legs and loss of accommodation can appear late in the course of the disease, even after delays exceeding a month. Activity should be authorized on the basis of the physical examination and serial electrocardiograms. If cardiac insufficiency occurs, digitalis should be used only with caution. Corticosteroids have been suggested, but their usefulness has not been established.

Paralysis of the soft palate can result in regurgitation and difficulty in swallowing that may lead to aspiration pneumonia. Therefore, it is preferable to feed these patients by esophageal tube. Postural drainage and aspiration of respiratory secretions are also recommended. In the rare patient in whom the paralysis extends to the respiratory muscles, respiratory assistance may also be necessary.

OTHER THERAPEUTIC MEASURES

Diphtheria is a reportable disease in all parts of the world. Isolation of patients is mandatory because the patient is a carrier. Two negative cultures, taken more than 24 hours apart after the cessation of antibiotic therapy, are required before the isolation precautions may be discontinued. If one of the cultures is positive, a new course of erythromycin should be prescribed.

Treatment of Contacts. Once diphtheria is microbiologically confirmed, a survey should be made of contacts in order to avoid further dissemination of the disease.

All persons in regular contact with the patient such as family members, friends, coworkers, and classmates are asked to submit to a clinical examination, a swab of the nose and throat, and a Schick test. All should receive erythromycin to eliminate any organisms that may be present.

Asymptomatic individuals should receive an injection of toxoid, either a first injection or a booster if they have already been immunized. If the culture is negative, erythromycin should be discontinued, and the decision to continue the immunization should depend on the result of the Schick test. If the culture proves positive, these individuals should be isolated and the erythromycin therapy continued. The tendency today is not to give prophylactic antitoxin to these asymptomatic people, but to follow them closely. In symptomatic contacts, antiserum should be given immediately after the cultures are taken, and these patients should be kept in isolation until the culture results are known.

All individuals with a positive culture, whether they are sick or not, should remain in isolation and should continue erythromycin therapy until they have had 3 negative cultures over 48 hours, after which the antibiotics are stopped. All patients with negative cultures who have not received antibiotics before culture can be considered free of the disease.

IMMUNIZATION

Immunization is the main preventive measure and is promoted even in countries where it is not mandatory. Although it does not offer complete protection against diphtheria, it does protect against the severe or malignant forms of the disease for approximately 10 years; and worldwide it has led to a considerable diminution in the prevalence of diphtheria.

The vaccine is a toxoid, that is, diphtheria toxin modified by the application of heat and formalin. A univalent vaccine, containing only the antigen and an adjuvant, does exist, but polyvalent preparations, which include the antigens for tetanus, whooping cough, and sometimes poliomyelitis, are more frequently used. Three injections of fluid toxoid (used in some European countries) or alum-precipitated toxoid are given subcutaneously or intramuscularly, respectively, at intervals of 4 to 8 weeks. A booster injection is given around a year later. Adults are given smaller doses than children because of the likelihood of febrile reactions; adult diphtheria toxoid is available. Individuals particularly exposed, such as physicians and nurses, are best protected by a booster shot every 10 years.

Immunization is generally well tolerated. Contraindications are patients with active infectious disorders or fever and immunosuppressed patients who may not be able to form antibodies.

> **Objective 3–8. Clinically distinguish infectious mononucleosis from other causes of viral pharyngitis.**

The majority of cases of pharyngitis are of viral origin and have no serious sequelae. As a general rule, knowledge of the precise viral origin is of little importance to the patient. Infectious mononucleosis is an exception. Once the diagnosis is made, the patient is in a better position to deal with the possibly protracted convalescence, and he can be informed of the most important risk, splenic rupture following trauma.

Infectious mononucleosis can often be diagnosed in the adolescent or young adult, the preferred target age group, during the initial physical examination. Fever, pharyngitis, lymphadenitis, and splenomegaly are often associated with this disease. The pharyngeal mucosa is inflamed and edematous, often secreting a large amount of exudate that can give the appearance of a false membrane (Fig. 3–6). Pharyngeal edema and hypertrophy of tonsils and adenoids can be considerable and can lead to a nasal voice and, occasionally, to true respiratory obstruction with dyspnea. Lymphadenopathy is seen in more than three-fourths of the patients. The lymph nodes are soft and are visible under the angle of the maxilla and in the posterior cervical and axillary areas. The patient complains most often of loss of appetite and energy and of excessive fatigue. The patient's temperature is generally under 102° F (39° C), but occasionally it is higher and may be associated with sweats and shaking chills during the first few days of illness.

The physical examination may also reveal other findings, listed in order of decreasing frequency:

1. Edema of the eyelids, in about 30% of patients.

THE SCHICK TEST

Goal: To identify the individuals with protective serum levels of diphtheria antitoxin.

Principle: Intradermal injection of toxin normally provokes a local inflammatory reaction in unprotected individuals. When the person is immune, antibody neutralizes the toxin, and the inflammatory reaction is not produced.

Technique: One should inject 0.1 ml diphtheria toxin intradermally on the volar surface of the forearm; 0.1 ml of a control solution (toxin heated to 65° C for 15 minutes) is given in the same fashion in the other arm.

Reading: The test is positive if a uniform zone of erythema of at least 1 cm is produced after at least 36 hours. Usually, a localized pigmentation and desquamation follow. The control serves to determine whether the individual is allergic to the bacterial proteins. This pseudoreaction begins during the first 18 hours, the maximum reaction being apparent in 24 to 36 hours. It is not followed by pigmentation or desquamation.

Interpretation:

Toxin	Control	Interpretation
(reactions)		
Negative	Negative	Protection against diphtheria
Negative	Positive	Protection; sensitivity to bacterial proteins
Positive	Negative	No protection
Positive	Positive	Sensitivity to bacterial proteins; Schick test difficult to interpret

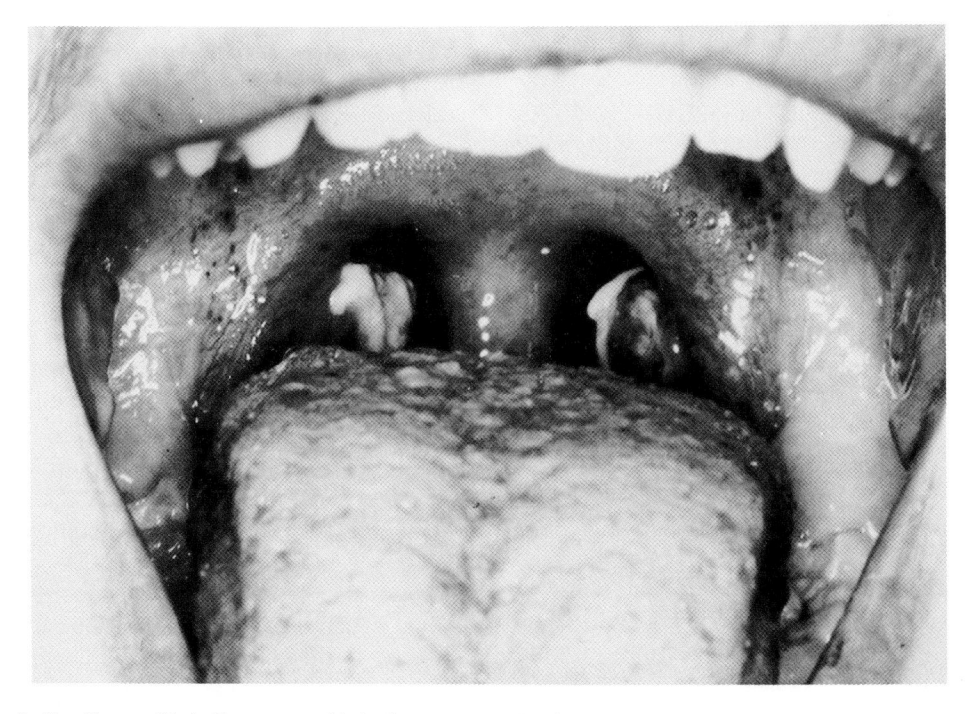

Fig. 3–6. Pharyngitis in the course of infectious mononucleosis. Note the false membranes and purpura of the soft palate; the uvula palatina is edematous.

2. Purpura of the soft palate, in about 25% of patients.
3. Hepatomegaly, in about 25% of patients.
4. Maculopapular rash, in 10% of patients, but in more than 50% when ampicillin has been given.
5. Jaundice, in 5% of patients, although the transaminase levels are elevated in nearly all cases.

The diagnosis of infectious mononucleosis is occasionally much more difficult than has just been suggested, particularly in the first few days of illness with an incomplete clinical picture and in the infant, in whom the infection does not always have the same characteristic appearance. The patient's blood count is often the first clue to the correct diagnosis.

> **Objective 3–9. Choose the appropriate laboratory tests to confirm the diagnosis of mononucleosis.**

If the disease is present, the patient's white blood cell count will reveal a mononuclear picture. The total number of white cells will be normal or slightly elevated, and the proportion of monocytes and lymphocytes will be slightly elevated. Large, basophilic, mononuclear cells and atypical lymphocytes may constitute more than 15% of the total white blood cell count. These cells are present at the time of the first symptoms and persist for several weeks. Although these hematologic findings have given their name to the illness, they are not entirely specific for it. Atypical lymphocytes are observed in the course of other infections, notably cytomegalovirus, rubeola, viral hepatitis, and typhoid fever, or even with drug or allergic reactions and various hematologic disorders. Contrary to a widely held opinion, mononucleosis is not always present when atypical lymphocytes are seen. Indeed, it is absent in close to one case in ten. Whether atypical lymphocytes occur or not, the serologic study confirms the diagnosis in the end.

Culture of the throat is not generally useful, but should be done to rule out a treatable cause of pharyngitis, such as group A hemolytic streptococcal pharyngitis.

SEROLOGIC TESTS

Two kinds of serologic tests are available: one type detects the heterophile antibody, which is the antibody directed against some antigen that is not part of the antigenic mosaic of the causative agent itself and cannot be detected in the host infected with the virus in question; the other tests are specific for the Epstein-Barr virus.

The heterophile antibodies found in mononucleosis agglutinate sheep or horse red blood cells. That these antibodies are absorbed by beef red blood cells, but not by guinea pig kidney cells, distinguishes them from similar heterophile antibodies seen in normal subjects or after a serum sickness. The complete procedure is the Paul-Bunnell and Davidsohn (PBD) reaction. Rapid slide tests, such as Monospot, Monotest, or Monosticon are also available. Although these commercial tests are convenient, they produce false-positive or, more rarely, false-negative reactions. The reference method, therefore, remains the PBD reaction.

The test for heterophile antibody is useful to the physician because it is positive in 88% of young adults with infectious mononucleosis. The percentage decreases with the decreasing age of the patient; the PBD test is rarely positive under 5 years of age.

MONONUCLEOSIS WITHOUT HETEROPHILE ANTIBODY

A patient with the clinical picture of mononucleosis, but without heterophile antibody, poses a diagnostic problem that has been resolved by the discovery of the etiologic agent, the Epstein-Barr virus (EBV), and by the development of specific serologic tests. Isolation of the virus from leukocytes or saliva, although theoretically possible, is difficult, time-consuming, and impractical. On the other hand, several types of antibodies can be detected in the serum (Fig. 3–7).

The most definitive serologic proof is the demonstration of a rising titer of neutralizing antibody, but it is technically simpler to detect, by indirect immunofluorescence, antibodies directed against antigens such as the viral capsid antigen (VCA) or against antigens that are not actually part of the viral structure, but are coded for by the virus and appear in infected cells. Examples of such antigens are the early antigen (EA), which consists of two types, D, diffuse, and R, restricted to the Golgi apparatus, and the Epstein-Barr nuclear antigen (EBNA). VCA antibody rises rapidly after infection, is normally present from the beginning of the clinical illness, and can persist for several years.

Only occasionally is it possible to demonstrate a significant increase in the titer of antibodies to EBV, with the exception of antibody to the nuclear antigen (EBNA). This antibody appears in 90% of cases, either late in the course of the illness or during convalescence. Consequently, the combination of an EBNA-negative and a VCA-positive reaction in the serum at the beginning of an illness supports the diagnosis of an active EBV infection likely to be associated with the clinical syndrome of infectious mononucleosis. As with all viral infections, however, many inapparent infections exist without attendant illness; thus, these serologic findings are occasionally noted in asymptomatic individuals. Antibody to EA of the diffuse type appears in 50 to 70% of patients with infectious mononucleosis. In contrast to EBNA and VCA antibody, EA antibody does not persist long. Because it is not present in all cases, EA is rarely useful in the diagnosis of mononucleosis and is only occasionally tested for in the laboratory.

IgM antibody to VCA appears in almost all patients with infectious mononucleosis or active EBV infection. This antibody does not last for more than 2 months and may reappear in exceptional circumstances, probably following recrudescence of an EBV infection, usually in the first year or so following the mononucleosis. It is, however, a difficult test to perform because of the rarity of anti-IgM-specific sera of adequate titer (1/16 to 1/32).

In summary, confirmation of the diagnosis of EBV infection with or without mononucleosis, if one has only a single specimen of serum, is determined by the following:

1. An EBNA-negative reaction combined with a VCA-positive reaction.
2. A titer of antibody to EA-D of 1/40 or more.
3. A VCA-IgM-positive test.

When 2 serum specimens, taken 25 or more days apart, are available, the diagnosis can be confirmed by an increase of 2 or more dilutions in the titer of EBNA antibody (VCA or, more rarely, EA).

> **Objective 3–10.** Take the proper precautions once the diagnosis of mononucleosis has been considered.

Even though no specific therapy for mononucleosis exists, several recommendations can certainly be made. Unfortunately, preventive measures are limited to reminding the patient that the saliva contains and can transmit the virus. The patient's enlarged, congested spleen is fragile, and its rupture is something to be concerned about. One tries to avoid traumatizing the spleen, notably by not palpating it too often or too insistently. If rupture occurs, rapid diagnosis and immediate surgical intervention are necessary. Dyspnea may also supervene because of laryngeal obstruction secondary to cervical edema and lymphadenopathy. In this circumstance, the patient should be hospitalized and corticosteroids should be prescribed (for example, 40 to 60 mg prednisone for 2 to 3 days, with rapidly decreasing doses thereafter). One should also recognize the possibility of neurologic complications, such as the Guillain-Barré syndrome, transverse myelitis, mononeuritis, or even encephalitis. Granulocytopenia, hemolytic anemia, and thrombocytopenia have also been reported as complications of mononucleosis. The most severe of these complications may respond to corticosteroid therapy of the type just mentioned. In exceptional circumstances, nearly any organ may be involved in the course of the disease.

Symptomatic infectious mononucleosis may last several months, in the form of fatigue or even low-grade fever. Unfortunately, no specific action is recommended—only rest and patience.

ATYPICAL LYMPHOCYTES

At least three types of atypical lymphocytes are seen, but the most common is a large lymphocyte with an abundant, basophilic (blue) cytoplasm that contains vacuoles with an irregular nucleus resembling that of a monocyte. The disease, mononucleosis, takes its name from that lymphocyte.

Most, if not all, atypical lymphocytes are blast-transformed T lymphocytes (NK, natural killer lymphocytes). These lymphocytes are probably reacting to the presence of the B lymphocytes that are parasitized by EBV, which, in turn, modifies their surface antigen mosaic and enables them to be identified by the T cells.

EPSTEIN-BARR VIRUS (EBV) AND CANCER

Epstein-Barr virus has been associated with polyclonal lymphoproliferative disorders in patients with congenital or acquired immunodeficiencies such as transplant patients or those receiving chemotherapy for cancer. In these patients, the lymphoproliferation, even if polyclonal, behaves like a malignant tumor, presumably because of immunosuppression. EBV has also been associated with two monoclonal malignant tumors, Burkitt's lymphoma and nasopharyngeal carcinoma.

EB nuclear antigen (EBNA) and the EBV genome are detected in more than 98% of African Burkitt's lymphomas and in almost 100% of the nasopharyngeal carcinomas of the anaplastic type (lymphoepitheliomas); virtually all these tumor patients possess antibodies to EBV-specific antigen at titers much higher than those in patients with other tumors of the same anatomic site. EBV is oncogenic in tissue culture and transforms leukocytes from the umbilical cord into permanent lymphoblastoid cell lines. In the monkey, EBV produces both lymphoproliferative disorders and lymphoid tumors. In the absence of human inoculation experiments, the only way to prove the cause-and-effect relationship in man would be an epidemiologic study of the efficacy of a hypothetic vaccine in preventing the development of these tumors.

EPSTEIN-BARR VIRUS (EBV)

Although infectious mononucleosis has been known for a long time, the etiologic agent has only been suspected since 1968. EBV belongs to the herpes family of viruses. Like all the viruses in this group, EBV is an enveloped icosahedral capsid, 100 mm in size, presenting 20 faces and 12 angles. EBV contains, like all viruses, only one kind of nucleic acid, DNA in this case. This virus was originally discovered in cell lines derived from a Burkitt's lymphoma, a malignant lymphoma that occurs in certain tropical regions of Africa. EBV has also been associated with certain nasopharyngeal cancers in South China and with a variety of less-common immunopathologic or lymphoproliferative syndromes.

EPIDEMIOLOGY

EBV infection is worldwide, but infectious mononucleosis is a disease of developed countries, whereas Burkitt's lymphoma and nasopharyngeal carcinoma are more prevalent in specific areas of Africa and Asia. Infectious mononucleosis is mainly seen in adolescents and in young adults who have escaped the infection during childhood, presumably because of better living conditions. The saliva of 10 to 20% of individuals in good health contains the infectious agent, clearly EBV, which is capable of transforming leukocytes from the umbilical cord into permanent lymphoblastic cell lines in which the virus can be identified. The virus is, therefore, probably transmitted orally, such as by kissing or similar close contact, although the transmission rate is only approximately 10% per year. The virus persists not only in saliva, but also in the circulating leukocytes of almost all children and adults after infection.

The incubation period of infectious mononucleosis is probably 30 to 45 days. Some authors have noted a peak of cases in February, but, in general, the incidence seems constant throughout the year. The incidence per 100,000 population per year is as follows: 45 on the whole in the United States; 66 for the group from 10 to 14 years; 343 for those from 15 to 19 years; and 123 for those from 20 to 34 years of age. It ranges from 316 to 2200 in various American universities and from 100 to 200 in the Canadian armed forces. The incidence of the illness seems thus to fluctuate according to the proportion of individuals from 17 to 25 years of age in the population studied.

PATHOLOGY

Within the lymph nodes and spleen, a nonspecific inflammatory reaction is found with hyperplasia of the reticuloendothelial cells and a predominance of both typical and atypical lymphocytes. The liver may show localized parenchymal necrosis in the periportal areas, which are distended by inflammatory cells consisting of both normal and atypical lymphocytes. The hepatic picture is sometimes difficult to distinguish from that of lymphocytic leukemia.

> **Objective 3–11.** Establish when a patient with sore throat and fever should be referred to a surgeon.

Most infectious processes involving the pharyngeal space resolve spontaneously or are easily cured with antibiotics. Although deep neck cellulitis or abscesses are infrequent, they may represent life-threatening situations in which surgical drainage should be considered.

Inadequate antibiotic therapy of a pharyngeal infection can lead to local encapsulation that spontaneously ruptures either in the pharynx, with flooding of the tracheobronchial tree, or in the peripharyngeal spaces. Aspiration of pus results in asphyxia, especially in babies, or in serious lung contamination. Parapharyngeal and retropharyngeal spaces communicate with all the connective tissues of the neck and with the mediastinum ("Lincoln Highway of the neck"). Peripharyngeal infection may thus be followed by mediastinitis.

Poor local defenses, as in babies, depressed host resistance against infection, as in patients with diabetes or debilitated immunity, as well as the presence of aggressive bacterial strains such as *Pseudomonas* or *Anaerobes* species facilitate the extension of infection.

PERITONSILLAR ABSCESS

The true *peritonsillar abscess* is usually easy to recognize. Common in adolescents or adults after an attack of acute tonsillitis due to a group A streptococcus, this abscess may also complicate the course of infectious mononucleosis. Fever and dysphagia may persist whether antibiotic therapy is initiated or not, but the presence of a referred otalgia, a *trismus* in the vicinity of the pterygoid muscles, or drooling with excessive and foul saliva leads one to suspect an abscess. In addition, the patient's speech has become muffled with some dyspnea. The neck may also be stiff, with tender lymph nodes.

Local applications of a cocaine solution on the posterior part of the middle turbinate bones can help to ease the trismus. When oral secretions have been drained by suction, uni- or bilateral inflammatory bulging of the soft palate close to the tonsil fossa becomes visible. The cardinal signs of abscess forma-

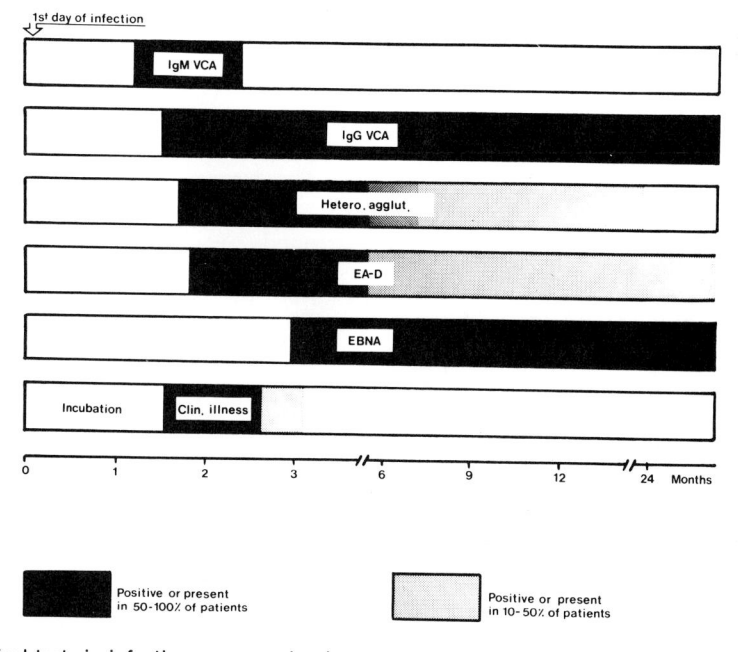

Fig. 3–7. Serological tests in infectious mononucleosis.

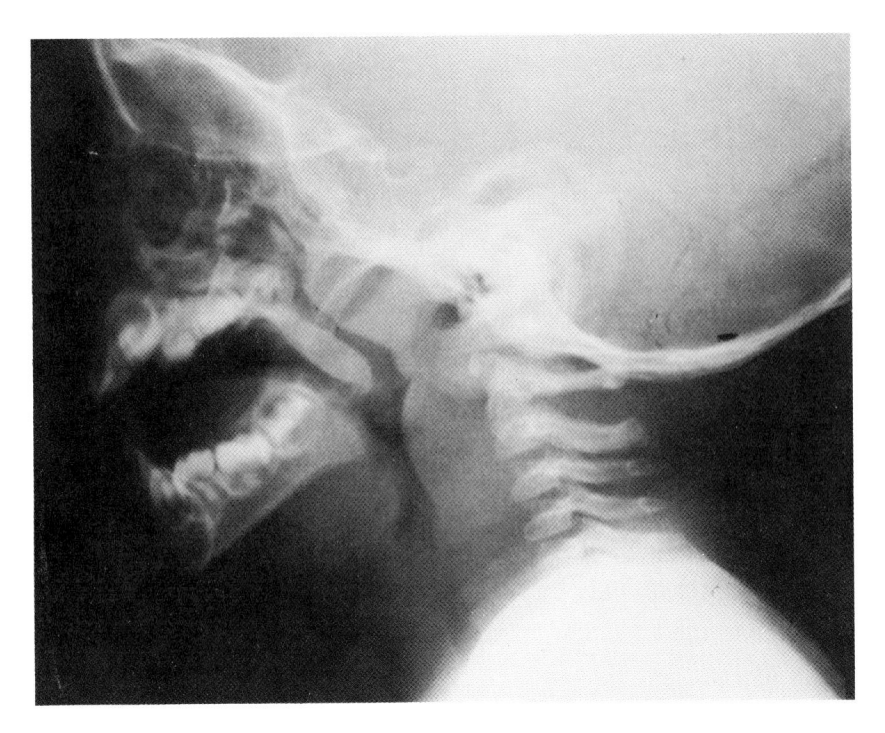

Fig. 3–8. Retropharyngeal abscess.

tion is *edema of the uvula*. Surgical drainage is, therefore, a definite asset, following administration of local anesthesia or, preferably, general anesthesia in a carefully intubated patient. A small incision of the mucosa is enlarged using hemostatic forceps, with rupture of all possible septations.

Medical treatment consists of intravenous administration of penicillin G until oral feeding is possible. A short course of parenteral corticosteroid therapy may help to alleviate the local postoperative swelling. Trismus should disappear within one day.

RETROPHARYNGEAL ABSCESS

The clinical presentation of this abscess is easy to recognize and must prompt the physician to perform surgical drainage as soon as possible. Retropharyngeal abscess usually affects the child under 3 years of age.

After an original attack of upper respiratory tract infection with nasal obstruction (adenoiditis), purulent rhinorrhea, and fever, the child rapidly shows signs of toxicity, dyspnea, and refusal to swallow. The patient's head is frequently in hyperextension. The absence of trismus allows one to identify a bulging mass behind the posterior pharyngeal wall extending inferiorly. Palpation or any other local manipulation can be hazardous and may result in a possible sudden rupture of the abscess and acute respiratory distress. The most helpful examination procedure is a lateral roentgenogram of the pharynx during inspiration. The laryngotracheal lucid image is pushed forward and thus the prespinal space is widened (Fig. 3–8).

Intravenous penicillin G should be administered without delay, and the child should be placed in an environment high in humidity for a few hours. If no improvement is noticed, surgical drainage should be considered. Anesthesia with endotracheal intubation may be dangerous. We prefer to incise the abscess promptly without anesthesia, with the child firmly wrapped in a blanket and immobilized in the Trendelenburg position. Pus is immediately suctioned out and is collected. Because the incision may be too small for adequate drainage, anesthesia is sometimes

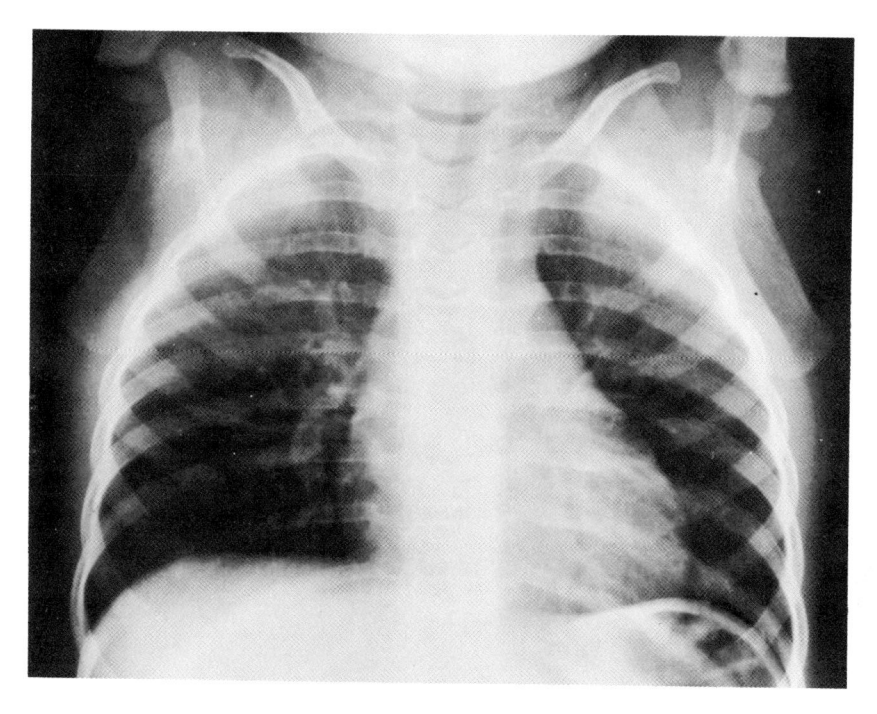

Fig. 3–9. Lateral pharyngeal abscess. Notice the lateral shift of the trachea to the left.

secondarily performed with intubation. Total debridement of the purulent pouch is therefore carefully performed. Intubation may be maintained for 48 hours if the patient's larynx appears edematous. Medical treatment is, of course, continued until recovery is complete.

These retropharyngeal suppurations in babies and young children are ordinarily the result of adenitis occurring in one of the retropharyngeal lymph nodes, the normal route for lymphatic drainage of the rhinopharynx before 3 years of age; however, these abscesses also occur secondary to accidental trauma such as hot milk burn or an enclosed foreign body. Although rare, osteoarthritis of the cervical spine must be ruled out by systematic roentgenographic studies of the patient's upper vertebrae.

LATERAL PHARYNGEAL ABSCESS

Diagnosis of *lateral superficial or deep pharyngeal abscesses* is frequently more difficult than that of retropharyngeal abscesses. These lateral abscesses can complicate common upper respiratory tract infections in children 3 to 10 years of age. The absence of trismus is the rule because the pterygoid muscles are not involved in the inflammatory process; this factor explains the frequent delay in diagnosis. Such abscesses develop at first deeply in the pharyngeal wall, displace the tonsil medially, and distort the soft palate.

The diagnosis can be suspected if an acute cervical adenitis along with fever and dysphagia persist despite adequate antibiotic therapy. When dysphagia worsens, examination of the throat reveals a large, bulging mass of the lateral part of the pharynx, extending inferiorly to the glossopharyngeal area. Frequently, some fluctuation of the ipsilateral neck adenitis indicates the formation of an intraganglionic abscess. In preference to simple incisions that offer poor drainage, surgical drainage is indicated to shorten the course of the disease and to avoid contamination of the parapharyngeal space. Such contamination results from cellulitis running through the superior constrictor muscle with free access to the mediastinum (Fig. 3–9).

With the patient under general anesthesia

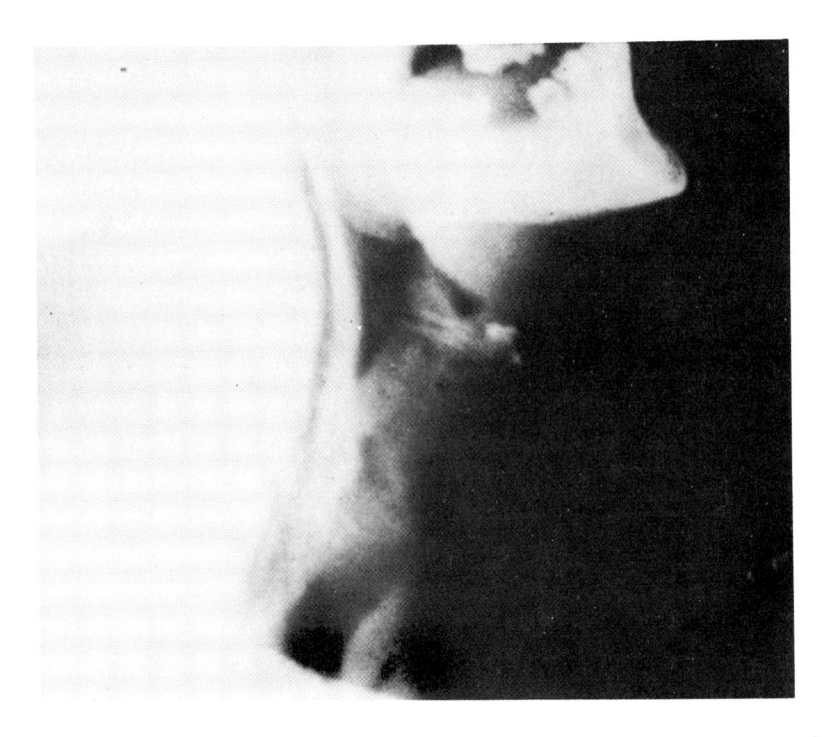

Fig. 3–10. Presence of air in the retropharyngeal space, indicating a deep cellulitis due to anaerobic bacteria.

with endotracheal intubation, the physician opens pus collection widely, and explores all inflammatory areas digitally. As a rule, the cervical abscess is drained simultaneously. A large suppuration involving most of the deep cellular spaces of the neck is sometimes discovered. External drainage must be maintained until recovery is complete.

The medical treatment of this abscess includes the intravenous administration of penicillin.

SPECIAL CIRCUMSTANCES

The presence of air, either in the retropharyngeal space or inside the neck soft structures, as demonstrated on lateral roentgenograms (Fig. 3–10), is due to contamination by anaerobic bacteria sometimes associated with a foreign body. External drainage is initiated behind the sternocleido-mastoid muscle, and a drain is inserted. The danger of mediastinitis is high in such instances.

Extensive necrotizing cellulitis involving all pharyngeal structures is possible in patients with diabetes or in those receiving immunosuppressive agents. Along with antibiotic therapy, which must include antipseudomonal drugs, local debridements should be performed regularly to remove all necrotic tissues. Orodermal fistulas may occur and may require plastic surgical procedures in the future. The substantial mortality rate with this condition stems from rupture of the carotid artery.

Repeated peritonsillar abscesses in a patient with chronic ulcerative tonsillitis or pharyngitis should lead one to suspect a carcinoma in adults. Biopsy is therefore necessary.

In summary, surgical drainage during the course of pharyngeal infections is rarely indicated if medical treatment is adequate and if host immunity is normal. Dangerous cellulitis and abscesses may arise, however, and should be surgically treated to avoid serious mediastinitis.

REFERENCES

1. James, L., and McFarland, B.: An epidemic of pharyngitis due to nonhemolytic group A streptococcus at Lowry Air Force Base. N. Engl. J. Med., 284:750, 1971.
2. Kaplan, E.L., et al.: Diagnosis of streptococcal pharyngitis: differentiation of active infection from the carrier state in the symptomatic child. J. Infect. Dis., 123:490, 1971.
3. Russel, W.T.: Med. Red. Counc. Spec. Rep. Ser., 247:9, 1943.

SUGGESTED READINGS

Denny, F.E., Wannamaker, L.W., and Hahn, E.O.: Comparative effects of penicillin, aureomycin and terramycin on streptococcal tonsillitis and pharyngitis. Pediatrics, 11:7, 1953.

Honikman, L.H., and Massell, B.F.: Guidelines for the selective use of throat cultures in the diagnosis of streptococcal respiratory infection. Pediatrics, 48:573, 1971.

Kaplan, M.H.: Rheumatic fever, rheumatic heart disease and the streptococcal connection: the role of streptococcal antigens cross-reactive with heart tissue. Rev. Infect. Dis., 1:988, 1979.

Krause, R.M.: Prevention of streptococcal sequelae by penicillin prophylaxis: a reassessment. J. Infect. Dis., 131:592, 1975.

Miller, L.W., et al.: Diphtheria carriers and the effect of erythromycin therapy. Antimicrob. Agents Chemother., 6:166, 1974.

Peter, G., and Smith, A.L.: Group A streptococcal infections of the skin and pharynx. N. Engl. J. Med., 297:311, 1977.

Reed, W.P., et al.: Streptococcal adherence to pharyngeal cells of children with acute rheumatic fever. J. Infect. Dis., 142:803, 1980.

Wannamaker, L.W.: Changes and changing concepts in the biology of group A streptococci and in the epidemiology of streptococcal infections. Rev. Infect. Dis., 1:967, 1979.

CHAPTER 4

Oral Infections

B.J. Mansheim

> **Objective 4–1. Manage a dental abscess.**

To diagnose and treat dental abscesses, it is important to understand the microbial ecology of the mouth. The oral cavity is colonized by many different bacterial species, including anaerobic and aerobic bacteria. Moreover, each of these species seems to adhere to certain epithelial surfaces with a surprisingly high degree of specificity. A list of the common bacterial species that colonize the mouth and their respective ecologic habitats is provided in Table 4–1. The numbers of bacteria that normally colonize the oral cavity depend on several factors: (1) their relative ability to adhere to a mucosal or tooth surface; (2) their ability to evade the cleansing action of saliva; and (3) their exposure to antibodies and other salivary constituents that inhibit bacterial adherence.

DENTAL ABSCESSES

Dental abscesses develop primarily in the two areas of the mouth where proliferation of bacteria continues unimpeded by the host defenses, namely, deep within the dental pulp and in the gingival crevice. Inflammation of the dental pulp arises from a severely carious tooth. Infected material spreads toward the tooth apex through the dental pulp (pulpitis) and can rupture into the adjacent tissues (periapical abscess). The patient complains of throbbing pain limited to the involved tooth; this pain is often worsened by heat, cold, or chewing. Fever may be present. Dental caries is obvious with minimal gingival swelling. Dental roentgenograms may show a radiolucent area at the tooth apex due to abscess formation. Treatment includes removal of the infected tooth to facilitate drainage or pulpectomy to remove the infected pulp. The infection is caused by mixed anaerobic bacterial flora. Therefore, penicillin V or tetracycline, in an oral dose of 500 mg 4 times daily for 5 days, is generally adequate.

PERIODONTAL ABSCESSES

Periodontal abscesses can develop from inflammation of the gingiva adjacent to an impacted, partially erupted tooth (pericoronitis) or as a late complication of periodontitis. Pericoronitis occurs most often at the mandibular third molar in young adults. Findings include severe localized pain, fever and limited jaw movement. Physical examination shows swelling, bleeding, and pus exuding from gingival tissue and partially obscuring the impacted tooth. Treatment includes analgesia, rinses with saline solution, extraction of the infected tooth, and a short course of oral antibiotics, either penicillin or tetracycline.

Periodontitis is generally a chronic, mixed

Table 4–1. Predominant Oral Bacterial Flora

Bacteria	Tooth surface	Tongue	Cheek	Saliva	Gingival Crevice
Streptococcus salivarius[b]	−[a]	+++	++	+++	−
Streptococcus mitis	+++	++	+++	++	+
Streptococcus sanguis	+++	++	++	+	−
Streptococcus mutans	+++	−	−	−	−
Gram-positive filaments[c]	−	++	−	−	+++
Veillonella[d]	−	++	−	−	++
Bacteroides[e]	−	−	−	−	++
Fusobacterium[e]	−	−	−	−	+
Spirochetes	−	−	−	−	+

[a]Relative concentrations ranging from low or absent (−) to high (+++)
[b]These four species of streptococci are alpha-hemolytic or so-called viridans streptococci
[c]Facultative anaerobes (Actinomyces and related species)
[d]Anaerobic gram-negative cocci
[e]Anaerobic gram-negative bacilli
(Modified from Gibbons, R.J., and van Houte, J.: Bacterial adherence in oral microbiology. Annu. Rev. Microbiol., 29:19, 1975. Reproduced with permission of Annual Reviews, Inc.)

anaerobic infection of the gingival tissues surrounding the teeth. When an obstruction to drainage develops, an abscess can result. Symptoms are typical of a localized suppurative process. Swelling, redness, fever, and pain are variable. Common findings include marked tenderness upon percussion of the adjacent tooth, lymphadenopathy, and sometimes mobility of the tooth if the periodontitis is advanced. Treatment is directed toward drainage of the abscess, followed by an appropriate periodontal surgical procedure and tooth extraction if necessary. Systemic signs such as fever and malaise suggest the need for a short course of oral antibiotic therapy with penicillin or tetracycline (1 to 2 g/day). Analgesia and rinses with saline solution are appropriate symptomatic treatment. Management of suppurative dental infections is best handled by a dentist or a periodontist.

LUDWIG'S ANGINA

Uncontrolled dental infections can spread through the soft tissues along fascial planes. These infections can take the form of an abscess or a diffuse cellulitis.

Ludwig's angina (Plate 3A) is a deep infection of the submandibular space. Infection spreads typically from the mandibular second and third molars to the floor of the mouth. The tongue becomes displaced superiorly from the marked swelling. The patient's airway may become compromised from distortion of the supraglottic larynx. Fever is characteristic. The neck may be swollen to a varying degree, but lymphadenopathy is not typical. Blood cultures should be taken. Aspiration of the edematous tissue is useful for Gram stain and culture, but drainage is usually not possible because the infection is not a walled-off abscess. Treatment includes maintenance of an adequate airway and antibiotics. Because of the potentially life-threatening nature of this infection, broad-spectrum antibiotics, including oxacillin (6 to 12 g/day) and gentamicin or tobramycin (3 to 5 mg/kg/day), are recommended until culture results are known. The most common bacterial pathogens are oral anaerobes sensitive to penicillin, which can be substituted if these bacteria have been identified.

> **Objective 4–2. Distinguish types of periodontitis and their treatment.**

Periodontitis or pyorrhea refers to the inflammation of the tissues that surround the teeth and also to the inflammation of the supporting structures of the teeth (periodontium). This chronic infection affects 90% of the adult population to some degree and is the major cause of tooth loss in adults.

Because of their varying severity, periodontal diseases are currently classified into several types. The most common periodontal disease, referred to as gingivitis, is limited to inflammation of the gingival margins. More severe forms include juvenile periodontitis (periodontosis), rapidly advancing periodontitis, chronic periodontitis, and acute necrotizing ulcerative gingivitis. Precise definition of each of these entities is difficult because they have overlapping characteristics, and each disorder typically has periods of inactivity interspersed with exacerbations.

Factors that predispose someone to periodontitis are numerous and include nutritional deficiencies, such as vitamin D deficiency and starvation, mechanical problems, such as failure to remove plaque by toothbrushing, congenital abnormalities, and trauma. The result is the same: overgrowth of mixed anaerobic bacterial species with release of toxic products and influx of inflammatory cells, antibodies, and other serum proteins. Finally, the supportive soft tissues of the tooth are destroyed as the infection spreads. The periodontal ligament and the alveolar bone are eventually resorbed, and the tooth loses its attachment.

GINGIVITIS

Mild gingivitis is characterized by friable, swollen gums. The patient may complain only of bleeding upon toothbrushing. Management of this early phase of periodontal disease is directed toward vigorous plaque control by frequent toothbrushing, use of dental floss, and mechanical plaque removal by a dental hygienist.

ADVANCED PERIODONTITIS

Advanced periodontitis can be remarkably silent in its clinical presentation. Complaints vary from mild gingival bleeding during toothbrushing to foul-smelling breath, spontaneous bleeding, and pain surrounding the teeth. Lymphadenopathy, fever, or other systemic symptoms are not typical. Physical examination requires the expertise of a dentist or periodontist. Grossly, the gingival tissue may appear pale, swollen, and friable (Fig. 4–1). Recession of the gingiva from its usual tight attachment to the tooth is characteristic.

The level of gingival detachment is measured with an instrument that probes the infected pocket to determine its depth. Roentgenograms are necessary to evaluate the degree of alveolar bone loss. Treatment depends upon the degree of periodontitis, the extent of involvement, and the activity of the disease. The first approach is removal of necrotic debris from the infected gingival pockets (plaque removal). Aggressive plaque control may reverse the process. If the periodontitis is advanced, antibiotics are sometimes given to enhance healing of the infection. The decision to use antibiotics is empirical because no large controlled trials have confirmed their value. Penicillin, tetracycline (1 to 2 g/day), or metronidazole (250 mg/day) for several weeks may help. Surgical therapy, which includes removal of the infected pocket by gingivectomy or, if necessary, tooth extraction, is often required for definitive control of advanced periodontitis.

ACUTE NECROTIZING ULCERATIVE GINGIVITIS

Acute necrotizing ulcerative gingivitis is an uncommon form of periodontal disease seen almost exclusively in young adults between 18 and 30 years of age. This disorder is characterized by marked inflammation of the interdental papillae, accompanied by severe, localized pain. The infection typically involves only certain areas of the gingiva, not the entire mouth. The old description of this entity, "trench mouth," dates back to its prevalence during World War I. Physical findings include inflamed, tender, interdental papillae. A gray pseudomembrane is often seen along the gingival margin. Fever and other evidence of systemic infection are not characteristic. Lymphadenopathy may be present. Vesicles along the margin have been described in association with this entity, but these are most likely aphthous ulcers, not a spreading bacterial infection. Treatment includes antibiotics, such as penicillin or erythromycin, effective against the probable fusospirochetal pathogens. The medication is administered as in other severe forms of per-

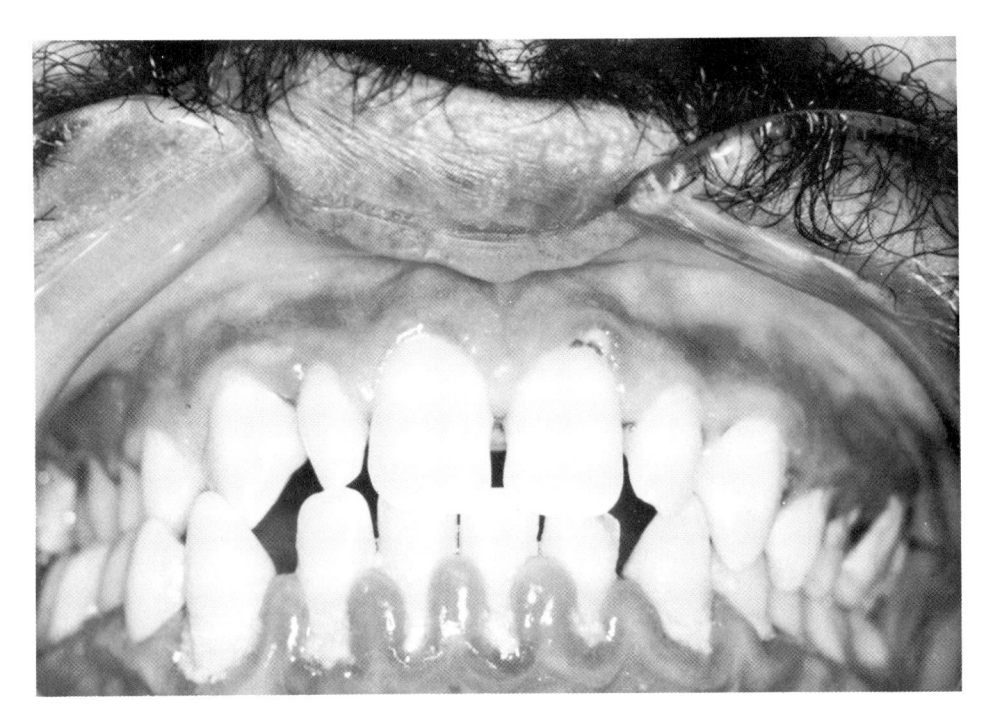

Fig. 4—1. Periodontitis. (Courtesy of W.B. Clark)

iodontitis; however, more important are debridement of infected, necrotic tissue and removal of plaque from the gingival crevice.

> **Objective 4–3. Recognize herpes simplex virus as a cause of oral ulceration.**

Herpes simplex virus (HSV) is a DNA virus that infects human populations throughout the world. Transmission of the virus occurs by direct contact with infected secretions; no animal vector has been identified. Measurements of serum antibody levels in various population groups around the world show that this virus infects the majority of mankind and is among the most prevalent of all infectious organisms. Two distinct virus types, known simply as HSV-1 and HSV-2, have been identified. Each has a characteristic pattern of infection, but either can apparently cause clinical syndromes characteristic of the other. Some of the major distinguishing features of these two types of HSV are listed in Table 4–2.

The manifestations of HSV in humans

Table 4—2. Distinctions between Herpes Simplex Virus Type 1 (HSV-1) and Type 2 (HSV-2)

	HSV-1	HSV-2
Location of Primary and Recurrent Infections	Mouth	Genitals
Type of infection	"Cold sores" of lip; corneal and hand (whitlow infection)	Commonly sexually transmitted disease, neonatal infection by direct vaginal contact
Mode of transmission	Generally nongenital	Sexual
Location of latent infections	Trigeminal ganglia	Sacral ganglia
Comment	Clinical lesions similar in appearance to, but serologically distinct from, HSV-2 lesions	

range from subclinical infections to life-threatening encephalitis. Epidemiologic studies support the notion that most humans develop either mild infection or none at all. Once the virus infects a person, it apparently persists for life in a latent form within sensory ganglia, especially the trigeminal or sacral ganglia. Symptomatic recurrences develop in approximately one-third of the population, usually in the form of herpes labialis or so-called cold sores.

PRIMARY HERPES SIMPLEX INFECTION

Primary herpes infections occur mainly in the perioral, ocular, or genital areas. The genital form is largely due to HSV-2, although it can infect the mouth through oral-genital sexual contact. The primary infection, when symptomatic, is usually much more severe than recurrent herpes infections. Primary infection with HSV-1 occurs most often in preschool children, but is occasionally seen in adults. The major clinical feature is the development of small (1- to 3-mm) vesicles scattered throughout the oral mucosa, following a short period of fever, sore throat, and lymphadenopathy. The vesicles involve the tongue, palate, buccal mucosa, and gingiva. Shortly after their development, the vesicles break and leave shallow, red-based, painful ulcers. Severe mouth pain is typical. Fever and cervical lymphadenopathy can persist for many days. Because of the extreme mouth pain, oral intake may be curtailed for an extended period, and dehydration is a potential complication. The presenting complaint with primary herpes infection in young adults may be pharyngitis, and it must be distinguished from streptococcal, diphtheritic, or other viral pharyngitis, especially that caused by infectious mononucleosis. The disease is self-limited, and recovery occurs within 1 to 2 weeks. Because of the typical clinical presentation in the young child, primary herpes infection does not present a difficult diagnostic challenge. Viral cultures of the saliva are invariably positive and serum antibody titers rise, but such diagnostic tools are usually unnecessary.

RECURRENT HERPES SIMPLEX INFECTIONS

Recurrent herpes infections often follow the primary infection, whether it be subclinical, mild, or severe. These recurrences can appear at sporadic intervals (months to years) for life. Most recurrent oral herpes infections manifest as a group of blisters, which cluster at the mucocutaneous junction of the lip. These lesions are called "cold sores" or "fever blisters" because they frequently appear concurrently with various febrile illnesses. The recurrence is attributed to reactivation of the latent virus, which travels down the nerve ending from its dormant focus in the trigeminal ganglion to reinfect the skin. The blisters coalesce, break down, and eventually heal after forming a scab. Their appearance is unpredictable. Besides an association with febrile illnesses, recurrent herpes infections sometimes follow prolonged exposure to sunlight or occur during a state of anxiety. Much less frequent is recurrent HSV-1 infection involving the intraoral mucosa.

DIFFERENTIAL DIAGNOSIS

Such recurrence can be confused with another cause of oral ulceration, namely aphthous stomatitis. The major distinguishing features of these two causes of oral ulceration are summarized in Table 4–3. Aphthous ulcerations, or canker sores, are larger and occur with much greater frequency than the lesions of recurrent herpetic gingivostomatitis (Fig. 4–2). Aphthous sores have yellow, necrotic bases that are deeper than herpetic ulcers. Aphthous ulcers are almost always found on movable mucosal surfaces, such as the cheek, tongue, and inner lip. No cause has been identified. Recurrent herpetic ulcers are almost always limited to small crops of tiny vesicles that rupture to form small, (1- to 3-mm) shallow ulcers and are localized to the firmly attached mucosa of the hard palate or the gingiva over the alveolar ridge. Recurrent herpes infection occurs as intraoral ulceration most frequently in the immunocompromised host, in whom the infection

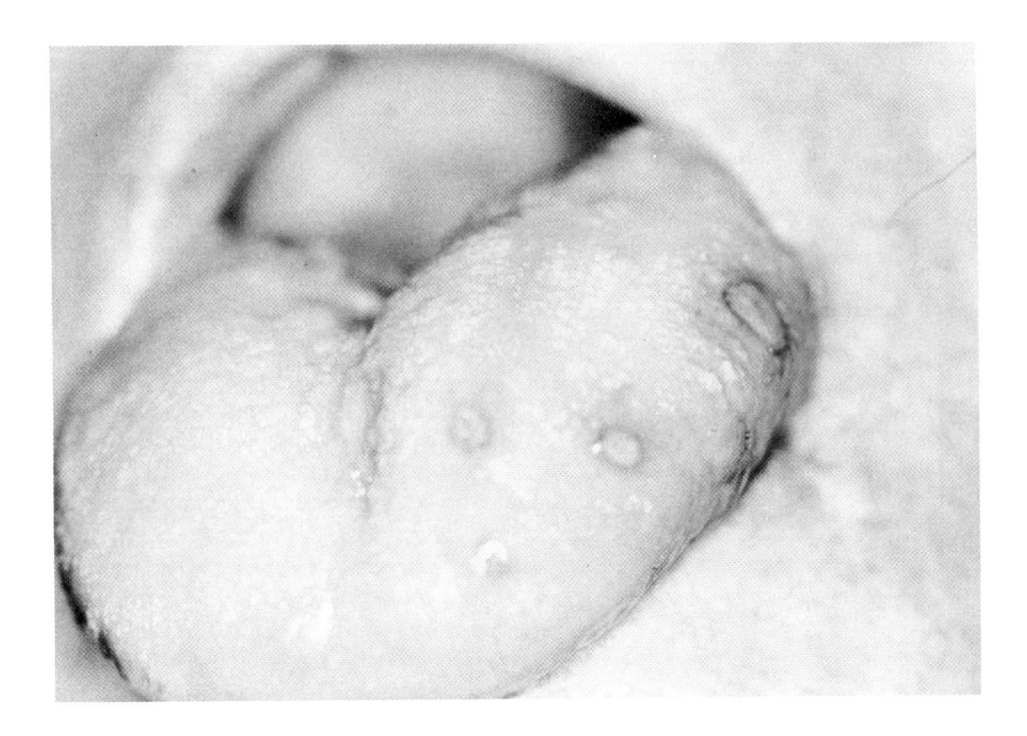

Fig. 4–2. Aphthous ulcers of the tongue. (Courtesy of R.A. Baughman)

may be associated with fever and other systemic symptoms.

Other less common causes of intraoral ulcerations, such as erythema multiforme and Behçet's disease (oculogenital-oral ulceration), are less apt to be confused with recurrent herpes gingivostomatitis.

Treatment of oral herpes ulcers is symptomatic. No antiviral compound, either topical or systemic, has yet been effective.

> **Objective 4–4.** Recognize inflammation of the salivary glands and identify mumps as a possible cause.

Three sets of salivary glands drain into the oral cavity. The largest are the parotid glands, which lie anterior and inferior to the external ear, superior to the mandible. Each parotid gland opens into the mouth through the

Table 4–3. Distinctions between Recurrent Intraoral Herpetic Ulcers and Aphthous Ulcers

	Recurrent Herpetic Ulcers	Recurrent Aphthous Ulcers
Age of incidence	Commonly adults	Wide range
Location	Hard palate and gingiva	Movable mucosa
Size	<3 mm in diameter	>3 mm in diameter
Number and configuration	Few, in cluster	Many; may coalesce
Ulcer base characteristics	Shallow; red center	Necrotic; yellowish
Rate of recurrence	Sporadic	Often within weeks to months
Histologic features	Multinucleated giant cells	Nonspecific inflammation

cheek (Stensen's duct). The second largest set of salivary glands are the submaxillary glands, which lie inferior to the mandible. These glands drain jointly into the mouth inferior to the tongue in the midline (Wharton's duct). A third set of salivary glands, the sublingual glands, are scattered along the floor of the mouth at the margin of the tongue. Their ducts are tiny and are generally not visible.

Inflammation of the salivary glands is characterized by swelling and pain in the area of the infected gland. The pain is commonly worsened by eating or chewing because saliva production is stimulated at such times. Parotid inflammation (parotitis) is most common. The swollen parotid gland distends the cheek and may displace the ear lobe outward and upward. The normal mandibular angle is lost if the swelling is marked. The area overlying the gland is typically tender when palpated and may be warm. The parotid duct may be inflamed, or it may show purulent drainage if suppurative parotitis exists. Submaxillary gland inflammation, characterized by swelling and pain beneath the mandible, is often difficult to distinguish from submandibular lymphadenitis. Ductal inflammation is an unreliable sign. Cervical or other lymphadenitis is not characteristically associated with salivary gland inflammation. Sublingual adenitis is uncommon.

MUMPS

Mumps, or epidemic parotitis, is the most common cause of acute salivary gland inflammation. It is caused by a paramyxovirus and is an infection seen predominantly in prepubertal children (85%). In all geographic regions, mumps is asymptomatic in 25% of cases; by adulthood, approximately 95% of the population have evidence of immunity to mumps from past clinical or asymptomatic infection.

Clinical infection has its onset after an incubation period of 16 to 18 days. The earliest symptoms include moderate fever, headache, anorexia, and malaise. The severity of these symptoms is variable. Within a day the patient may complain of an "earache" that becomes worse with chewing. For the next 1 to 3 days, bilateral parotid swelling develops. In a minority (25%) of cases, the swelling is unilateral. Parotid pain is associated with the swelling, and eating frequently makes it worse. Tenderness over the inflamed gland is common, but inflamed ductal orifices are an inconstant finding. Presternal pitting edema is commonly seen in association with mumps parotitis. The symptoms gradually resolve over several days, and parotid swelling diminishes with resolution of the symptoms. The disease is self-limited, and sequelae are uncommon. Mumps orchitis is mostly limited to adults. Meningoencephalitis may complicate mumps in 5 to 10% of cases. Most meningeal involvement is limited to headache. Aseptic meningitis may occur, sometimes prior to, or in the absence of, parotitis. Mumps is a major cause of aseptic meningitis in the winter or spring.

Diagnosis of mumps is based primarily on a history of exposure to an infected person, as well as a compatible clinical presentation. Serologic tests such as complement fixation are available, but are generally unnecessary. Virus isolation is impractical. The peripheral blood leukocyte count may be normal or slightly elevated with a predominance of lymphocytes. Serum amylase is usually elevated, even in the absence of clinical parotitis.

The differential diagnosis is straightforward. Rarely, parotitis may be caused by parainfluenza or cytomegalovirus infection. Impaction of a salivary gland stone may occasionally cause submaxillary or parotid gland inflammation in adults. Purulent parotitis is a much more severe infection, usually caused by *Staphylococcus aureus* and mainly limited to postoperative or debilitated patients. Systemic toxicity is marked; pus is frequently expressible from the duct orifice. Mumps that is limited to the submaxillary glands may be difficult to distinguish from cervical adenitis.

Treatment of mumps is supportive. Oral intake is limited during the acute symptomatic period. Aspirin may be useful for its antipyretic and anti-inflammatory properties. The infection is self-limited.

Objective 4–5. Recognize and treat oral moniliasis.

Moniliasis, or candidiasis, is a fungal infection caused by *Candida albicans* or other *Candida* species. Such infection is rarely disseminated throughout the body. When it is, the condition is almost always related to immunosuppression. Most commonly, however, *Candida* infection is localized to a particular body site, as in vulvovaginitis, intertrigo, or oral moniliasis.

Candida species are considered part of the normal indigenous mouth flora and can be isolated from up to 50% of normal human mouths. Under certain conditions, the fungus may proliferate at this site and may cause invasive oral infection. Many factors predispose patients to this type of infection, including the following: extremes of age; pregnancy; medical therapy with steroids, antibiotics, or immunosuppressive drugs; deficiency states; endocrine disorders; blood dyscrasias; or the use of dentures. Each of these situations alters the host-parasite relationship is such a way that oral infection with *Candida* species can result.

ORAL MONILIASIS

Oral moniliasis may be acute or chronic. Acute infection, known as thrush, is characterized by creamy-white, discrete patches on the tongue and mucosal surfaces (Fig. 4–3). These patches consist of a pseudomembrane of desquamated epithelial cells, leukocytes, and necrotic debris. Removal of the patches by scraping reveals a raw, bleeding surface. The patient may complain of burning pain in the involved area. A scraping of the lesion shows yeast forms and pseudohyphae on Gram stain or potassium hydroxide preparation.

Long-standing oral moniliasis manifests itself in several ways. Chronic atrophic candidiasis is most often associated with the use of dentures and is one cause of denture stomatitis. The mucosa of the hard palate may

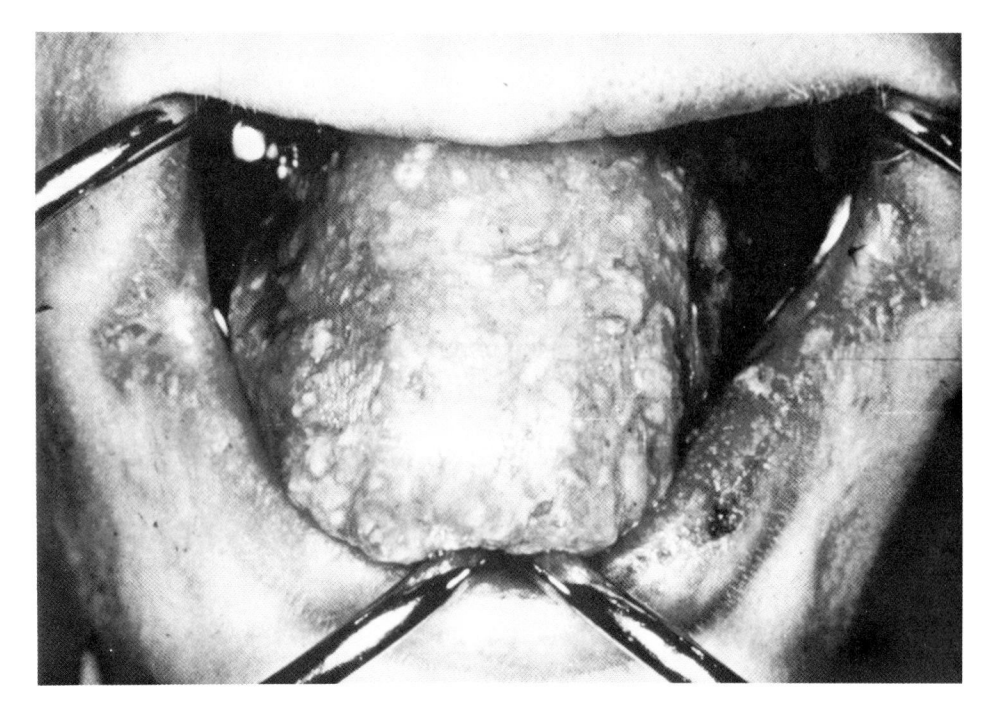

Fig. 4–3. Severe oral moniliasis with white plaques on the tongue and angular cheilitis. (Courtesy of R.A. Baughman)

be red and inflamed, with multiple small ulcerations covered with white, friable, curd-like flecks. Chronic oral moniliasis may be accompanied by angular cheilitis (Fig. 4–3). Another form of oral moniliasis, called chronic hyperplastic candidiasis, is characterized by a burning, tender, and dry tongue. The tongue may be deeply fissured and covered with white plaques, or it may be intensely red, glistening, and slightly swollen. As in other forms of oral candidiasis, scrapings are positive for yeast forms and pseudohyphae, and fungal cultures grow *Candida*.

Symptomatic relief from the discomfort of oral moniliasis is sometimes possible with saline rinses or anesthetic-containing lozenges. Specific antifungal therapy is essential to treat the infection effectively, however. Topical gentian violet (1%), applied to the lesions twice daily for several days, is often adequate therapy for acute moniliasis. Oral irrigation with 0.2% chlorhexidine gluconate has been successfully used. Nystatin is the most common antifungal agent used to treat oral candidiasis. It can be given either as an oral suspension 100,000 U (5 ml) 4 times daily, or more effectively as tablets, 4 daily, which are sucked. The tablets are more effective because of prolonged exposure to the infected mucosa, but they have the disadvantage of an unpleasant taste. Other antifungal agents, such as miconazole, clotrimazole, and, most recently, ketoconazole, are also effective. Eradication of chronic candidiasis may require therapy for several weeks or even longer. Any underlying predisposing factor that is reversible must be corrected to minimize the likelihood of recurring infection.

SUGGESTED READINGS

Anonymous: Mumps vaccine. Morbid. Mortal. Weekly Rep., *31*:617, 1982.

Chow, A.W., Roser, S.M., and Brady, F.A.: Orofacial odontogenic infections. Ann. Intern. Med., *88*:392, 1978.

Cohen, L.: Oral candidiasis: its diagnosis and treatment. J. Oral Med., *27*:7, 1972.

Finegold, S.M.: Anaerobic Bacteria in Human Disease. New York, Academic Press, 1977.

Gibbons, R.J., and Van Houte, J.: Bacterial adherence in oral microbiology. Annu. Rev. Microbiol., *29*:19, 1975.

Greenberg, M.S., Brighton, V.J., and Ship, I.I.: Clinical and laboratory differentiation of recurrent intra-oral herpes simplex virus infections following fever. J. Dent. Res., *48*:385, 1969.

Holmberg, K.: Oral mycoses and antifungal agents. Swed. Dent. J., *4*:53, 1980.

Krugman, S., Ward, R., and Katz, S.L.: Infectious Diseases of Children. St. Louis, C.V. Mosby, 1977.

Page, R.C., Engel, L.D., Narayanan, A.S., and Clagett, J.A.: Chronic inflammatory gingival and periodontal disease. JAMA, *240*:545, 1978.

Page, R.C., and Schroeder, H.E.: Pathogenesis of inflammatory periodontal disease. Lab. Invest., *34*:235, 1976.

Travis, L.W., and Hecht, D.W.: Acute and chronic diseases of the salivary glands: diagnosis and management. Otolaryngol. Clin. North Am., *10*:329, 1977.

Weathers, D.R., and Griffin, J.W.: Intraoral ulcerations of recurrent herpes simplex and recurrent aphthae: two distinct clinical entities. J. Am. Dent. Assoc., *81*:81, 1970.

CHAPTER 5

Influenza Syndrome

G. Murray

Objective 5–1. Diagnose a real case of influenza virus infection with an influenza syndrome.

Influenza, or the grippe, is an infection caused by *Myxovirus influenzae*. The terms are often used loosely to designate all infections producing the nonspecific symptoms of the grippe or the "flu syndrome," which are fever, headache, arthralgia, myalgia, cough, and some signs of upper respiratory infection that remain mild, however, during the course of a true grippe.

The influenza or flu syndrome can be caused by a great variety of agents. Some are responsible for interstitial pneumonia, and it is important to recognize these agents because some specific treatment is available (see Table 6–5). Other causes of the syndrome include: leptospira, which can cause hepatitis, meningitis, and renal impairment; the adenoviruses, which cause marked symptoms of conjunctivitis, catarrh, or rhinorrhea; the echo- and coxsackieviruses, which often produce diarrhea and skin eruptions; and the paramyxoviruses and respiratory syncytial viruses (RSV), which primarily affect young children. Even malaria, typhoid fever, histoplasmosis, or coccidioidomycosis may resemble the flu syndrome in their initial stages.

The incubation period is short (1 to 3 days), and the onset is abrupt. The disease begins with shaking chills. Fever then rises rapidly and reaches a plateau for 24 to 48 hours. Later, after a sudden fall in temperature, a low-grade fever can be observed. Fronto-orbital headaches, photophobia, prostration, and myalgias often accompany the fever. Respiratory signs remain limited to rhinorrhea, dryness of nasopharyngeal mucosa, and dry cough. One can observe some hyperemia of the conjunctiva and pharynx. More rarely, crepitant rales can be heard over a localized area of the lung.

In an epidemic period, the diagnosis of influenza can be considered solely on the basis of the clinical picture, but in an interepidemic period the clinical appearance alone does not really permit such an identification because the manifestations are similar to those seen in the infections previously mentioned.

Confirmation of the diagnosis of influenza then rests upon the demonstration of the causative agent or the elevation of specific antibodies. Both approaches generally leave the practitioner unsatisfied. The isolation of the virus in cell culture can be made from sputum, throat washings, or nasopharyngeal swabs taken during the first 3 days of illness. Unfortunately, this method requires time and money. A rapid diagnosis is possible by direct

INFLUENZA VIRUSES

The influenza viruses are classified into three types: A, B, and C. Type A is the epidemic variety; type B is more often endemic, causing only localized epidemics; and type C does not cause epidemics, but produces primarily inapparent infections. Influenza virus type A is extremely contagious through the respiratory tract. It is classified into subtypes on the basis of 2 antigens: hemagglutinin (H) and neuraminidase (N) (Fig. 5–1 and Table 5–1). Immunity to these antigens confers protection against influenza. The RNA of type A influenza virus is unstable, however. Thus, the antigens are subject to continual mutation. Because of these so-called minor changes, the virus partially escapes the mass immunity and produces localized epidemics every 2 or 3 years. These epidemics always occur in the winter and reach their peak in about 2 weeks. Their spread and the seriousness of the illness they produce in the population are inversely proportional to the immunity of the population: that is, a morbidity rate of about 2 to 7% and an infection-to-sickness ratio ranging from 9:1 to 3:1. The nature of these minor variations depends on immunologic resistance pressure. Each new viral strain reacts strongly with a specific homologous antibody, but only weakly with antibodies developed against previous strains.

After 10 to 20 years of antigen drift, a major variation of one or both antigens, H and N, occurs, and a pandemic sweeps the globe for several months. The pandemic of 1918 left 20 million dead, 400,000 in the United States alone. In 1957, such a major variation killed 40,000 in the United States.

The virus of type B influenza is much more stable than that of type A. Nevertheless, every 2 to 6 years, localized epidemics occur, the severity and clinical signs of which are indistinguishable from those of type A. Influenza primarily affects the elderly, young children, and debilitated individuals by causing pneumonias or decompensation of any underlying disease. Thus, in each epidemic a corresponding excess in mortality is seen, not only under the heading of pneumonia, but also under all other categories of cardiorespiratory death (Fig. 5–2).

Table 5–1. Different Kinds of Type A *Myxovirus influenzae* (since 1889)

Subtypes	Surface antigens*	Present nomenclature	Pandemics	Years of prevalence
A_2**	H_2N_2	H_2N_2	1889	1889–1917
A_0	$H_{sw}N_1$***	H_1N_1	1918 (Spanish influenza)	1918–1956
A_0	H_0N_1		None	1933–1946
A_1	H_1N_1		Minor	1947–1957
A_2	H_2N_2	H_2N_2	1957 (Asiatic flu)	1957–1967
A_3	H_3N_2	H_3N_2	1968 (Hong Kong flu)	1968–?
A_1	H_1N_1	H_1N_1	Minor	1979–?

*Three types of hemagglutinins (H_1, H_2, H_3) and 2 types of neuraminidases (N_1, N_2) in type A influenza virus are presently recognized as the causes of epidemics in humans. However, the new classification of the World Health Organization encompasses 12 subtypes of hemagglutinins (H_1 to H_{12}) and 9 subtypes of neuraminidases (N_1 to N_9) by including the equine and avian strains.
**Determined by studies of antibody against each subtype in populations of different age.
***H_{sw} (swine) strain related to that isolated in pigs since 1931 and again in man in 1976 (A/New Jersey, 1976 [$H_{sw1}N_1$]), which led to the fear of a new pandemic.

immunofluorescence of nasal cells obtained during the first 3 days of the illness, but this promising technique is not commonly available. The serologic diagnosis is achieved primarily by means of complement fixation with the type-specific nucleocapsid antigen. A titer of 1/80 in a serum drawn late in the course of the illness is presumptive evidence, but as always, complete confirmation depends on a rise in titer between early and late specimens, 2 or 3 weeks apart. The hemagglutination inhibition and neutralization tests, using the surface antigens, detect only subtype or strain-specific antibodies and are not clinically useful for the individual patient. Thus, the serologic studies confirm the diagnosis only late in the course of influenza and are useless in directing treatment.

For the community, however, exact antigenic identification of the strains in circulation each year is an important step in the defense against influenza virus, because public health consists in foreseeing, a year in advance, the epidemic strain of the following year with a view to producing a vaccine. The gamble seems worth the effort, but errors in

Influenza Syndrome

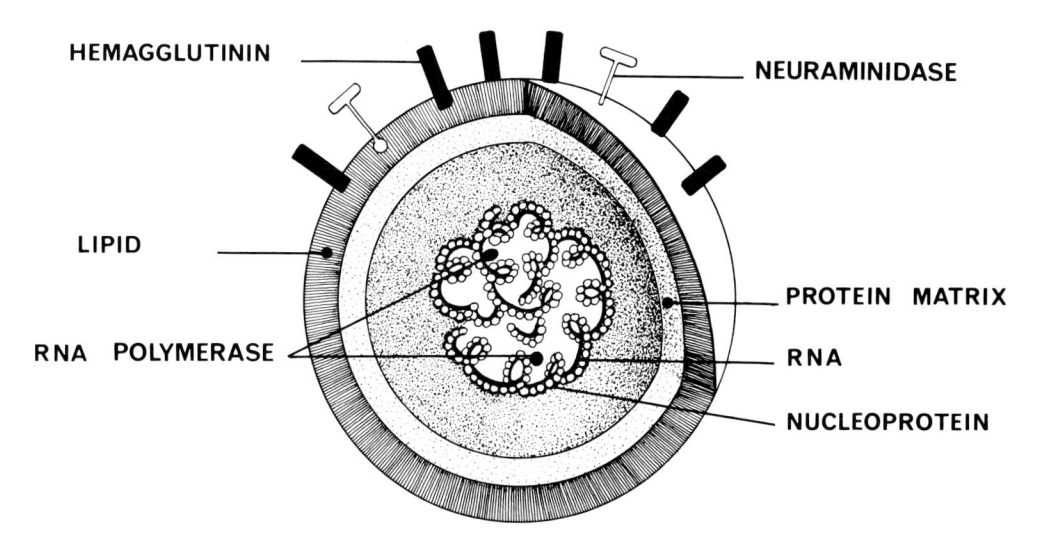

Fig. 5–1. Schematic diagram of type A *Myxovirus influenzae*. The envelope has a helicoid symmetry. The RNA is distributed among eight segments, a division which results in a great plasticity and propensity for recombination. The hemagglutinin, which takes its name from its property of agglutinating red cells, affixes itself to the mucoprotein cellular receptors. The neuraminidase is necessary for the liberation of the virus from the cell during propagation and facilitates the spread from one cell to the other.

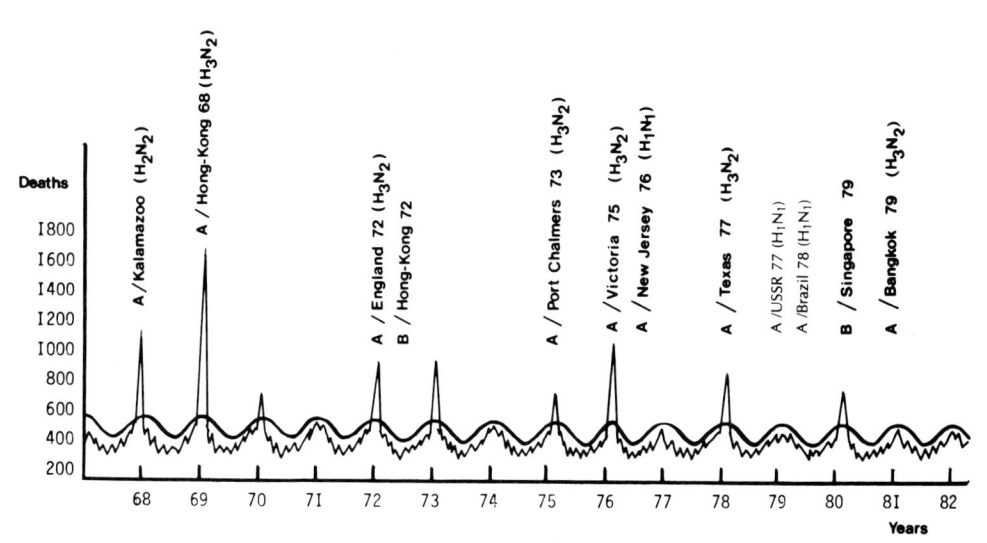

Fig. 5–2. Number of deaths by pneumonia as a complication of influenza in 121 cities in the United States (1968 to 1981). Name indications on the peaks correspond to minor variations. The most important peak indicates a major variation of antigen H. The name of an influenza virus includes its type and family (A_1), the place and year in which it was isolated (USSR 77), and the surface antigens (H_1N_1).

guessing do occur. In 1976, following the isolation of a virus that seemed to be that of the "Spanish flu," 40 million people were immunized against a virus that never spread. The story would have been more dramatic, however, if an epidemic of another subtype had occurred against which the vaccine offered no protection.

Objective 5–2. Recognize the complications of influenza.

Uncomplicated influenza lasts 3 to 7 days. Some individuals may feel a residual fatigue for several weeks. In certain cases, a severe and prolonged cough is evidence of tracheobronchitis, sometimes accompanied by dyspnea and thoracic pain. The major fatal complication is pneumonia, which can be either viral or secondary to bacterial superinfection.

Viral pneumonia develops early, at the beginning of the illness. The frequency varies with each epidemic. The chest roentgenogram is characteristic of an interstitial pneumonia. Gram staining and cultures show normal flora. Death can be caused by pulmonary edema and anoxia, most commonly in individuals with pre-existing cardiopulmonary diseases.

Bacterial pneumonia is the most frequent complication in the previously healthy patient, as well as in the debilitated host. This pneumonia may graft itself onto a beginning viral pneumonia and may worsen an already serious prognosis. It usually develops at the end of the influenza, however, often after one or several days of improvement. The bacteria usually implicated are *Streptococcus pneumoniae, Staphylococcus aureus, Haemophilus influenzae* (from which influenza received its name at the turn of the century), and other gram-negative bacteria. The clinical and radiologic signs are those of an alveolar or lobular pneumonia.

The possible extrapulmonary complications of influenza are as follows: postinfectious encephalitis (1/1,000 cases at the time of the 1957 epidemic), radiculoneuritis, myocarditis, pericarditis, abortion, and fetal malformations. More frequent, however, is the aggravation of already existing debilitating illnesses and otorhinolaryngeal superinfections, such as otitis and sinusitis.

Objective 5–3. Treat influenza with antimicrobial agents when required.

The treatment of uncomplicated influenza is symptomatic and includes bed rest, hydration, and administration of antipyretics, analgesics, and cough suppressants. Amantadine hydrochloride, at a dose of 200 mg/day in the adult and 5 mg/kg/day in the infant, is effective in the treatment of influenza, provided the administration is not initiated more than 48 hours after the onset of symptoms and is continued for 2 to 3 days after their disappearance. The drug blocks both the cellular entry of the virus and its multiplication. Its use is recommended for the following target groups:

1. Those at high risk, such as those listed in Table 5–2.
2. Normal patients with severe infections.
3. Infants with infection complicated by severe laryngitis.
4. Certain individuals who supply essential community services during an epidemic; for example, physicians, policemen, firemen, and those working on electrical or water supplies.

The central nervous system side effects, such as insomnia, nervousness, and loss of

Table 5–2. Diseases or Conditions in Which Influenza Immunization is Indicated

1. Cardiac disease, congenital or acquired (mitral stenosis, cardiac insufficiency)
2. Chronic obstructive pulmonary diseases, bronchiectasis, asthma, cystic fibrosis, neuromuscular disease with respiratory difficulties
3. Chronic renal disease (uremia, nephrotic syndrome)
4. Diabetes and other metabolic diseases
5. Chronic anemias, such as sickle cell anemia
6. Immunocompromise (neoplasia, immunosuppression, chemotherapy)
7. Age over 65 years

concentration, can occur in 5 to 10% of individuals at the beginning of treatment. Amantadine has no action against influenza B or viruses other than influenza A that cause the grippe syndrome.

Ordinarily, antibiotics have no place in the treatment of influenza; however, a pulmonary superinfection requires an antibacterial agent. When the exact cause of the illness is unknown, a cephalosporin type of antibiotic is a logical first choice, but sputum should be obtained first for smear and culture. If necessary, antibiotic therapy can be subsequently adjusted according to the laboratory results.

> **Objective 5–4. Identify the individuals who might benefit from influenza prophylaxis.**

The most common preventive measure is vaccination. As can be seen from the previous discussion, however, it is necessary to adapt the vaccine to the particular epidemiologic situation. For example, in North America in 1980 and 1981, the preparation used contained the following 3 strains, which were expected to recur at a later date: A/Brazil/78 (H_1, N_1), A/Bangkok/79 (H_3, N_2), and B/Singapore/79. This killed virus vaccine, administered by nasal instillation, has been used experimentally in several countries, but is not in general use. Influenza vaccine is strongly recommended in certain compromised hosts (Table 5–2) and for people over 65 years of age because of their excessive mortality rates during an influenza epidemic.

Local secondary reactions to the vaccines such as redness and induration are frequent. Fever and myalgias also occur, particularly in infants who are having their first contact with influenza antigen. A fractionated vaccine that causes fewer secondary side effects than the whole virus vaccine is therefore recommended for children. Immediate allergic reactions to the vaccine's constituents are always possible, but they are extremely rare. The Guillain-Barré syndrome, for example,

appeared to accompany the "swine flu" immunization; it has occurred once in every 100,000 to 1,000,000 vaccinations.

Amantadine hydrochloride, 200 mg/day for an adult, has been shown to be 70% effective in the prophylaxis of influenza A. The dosage should be maintained for a period of 4 to 6 weeks or until the appearance of antibodies if the vaccine is given concurrently in the context of a proved virologic epidemic of influenza A. The drug should be given for 10 days if the patient has already been immunized with a related strain or for 4 to 6 weeks if the individual has never been vaccinated or if a possibility exists that a strain may have different surface antigens.

SUGGESTED READINGS

Blumenfeld, H.L., Kilbourne, D.E., and Rogers, E.R.: Studies on influenza in the pandemic of 1957–1958. I. An epidemiological, clinical, and serologic investigation of an intrahospital epidemic, with a note on vaccination efficacy. J. Clin. Invest., 38:199, 1959.

Chain, A.: Influenza: vaccines or amantadine? JAMA, 237:1445, 1977.

Clinical Studies on Influenza Vaccines: J. Infect. Dis., 136 (Suppl.), 341, 1977.

Dolin, R., Reichman, R.C., and Maldore, H.P.: A controlled trial of amantadine and rumantadine in the prophylaxis of influenza A infection. N. Engl. J. Med., 307:580, 1982.

Douglas, R.G., and Betts, R.F.: Influenza virus. In Principles and Practices of Infectious Diseases. Edited by G.L. Mandell, R.G. Douglas, Jr., and J.C. Bennet. New York, John Wiley and Sons, 1979.

Dowdle, W.R., Coleman, M.I., and Gregg, M.B.: Natural history of influenza type A in the United States, 1957-1972. Progr. Med. Virol., 17:91, 1974.

Elliot, J.: Consensus on amantadine use in Influenza A. JAMA, 242:2383, 1979.

Fishaut, M.: Amantadine for severe influenza A pneumonia in infancy. Am. J. Dis. Child., 134:321, 1980.

Kaplan, M.M., and Webster, R.G.: The epidemiology of influenza. Sci. Am., 237:88, 1977.

Kilbourne, E.D.: The Influenza Viruses and Influenza. New York, Academic Press, 1975.

Kilbourne, E.D.: The molecular epidemiology of influenza. J. Infect. Dis., 127:478, 1973.

Lamontagne, J.R., and Galasso, G.J.: From National Institutes of Health. Report of a workshop on clinical studies of the efficacy of amantadine and rimantadine against influenza virus. J. Infect. Dis., 138:928, 1978.

Louria, D.B., et al.: Studies on influenza in the pandemic of 1957–1958. II. Pulmonary complications of influenza. J. Clin. Invest., 38:213, 1959

Monto, A.S., Gunn, R.A., Bandyk, M.G., and King,

C.L.: Prevention of Russian influenza by amantadine. JAMA, 241:1003, 1979.

National Institutes of Health: Epidemiology of influenza. Summary of influenza workshop IV. J. Infect. Dis., 128:361, 1973.

Parkman, P.D., Galasso, G.J., Top, F.H., and Noble, G.R.: Summary of clinical trials of influenza vaccines. J. Infect. Dis., 134:100, 1976.

Schwarzmann, S.W., Adder, J.L., Sullivan, R.J., and Marine, W.M.: Bacterial pneumonia during the Hong-Kong influenza epidemic of 1968-1969. Arch. Intern. Med., 127:1037, 1971.

Symposium on Amantadine: Does it have a role in the prevention and treatment of influenza? A National Institutes of Health consensus development conference. Ann. Intern. Med., 92:256, 1980.

United States Department of Health and Human Services: Influenza vaccine. Recommendation of the Public Health Service Advisory Committee on Immunization Practices. Morbid. Mortal. Weekly Rep., 29:225, 1980.

Webster, R.G., Campbell, R.H., and Granoff, A.: The "in vivo" production of "new" influenza viruses. III. Isolation of recombinant influenza viruses under simulated conditions of natural transmission. Virology, 51:149, 1973.

Weinstein, L.: Influenza-1918, a revisit? N. Engl. J. Med., 294:1058, 1976.

World Health Organization: International conference on Hong-Kong influenza. W.H.O. Bull., 41:335, 1969.

World Health Organization: A revision of the system of nomenclature for influenza viruses: a W.H.O. Memorandum. W.H.O. Bull., 58:585, 1980.

Wright, P.F., Dolin, R., and Lamontagne, J.R.: Summary of clinical trials of influenza vaccines. II. From the National Institute of Allergy and Infectious Diseases of the National Institutes of Health, the Center for Disease Control and the Bureau of Biologics of the Food and Drug Administration. J. Infect. Dis., 134:633, 1976.

CHAPTER 6

Acute Pneumonias in Adults

J.C. Pechère and J. Joly

> Objective 6-1. Decide when a chest roentgenogram is necessary in patients with fever and cough.

It is mainly at the coldest time of the year that large numbers of patients with fever and cough consult a physician. In most cases, these individuals have contracted a benign viral infection, such as bronchitis, tracheitis, or an upper respiratory infection. They may also have a far more serious infection of the pulmonary parenchyma, pneumonia, which must be diagnosed promptly. In North America alone, 2 to 3 million cases of pneumonia are reported each year, resulting in 40 million days of illness. This disease is the leading infectious cause of death in industrialized countries and ranks fifth among all causes of death in populations in which the annual death rate ranges from 18 to 100 per 100,000. The mortality rate is even higher in developing countries.

One of the keys to the diagnosis of pneumonia is the chest roentgenogram. From a practical standpoint, however, it is not possible to provide x-ray examinations for the multitudes of patients with fever and cough. Therefore, the difficulty lies in selecting those who should be referred to a radiologist.

RISK FACTORS IN PNEUMONIA

The first step in this selection process is to recognize the patient at risk. The normal lung defends itself well against infection; a succession of natural barriers prevents pathogenic organisms from penetrating the alveoli. The anatomic arrangement of the upper airways filters and humidifies the inspired air, and only particles 0.3 to 5 µ in diameter are likely to reach the alveoli. Smaller particles remain in suspension and are expired; larger ones are precipitated on mucosal secretions and then, propelled by the cough reflex and ciliary bronchial epithelium, they are swallowed or expectorated. In addition, several immunologic mechanisms of defense exist, such as local secretory antibodies, alveolar macrophages, lymphocytes, polymorphonuclear cells, and humoral antibodies. Some individuals have incomplete defenses. For example, tracheostomy or intubation bypasses the supralaryngeal barriers to infection. Loss of consciousness, even of short duration, for example from alcohol consumption, epilepsy, drug overdose, stroke, or anesthesia, favors aspiration in the bronchi and can result in aspiration pneumonitis. Heavy smokers and patients with chronic bronchitis and emphysema have an altered bronchial mucosa with a reduced capacity for eliminating bacteria, but diagnostic decisions are always difficult in these persons because cough and expectoration are habitual symptoms. Furthermore, persons at risk include those with pulmonary obstructive disease, paralysis of the respiratory muscles, pneumoconiosis, cystic fibrosis, pulmonary edema, and bronchial cancer, as well as all patients who are immunodepressed, including alcoholics, the malnourished, and the aged. One ancient idea remains valid today; pneumonia is facilitated by exposure to cold.

OTHER INDICATIONS FOR A CHEST ROENTGENOGRAM

Another indication for x-ray examination is the possible presence of septicemia. Both the filtering function of the lung and the richness of its capillary bed favor hematogenous pulmonary seeding. Thus, a patient with a cough in whom septicemia is suspected, for instance, because of a high fever and shaking chills, should definitely have a chest roentgenogram.

Even people in apparently good health may develop pneumonia. In approximately one of every five cases of pneumonia, no risk factors can be found in the patient. The best clinical criterion for alveolar involvement is the presence of tubular breath sounds with bursts of crepitant rales at the end of inspiration in one or more localized areas of the chest. A chest roentgenogram should also be ordered on the following grounds: when the patient has (1) a toxic appearance, (2) chest pain, (3) expectoration of purulent or bloody sputum, (4) short and rapid respiration, (5) splinting of one side on inspiration, or (6) cyanosis.

In the aged, the onset of a pneumonia can be insidious. The disease may manifest itself in a misleading fashion, with mental confusion or even cardiac failure. Fever may not necessarily be high, or it may not be present. When the pneumonia involves the lower lobes, the findings of abdominal pain, distension, or even paralytic ileus may wrongly suggest a surgical abdomen.

> **Objective 6–2.** Make the diagnosis in the presence of fever, dyspnea, and roentgenographic evidence of pulmonary infiltrates a few days after a surgical procedure.

The physician's skill is put to the test in this situation because the problem is often severe enough to necessitate admitting the patient to a hospital's intensive care unit. The four most frequently considered diagnoses are pneumonia, pulmonary embolism, pulmonary edema, and atelectasis.

PNEUMONIA

A fever present at the beginning of the disease is indicative of pneumonia. The sputum is then purulent, sometimes containing flecks of blood, and shows, on Gram staining and culture, a predominant microbial flora (see Objective 6–3), most often of gram-negative bacilli or staphylococci. The chest roentgenogram reveals either bronchopneumonia or alveolar (lobar) pneumonia (see Objective 6–3); one or several cavitations within the infiltrate are characteristic. A leukocytosis with neutrophils and juvenile cells is seen. The blood cultures may be positive, as may be an aspirate of pleural fluid, when present.

PULMONARY EMBOLISM

Clinical signs of pulmonary embolism include initial thoracic pain in the absence of fever at that moment, peripheral thrombophlebitis or a predisposing underlying disease, and hemoptysis with a normal sputum flora visible on microscopic examination. Radiologically, one or more opacifications with vascular distributions can be seen, for example, segmental, often with an engorgement or an abrupt cutoff of the corresponding pulmonary vessels. Hypoxemia is a constant and is surprising in degree when one considers the chest film. Neither the right ventricular overload on the electrocardiogram (the classic $S_1 Q_3$ pattern) nor the increase in the glutamic aminotransferases (SGOT) or the lactic dehydrogenases (LDH) is sufficiently specific.

When available, a lung scan can be useful in revealing one or several "cold areas" of vascularly distributed cutoffs in infusion. Characteristically, these cold areas should appear where no infiltrate is seen on the regular chest film. A normal lung scan rules out the diagnosis. A balloon catheter (Swan-Ganz) introduced into the right heart can measure the clearly elevated pulmonary artery pressures. The pulmonary wedge pressure, however, remains normal.

PULMONARY EDEMA

Pulmonary edema occurs principally following fluid overload or cardiac insufficiency. One should be able to obtain corroborating evidence for this condition. Loud crepitant rales are generally heard at the lung bases, and the patient's sputum is frothy. On the chest roentgenogram, one sees bilateral, fluffy infiltrates spreading from the hilum, more accentuated in the lower lobes, and perhaps blunting of the costophrenic angles. Cardiomegaly can be added to this picture if the disease is of long standing. With the hypoxemia, one often sees marked hypercapnea. The pulmonary wedge pressure, measured with the aid of a balloon catheter, is elevated. If in doubt about the existence of a fluid overload, the physician may administer a trial dose of furosemide and order a new chest film after the ensuing diureses. In the case of pulmonary edema, the opacities are diminished.

ATELECTASIS

Atelectasis is primarily diagnosed radiologically by the presence of linear or triangular infiltrates with a loss of lung volume on that side. Unfortunately, this precise sort of evidence may be lacking, and the overall complexities of the presentation of this disorder may confuse the diagnostic picture.

Pneumonia can complicate an edema or an embolism. Atelectasis and infection are often associated, as in aspiration pneumonia for example. Thus, the precise diagnosis may remain unclear. Because it is dangerous to wait with these severely ill patients, decisions must be based on a presumptive diagnosis, to give the patient every chance of recovery. Therefore, it is acceptable to prescribe antibiotic therapy, according to the regimen discussed in Objective 6–8, even when the diagnosis of pneumonia is not yet firmly established.

> **Objective 6–3. Outline the particular steps in making the etiologic diagnosis of pneumonia.**

Once pneumonia is diagnosed, it is necessary to identify the responsible organism. This difficult step does not always lead to a definitive conclusion, but it nevertheless remains helpful for directing appropriate therapy. Numerous causes are possible, and only the most frequent are shown in Table 6–1. The most important elements in identifying possible causes are the determination whether the pneumonia is (1) hospital- or community-acquired; (2) alveolar, lobular, or interstitial; and (3) related to a state of immunodeficiency.

CLINICAL FINDINGS

Once the antecedents of the illness have been identified (Table 6–2), the patient's medical history may provide valuable aid in the diagnosis when a specific epidemiologic context is found, such as illnesses in contacts, in patients in the same hospital room, and in the population outside the hospital. The physical examination is often disappointing, but finding one or more foci of consolidation, such as crepitant rales, dullness, or tubular breath sounds, suggests bacterial pneumonitis.

RADIOLOGIC FINDINGS

The chest roentgenogram is also helpful in making the diagnosis. Schematically, there are three types of infiltrates seen in pneu-

Table 6–1. Major Causes of Pneumonias (excluding Immunosuppressed Patients, Infants, and the Newborn)

Community-acquired		Hospital-acquired
Alveolar or Lobular Pneumonias	Atypical Pneumonias	Alveolar or Lobular Pneumonias
Streptococcus pneumoniae	*Mycoplasma pneumoniae*	Klebsiella, Enterobacter, Serratia
Haemophilus influenzae	*Legionella pneumophila*	*Escherichia coli*
Klebsiella pneumoniae	*Coxiella burnetii*	*Pseudomonas aeruginosa*
Staphylococcus aureus	*Chlamydia psittaci*	Acinetobacter
Anaerobic bacteria	Various viruses (see Table 6–6)	Anaerobic bacteria
Mycobacterium tuberculosis		

monia, as discussed in the following paragraphs.

Alveolar Pneumonia. Also termed lobar pneumonia, although this term is anatomically incorrect, alveolar pneumonia is characterized by an extensive, but delineated, homogeneous density, unless an abscess has formed. An associated air bronchogram sign is an excellent indication of alveolar involvement (Fig. 6–1). A bacterial origin is probable in such a case, most likely with a pneumococcus. The infection is considered to start within the alveolus and to propagate itself from alveolus to alveolus and then from acinus to acinus through the pores of Kohn and Lambert's canals. This means of spreading explains the sharply limited borders.

Bronchopneumonia (Lobular Pneumonia). Bronchopneumonia or so-called lobular pneumonia (Fig. 6–2) is characterized by poorly delimited nodules of varying diameter that tend toward confluence. The nodules are numerous and predominate in the parahilar area. Some air-filled blebs seen within the opacification produce an "air alveologram," the significance of which is similar to that of the air bronchograms. In this case, the pathogenic organisms penetrate the lung through the bronchi and the bronchioles and then infect the neighboring parenchyma, as in staphylococcal pneumonia. A similar radiographic image, but with a distribution of opacities farther from the hilum and predominantly in the lower lobes, is observed in pneumonias that complicate septicemias. The dissemination is then hematogenous and not bronchogenic, as in staphylococcal tricuspid endocarditis in addicts (Fig. 6–3).

Interstitial Pneumonia. This type of pneumonia results from a primary lesion in the pulmonary connective tissue. It is characterized by the reticular or honeycomb appearance of the infiltrate, with or without the presence of tiny nodules (granuloma) of nearly uniform diameter, often distributed at both bases. Alveolar involvement may be associated with this type of pneumonia and may be seen on the chest roentgenogram as a larger and more irregular nodularity. What is usually called an atypical pneumonia is a mainly interstitial infiltrate spreading out from the hilum. The greatest accentuation of the interstitial markings is visible at the bases (Fig. 6–4), where it is occasionally mixed with patches of alveolar infiltrate. Such roentgenograms chiefly suggest a mycoplasma infection, but they are also compatible with legionellosis, psittacosis or ornithosis, Q fever, various viruses, and tularemia. Another interstitial picture is composed of widely disseminated small granulomas, often barely visible and sometimes requiring an expiratory film to make them stand out. These granulomas indicate miliary pulmonary involvement, which can have several noninfectious causes, such as sarcoid, as well as a tubercular or histoplasmic origin.

Other Radiologic Findings. In addition to these 3 large categories of pulmonary infiltrates—alveolar, lobular, and interstitial pneumonias—one sees necrotizing and abscess-forming pneumonias, possible causes of which are given in Table 6–3. Major pleural reactions are noted in more than half the gram-negative pneumonias and in 10 to 25%

Table 6–2. Possible Responsible Organisms in Pneumonia, as Suggested by the Clinical Findings

Clinical Findings	Likely Organism
History, Antecedents	
Sudden onset with shaking chills	*Streptococcus pneumoniae*
Recent travel (to endemic region)	*Coccidioides immitis, Histoplasma capsulatum, Pseudomonas pseudomallei, Ancylostoma duodenale,* schistosoma, *Paragonimus westermani*
Contact with animals	*Coxiella burnetii* (Q fever), *Chlamydia psittaci, Francisella tularensis, Pasteurella multocida, Bacillus anthracis, Echinococcus granulosus*
Epidemic disease (closed communities)	Viruses, *Mycoplasma pneumoniae, Streptococcus pneumoniae, Staphylococcus aureus* (hospital)
Complication of influenza	*Staphylococcus aureus, Haemophilus influenzae, Streptococcus pneumoniae*
Alcoholism	*Streptococcus pneumoniae, Klebsiella pneumoniae, Mycobacterium tuberculosis,* mixed anaerobes
Loss of consciousness (aspiration pneumonia)	Mixed anaerobes, enteric bacteria
Chronic pulmonary obstructive disease	*Streptococcus pneumoniae, Haemophilus influenzae*
Cystic fibrosis	*Pseudomonas aeruginosa, Staphylococcus aureus*
Absence of spleen	*Streptococcus pneumoniae, Haemophilus influenzae*
Recent immigration to North America	*Mycobacterium tuberculosis*
Immunosuppression	All the agents mentioned and nocardia, mycobacterium, "Pittsburg agent," aspergillus, candida, zygomycetes, cryptococcus, *Pneumocystis carinii, Toxoplasma gondii, Strongyloides stercoralis,* herpes simplex and herpes zoster viruses, cytomegalovirus
Age: Young child	*Streptococcus pneumoniae, Haemophilus influenzae, Staphylococcus aureus,* respiratory syncytial virus, parainfluenza virus, measles virus
Elderly	Gram-negative bacteria
Signs and Symptoms	
Diarrhea, abdominal pain	*Legionella pneumophila, Mycoplasma pneumoniae, Salmonella typhosa*
Impairment of consciousness	*Legionella pneumophila*
Herpes labialis	*Streptococcus pneumoniae*
Furuncle, pyoderma	*Staphylococcus aureus*
Pyorrhea, carious teeth	Anaerobic bacteria
Upper respiratory infection ("cold")	Viruses, *Mycoplasma pneumoniae*
Bullous myringitis	*Mycoplasma pneumoniae*
Rash	Measles virus, herpes varicella zoster virus, echovirus, coxsackievirus, adenovirus, *Mycoplasma pneumoniae, Chlamydia psittaci*
Clearly seen pulmonary infiltrate	Bacteria
Appearance of Sputum	
Mucopurulent	All origins
Clear mucous	*Mycoplasma pneumoniae,* viruses
"Rusty"	*Streptococcus pneumoniae*
"Gooseberry jelly"	*Klebsiella pneumoniae*
Nauseating	Anaerobic bacteria

of the pneumococcal. On careful examination, small effusions can be detected in up to 20% of hospitalized patients with mycoplasmal pneumonias. Labile infiltrates with transitory hazy opacities that change nearly from day to day also occur and are accompanied by eosinophilia. Among the causes of this pulmonary infiltrate-eosinophilia syndrome are several parasitic infections with ascaris, strongyloides, and hookworm. The tropical eosinophilia seen in India is probably yet another parasite-associated part of the syndrome.

LABORATORY TESTS

Blood Count. The blood count reveals this eosinophilia, but the principal importance of

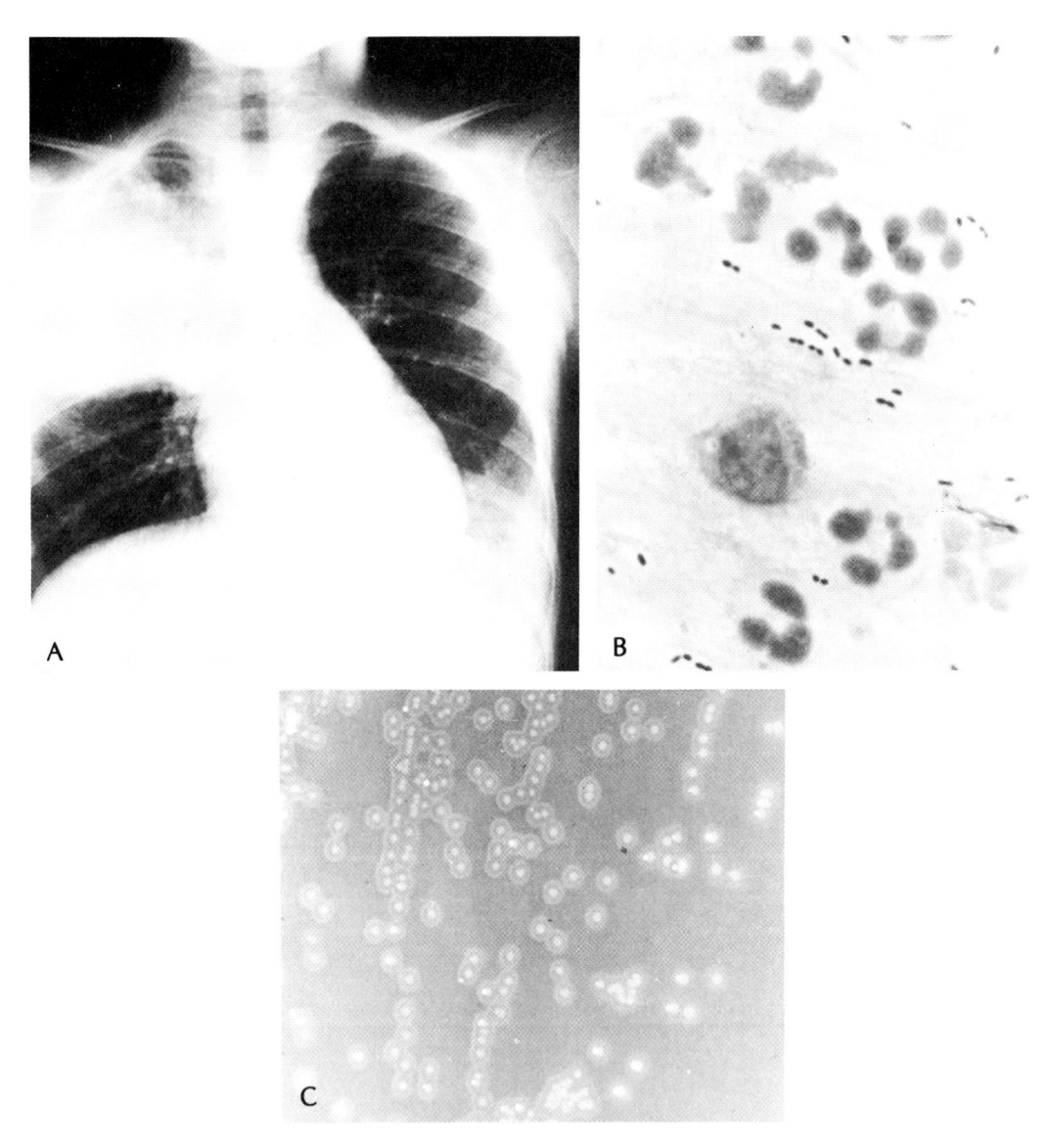

Fig. 6–1. *A,* Pneumococcal pneumonia. Two lobes (right superior and left inferior) are involved. Notice the air bronchogram on the right side. *B,* Same patient as in *A.* Gram-stained smear of the sputum. *C,* Typical colonies of *Streptococcus pneumoniae* on blood agar. Note the complete hemolysis around the colonies.

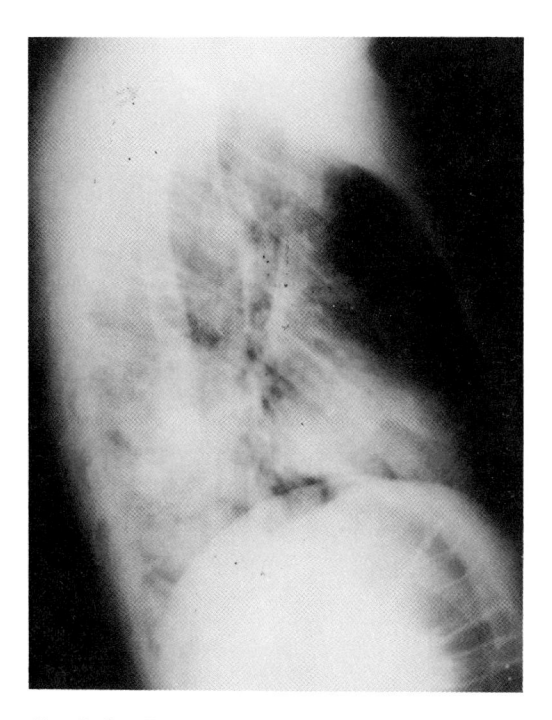

Fig. 6–2. Bronchopneumonia (lobular pneumonia) due to *Klebsiella pneumoniae*.

this test lies in establishing the presence of a polymorphonuclear leukocytosis. Although the total leukocyte count is less than 15,000 in 95% of cases due to a virus or mycoplasma, it is above this limit in 50% of cases due to pneumococci.

Sputum Examination and Culture. The sputum should be examined briefly at the patient's bedside (Table 6–3), but this specimen is difficult for the laboratory to interpret because it is usually contaminated with saliva to some extent. Indeed, after the intestine, the mouth is the most highly contaminated body site. One milliliter of saliva contains more than 10 million bacteria, which likely mask the true pathogen. To improve the quality of test results, it is necessary to obtain a sputum specimen obtained from the lung by means of a cough. Whenever possible, one should instruct the patient how to proceed instead of merely leaving a sputum cup with no explanation. In certain cases, the patient can be assisted by thoracic percussion, postural drainage, or the inhalation of hypertonic aerosols. Once a proper specimen is obtained, it should be rushed to the laboratory and examined as soon as possible.

In order to avoid contamination with saliva, a number of methods, including washing the sputum, homogenization, and counting the bacteria, have been tried, but without tangible, practical results. A gram-stained smear of the purulent material, on the other hand, is of prime importance and is much underused. The predominance of specific bacterial morphologic features is rapidly revealed, and a presumptive diagnosis of staphylococcal, pneumococcal, *Haemophilus influenzae,* or gram-negative pneumonia can often be quickly established. The culture results are then only a confirmation of a diagnosis already suspected. In fact, some authors consider that bacterial culture, even of potential pathogens, has scarcely any diagnostic importance for bacteria not seen previously on the smear.

Microscopic examination also permits grading of the quality of the specimen. The presence of more than 25 polymorphonuclear leukocytes and fewer than 10 epithelial cells from the buccal mucosa, under a low power field, (100×) suggests that the specimen is adequate. If the specimen is inadequate, however, it is better to obtain a new one rather than to rely on the existing sample. After culture, despite these precautions, the difficulty of interpretation persists. False-negative results are obtained at least 33 to 50% of the time with pneumonias caused by the fragile pneumococcus and *Haemophilus influenzae.* Contamination, particularly with enteric bacteria, is also a frequent occurrence.

Blood Culture. Blood cultures are usually positive, from 5 to 40% of the time, depending on severity, in pneumococcal pneumonia, if they are taken early in the course of the disease. Cultures are less often positive in pneumonias caused by other agents. Because a positive blood culture easily confirms the etiologic agent, the culture should always be taken.

Pleural Fluid Examination. Examination of the pleural fluid can also greatly simplify the

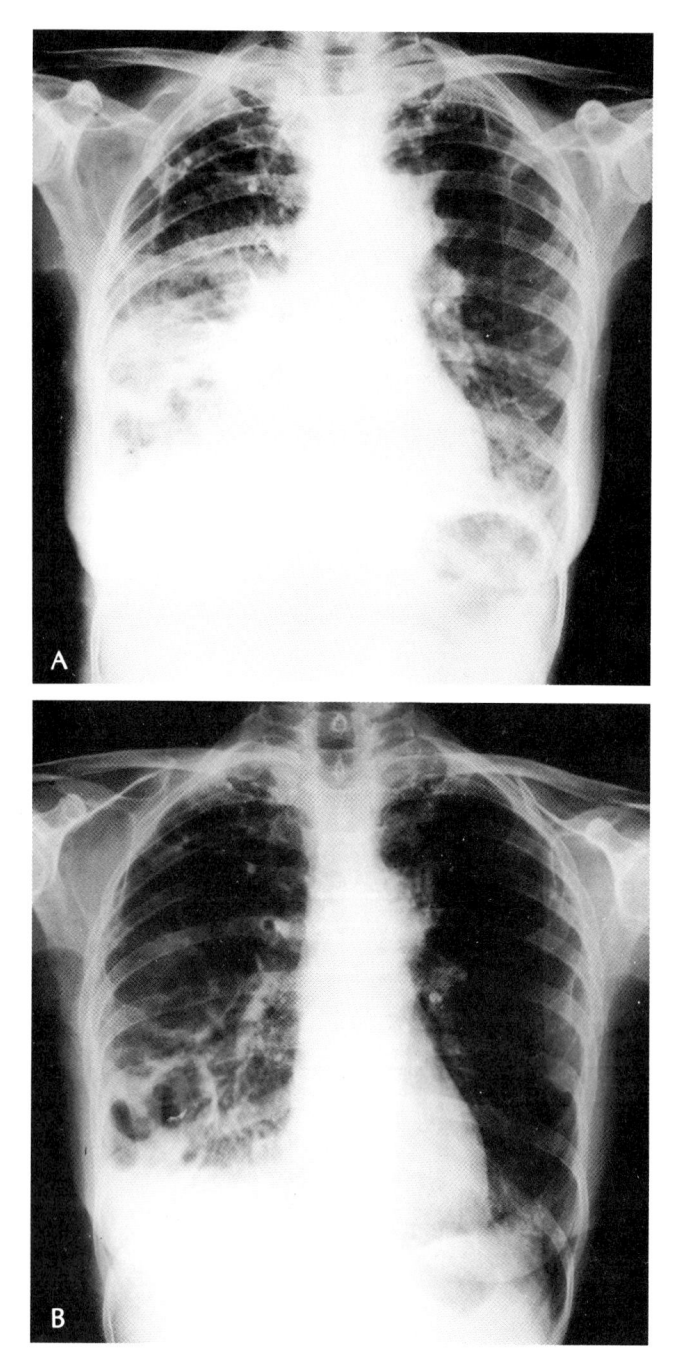

Fig. 6–3. *A* and *B*, Staphylococcal pneumonia complicating a tricuspid endocarditis due to *Staphylococcus aureus (A)*. Four days later, note the typical appearance of bullae-like pneumatoceles *(B)*.

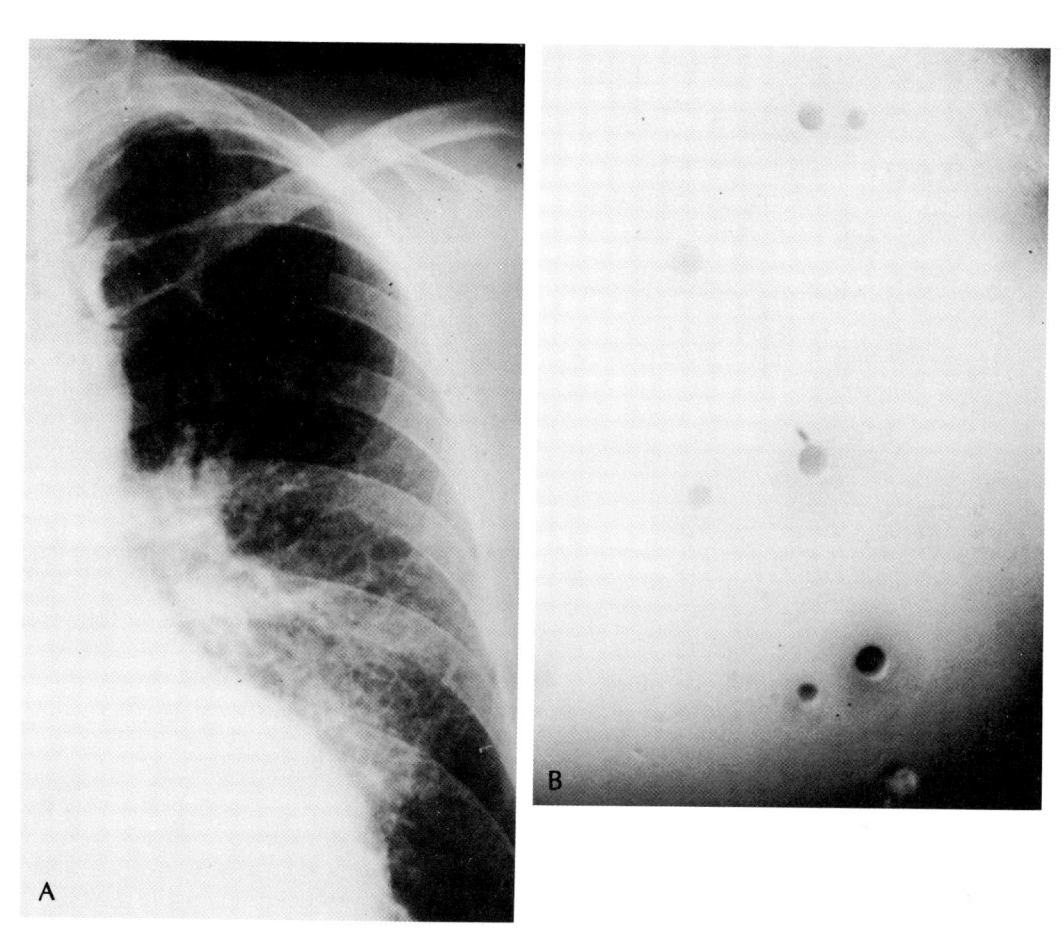

Fig. 6–4. *A,* Showing the reticular appearance of an interstitial pneumonia due to *Mycoplasma pneumoniae. B,* Colonies of *Mycoplasma pneumoniae* on special media.

Table 6–3. Principal Bacteria Responsible for Necrotizing Pneumonias

Anaerobic Bacteria (70–90% of Cases)	Other Frequent Causes	Rarer Causes
Bacteroides melaninogenicus	*Staphylococcus aureus*	Nocardia
Fusobacterium nucleatum	*Klebsiella pneumoniae*	Actinomycetes
Peptococcus	*Pseudomonas aeruginosa*	*Pseudomonas pseudomallei*
Peptostreptococcus	*Mycobacterium tuberculosis*	Aspergillus
Bacteroides fragilis		*Entamoeba histolytica*
Spirochetes		

search for the bacterial origin of a pneumonia by isolating the responsible organism.

Serologic Study. The serology in bacterial pneumonias is disappointing. For mycoplasma, viruses, and fungi, serologic means of diagnosis are occasionally available, but these tests generally require two samples, taken 10 to 15 days apart, for interpretation; this delay makes the tests entirely useless at the crucial moment of choosing therapy.

The detection of cold agglutinins suggests the possibility of a mycoplasmal infection. The presence of capsular antigen, detectable from the onset of the illness by counterimmunoelectrophoresis, mainly for pneumococcus, may become an important element in the diagnosis of pneumonia in the future.

Even after considering all the evidence, the cause of pneumonia may not always be apparent, especially when results from the sputum samples have not been satisfactory. Because pneumonia is clearly a life-threatening illness in many patients, the physician may opt for a more aggressive form of investigation while deciding upon the specific therapy.

INVASIVE INVESTIGATIONS

Transtracheal Aspiration. Transtracheal aspiration consists of piercing the cricothyroid membrane under local anesthesia with a large-caliber needle through which a polyethylene catheter is inserted into the trachea. The needle is then withdrawn. Several milliliters of saline solution are injected through the catheter into the trachea; this maneuver produces a cough reflex. The tracheal secretions are then aspirated through the catheter by means of a syringe. This technique permits the collection of pulmonary secretions without pharyngeal or buccal contamination. Although the yield is small in an interstitial pneumonia, this procedure is significant in the diagnosis of alveolar pneumonia and of bronchopneumonias of bacterial origin. As soon as the microscopic examination of the sputum is made, a presumptive diagnosis is often possible because the morphologic features of the individual pathogens are distinctive: encapsulated gram-positive diplococci (pneumococci), gram-positive cocci in clusters (staphylococci), small coccobacillary gram-negative organisms (*Haemophilus influenzae*), or thick gram-negative bacilli (enteric bacteria) (Figs. 6–5 to 6–7). Minor complications, such as minor hemoptysis or subcutaneous emphysema that reabsorbs spontaneously, occur in about 10% of transtracheal aspirations. Major problems, such as large hemorrhages, pneumothorax, and hypoxia, rarely occur. The indications for this procedure are, therefore, severe alveolar or lobular pneumonias when other methods, such as sputum culture, blood culture, thoracentesis, or even serologic methods, have not provided the needed information.

Fiberscopic Bronchoscopy. Fiberscopic bronchoscopy, with or without brushing, is generally less useful in the diagnosis of pneumonia than transtracheal aspiration because of the greater likelihood of bacterial contamination and because of false-negative results caused by the antibacterial effects of preservatives in local anesthetics.

Lung Biopsy. Needle biopsy of the lung is sometimes used in pediatrics when transtracheal aspiration is inadvisable. This method confirms a bacterial diagnosis in about a third of patients. In the adult, open surgical or needle biopsy is considered mainly in interstitial pneumonias in the immunosuppressed patient. Direct lung puncture can also be an important diagnostic tool in lung abscess.

> Objective 6–4. Establish the etiologic diagnosis of a community-acquired pneumonia with an evident alveolar infiltrate and choose the proper therapy.

In pneumonia in which an alveolar infiltrate is noted, a bacterial origin should be suspected (see Table 6–1).

STREPTOCOCCUS PNEUMONIAE

Streptococcus pneumoniae (pneumococcus) is responsible for more than 90% of bac-

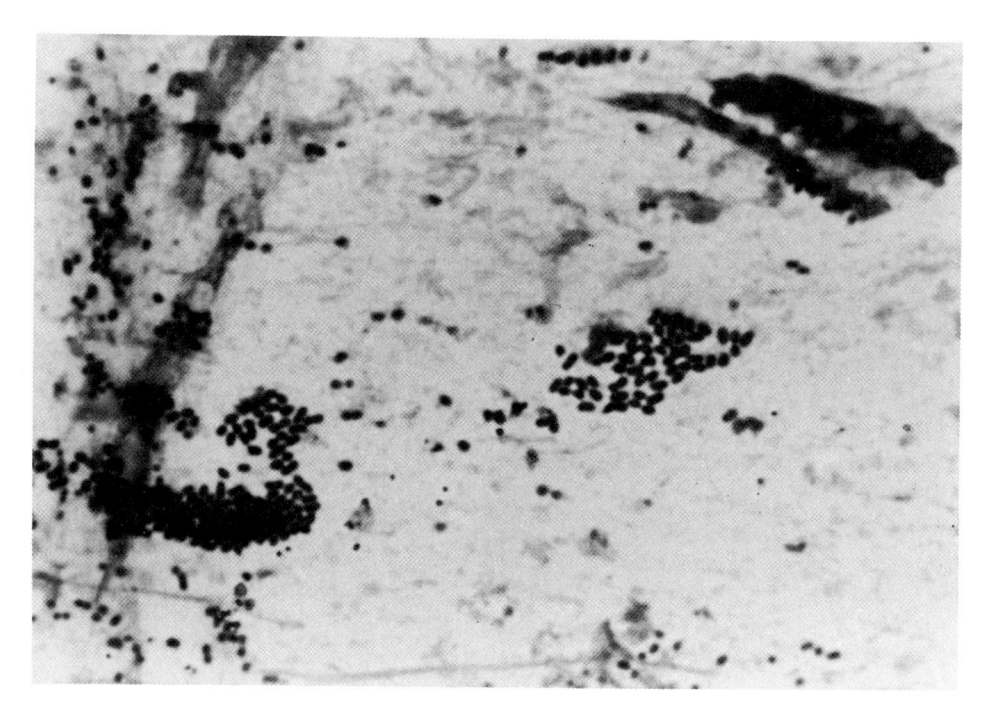

Fig. 6–5. Gram-stained smear of transtracheal aspirate showing *Haemophilus influenzae*.

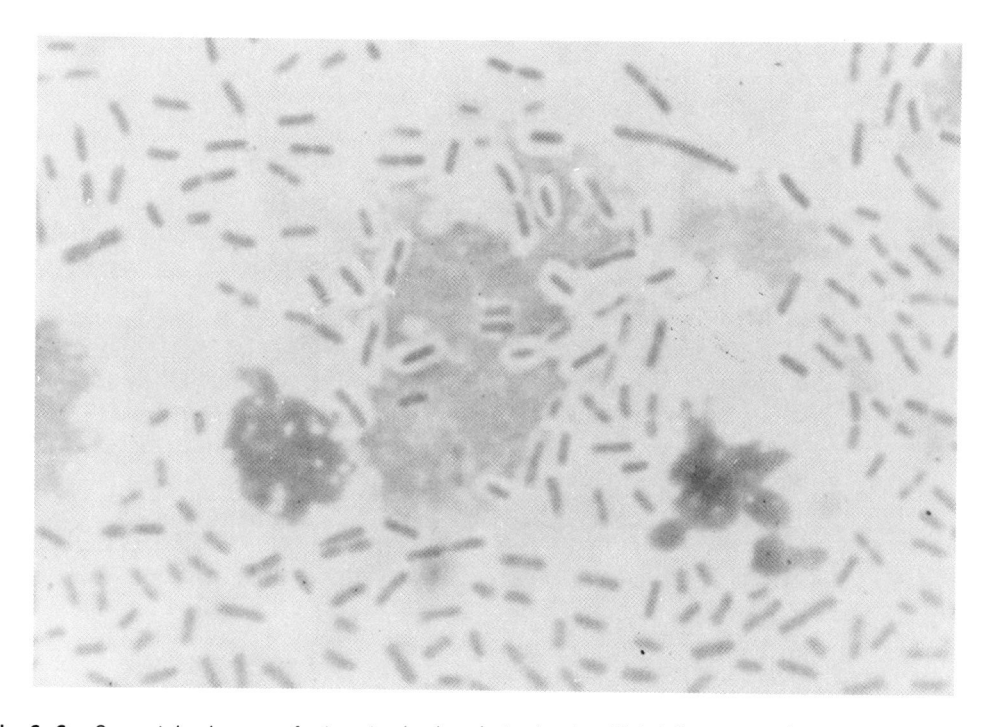

Fig. 6–6. Gram-stained smear of a transtracheal aspirate showing *Klebsiella pneumoniae*.

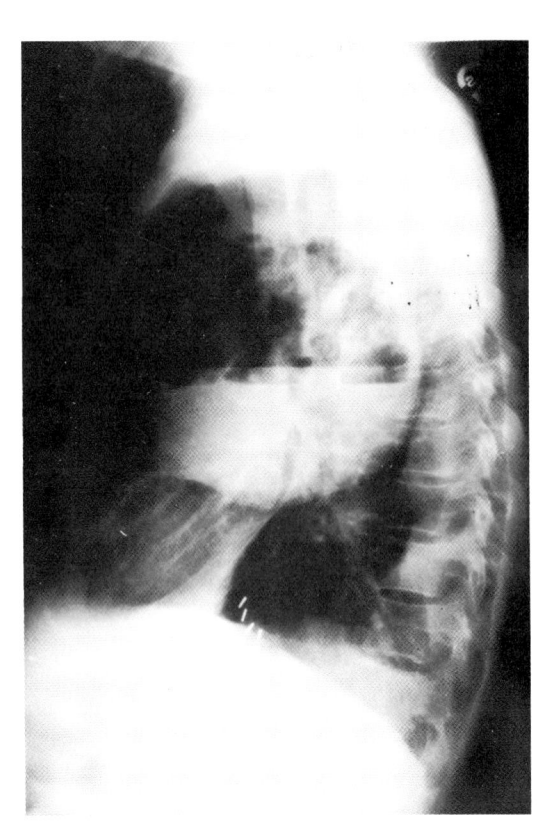

Fig. 6–7. Lung abscess showing two fluid levels. *Escherichia coli*, staphylococcus, and pneumococcus were isolated after needle biopsy in this 50-year-old patient.

terial pneumonias. This illness occurs all year round, in sporadic fashion, with a peak in the winter months. Underlying factors that have been identified are cold, wet weather, prior viral infection (the fluctuation in prevalence parallels that of "flu" or "grippe"), ages of less than 5 or more than 50 years, alcoholism, absence of the spleen, qualitative or quantitative insufficiency of immunoglobulins, and underlying pulmonary disease such as chronic bronchitis or emphysema. Both morbidity and mortality rates are higher in males, in particular men over the age of 50.

The typical patient experiences a sudden, shaking chill and an elevated fever 1 to 3 days after an infection of the upper airways. Nausea or vomiting, myalgia, weakness, and sharp thoracic pains are often associated symptoms. Sputum is generally copious and is rusty or frankly bloody. The physical examination may reveal a cluster of herpetic lesions on the patient's lip and a typical area of pulmonary consolidation, as well as a pleural friction rub. Evidence of associated bacterial meningitis or arthritis suggest the presence of pneumococci.

The chest roentgenogram shows a picture of homogeneous alveolar infiltrate (see Fig. 6–1A) that is generally confined to one lobe, but more rarely affects two or three. Abscess formation is rare, but pleural reaction is present in more than half the cases. Microscopic examination of the sputum shows typical, gram-positive, lancet-shaped, "willow leaf blade" diplococci, sometimes in short chains surrounded by a capsule (see Fig. 6–1B). These microscopic findings are neither constant nor conclusive, however, except when the predominance of the organism is marked. Positive blood cultures, seen in more than a quarter of cases, are diagnostically and prognostically important (Table 6–4). In three quarters of patients, counterimmunoelectrophoretic techniques allow one to detect pneumococcal capsular antigens from sputum, urine, or blood. A polymorphonuclear leukocytosis is usual. Hyperbilirubinemia and various anomalies of hepatic function are observed in patients with bacteremia.

Pneumococcal pneumonia requires immediate therapy. The mortality rate, on the average, is around 10%, with death nearly always occurring in the first few days. Among the factors in the gravity of the prognosis are aging, bacteremia (Table 6–4), late treatment, the involvement of several lobes, leukopenia, and certain specific pneumococcal types, such as type III, a producer of a large amount of capsular material. Cirrhosis, diabetes, arteriosclerosis, and chronic obstructive lung disease also worsen the patient's outlook.

The treatment of choice, in the absence of aggravating conditions, is procaine penicillin, 600,000 U every 12 hours intramuscularly, for 5 to 10 days. If the pneumonia is mild, or after a favorable therapeutic response, penicillin V, 250 mg every 6 hours, can be pre-

Table 6–4. Pneumococcal Pneumonia: Mortality Rates According to Age and to the Presence of Bacteremia

Age (years)	Cases with Positive Blood Cultures (%)	Positive Blood Cultures (%)*	Negative Blood Cultures (%)*
12–29	13	8	1
30–49	29	9	3
50 and up	32	30	20

*Mortality rates.
(From Austuan, R., and Gold, J.: Ann. Intern. Med. 60:759, 1964.)

STREPTOCOCCUS PNEUMONIAE

Streptococcus pneumoniae is part of the normal flora of the upper airways. More than half of normal individuals are carriers of this organism. The lung parenchyma is generally infected from this endogenous flora, even though the types most commonly found in the throat (3, 8, 9, 18, 19, 23) do not completely correspond to the serotypes usually responsible for pneumonias (1, 3, 4, 6, 7, 8, 12, 14, 19, and 23). Evidently, an exogenous type of infection also occurs in the form of small outbreaks within densely populated communities.

Along with other streptococci, *Streptococcus pneumoniae* shares the morphologic features of a gram-positive coccus and has an anaerobic metabolism that does not exclude a broad tolerance for atmospheric oxygen. Typically, under the microscope, the organism forms into groups of 2, which are like a figure 8 and surrounded by a generally visible capsule (see Fig. 6–1B). In pathologic specimens, however, these characteristics may be lacking, and they can be arranged instead into short chains similar to the other streptococci. These fastidious organisms do not grow on ordinary agar. On blood agar, they form small, clear colonies in 24 hours, surrounded by a halo of alpha hemolysis (see Fig. 6–1C). Identification is based on several particular properties: presence of a capsule, fermentation of inulin, bile solubility, sensitivity to Optochin (ethylhydrocupreine), and, at one time, its remarkable pathogenicity for mice, which it killed by septicemia within 24 hours after intraperitoneal inoculation.

The capsule, formed of polysaccharides, seems to play a pre-eminent role in the organisms' pathogenicity. Thus, mutants lacking a capsule become incapable of producing experimental disease in mice, and a relationship can be demonstrated between the quantity of capsular material produced and the virulence of the organism, at least with some pneumococcal types. In the absence of anticapsular antibody, this material impedes phagocytosis and allows the pneumococcus to multiply freely. In turn, pneumococci without a capsule, or those covered by anticapsular antibody, can be detected and ingested rapidly by the polymorphonuclear leukocytes. The capsule possesses some antigenic properties. More than 80 different types have been distinguished serologically. These reactions are remarkably specific, aside from a few cross-reactions among types and with other streptococci, such as *Klebsiella pneumoniae* and salmonella.

Several somatic antigens also exist. Substance C, a glucoside, is part of the cell wall. It has the property of forming a precipitate in the presence of a serum beta globulin, that is, the C-reactive protein. This protein is not an antibody, but appears in the blood only in certain acute inflammatory diseases particularly acute rheumatic fever. An M antigen, a protein, is also found and is similar to the specific M proteins of different types of group A streptococci, but the pathogenic role for it appears less evident than for the group A streptococci.

---

scribed. When aggravating conditions do exist, however, it may be necessary to increase the dose: penicillin G, 600,000 U every 4 to 6 hours intravenously for 7 to 10 days. In patients showing signs of shock, purulent pleural effusions, and lung abscess, 6 to 12 million U/day are given, reaching 18 to 20 million U/day with an associated bacterial meningitis or septic arthritis. If the patient is allergic to penicillin, the alternatives are either a first-generation cephalosporin, 1 g every 4 to 6 hours (caution is advised if the previous reaction was anaphylaxis), or erythromycin, 500 mg every 6 hours.

Some pneumococcal isolates, belonging to a number of different capsular types, have a minimal inhibitory concentration (MIC) to penicillin that is moderately high, 0.16 to 0.32 mcg/ml, instead of a median MIC of .02 mcg/ml for sensitive isolates. Originally described in New Guinea in 1967 and since seen the world over, these isolates generally remain responsive to the usual therapy. Since 1977, however, first in South Africa and then elsewhere in the world, truly resistant pneumococci have been isolated for which the MIC is 4 mcg/ml or greater. An associated cross-resistance is noted with other antibiotics in common use: tetracycline, chloramphenicol, erythromycin, clindamycin, and occasionally, rifampicin. In such cases, vancomycin, 500 mg every 6 hours intravenously, or possibly a third-generation cephalosporin (clinical data not yet available) can be recommended.

HAEMOPHILUS INFLUENZAE

For reasons that remain unclear, pneumonias due to *Haemophilus influenzae* seem to be increasing. Pediatricians have long recognized this entity in children under 5 years of age. It is seen today in adults as well when predisposing factors exist, such as chronic obstructive disease, alcoholism, and preceding "flu" infection. *H. influenzae* is also an important cause of pneumonia in the immunosuppressed patient. The clinical picture includes fever, chills, cough, purulent sputum or hemoptysis, and pharyngeal and thoracic pain. Radiologically, the pulmonary infiltrates are of the alveolar type or have the appearance of bronchopneumonia in the lower lung fields. A pleural reaction is seen in nearly half these patients, although abscess formation is rare. On Gram stain of the sputum, this origin is suggested by the finding of numerous pleomorphic coccobacillary gram-negative organisms, or gram-variable organisms sometimes resembling pneumococci if decolorization has not been sufficient (see Fig. 6-5). Culture requires specific media, namely chocolate agar and an atmosphere enriched with CO_2. A positive culture is not in itself diagnostic because 0.4 to 6% of healthy individuals are carriers of encapsulated virulent organisms. The percentage of carriers may reach 50 to 60% in patients with chronic bronchitis (nonencapsulated forms). Blood cultures may be positive and may thus establish the diagnosis. In bacteremic patients, the blood isolates of *H. influenzae* are generally encapsulated and nearly always belong to type B. On the other hand, in nonbacteremic cases, the *H. influenzae* strain is occasionally nonencapsulated and is not typeable. A polymorphonuclear leukocytosis is usual.

The mortality rate has been estimated at between 6 and 33%. It is over 50% in the elderly, when the underlying disease is serious, and in bacteremic cases.

The traditional antibiotic therapy is ampicillin, 1 g every 4 to 6 hours intravenously or intramuscularly, or amoxicillin, 250 to 500 mg every 8 hours orally. The appearance of beta-lactamase-secreting strains, which are more appropriately detected by directly testing for the production of the enzyme than by antibiotic sensitivity testing, however, has required the use of chloramphenicol, 500 mg every 6 hours intravenously or orally, or one of the new beta-lactamase-resistant cephalosporins (see Table 13-7). Naturally, once treatment is started with either chloramphenicol or a beta-lactamase-resistant cephalosporin and the isolate of *H. influenzae* is shown not to secrete a beta lactamase, therapy can revert to ampicillin.

KLEBSIELLA PNEUMONIAE

Pneumonias caused by klebsiella, when community acquired, mainly attack persons over 50 years of age. The representative profile is that of a male, chronic alcoholic, retired, and living in an institution, although individuals with cardiac disease, diabetes, or cancer, may also be victims. Characteristically, the disease begins suddenly and becomes severe, with the following symptoms: toxicity, prostration, high fever, shaking chills, dyspnea, cyanosis, chest pain, cough, and "gooseberry jelly" sputum, which is a mixture of purulent sputum, mucus, and blood. The area of consolidation, often localized on physical examination, is usually seen on chest roentgenograms as an alveolar infiltrate, with several to numerous small cavities, in the inferior segment of the right upper lobe.

Less characteristic is the picture of bronchopneumonia. In the sputum, klebsiella are seen as large, plump, gram-negative rods, sometimes in dividing pairs, with a capsule (see Fig. 6-6). The organism grows rapidly on ordinary agar plates as large, mucoid colonies and comprises three different species: *Klebsiella pneumoniae*, by far the most frequent, *K. ozaenae*, and *K. rhinoscleromatis*.

The organism can also be isolated from blood in 20 to 66% of cases or from pleural effusions. The prognosis is grave, with a mortality rate that exceeds one-third of the cases.

Klebsiella species have a facility for rapidly acquiring resistance to antibiotics; therefore, the definitive treatment should be based on sensitivity tests. Ampicillin is nearly always inactive. An aminoglycoside, such as gentamicin, tobramycin, or netilmicin (1.5 mg/kg every 8 hours intravenously), amikacin (7.5 mg/kg every 12 hours intravenously), or a newer cephalosporin (see Table 13-7) are most often used. Chloramphenicol represents only a second choice. The duration of therapy depends on the clinical response.

STAPHYLOCOCCAL PNEUMONIAS

Staphylococcal pneumonias comprise between 3 and 10% of the total group of bacterial pneumonias. Various modes of acquisition have been noted. Staphylococcal pneumonitis can occur in an infant under 6 months of age, sometimes in the course of a hospital nursery outbreak. Other cases in children can complicate the course of cystic fibrosis or can occur after measles. In the adult, this type of pneumonia is observed in the course of a respiratory virus infection, such as an influenza. Other predisposing causes that have been identified are chronic obstructive pulmonary disease, antibiotic therapy not directed at or ineffective against staphylococci, long-term hemodialysis, neutropenia, and in a more general way, the immunosuppressed patients.

Finally, staphylococcal pneumonia is frequently seen in the course of a right-sided staphylococcal endocarditis, notably in drug addicts, from pulmonary septic emboli. The clinical presentation varies from case to case. Radiologically (see Fig. 6-3), the multiple alveolar infiltrates, which involve several lobes, are not diagnostic in themselves, unless one also sees multiple microabscesses, the appearance of the bullae-like pneumatoceles, a rapidly developing empyema, or pneumothorax. The staphylococcal exotoxins, in effect, favor tissue necrosis, affecting first the bronchioles and then the alveolus. When one of the abscesses communicates with an airway, the air inflates the cavity to form a pneumatocele, which may then rupture through into the pleural space to produce a pneumothorax.

In the bacteriologic analysis of sputum or of tracheal aspirate and pleural fluid, direct microscopic examination is of major importance. One should expect to see numerous gram-positive cocci in grapelike clusters; without this sign, the diagnosis is seriously in doubt. Staphylococci do not conceal themselves. Positive culture without such preliminary observation is of questionable value. Blood cultures are positive in about 20% of cases.

Therapy usually involves a penicillin, such as penicillin G, 1 million U every 2 to 4 hours intravenously, if the isolate happens to be one of the 5% of penicillin-sensitive strains. When the results of antibiotic susceptibility tests are not available, oxacillin or nafcillin, 1 to 3 g every 4 hours intravenously, is usually preferred. If the patient is allergic to penicillin, one can administer cephalothin, 2 g every 4 hours intravenously, or vancomycin, 500 g every 6 hours intravenously. Vancomycin is also the agent of choice when the strain is methicillin-resistant. The duration of treatment has to be judged in each case. Two weeks appears to be the minimum. A purulent pleuritis or an abscess demands longer therapy, and a patient with septicemia, suggesting the possibility of endocarditis, requires at least 4 weeks of antibiotic therapy.

OTHER CAUSES OF PNEUMONIA

Among the other important causes of conspicuous alveolar pulmonary infiltration are certain forms of *Legionella* (see Objective 6-6), aspiration pneumonia (see Objective 6-7), and tuberculosis (see Chap. 8).

> **Objective 6-5.** Establish the etiologic diagnosis of hospital-acquired pneumonia with an obvious alveolar infiltrate and choose the appropriate antibiotic.

It is difficult to identify the cause of this type of pneumonia because, in addition to the possible causes already described in Objective 6–4, a number of gram-negative organisms may be responsible. Among them, *Klebsiella pneumoniae* figures prominently (see Objective 6–4). Enterobacter can cause similar infections, but they are less serious.

Serratia marcescens is a typical nosocomial organism, which contaminates nebulizer reservoirs, respirator aerosols, inhalators, respirators, drainage tubes, and intravenous lines. The pneumonias it produces have a mortality rate of up to 80% in certain series, probably because of the underlying condition of these patients.

Pseudomonas aeruginosa, like *Serratia marcescens*, grows easily in water and colonizes and contaminates the same sorts of apparatus. Among the factors favoring the development of this infection are chronic lung disease, cystic fibrosis, and immunosuppressive therapy with its attendant neutropenia, and possible preceding antibiotic treatment (this organism is resistant to most antibiotics and outgrows other bacteria in such a situation). Radiologically, one usually sees a picture of bronchopneumonia with numerous microabscesses (necrotizing pneumonitis), although the organism can exist even if these foci are not present. When a respirator is the mechanical vector of this organism, the infiltrate is usually bilateral, butterfly-shaped, and often resembles pulmonary edema. Prognosis is grave, with a mortality rate of over 50%.

Pseudomonas cepacia has also been implicated in hospital-acquired pneumonias. Differing from *P. aeruginosa*, this organism is usually resistant to aminoglycosides, but chloramphenicol or trimethoprim-sulfamethoxazole can be effective against it. The list of organisms responsible for hospital-acquired pneumonia also includes *Escherichia coli*, proteus, and acinetobacter.

The bacterial results obtained from sputum or from tracheal secretions by tracheostomy, cannulation, or endotracheal intubation must be examined in light of observations, too often forgotten, that gram-negative bacteria frequently colonize the oropharynx and trachea of hospitalized patients and do not necessarily produce pneumonia.

TREATMENT OF HOSPITAL-ACQUIRED PNEUMONIA

The main therapy is administration of the aminoglycosides, then secondarily, one of the antipseudomonal penicillins such as carbenicillin, ticarcillin, mezlocillin, and piperacillin, and certain third-generation cephalosporins. The seriousness of these infections and the variability of their antibiotic sensitivities justifies the initial use of a combination of an aminoglycoside and a beta-lactam antibiotic, especially in pneumonias likely to be due to *Serratia marcescens* and to *Pseudomonas aeruginosa*. *P. cepacia* is resistant to aminoglycosides and beta-lactams; chloramphenicol may be the drug of choice.

Objective 6–6. Outline the diagnosis and treatment of an atypical pneumonia.

An atypical pneumonia is defined, first of all, by its appearance on the roentgenogram, as described in Objective 6–3. The clinical profile may be distinct from that of an alveolar or lobar pneumonia in that the onset of an atypical pneumonia is more insidious, the appearance of the patient is less toxic, and auscultation findings are surprisingly poor in comparison with the radiologic signs. Moreover, entirely different organisms are responsible for the illnesses (see Table 6–1).

The principal bacterial agents are presented in Table 6–5. *Mycoplasma pneumoniae* and *Legionella pneumophila* are described here in detail because of the frequency of the former and the importance of the choice of therapy in the latter.

MYCOPLASMA PNEUMONIAE

Once considered to strike mainly individuals between 5 and 20 years of age, *Mycoplasma pneumoniae* infection is now known to affect children and adults of all ages. The persons most at risk are those who live together in groups: families of 4 or more,

Table 6–5. Useful Features in the Diagnosis of Atypical Pneumonias of Bacterial Origin

Organism	*Mycoplasma pneumoniae*	*Legionella pneumophila*	*Francisella tularensis*	*Chlamydia psittaci*	*Coxiella burnetii*
Disease	Atypical Pneumonia	Legionnaire's Disease	Tularemia	Ornithosis, Psittacosis	Q Fever
Origin of infection	Human	? Ground water, air conditioning	Rabbits, ticks	Parakeets, pigeons, turkeys, ducks	Cattle, sheep, goats
Age, most usual	5–40 years	>50 years	Adults	All	All
Special clinical signs	See text	Myalgia, diarrhea, mental confusion, relative brachycardia	Chest pain, splenomegaly, adenopathy	Chest pain, myalgia, headaches, macular rash (face), relative brachycardia	Myalgia, headache, splenomegaly
Special x-ray signs	Generally interstitial	Alveolar, sometimes major	Hilar adenopathy, pleuritis	Infiltrate, often large	Interstitial hilar infiltrates
Laboratory features	Cold agglutinins	Hematuria, microscopic, renal insufficiency	—	Leukopenia	Hepatitis (30%)
Serologic test	Complement fixation	Immunofluorescence	Agglutination	Complement fixation	Complement fixation
Usual antibiotic therapy	Nothing or erythromycin or tetracycline (500 mg q6h, po for 10 days)	Erythromycin (500–1000 mg IV or po q6h for 14 days)	Streptomycin (500 mg q6h IV for 2–3 days, then 500 mg q8h IM for 3–5 days)	Tetracycline (500 mg q6h po for 10–14 days)	Tetracycline (500 mg q6h po for 10–14 days)

schoolchildren, military personnel, and those in prison. The infection occurs all year round, with a slight increase in incidence at the beginning of the colder months. Fewer than 10% of patients infected suffer a pneumonia; the others have an upper respiratory infection or a simple bronchitis. In the first instance, fever, chills, headache, and above all, a dry, persistent cough dominate the clinical picture. Mucous or purulent sputum is seen in only about one-third of the these patients. Hemoptysis and pleuritic pain are rare. Rales and rhonchi may be heard on auscultation without an infiltrate visible on the chest roentgenogram. Signs of an upper respiratory infection are also present. Ear pain rarely means a bulbous otitis media, but it is often mentioned in texts. Still less frequent are conjunctivitis, muscle pain, diarrhea, or a rash ranging from maculopapular to pustular. Radiologically, most patients have interstitial pneumonia with a hilar distribution; alveolar-type involvement is limited to several small patches, localized in the lower lobes (75 to 90%) and limited to one side (60 to 90%).

Pleural effusion, traditionally considered rare, is observed in up to 20% of patients when decubitus roentgenograms are taken. Frank consolidation or an abscess is unusual.

On the whole, this illness is benign, and even without specific treatment it nearly always resolves favorably; the mortality rate is less than 0.1%. The period of symptoms, however, and above all, a persistent cough, can last beyond 3 weeks, and prolonged fatigue may delay full recovery. Although complications are rare, *Mycoplasma pneumoniae* infections have been associated with hemolytic anemia with high titers of cold agglutinins, erythema multiforme, and even Stevens-Johnson syndrome, meningoencephalitis, Guillain-Barré syndrome, arthritis, myocarditis, and pericarditis.

A precise microbiologic diagnosis is often difficult because none of the individual elements previously cited are pathognomonic, and the laboratory tests either lack specificity or take a discouraging length of time. In practice, the clinical impression is of primary use. An accurate presumptive diagnosis can be made on the basis of elevated cold agglutinins, present in about 50% of ambulatory cases. The test for MG streptococcal agglutinins is now obsolete.

Isolation of the organism takes 2 to 3 weeks and requires special media. The specific serologic response, 2 samples of blood taken 2 weeks apart, permits a late but certain and easy diagnosis; complement fixation and inhibition, indirect hemagglutination, and immunofluorescence tests are most often used, especially complement fixation. Tetracycline and erythromycin, at a dose of 500 mg every 6 hours orally for 10 days, hasten the resolution of the fever, the cough, and the radiologic abnormalities. Fifty percent of the patients remain carriers of *Mycoplasma pneumoniae*. Before prescribing an antibiotic, however, remember that spontaneous resolution occurs in the majority of patients; therefore, in practice, one should prescribe a drug only when a patient appears more ill than usual. When the differential diagnosis lies among *M. pneumoniae*, *Legionella pneumophila*, and pneumococci, then the logical choice of therapy is erythromycin, which is active against all these organisms.

LEGIONELLA PNEUMOPHILA

Legionellosis is an acute infection caused by *Legionella pneumophila*. It was first identified in 1976, 5 months after an explosive epidemic in Philadelphia, where 221 people who attended an American Legion Congress were affected and 34 died.

Actually, two general forms of legionellosis are known. Pontiac fever, a benign infection with a short incubation period (1 to 2 days), is characterized by a high fever, chills, myalgias, headaches, and on occasion, cough, some diarrhea, obtundation, and spontaneous recovery. Legionnaire's disease, the other, more serious form of legionellosis, usually entails a pneumonia (80% of the Philadelphia cases). This disease, at least at its outset, often has the appearance of an atypical pneumonia, but with an alarming degree of gravity. On the other hand, 20% of patients have infiltrates that could be considered alveolar, as noted in Objective 6–4. The infection is seen in epidemic form mainly during the summer and autumn, especially in hospitals, but it occurs sporadically all year round. The average age of the patients in these outbreaks is 50 to 60 years, but cases have been noted in infants. Men are affected 2 to 4 times more often than women. Among the predisposing factors are heavy smoking, alcoholism, cancer, or other immunodepressant diseases and conditions, particularly renal transplantation. The illness seems to be airborne; in most outbreaks, the ventilation or air conditioning systems have been incriminated.

Clinical Features. Despite a great variability in clinical features, the incubation period lasts 2 to 10 days, after which the patient has fever, chills, malaise, and myalgias. Diarrhea may be added to this picture; it can predominate and even precede the other symptoms. Vomiting and abdominal pains are not generally present. The patient's cough remains nonproductive and rarely leads to a purulent or bloody sputum. Nearly 40% of patients with Legionnaire's disease becomes dyspneic. Some chest pain and headaches are noted, but the mental confusion, even delirium and coma, have attracted far more attention. The symptomatic picture progressively worsens and toward the third to fifth days hospitalization often becomes necessary.

On examination, a remarkable alteration in the patient's general health is seen, and in more than one out of every two cases, relative brachycardia is present. Leukocytosis is rarely absent (50% of patients in Philadelphia had more than 10,000 WBC/mm^3). The sedimentation rate is elevated, as are the transaminases; the blood urea nitrogen and creatinine levels may also be higher than normal. More rarely, microscopic hematuria is seen; but the cerebrospinal fluid remains normal. On the chest film, no precisely characteristic features are visible. Soft, fluffy infiltrates are found, segmented or even lobar, and bilateral in a third of cases. A small pleural reaction may be observed, although abscess formation is unusual and is mainly seen in the immunosuppressed.

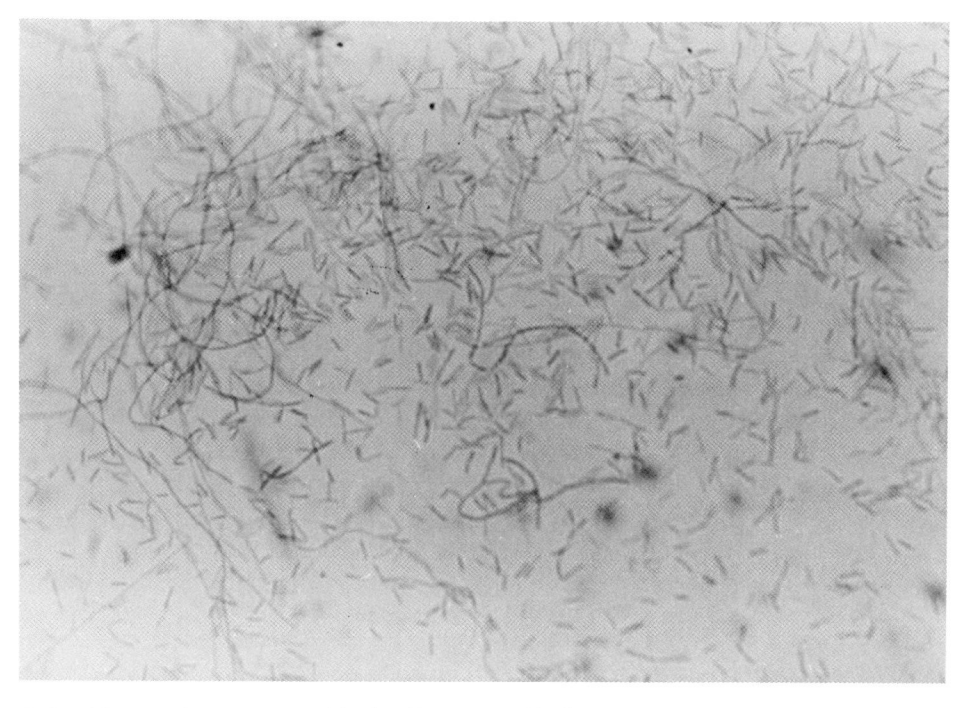

Fig. 6–8. Microscopic appearance of *Legionella pneumophila* from a culture.

Diagnosis. One should think of the diagnosis when a pneumonitis fails to respond despite apparently adequate therapy with a beta-lactam antibiotic. Immediate confirmation is difficult. In general, legionella is not seen on a sputum Gram stain, even though other potential pathogens are visible. Sputum and blood cultures are usually negative; cultures of material from bronchoscopy, lung biopsy, pleural fluid, and tracheal aspirate may yield legionella (Fig. 6–8); isolation and identification on special media takes 5 to 10 days. For the most part, the diagnosis is confirmed serologically. Because it sometimes takes 6 weeks for a clear seroconversion, however, the diagnosis is necessarily retrospective. With indirect fluorescence, a fourfold rise or a titer of $1 \geq 128$ is considered significant. A more immediate diagnosis by direct immunofluorescence is possible; this technique detects legionella in sputum, pleural fluid, bronchial aspirate, or on a pulmonary biopsy.

Treatment. Erythromycin seems to be the treatment of choice, even if several agents are active, although the optimal dose and duration of therapy are unknown. Empirically, the most seriously ill patients should receive 500 to 1000 mg intravenously every 6 hours (children should receive 15 mg/kg every 6 hours) for at least 14 days; in less severe pneumonias, a dose of 500 mg every 6 hours orally for 2 weeks is recommended. A relapse should be treated in the same fashion. Rifampin is another possible choice, but one with which physicians have far less experience. A combination of erythromycin and rifampin has been suggested in the most serious cases, that is, in patients who have responded poorly to erythromycin or in immunosuppressed patients with abscess formation.

Response to treatment is gradual. The fever can take up to 7 days to disappear, and the chest films do not begin to improve for 2 weeks in most patients. In addition, some are left with a reduced pulmonary capacity. Without treatment, the reported mortality rate is 15 to 20%; this rate falls to 5 to 10% with erythromycin administration.

VIRAL PNEUMONIAS

A number of viruses are capable of causing a pneumonia in man (Table 6–6). Most of the

Table 6-6. Major Viral Pneumonias

Frequent Causes		Less Frequent Causes	
Virus	Clinical Findings	Virus	Clinical Findings
Respiratory syncytial	Bronchopneumonia in infants	Adenovirus Type 4,7,3 (14,21)	Sporadic upper respiratory infections, occasionally with mild pneumonitis
	Bronchitis sometimes complicated by pneumonia in the elderly	Type 3,7	Severe pneumonia, often fatal in young children
Parainfluenza 1,3	Bronchiolitis sometimes with pneumonia, chiefly in children	Coxsackie virus A_{12}	Pneumonias in institutions or in dense populations (military)
Influenza A, B, C	Pneumonias complicating a "flu" or "grippe"	Varicella	10-15% of cases in the adult, rarer in children
		Measles	Bronchopneumonia in 3-5% of cases of rubeola
		Cytomegalovirus	Pneumonia in the immunosuppressed

time, the pneumonia has the appearance of interstitial pneumonitis, with or without alveolar involvement. Bacterial superinfections, especially pneumococcal, may complicate the course of the illness.

The clinical picture of viral pneumonia is hardly distinguishable from influenza or a mycoplasma infection, except in the case of pulmonary involvement in infectious mononucleosis, varicella, or measles; the characteristic signs of these illnesses usually permit easy identification. In other cases, the physician depends more often on the epidemiologic context or on the presence of simultaneous clinical signs, such as conjunctivitis, rhinitis, pharyngitis, laryngitis, myringitis, and rash. The white blood cell count is less than 15,000/mm^3 in the absence of superinfection. The diagnosis may be confirmed by isolation of the virus from the throat, blood, stools in tissue culture or by serologic study such as complement fixation, hemagglutination inhibition, or neutralization. The prognosis is generally good, except when pre-existing illnesses are present, such as respiratory or cardiac insufficiency, lipoid nephrosis, or debilitation, and for certain causes; for example, varicella pneumonia in the adult has been reported to have a mortality rate close to 20%.

Objective 6-7. Recognize an aspiration pneumonia.

A single milliliter of oropharyngeal secretions in a normal adult contains about 10^7 aerobic and 10^8 anaerobic bacteria; this bacterial flora can be even more dense, particularly when dental hygiene is poor. The aspiration of several droplets of saliva into the trachea or bronchi carries a considerable inoculum into the lungs. By way of comparison, inhaled ambient air containing 15 bacteria per m^3 introduces only 10 bacteria per hour. Thus, aspiration of saliva may overwhelm the host defenses and may produce a life-threatening pneumonia. This situation can occur in persons who have a profound alteration of consciousness, whether due to coma, general anesthesia, acute alcoholic intoxication, epileptic seizure, or even a sedative overdose, because the cough reflex is diminished or abolished in these cases. The risk also exists after dental manipulation and in the severely mentally retarded.

Aspiration into the airways can induce a chemical alveolitis and bronchitis with introduction of gastric juice (Mendelson's syndrome, which has a grave prognosis), an atelectasis when foreign bodies, such as undigested food, obstruct the bronchi or bronchioles, and about four different types of

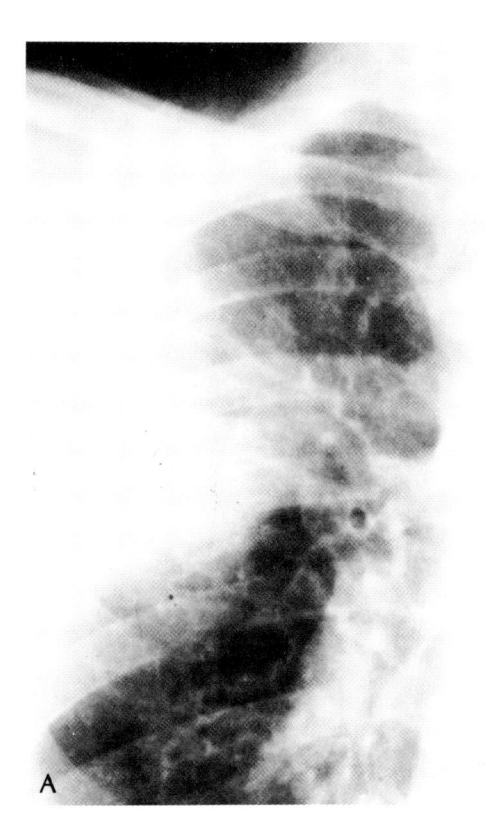

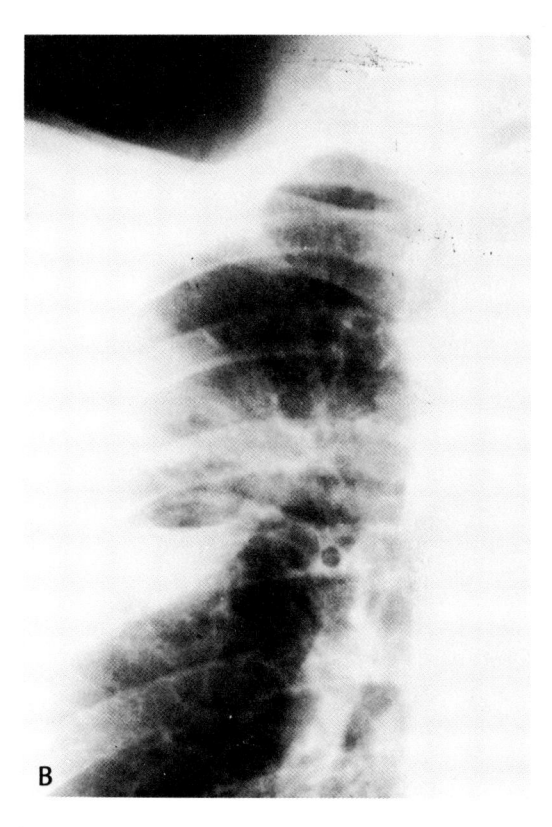

Fig. 6–9. Pneumonia due to *Bacteroides melaninogenicus*. A, Appearance before suppuration. B, After 3 days, note the development of an abscess with fluid level.

infection. The first type is simple pneumonia with a consolidation and fever. If quickly treated, patients with this illness respond rapidly and completely. Next is necrotizing pneumonitis, a more severe toxic illness characterized by the formation of multiple abscesses within the zone of consolidation and often involving more than one lobe. A large solitary abscess (Fig. 6–9) and empyema, both with a mixed bacterial flora, represent the two other possibilities.

DIAGNOSIS OF ASPIRATION PNEUMONIA

Whatever the clinical presentation, the diagnosis rests mainly on the patient's medical history. The instant one of the predisposing circumstances is discovered, the diagnosis of an aspiration pneumonia should be considered.

Bacteriologic diagnosis from sputum is difficult if not impossible in most circumstances because contamination with saliva complicates the interpretation, and further, the usual methods of obtaining a specimen are not suitable for anaerobic bacteria. Blood cultures and pleural aspirates may provide the key to the diagnosis, however. When aspiration pneumonia is community-acquired, strict anaerobes are found in more than 90% of cases, either alone (50 to 60%) or mixed with aerobes. The species most frequently implicated include *Bacteroides melaninogenicus*, gram-positive anaerobic cocci, *Fusobacterium* species, and *Bacteroides fragilis*. On the aerobic side, the streptococci are most commonly implicated. When the infection is nosocomial, more aerobes and facultative aerobes are identified (close to one-third in culture by themselves, and close to half in association with anaerobes). In this case, the organisms belong to different species. *Staphylococcus aureus*, the Enterobacteriacae, and pseudomonas reflect a parallel modification in the oropharyngeal flora during hospitalization of a patient.

TREATMENT OF ASPIRATION PNEUMONIA

Initial treatment depends mainly on penicillin G, 1 to 2 million U every 4 hours intravenously, especially if the pneumonia is acquired outside the hospital. This regimen seems effective even in the presence of *Bacteroides fragilis*, although this bacterium usually produces a beta-lactamase. If *B. fragilis* is found in pure culture, however, conservative wisdom suggests the use of cefoxitin, 1 to 1.5 g every 4 hours intravenously, or clindamycin, 600 to 800 mg every 8 hours intravenously, instead of penicillin. Moreover, these agents, as well as chloramphenicol at a dose of 500 to 1000 mg every 6 to 8 hours intravenously or orally, represent the best therapeutic alternatives to penicillin.

When the disease is hospital-acquired, *Staphylococcus aureus* and gram-negative aerobes are also likely to be responsible for the infection. Consequently, when we deal with a severely ill patient, our policy consists of combining penicillin G and an aminoglycoside or administering one of the newer cephalosporins, such as cefoxitin, cefotaxime, or ceftazidime. If the pneumonia is not severe, we initiate therapy with penicillin G alone, and we may continue with this agent or change the therapy, depending on the bacteriologic results and the patient's response.

> **Objective 6–8.** Choose the antimicrobial therapy for a bacterial pneumonia in the absence of the precise causative agent.

The therapy suggested up to now presupposes that the organism responsible for the pneumonia is known. At the beginning of an illness, once the cultures have been taken and before the results are on hand, however, the seriousness of the infection commonly requires that an antimicrobial agent be given without further delay.

In the case of a community-acquired, alveolar pneumonia, the most likely cause is pneumococcus, especially when the onset of the illness is abrupt and the infiltrate is clearly marked with lobar or segmental distribution, particularly in the lower lobes. In this instance, penicillin G is the therapy of choice and covers aspiration pneumonias as well.

Sometimes, however, another organism produces a similar picture: in the aged, *Haemophilus influenzae* and various gram-negative bacilli, especially klebsiella; after a "flu" or "grippe," *H. influenzae* and staphylococci are possible as well as pneumococci, in the presence of underlying lung disease such as chronic bronchitis, klebsiella and pseudomonas can be added to the three preceding organisms. A properly done Gram stain may provide the required basic information because gram-positive diplococci, suggesting pneumococci, are not the clearly predominant organism on the slide, then other causes have to be considered. In these cases, one of the recently introduced cephalosporins, such as cefotaxime or ceftazidime, is probably the most effective, inasmuch as clinical experience bears out our initial favorable impressions.

When a hospital patient develops a radiologically visible infiltrate, the treatment necessarily consists of compounds active against gram-negative organisms: aminoglycosides and cephalosporins. Some physicians prefer a penicillinase-resistant penicillin in combination with an aminoglycoside.

In an atypical pneumonia in a patient not known to be immunosuppressed, one must first consider whether antibiotic therapy is necessary at all. A virus could be responsible for the illness. Even if *Mycoplasma pneumoniae* is responsible, the pneumonia generally resolves spontaneously. In a severely ill patient or one showing signs of toxicity, or when the clinical possibility of legionellosis exists, one should probably administer erythromycin, which is also active against the pneumococcus, an organism sometimes considered in the differential diagnosis of what appears to be a questionable interstitial infiltrate.

If the patient is an active male homosexual, then one must consider the possibility of *Pneumocystis carinii* in the context of an atypical pneumonitis (see Objective 33–6).

Objective 6–9. Recognize the failure of therapy during the course of a bacterial pneumonia and identify its cause.

Confident in the habitual sensitivity of the pneumococcus, the physician becomes impatient when a clear-cut improvement is not apparent within hours of initiating penicillin therapy in a presumptively diagnosed pneumococcal pneumonia. The majority of patients are indeed better in a day or so, but fever may persist for 3 to 5 days or more, with cough, sputum, and continued chest pain, as well as with clinical signs of infiltration and an unchanged radiologic opacification. This situation does not necessarily mean a failure of therapy. Confusion is all the easier because chest roentgenograms resolve slowly. One should not expect to see complete resolution any earlier than 2 to 3 weeks. The time lag between the clinical and radiologic signs occurs even after the start of therapy. Initial worsening of the infiltrate is compatible with a favorable response. Actually, the clinical factor that should guide the physician is the general condition of the patient: his appetite, activity, pulse rate, and ease of breathing. The physician should keep in mind the factors that ordinarily retard a "normal" response, such as pleural fluid, advanced age, underlying disease, and alcoholism. Certainly, pneumonias due to staphylococci, klebsiella, or pseudomonas respond even less readily to therapy than those due to the pneumococci.

In certain patients, however, daily observation leads to the conclusion of a therapeutic failure. The patient's fever persists and even

Table 6–7. Causes of Therapeutic Failures during Pneumonias

Causes of Failure	Clinical Examples	Diagnostic Procedures	Therapeutic Responses
Empyema	Pneumonia due to anaerobes or staphylococci	Thoracocentesis	Pleural drainage
Improperly drained pulmonary abscess(es)	Pneumonia due to anaerobes, staphylococci, klebsiella, pseudomonas	Looking for fluid levels on the chest film (Figure 6–7A and B); tomographies	Proper bacteriologic diagnosis (70–90% of necrotizing pneumonias are due to anaerobic bacteria)
			Drainage, postural, inhalation, aerosols
			Some failures may force surgical cure
Bronchial obstruction	Pneumonia complicating bronchial cancer or foreign body ingestion	Bronchoscopy	Treatment of the cause
Sustaining septic pulmonary emboli	Pneumonia after tricuspid endocarditis in a drug addict	Blood cultures	High doses of properly chosen antibiotics
Associated chemical pneumonitis	Mendelson's syndrome (aspiration pneumonia with gastric fluid)	History	
Superinfection of the pneumonia	Gram-negative bacteria superinfection in a hospitalized patient treated for pneumococcal pneumonia	Repeat of the bacteriologic procedures (sputum, etc.)	Change of antibiotic treatment
Spurious bacteriologic diagnosis	Misleading pneumonias; tuberculosis, pulmonary mycosis, legionellosis	Correct bacteriologic procedures	Appropriate treatment

increases, the pulse is more rapid, the general condition worsens, and leukocytosis continues. Table 6–7 lists some causes of therapeutic failures during pneumonias.

Objective 6–10. Select the individuals for whom pneumococcal immunization is indicated.

In the United States alone, *Streptococcus pneumoniae* annually produces 500,000 cases of pneumonia, 1,200,000 cases of otitis, and 5000 cases of meningitis. Some of these infections lead to rapid death. The mortality rate for pneumonia, reduced by two-thirds after the introduction of antibiotics, remains at an apparently irreducible level of about 10%; 60% of the deaths occur in the first 5 days of illness. To this high toll of morbidity and mortality, the threat of the appearance of antibiotic-resistant pneumococci must now be added.

All these factors were arguments for the production of a vaccine in 1977. The vaccine contains the capsular polysaccharides of the 14 types of organisms implicated in 80% of the pneumococcal infections. A single injection of the vaccine leads to the formation of detectable antibody in the blood in about 2 weeks, antibodies that persist for at least 4 years. Side effects are frequent but minor: local pain and erythema (40%) and low-grade fever (3%). The vaccine does not provide absolute protection and is certainly of no use against the types of pneumococcus that it does not contain. Furthermore, antibody is not always elaborated against these 14 vaccine types, and the expected immunologic responses are actually observed in only 90% of normal adults. The proportion of responders is even lower in some groups, such as young children or persons under treatment for Hodgkin's disease; immunization seems to be an outright failure below the age of 2 years. Clinical proof of vaccine efficacy has not yet been effectively shown for children of 10 years or less. The vaccine's effectiveness has been estimated at 75 to 95% in clinical trials among older volunteers, and at 60% in older individuals to whom the vaccine was admin-

---

LEGIONELLA

The different bacterial species responsible for the clinical syndrome known as Legionnaire's disease are all members of a new bacterial family, the Legionellaceae. Seven species are currently included in this family, and some contain as many as 6 serogroups. The actual number of serogroups or species within the family will probably continue to grow rapidly in the near future. Although the DNA homology of these bacterial species is low, usually 25% or less, all share common phenotypic characteristics: they are gram-negative rods, with polar flagella, and they measure 1 to 3 μm long by 0.3 to 0.7 μm wide, although coccobacillary as well as filamentous forms have been described. Legionellaceae grow not on the usual blood agar plates, but on more complex medium containing cysteine and iron. These organisms are inert biochemically when tested on the standard medium used in bacterial identification.

The laboratory diagnosis of legionellosis remains difficult because of the unusual nutritional requirements of these organisms, their slow growing time, and the frequent overgrowth by normal pharyngeal flora. Different bacteriologic media have been described, but the most common is the charcoal yeast extract (CYE) medium. Numerous selective and semiselective media have been recently described, but no comparative evaluation of these media has been done. Under the best conditions, the standard CYE medium has a sensitivity of 65% when compared to serologic study and direct fluorescent antibody testing. Currently, only direct fluorescent antibody testing can provide a rapid diagnosis of legionellosis, but its sensitivity is low.

Most cases of legionellosis are identified by serologic study (indirect fluorescent antibody testing). When carefully performed, this technique is highly specific, but it does present some problems with regard to sensitivity. In 2 studies in which Legionnaire's disease was diagnosed by culture or direct fluorescent antibody testing, seroconversion was observed in 75% and in 64% of these cases respectively. Other diagnostic procedures have been described, but none is superior to the indirect fluorescent antibody testing.

In vitro sensitivity testing of the Legionellaceae has shown that these bacteria are generally sensitive to erythromycin, rifampin, and tetracycline. Although Legionellaceae are susceptible in vitro to aminoglycosides, patients with Legionnaire's disease who were treated with these drugs during the Philadelphia outbreak did not respond favorably. Currently, the drug of choice for the treatment of legionellosis is erythromycin.

istered because underlying disease was an apparent indication.

Despite these reservations, the seriousness and frequency of pneumococcal infections in high-risk groups require an immunization program. The vaccine is contraindicated in pregnant women, in children under 2 years of age, and in individuals incapable of producing antibodies, such as those with hypogammaglobulinemia. Vaccination merits consideration when age or underlying disease exposes the individual to a higher risk of pneumococcal disease, as in the following examples: absence of the spleen or splenic dysfunction; renal, hepatic, or cardiac insufficiency; old age, especially if such persons live in an institution. If even one of these conditions affects a child between 2 and 10 years of age, the vaccine can be given the benefit of the doubt without neglecting the other precautions. Thus, from the time a splenectomy is performed on a child under the age of 5, antibiotic prophylaxis should be administered, and a prescription should always be available to be filled in case of an acute febrile episode. Which antibiotic should be chosen? Penicillin is traditional, but the increasing importance of resistant isolates could be a problem; the trimethoprim-sulfamethoxazole combination has the advantage of protecting against *Haemophilus influenzae*, the other pathogen dangerous in these circumstances.

Other questions remain to be answered with regard to the vaccine: How long does immunity last? Are booster injections necessary, and if so, how often should they be given? Should we immunize patients with repeated pneumococcal meningitis? The answers await further studies.

SUGGESTED READINGS

Ammann, A.J., et al.: Polyvalent pneumococcal-polysaccharide immunization of patients with sickle-cell anemia and patients with splenectomy. N. Engl. J. Med., 297:897, 1977.

Blackmon, J.A., et al.: Legionellosis. Am. J. Pathol., 103:429, 1981.

Broome, C.V., Facklam, R.R., and Fraser, D.W.: Pneumococcal disease after pneumococcal vaccination. An alternative method to estimate the efficacy of pneumococcal vaccine. N. Engl. J. Med., 303:549, 1980.

Center for Disease Control: Pneumococcal polysaccharide vaccine. Recommendation of the immunization practices advisory. Ann. Intern. Med., 96:203, 1982.

Cunha, B.A., and Quintiliani, R.: The atypical pneumonias. A diagnostic and therapeutic approach. Postgrad. Med., 66:95, 1979.

Donowitz, G.R., and Mandell, G.L.. Acute pneumonia. *In* Principles and Practice of Infectious Diseases. Edited by G.L. Mandell, R.G. Douglas, Jr., and J.E. Bennett. New York, John Wiley and Sons, 1979.

Fine, N.L., Smith, L.R., and Sheedy, P.F.: Frequency of pleural effusions in mycoplasma and viral pneumonias. N. Engl. J. Med., 283:790, 1970.

Follansbee, S.E., et al.: An outbreak of Pneumocystis carinii pneumonia in homosexual men. Ann. Intern. Med., 96:705, 1982.

Garb, J.L., et al.: Differences in etiology of pneumonias in nursing home and community patients. JAMA, 240:2169, 1978.

Gerding, D.G.: Etiologic diagnosis of acute pneumonia in adults. Postgrad. Med., 69:136, 1981.

Hausmann, W., and Karlish, A.J.: Staphylococcal pneumonia in adults. Br. Med. J., 2:845, 1956.

Helms, C.M., et al.: Comparative features of pneumococcal, mycoplasmal and legionnaire's disease pneumonias. Ann. Intern. Med., 90:543, 1979.

Johanson, W.G., and Harris, G.D.: Aspiration pneumonia, anaerobic infections and lung abscess. Med. Clin. North Am., 64:385, 1980.

Jonas, M., and Cunha, B.A.: Bacteremic Escherichia coli pneumonia. Arch. Intern. Med., 142:2157, 1982.

Mimica, I., et al.: Lung puncture in the etiological diagnosis of pneumonia. A study of 543 infants and children. Am. J. Dis. Child., 122:278, 1971.

Rein, M.F., et al.: Accuracy of the Gram's stain in identifying pneumococci in sputum. JAMA, 239:2671, 1978.

Reyes, M.P.: The aerobic gram negative bacillary pneumonias. Med. Clin. North Am., 64:363, 1980.

Schwartz, J.S.: Pneumococcal vaccine: clinical efficacy and effectiveness. Ann. Intern. Med., 96:208, 1982.

Sthapatayavongs, B., et al.: Rapid diagnosis of legionnaire's disease by urinary antigen detection. Am. J. Med., 72:576, 1982.

Swartz, M.N.: Clinical aspects of legionnaire's disease. Ann. Intern. Med., 90:492, 1979.

Thorsteinsson, S.B., Musher, D.M., and Fagan, T.: The diagnostic value of sputum culture in acute pneumonia. JAMA, 233:894, 1975.

Yu, V.L., Kroboth, F.J., Shonnard, J., and Brown, A.: Legionnaire's disease: new clinical perspective from a prospective pneumonia study. Am. J. Med., 73:357, 1982.

CHAPTER 7

Acute Pneumonias in Infants

J.C. Rolland

> **Objective 7–1.** Combine the clinical and epidemiologic evidence for a diagnosis of bronchiolitis in an infant with dyspnea.

Acute bronchiolitis is observed almost exclusively in children under 2 years of age. It is usually caused by respiratory syncytial virus (RSV) but it may also be due, much less often, to parainfluenza type 3 virus, adenovirus, rhinovirus, or influenza virus, in decreasing order of frequency. The often spectacular acute dyspnea may progress even to respiratory insufficiency. The physician's task, therefore, is to prevent or to detect and correct the patient's hypoxemia.

After 2 or 3 days of rhinopharyngitis, an infant quickly develops fever, cough, and polypnea. The patient's fever is variable but has no prognostic value. The cough is dry, persistent, sometimes has a whooping quality, and induces vomiting. Generally, the respiratory difficulty causes concern and is the reason for consulting a physician. The patient has rapid, shallow respiration at a rate of 60 to 80 breaths per minute, nasal flaring, subcostal and intercostal retraction, and often loud and prolonged expiration, accompanied by wheezing. The chest is hyperinflated and is resonant on percussion. Auscultatory signs are variable. The patient may have diminished breath sounds with prolonged expiration, no rales, disseminated rhonchi, or sibilant rales of bronchial origin, or more or less dry, fine rales of alveolar origin. It is not uncommon for these varying signs to be present successively in the same child. The severity of the disease is not proportional to the spectacular character and intensity of the dyspnea and auscultatory findings. On the contrary, children whose breath sounds are extremely attenuated must be watched even more closely because this sign indicates a particularly diffuse and intense obstruction.

The chest roentgenogram shows the following signs of diffuse dilatation: position of the diaphragm below the tenth rib, widened intercostal spaces with horizontal configuration of the ribs, and diffuse hyperlucency predominating at the bases and in the retrosternal region. The roentgenographic changes of the bronchi themselves are usually slight: a simple accentuation of the hilar opacities and bronchovascular markings. These changes may be associated with variable diffuse macronodular densities, increased pleural markings, and transitory segmental density.

> **RESPIRATORY SYNCYTIAL VIRUS**
>
> Respiratory syncytial virus (RSV) is a paramyxovirus (see Table 2–1) with helical symmetry whose capsid measures 80 to 120 nm. This virus is unstable at temperatures above 38° C. Its infectiousness is destroyed by slow freezing, but is preserved by rapid freezing to −70° C. Although it infects many laboratory animals, RSV produces clinical signs only in the chimpanzee; this property accounts for the original name of this virus, chimpanzee coryza agent (CCA). When RSV is cultivated in continuous human cell lines (HeLa, HEp_2, KB) or in diploid human cells, large characteristic syncytia and multinucleate giant cells appear in 3 to 7 days. RSV has no hemagglutinin, no neuraminidase, and no hemolysin. Serologic diagnosis of RSV is based on the demonstration of complement-fixing antibodies and, sometimes, neutralizing antibodies. The soluble nucleocapsid antigen in all these reactions is common to all strains of RSV and is specific.
>
> After a short phase of growth in the epithelial cells of the upper respiratory tract, RSV becomes localized and multiplies in the cells of the ciliated epithelium of bronchioles. There it produces an inflammatory hyperplasia of the epithelium and an exudate that obstruct the bronchiolar lumen either completely, resulting in atelectasis of the underlying alveoli or, more often, incompletely, resulting in progressive local emphysema due to the accumulation of air behind the block.
>
> Because of the different aspects of the infection produced by RSV, an immunologic reaction is suspected to be responsible for the bronchiolitis of infancy. The most severe bronchiolitis is seen in infants under 3 months of age, even though they all possess maternally transmitted antibodies to RSV. In addition, trials with a killed RSV vaccine have demonstrated that cases of bronchiolitis were more numerous and more severe in vaccinated infants than in controls. Older children and adults generally have inapparent infections or infections limited to the upper airways.
>
> Two mechanisms have been suggested to explain this bronchiolitis: (1) the formation in the bronchioles of immune complexes between the viral antigen and the circulating antibodies (of maternal or vaccinal origin), or (2) a local anaphylactic reaction during a second contact with the virus. Neither of these hypotheses has been fully confirmed.
>
> RSV also causes other forms of respiratory infections, such as rhinopharyngitis, laryngitis, bronchitis, and pneumonia.

RSV bronchiolitis occurs in short, sudden, annual epidemics in late winter and in spring. It is nearly twice as frequent in boys as in girls and is particularly evident between the ages of 3 and 12 months.

For the practitioner, the essential problem of bronchiolitis in infancy is not a matter of diagnosis, but of treatment. The syndrome is easily recognized on the basis of clinical and sometimes radiologic findings. Because RSV is likely to be the causative agent in children under 18 months of age in epidemic periods, confirmation of this fact by isolating the virus in pharyngeal specimens has no practical value. In addition, serologic tests are difficult to interpret before the age of 6 months because of the presence of maternal antibodies.

> **Objective 7–2. What determines the prognosis of bronchiolitis?**

Several complications make bronchiolitis a serious condition. Respiratory insufficiency, for example, may be life-threatening, but the prognosis of bronchiolitis has been improved via ventilatory assistance. Throughout the course of bronchiolitis, the physician must watch for the following signs of incipient cardiorespiratory decompensation:

1. *Hypercapnia*: sweating, anxiety, reduced respiration and heart rate, hypertension.
2. *Hypoxemia*: cyanosis, agitation, weakness, hypotonicity, confusion.
3. *Congestive heart failure:* tachycardia, muffling of heart sounds or gallop rhythm, rapidly progressive hepatomegaly, reduced output of urine. (Because of the bronchiolitis, crepitant rales at the bases can be difficult to interpret.)

Young infants should be particularly watched for the following: color of face and nails, heart and respiration rate, quality of alertness and contact, feeding behavior (refusal to drink, vomiting, diarrhea), and state of hydration. The following figures are considered "normal" in uncomplicated bronchiolitis of infancy: heart rate 140 to 180 beats/min., respiration rate 40 to 80 breaths/min., lower border of liver 3 cm below the costal margin.

The average duration of bronchiolitis of infancy is from 5 to 7 days, but the risk of respiratory decompensation is greatest during the first 2 days.

TREATMENT

Because the main danger in this disease is the development of hypoxia, treatment is based on supplying oxygen in an effective way, according to the condition of the child. Spontaneous respiration in a normal atmosphere is sufficient in the majority of cases; concentrated and humidified oxygen with monitoring of blood gases is indicated in severe cases; intubation and assisted ventilation, in a case with clinical aggravation (progressive exhaustion, apnea) or biochemical aggravation (acidosis, hypoxemia), are recommended in exceptionally severe cases.

Digitalization (digoxin 30 µg/kg/day), combined, in case of emergency, with a diuretic (furosemide, 1 mg/kg intravenously or intramuscularly) is instituted when the patient shows signs of incipient congestive heart failure.

The efficacy of corticosteroids has not been demonstrated. The effectiveness of bronchodilators is generally nil and can be tested by giving the patient a single injection of 0.1 ml epinephrine subcutaneously or theophylline, 4 mg/kg intravenously.

Antibiotic treatment is indicated only if a bacterial superinfection exists, based on the bacteriologic findings from bronchial aspirates, pleural puncture, or even needle aspiration of the lung.

In every patient, it is essential to provide an adequate fluid and caloric intake by normal or parenteral means, according to the child's condition. Administration and supervision of this therapy require that the patient be hospitalized in a specialized unit.

> **Objective 7–3.** Collect relevant evidence for pertussis in an infant with cough and determine appropriate management.

The complications of pertussis are especially frequent and severe in a child under the age of 6 months. This risk justifies hospitalization for intensive care observation in a specialized unit and is the major argument for continuing the practice of vaccination, despite its less-than-perfect effectiveness and its rare, but severe, neurologic reactions.

CLINICAL FEATURES OF PERTUSSIS

The disease begins insidiously enough with an apparent common cold and little or no fever, but the persistent cough becomes more frequent, is spasmodic, and occurs predominantly at night. This catarrhal stage lasts 7 to 10 days. At this stage the disease is most communicable, although in the absence of a known contact, the diagnosis is rarely made at that time. The characteristic paroxysms appear progressively. First is a series of coughs in increasingly rapid succession during a single expiration. The patient's face is red at first, and then cyanosed, the eyes bulging and watery, and the jugular veins and veins of the scalp dilated. After 10 to 20 explosive coughs, a period of apnea lasts a few seconds, followed by a long-drawn sibilant inspiration with a crowing sound, the whoop. The end of the paroxysm is sometimes marked by the expectoration of ropy mucus or, more often at that age, by vomiting. The number of paroxysms varies from just a few to 50 or more per day; they increase for 2 or 3 weeks and then diminish gradually. Altogether, the cough may last for 2 or 3 months. The disease basically consists of the cough and its consequences. No fever is present. If fever does occur, a superinfection must be suspected. Auscultation of the lung and the rest of the clinical examination are usually normal between paroxysms.

Even when the paroxysms are free and uncomplicated, whooping cough of infancy is a distressing and trying condition, both for the child and his family. The frequent paroxysms interfere with sleep and feeding because they produce repeated vomiting. The child often fails to gain weight during the entire course of the illness. In addition, the unavoidable and unpredictable occurrence of the paroxysms, which continue day and night for weeks on end, bring fear of asphyxiation and are a source of anxiety.

Respiratory and neurologic complications are observed almost exclusively in infants under 6 months of age.

The finding of one or more of the following criteria is a probable indication of serious pertussis:

1. The patient is less than 6 months of age.
2. Periods of apnea are prolonged, cyanosis between paroxysms is persistent, or vasomotor disorders are present (transitory marbling of the skin over the whole body is a sign of peripheral circulatory failure).
3. Convulsive seizures or disorders of consciousness are seen.
4. Tachycardia of more than 200 beats/min. present in the absence of fever.
5. Abdomen is grossly distended with air.
6. One of the following laboratory findings is present: leukocytosis of more than 50,000/mm^3, thrombocytosis of more than 500,000/mm^3, and hyponatremia of less than 130 mmol/L.

PAROXYSMAL RESPIRATORY INSUFFICIENCY

Asphyxiating paroxysms are particularly intense and prolonged, lead to apnea without an inspiratory whoop, and produce bradycardia and the risk of circulatory arrest. Syncopal apnea is rarer; as a rule, it is seen only under the age of 3 months and occurs early in the disease. It consists of an unexpected respiratory arrest without a prior coughing fit. Even when they resolve spontaneously, these types of episodes are serious because of the risk of cerebral anoxia. Both require immediate hospitalization in a specialized unit with facilities for cardiac and apnea monitoring, an effective aspiration system, and intubation and ventilation equipment. In most cases, the permanent monitoring and immediate treatment of apnea by gentle aspiration, mask oxygenation, and ventilation make it possible to avoid endotracheal intubation with its risks of superinfection.

PULMONARY COMPLICATIONS

A syndrome of interstitial pneumonia in infants occurs early, at the beginning of the paroxysmal stage, and is characterized by moderate fever, polypnea, disseminated bullous rales, accentuation of hilar shadows, and a reticular appearance of the lung markings. This condition is a bronchoalveolitis, seemingly an extension of the symptomatic bronchitis of pertussis. Interstitial bronchopneumonia, formerly the principal cause of death in this disease, has now fortunately become much less common and less serious. Although bordetella has been incriminated on occasion, this type of pneumonia is generally caused by a bacterial superinfection with beta-hemolytic streptococcus, pneumococcus, *Haemophilus influenzae*, and also, in a hospital setting, staphylococcus, the Enterobacteriaceae, and pseudomonas. The disease produces steady respiratory distress with high fever, impaired general health, shallow polypnea with retraction and cyanosis, less-frequent and less-intense cough, fine, moist, disseminated rales, and homogeneous and widely scattered multiple opacities within the lung. Treatment consists of a combination of antibiotic therapy adapted to the causative organism, or a broad-spectrum bactericidal combination, and symptomatic treatment of the respiratory insufficiency. Lobar or segmental atelectasis is less frequent in infants than in older children. Both forms of atelectasis are often discovered by chance and resolve spontaneously in a few days. They do not appear to promote the subsequent development of bronchiectasis and are localized mainly in the upper lobes, sometimes in the middle lobe and lingula, and rarely in the inferior lobes. Pneumothorax and pneumomediastinum, as direct consequences of the cough, are even more uncommon today. Emphysema is a common postmortem finding and probably exists in the lungs of many patients.

NEUROLOGIC COMPLICATIONS

These complications are rarely observed in patients under a year of age. They are a consequence of cerebral anoxia, and their severity primarily depends on the intensity and duration of oxygen deprivation. The manifestations generally consist of brief, transient, convulsive seizures following an ordinary paroxysm or one that causes more than usual cyanosis. Prolonged apnea may cause repeated convulsions, however, with coma and possibly severe sequelae of motor deficit, epilepsy, and mental retardation. Close and systematic monitoring of pertussis in infants and immediate treatment of periods of apnea have reduced the frequency of these complications and have thus confirmed that they were the result of anoxic injury.

DIAGNOSIS

Pertussis is easy to recognize in the presence of a typical paroxysm, which can sometimes be elicited by an examination of the throat. This diagnosis should be suspected in an infant with an unexplained cough, which is persistent, that produces no fever and vomiting. Epidemiologic evidence, although useful, is rarely decisive. Although it is more frequent in the winter, pertussis occurs all year round, sporadically or in small epidemics. Unlike the other respiratory diseases of childhood, it is more frequent and severe in girls than in boys. The history of contact may be lacking, even in infants whose contacts are limited indeed. A known previous vaccination does not rule out the diagnosis because the vaccination may be incomplete, too recent, or ineffective. The finding of leukocytosis (15,000 to 50,000 or more per mm^3) with lymphocytosis (the normal value is 60 to 75% before the age of a year), though not constant, constitutes valuable evidence that can be obtained simply and rapidly. In infants, the risks of pertussis are such that the disorder should be confirmed as rapidly as possible by identifying the organism from a nasopharyngeal swab, through culture requiring special media, or by a direct smear of fluorescent antibodies. This last is the fastest and simplest method. Serologic tests, on the other hand, are not useful because antibodies only appear after 2 to 3 weeks, as is common in other illnesses.

TREATMENT

In severe forms of pertussis and routinely if the child is under the age of 3 months, hospitalization is required. The patient should be isolated in a unit where he can be monitored continuously and where episodes of apnea can be treated immediately.

Bordetella pertussis, the causative agent of pertussis, is susceptible to many antibiotics, such as aminoglycosides, macrolides, chloramphenicol, and tetracyclines. Even though these drugs can eliminate the bacterium from nasopharyngeal secretions in a matter of days and can reduce the incidence and severity of infectious bronchopulmonary complications, none of these antibiotics alter the course of the illness itself, in terms of either its duration or the frequency and intensity of the paroxysms. The antibiotic of choice is erythromycin, 35 to 50 mg/kg body weight/day in 4 divided oral doses for 14 days. Ampicillin, although active in vitro, is unable to eradicate *B. pertussis* from the nasopharyngeal mucus because of the weak penetration of this antibiotic in the respiratory mucus.

Controlled studies have shown that even when administered after the onset of the paroxysmal phase, corticosteroids reduce the frequency, intensity, and duration of the paroxysms, especially in infants. Recommended are betamethasone, 0.075 mg/kg/day orally, or hydrocortisone sodium succinate, 30 mg/kg/day intramuscularly; these doses should be given for the first 2 days, followed by decreasing doses until the seventh or eighth day.

The usefulness of specific hyperimmune gamma globulin is controversial. It is probably ineffective.

The prophylactic treatment of contacts, particularly young infants in contact with older siblings in whom pertussis has just been diagnosed, is difficult because the diagnosis of whooping cough is often made late, and the disease is most contagious during the catarrhal phase, which generally occurs before the diagnosis is confirmed. Seroprophylaxis with specific hyperimmune gamma globulin is probably ineffective. Usually, the prescription of prophylactic antibiotic therapy with oral erythromycin or spiramycin (in Europe), 50 mg/kg/day for 5 days, is recommended.

Objective 7-4. Evaluate the arguments for and against pertussis vaccination.

Pertussis vaccine is a preparation of the killed phase I of *Bordetella pertussis*. The antigenicity is increased by adsorption on aluminum hydroxide or calcium phosphate. It is generally used in combination with tetanus and diphtheria antitoxins. The usual protocol calls for an intramuscular or subcutaneous injection at the beginning of the third, fourth, and fifth months of life, with booster injections 1 year and then 5 years later. Infants without maternally transmitted antibodies to pertussis are not protected during the first weeks of life, the period when the disease is most serious. For this reason, in countries with a high incidence of pertussis, it is considered useful to give older siblings booster injections when a birth is expected, to reduce the likelihood of their being carriers.

The spectacular reduction in the frequency of pertussis has proved the effectiveness of the vaccine. This vaccine is incomplete, however, and it is not unusual for the disease to occur, generally in attenuated form, even after adequate vaccination.

This vaccine is not harmless. It may produce three types of complications:

1. Minor reactions in 20% of patients: fever, pain, and induration at the injection site, malaise, and generalized aches for a day or so.
2. Major reactions in 1 case out of 3000: cries and disordered agitation for a few hours to 2 days, high fever for 3 to 5 days, and hyperthermic convulsive seizure.
3. Severe complications in 1 out of 34,000 vaccinations: circulatory failure with collapse, shock, and loss of consciousness, for 30 to 40 minutes, repeated convulsions, meningeal reaction, encephalopathy, and massive myoclonic spasms with hypsarrhythmia; injection of the vaccine has even been alleged to cause a few cases of sudden infant death.

Because of the existence of these complications, the risks of the vaccination have to be weighed against those of the disease. In view of these risks, pertussis vaccination has been found inadvisable in children suffering from encephalopathy and cerebral palsy, in those who have manifested one or more hyperthermic convulsive seizures, and in those who have had a major reaction to the first injection. When these precautions are taken, however, pertussis vaccination certainly remains useful.

Objective 7-5. What are clinical and laboratory evidence of neonatal bronchopulmonary infection caused by *Chlamydia trachomatis*?

When rapidly progressive respiratory disorders appear in an infant aged 1 to 3 months, 3 principal causes should be investigated first:

1. Cardiac decompensation from congenital heart disease, or acute myocarditis.
2. A bronchopulmonary lesion caused by repeated inhalation of food products, swallowing disorders, or gastroesophageal regurgitation.
3. An infection, in particular a neonatal infection caused by *Chlamydia trachomatis*.

The probability of neonatal *C. trachomatis* infection can be determined on the basis of the following information:

1. The prevalence of maternal genital infection. Contamination of the child occurs during birth, in contact with maternal infection. *C. trachomatis* as a genital maternal infection is observed in 30 to 60% of women whose partner has or has recently had urethritis, in 10 to 20% of asymptomatic women who at-

> **BORDETELLA PERTUSSIS**
>
> Pertussis is caused by *Bordetella pertussis* and, much more rarely, by *Bordetella parapertussis*. Cases of clinically indistinguishable "pertussis" caused by adenoviruses have been reported.
>
> *B. pertussis* is a small, gram-negative, nonmotile, encapsulated bacillus. It is fragile and must be inoculated immediately on Bordet-Gengou medium (fresh sheep blood agar to which penicillin is added to inhibit contaminating organisms). After 2 to 3 days of incubation at 37° C, small, pearly, glistening colonies appear, surrounded by a zone of hemolysis. Identification is based on agglutination of the organism by specific antiserum. In phase I of the culture (equivalent to the S state), *B. pertussis* has many antigenic substances: several agglutinating antigens, a heat-labile exotoxin lethal to the mouse, a lipopolysaccharide heat-stable endotoxin, and the protective antigen, which is not isolated but is specific for that phase.
>
> The pathogenic processes are poorly known. In the animal, *B. pertussis* is much more virulent when injected intranasally than intraperitoneally. The bacterium multiplies selectively on bronchial ciliated epithelium. Inoculation of cells containing phase I organisms produces lymphocytosis and increases sensitivity to histamine and serotonin. The diffuse inflammatory lesions and areas of necrosis in the bronchial epithelium are attributed to the action of the exotoxin. Cerebral lesions that may occur during the course of the disease have nothing in common with the lesions of viral encephalitis; rather, they are nonspecific changes induced by anoxia and ischemia.

tend a gynecologic or birth-control clinic, and in 5 to 13% of women at the end of pregnancy.

2. The risk of neonatal infection. Among children born of a mother infected with *C. trachomatis*, the risk of perinatal infection is high: 60 to 70% of these children develop a serologic infection; 40 to 50% have a clinical infection. This risk is even higher with prolonged rupture of amniotic sac.

3. The presence of neonatal conjunctivitis. This disorder appears in 50% of cases and is the earliest and most frequent clinical manifestation of *C. trachomatis* infection in the neonate. It is not completely prevented by the routine instillation of drops of silver nitrate solution. The conjunctivitis appears between the fifth and the fourteenth day after birth, may be moderate or purulent, and is self-limited after a few weeks or months. The diagnosis can be made by direct examination, not of the purulent exudate, but of scrapings of conjunctival epithelial cells. After staining these cells by Giemsa's method, the physician can observe the characteristic inclusions next to the nucleus.

Signs of pulmonary infection appear progressively 1 to 3 months after birth with a cough that becomes repetitive and paroxysmal, but without a crowing inspiration, and with tachypnea. No fever is present. Auscultation of the patient's chest is normal or reveals inspiratory, and a few sibilant, rales. The chest roentgenogram shows increased radiolucency of the lung or diffuse, reticulonodular, bilateral opacities as signs of interstitial pneumonia. Other indications of infection are leukocytosis with eosinophilia of more than 300 per mm^3 and an elevation of the plasma levels of IgG and IgM.

The diagnosis of chlamydial infection can be confirmed by the following:

1. Direct examination of nasopharyngeal cells after Giemsa staining.
2. More rarely, culture of *C. trachomatis* from nasopharyngeal secretions collected and transported in a special medium.
3. Specific serologic response, with a titer of anti-*C. trachomatis* IgM of 1:32 or higher.

The disease resolves spontaneously after a prolonged course of several weeks; its clinical appearance is often alarming.

Treatment is based on the oral administration of sulfisoxazole, 150 mg/kg/day, or erythromycin, 50 mg/kg/day for 2 weeks. Usually, the eradication of *C. trachomatis* is observed within 3 days, a frank clinical improvement is noted within 5 days, and the chest roentgenogram returns to normal within 20 days.

> **Objective 7–6. Collect clinical, radiologic, and bacteriologic evidence for a staphylococcal pleuropulmonary infection in a sick infant.**

Staphylococcal pleuropulmonary infections (SPPI) have become rare in developed countries, although they were common 20 years ago.

This disease is primarily found in infants and generally occurs before the age of 6 months, nearly always before the age of a year. It is more frequent in institutionalized and malnourished children, in those with an underlying condition, such as cystic fibrosis, that favors the development of SPPI, and following a viral pneumonia, such as from influenza, or measles.

CLINICAL FEATURES AND DIAGNOSIS

Initially, the picture is that of a common nasopharyngeal infection. Then, in a matter of hours, the infant's condition worsens. In most cases, fever is above 39° C, but it may be slight or absent. The respiratory signs are not spectacular, but are always present and should nevertheless attract attention. They are rapid respirations, nasal flaring, subcostal retraction, and grunting respirations. Diarrhea and vomiting, especially vomiting, are frequent and may suggest a gastrointestinal obstruction, particularly because abdominal distension is nearly always associated with the disease. Also characteristic is a gray and pallid skin color.

SPPI is often confirmed by physical examination of the chest, not so much by auscultation, which may be normal or nonspecific, but by percussion, which reveals a greater or lesser diffuse dullness of a hemithorax early in the course of the illness. In this context, the dullness is practically synonymous with staphylococcal purulent pleurisy. I must emphasize the diagnostic value of this simple procedure. Percussion of the chest *must* be carried out in any infant suspected of infection, even if the "respiratory" signs are slight. The hematologic laboratory results usually show anemia with a suggestive polymorphonuclear leukocytosis, but may show leukopenia.

Even at this stage, the chest roentgenogram may reveal one of the associated types of pulmonary findings, most commonly one or more macronodular parenchymal opacities with well-defined borders, either lobar or segmental. Bullae or pneumatoceles are rare at this point, but they are specific for staphylococcal pneumonia (Fig. 7–1). One should search for signs of pleurisy, sometimes large, but more often small, in the form of pleural thickening or the blunting of a costophrenic angle. In all possible cases, thoracentesis should be performed, thus making it possible to isolate the organism. The pleural fluid, whether resembling frank pus or serous fluid, teems with gram-positive cocci on direct examination. *Staphylococcus aureus* is rapidly grown from the culture. Antibiotic treatment is begun immediately while the physician awaits the results of sensitivity testing.

> **Objective 7–7. Direct the treatment and the continuing care of an infant with a staphylococcal pleuropulmonary infection.**

An infant who is suspected of having SPPI must be hospitalized in a pediatric unit immediately, both for isolation and for institution of antibiotic treatment.

In view of the urgency of this situation and because vomiting is frequently associated with the disease, parenteral administration of antimicrobial agents is begun immediately, with a penicillinase-resistant beta-lactam (for example, oxacillin, 100 to 200 mg/kg/day in intravenous infusion over a period of an hour, every 6 hours), perhaps in combination with an aminoglycoside (gentamicin, 2 mg/kg via 2 intramuscular injections BID). This treatment should be adapted to the sensitivity of the organism.

Equally important is continuous surveillance of the child, so that the various pul-

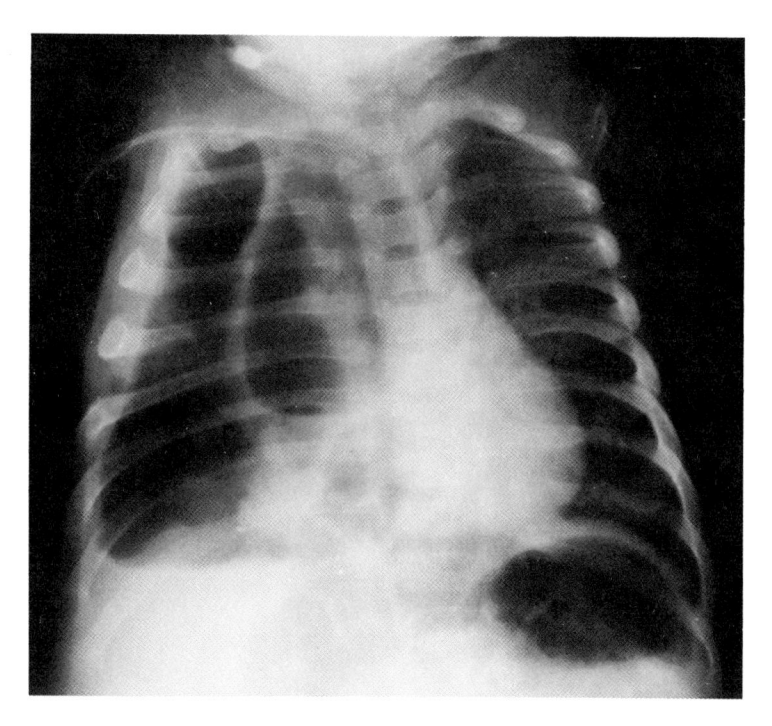

Fig. 7–1. In a febrile and polypneic infant, an impressive pneumatocele and pyopneumothorax typical of a pleuropulmonary infection.

monary complications can be treated as quickly as possible.

Despite early diagnosis and the immediate institution of appropriate antibiotic treatment, the pleural and pulmonary lesions may continue to evolve for several days. It is not unusual to see a purulent pleural effusion increase. Within the parenchyma, distended bullae often evolve rapidly and unpredictably and may rupture at any time in the pleura, to produce a pyopneumothorax or a simple pneumothorax. This development is serious in the infected and fatigued infant, especially when the lesions are bilateral, and the resultant pneumothorax must be treated immediately. Therefore, thoracic drainage and aspiration equipment, as well as trained personnel, must be available to the patient at all times.

When this critical stage has passed, several days into the illness, the pneumonia will not progress much further. Recovery takes about 3 to 4 weeks, with almost complete resolution of the pulmonary and pleural changes.

SUGGESTED READINGS

Danus, O., Casar, C., and Larrain, A.: Esophageal reflux: an unrecognized cause of recurrent obstructive bronchitis in children. J. Pediatr., 89:220, 1976.

Harrison, H.R., English, M.G., Lee, C.K., and Alexander, E.R.: Chlamydia trachomatis infant pneumonitis. Comparison wih matched controls and other infant pneumonitis. N. Engl. J. Med., 298:702, 1978.

Lipson, A., Marshall, W.C., and Hayward, A.R.: Treatment of Pneumocystis carinii pneumonia in children. Arch. Dis. Child., 52:314, 1977.

Macasaet, F.F., Kidd, P.A., Bolano, C.R., and Wenner, H.A.: The etiology of acute respiratory infections. III. The role of viruses and bacteria. J. Pediatr., 72:829, 1968.

McIntosh, K.: Bronchiolitis and asthma: possible common pathogenetic pathways. J. Allergy Clin. Immunol., 57:595, 1976.

Moffet, H.L.: Pediatric infectious diseases. A problem-oriented approach. Philadelphia, J.B. Lippincott, 1975.

Stewart, G.T.: Vaccination against whooping-cough: efficacy versus risks. Lancet, 1:234, 1977.

Taylor, B., Abbott, G.D., Kerr, M. McK., and Fergusson, D.M.: Amoxycillin and cotrimoxazole in presumed viral respiratory infections of childhood: placebo controlled trial. Br. Med. J., 2:552, 1977.

CHAPTER 8

Pulmonary Tuberculosis

M. Desmeules, Y. Cormier, J. Laforge,
J.C. Pechère, and P. Solal-Céligny

> Objective 8–1. Recognize pulmonary tuberculosis.

MODE OF PRESENTATION

Pulmonary tuberculosis can become manifest in different ways.

Primary Tuberculosis. This form of tuberculosis results from the patient's initial contact with *Mycobacterium tuberculosis* (Table 8–1) and is generally acquired by inhaling microdroplets of sputum from a tuberculosis carrier. By definition, primary tuberculosis occurs only in a nonimmune individual. The risk of infection depends both on the number of microorganisms in the pulmonary secretions of the carrier during coughing and sneezing and on the closeness and duration of the patient's contact with the carrier. Many cases of primary tuberculosis are identified in the circle of contacts of a tuberculous patient.

Primary tuberculosis is clinically silent in 95% of the cases. Conversion of a negative tuberculin test to a positive test is then the only evidence of the disease. An old primary infection can be revealed both by a positive purified protein derivative (PPD) reaction or by hilar calcifications and pulmonary "scars."

Clinical manifestations occur in approximately 5% of primary infections. These features include a mild, nonspecific, infectious syndrome with cough, moderate fever, sweating, and asthenia. Erythema nodosum and a phlyctenular conjunctivitis, although rare, are considered classic manifestations. The x-ray examination of the lung sometimes reveals hilar or mediastinal adenopathies or a dense area often situated at the bases or the midlung (Figs. 8–1 and 8–2).

The natural course of an untreated primary infection is usually an apparent cure with the concomitant development of a state of relative immunity. Several complications are related to tuberculous lymphadenopathy, however. During the course of the acute infection, the lymph nodes may drain through fistulas and may communicate with a bronchus, to produce a tuberculous bronchopneumonia. The lymph nodes also may compress a lobar bronchus and may thereby cause chronic atelectasis or bronchiectasis, which most often affects the lung's middle lobe or lingula. Eventual calcification of these hilar lymph nodes may result in later hemoptysis, broncholithiasis, or bronchopleural fistulas.

Even when the untreated primary infections remain clinically silent, however, *M. tuberculosis* may disseminate through the blood. When dissemination occurs, several events are possible: (1) the development of a

Table 8-1. Mycobacteria of Medical Importance

Classification and Species	Illness in Man
Obligate intracellular parasites	*Mycobacterium leprae:* leprosy
Facultative intracellular parasites	*Mycobacterium tuberculosis:* tuberculosis
	Mycobacterium bovis: tuberculosis, chiefly intestinal
	Atypical *Mycobacteria* species
	Group I: Photochromogens (forms a pigment when exposed to light)
	M. kansasii: adenopathy, pneumonia
	M. marinum: cutaneous ulcerations from swimming
	Group II: Scotochromogens (forms a pigment in the dark)
	M. scrofulaceum: adenopathy
	Group III: Nonchromogens (nonpigmented)
	M. avium: adenopathy, pneumonia
	M. intracellulare (includes Battey bacillus): adenopathy, pneumonia
	Group IV: Rapid growers
	M. fortuitum: saprophytes, generally; can be pathogenic in immunosuppressed patients

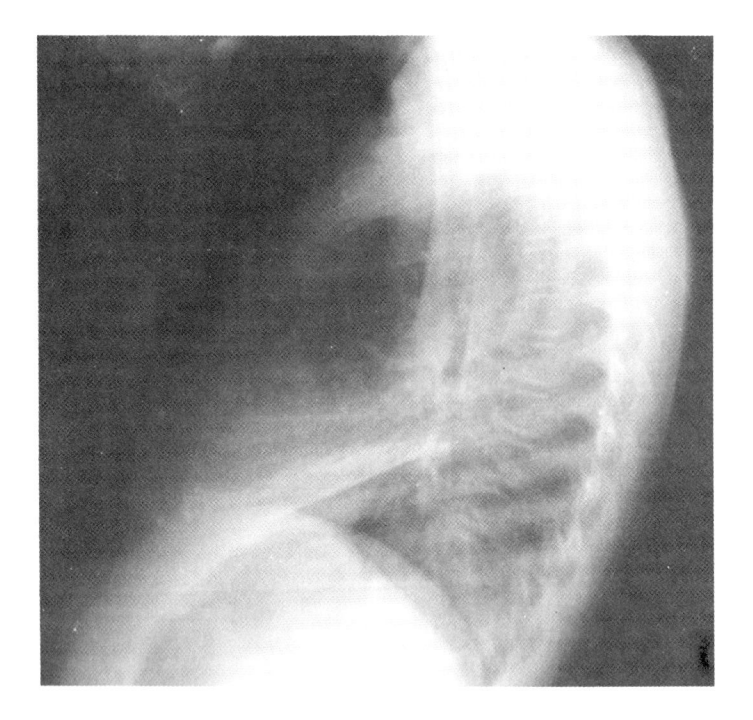

Fig. 8-1. Infiltration of the medial lobe in tuberculosis.

miliary tuberculosis, tuberculous pleurisy, or tuberculous meningitis (postprimary tuberculosis); or (2) the formation of microfoci of viable bacilli that remain latent in different organs. The sites of predilection for these microfoci are regions of high oxygen tension, namely the apexes of the lungs, the extremities of the long bones, and the renal cortex. From these foci reactivated pulmonary, osseous, or renal tuberculosis develops.

Abnormal Chest Roentgenogram. From 25 to 50% of cases of tuberculosis are detected by routine radiograms obtained during hospitalization or as part of a pre-employment examination or screening program. These individuals are generally asymptomatic and their physical examination is normal. On the chest film, two types of lesions should attract attention, as discussed in the following paragraphs.

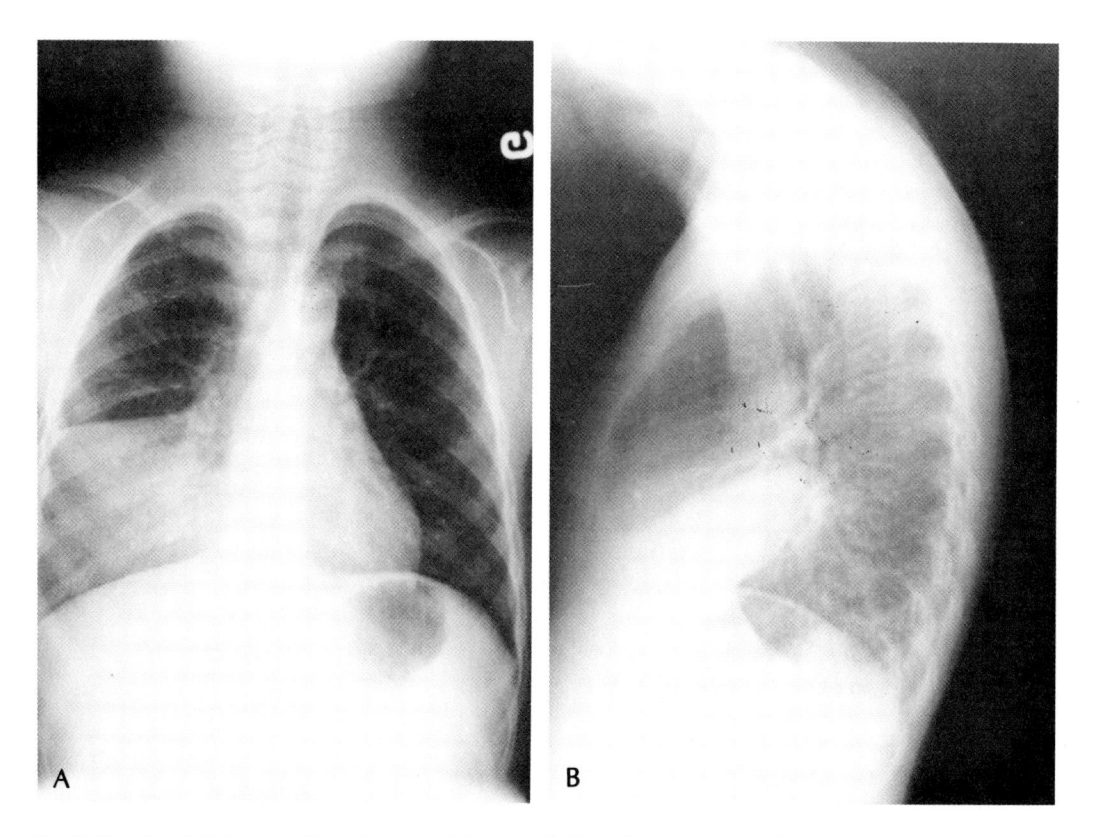

Fig. 8–2. A and B, Adenopathy and pneumatelectasis during primary tuberculosis.

First are nonsegmental infiltrations in the apical regions of the lungs, often accompanied by retraction of the parenchyma and adjacent structures, such as the lobar fissures, the hilum, or the primary bronchi. It is often difficult to distinguish between purely cicatricial, old, healed lesions and active ones. Only a comparison with previous roentgenograms makes it possible to demonstrate a change in the extent and distribution of the lesions, a sign of active disease. The presence of cavitation within these lesions is an indication of active tuberculosis (Fig. 8–3) although cavitation can also be seen in old, stable lesions.

An isolated nodular lesion is sometimes observed in the lung. The presence of a lesion of under 2 cm in diameter, with a well-defined outline, and with calcification and satellite lesions is evidence of a tuberculous granuloma. Again, comparison with previous roentgenograms is necessary for one to judge the time of appearance and rate of growth of the lesion. A search for *M. tuberculosis* in the sputum is rarely productive in a patient with a solitary pulmonary nodule. A transthoracic needle biopsy of the lung sometimes makes it possible to demonstrate the origin of the lesion, but the diagnosis may require a biopsy after thoracotomy.

Miliary Tuberculosis. This form of tuberculosis is defined as the presence of multiple small granulomas spread through many organs as the result of hematogenous dissemination. The discovery of a reticulomicronodular picture on the chest roentgenogram (Fig. 8–4) and a febrile syndrome accompanied by asthenia, anorexia, weight loss, and cough suggest this diagnosis. Typically, this form of tuberculosis occurs 3 to 6 months after the primary infection. Examination reveals a seriously ill patient with tachycardia, rapid respiration, and sometimes, crepitant rales.

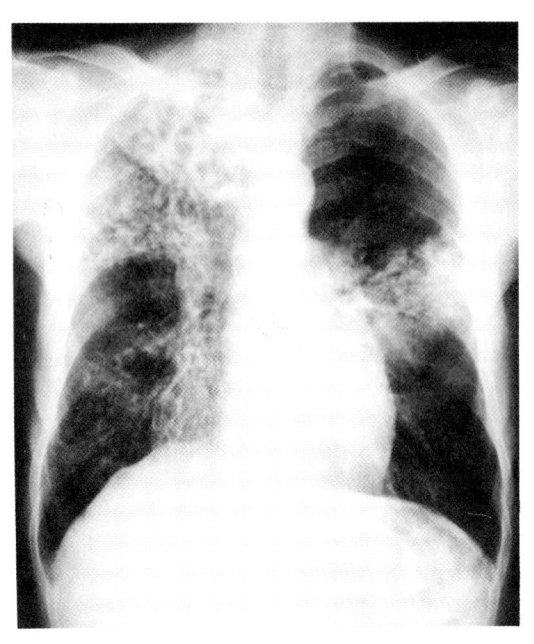

Fig. 8–3. Bilateral ulcerocaseous tuberculosis.

Hepatosplenomegaly is a frequent finding, notably in children. The discovery of tubercles on the choroid by funduscopy is infrequent, but suggests the diagnosis. Lesions of miliary tuberculosis may also involve the meninges, pleura, pericardium, peritoneum, and bone marrow.

It is worth mentioning that the typical reticulomicronodular radiologic aspect of the lung that represents the usual clue for the diagnosis often appears several weeks after the clinical onset of this disease, so the patient may have a fever of unknown origin in the meantime.

In laboratory tests, involvement of the liver is noted by a rise in the alkaline phosphatase level in most cases. One may note a reduction in the patient's pulmonary diffusion capacity, as well as hypoxemia and arterial hypocapnia. Respiratory insufficiency, rare today, killed many patients before the era of antibiotics. Acid-fast bacilli culture of the sputum or urine is seldom positive. Needle biopsy of the liver makes it possible to demonstrate noncaseating granulomas in more than two-thirds of patients. Aspiration of bone marrow or bone marrow biopsy is less-often positive. Because untreated miliary tuberculosis is invariably fatal, aggressive investigations are sometimes required, including surgical biopsy of the

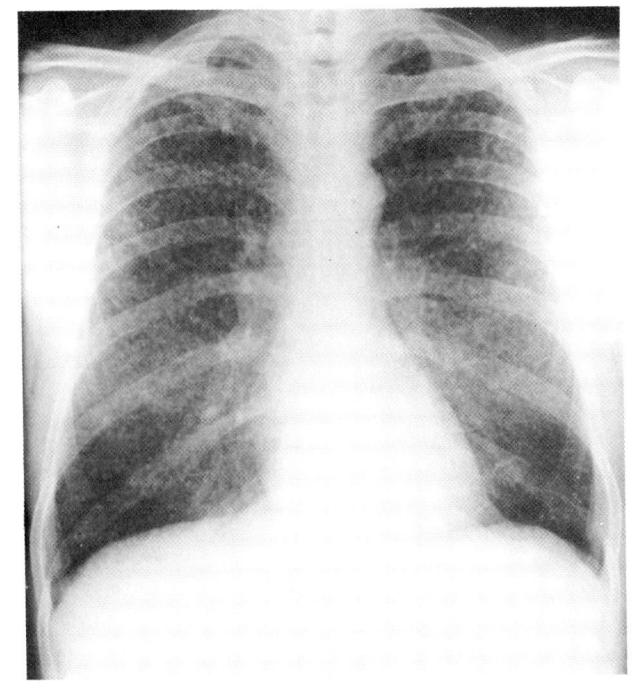

Fig. 8–4. Miliary tuberculosis.

lung. Part of the material taken by biopsy should always be cultivated for mycobacteria.

Tuberculous Pleurisy. In its classic form, tuberculous pleurisy occurs in young adults and follows a primary infection by a few months or several years. It may be caused by direct infection of the pleural space, by a subpleural pulmonary focus, or by hematogenous spread. The pleural disease, marked by chest pains and dyspnea, is often preceded by a general syndrome of asthenia, fever, and weight loss. Radiologic signs of effusion are not specific for this diagnosis. The underlying lung parenchyma is usually normal in appearance.

Tuberculous pleurisy of late onset, however, which occurs in individuals over 50 years of age and is often associated with old parenchymal foci, is increasingly observed today. The pleural fluid is serous or serohemorrhagic. The exudative fluid is high in proteins (3 g/dl or more) and is low in glucose (under 25 mg/dl). The differential white blood cell count shows a preponderance, if not a monotony, of small lymphocytes, with rare mesothelial cells. The culture of the sputum is generally negative in the absence of radiologic signs of parenchymal pulmonary tuberculosis. A culture of pleural fluid is seldom productive, unless many inoculations of large quantities of fluid are made. Pleural needle biopsy permits the demonstration of granulomas in 60 to 80% of patients.

Reactivated Pulmonary Tuberculosis. A late reactivation of tuberculous lesions often occurs years to decades after the primary infection. The site of predilection is the apex of the lung. This reactivation is favored by certain factors, such as alcoholism, malnutrition, gastrectomy, pregnancy, overwork, immunologic suppression, and possibly racial origin. The classic presentation is marked by a progressive weakness, a fever highest in the late afternoon, night sweats, and weight loss. Classic pulmonary symptoms include cough, purulent expectoration, and less frequently, chest pains and hemoptysis.

The physical examination provides little specific information. Sometimes, the presence of rales, bronchial breath sounds, an intense, low-pitched, hollow and predominantly inspiratory murmur, or signs of localized consolidation may be observed. The patient's differential leukocyte count may show some increase in monocytes, and the sedimentation rate is usually elevated. Sputum smears and culture are usually positive when the radiologic lesions are extensive or when cavities are present. When the lesions are minimal, results are far less constant.

METHODS OF DIAGNOSIS

Whatever the mode of presentation, some investigations are required.

Tuberculin Skin Test. A positive tuberculin skin test indicates a past infection if the patient has no history of bacille Calmette Guérin (BCG) vaccination. The test itself provides no information on the activity of the disease. Old tuberculin has been replaced increasingly by purified tuberculins: PPD, containing 5 U, or the Pasteur Institute purified tuberculin (IP-48), at a dose of 10 U for intracutaneous injection. The appearance of an induration of 10 mm or more in diameter 48 hours after the test is considered a positive reaction. A reaction of 5 to 9 mm is doubtful and nonspecific, especially in regions with a high prevalence of atypical mycobacterial infections. If the patient's reaction is negative, it is necessary to distinguish between the absence of infection and anergy. Anergy may be demonstrated by means of a series of skin tests with other antigens, such as candidin, trichophytin, or a 1/1000 dilution of streptokinase-streptodornase (Varidase). In the presence of anergy, a negative tuberculin reaction does not exclude a diagnosis of tuberculosis, for one of the following reasons:

1. The infection is recent (within the past 8 weeks) and tuberculin allergy has not yet appeared.
2. A technical error has been made. (Such errors account for up to 20% of false-negative reactions.)
3. Anergy is produced by an intercurrent

disease; such as measles, sarcoidosis, lymphoma, or severe debilitation.

Although tuberculosis may be observed in the presence of a negative skin test, the reaction is usually positive.

Bacteriologic Studies. Microbiologic tests constitute the major means for establishing the diagnosis of tuberculosis. With a freely coughing and expectorating patient, collection of adequate specimens is easy. Fresh morning sputum should be collected 3 days in a row. If sputum production is inadequate, expectoration should be stimulated by the administration of warm, hypertonic aerosols. It is sometimes necessary to obtain swallowed sputum by using a stomach tube when the patient is fasted (gastric aspiration). The importance of obtaining an adequate sample of bronchial secretions may even justify the use of a bronchoscope.

Direct microscopic examination of sputum smears is important for immediate diagnosis, for deciding whether to isolate the patient, and for initiating therapy. Direct examination of gastric aspirates is of lesser value because of the frequency of saprophytic mycobacteria in the gastric fluid. Auramine-rhodamine staining and fluorescent microscopy are sensitive but nonspecific because certain contaminating bacteria may also take up the fluorescent dye. For confirmation of the diagnosis, the classic Ziehl-Neelsen sputum stain is still the most specific means of demonstrating the presence of mycobacteria. To obtain a culture, the specimen is inoculated on the Löwenstein-Jensen medium and is incubated in a carbon-dioxide-enriched atmosphere. The culture may be positive after 2 or 3 weeks, but it generally takes about 3 to 4 weeks to obtain definitive diagnostic results. A positive niacin test on the bacterial colonies makes it possible to distinguish *M. tuberculosis* from atypical mycobacteria and saprophytes. With a positive culture, sensitivity studies on antituberculous drugs should be made to determine whether the patient is resistant to first-line drugs.

Table 8–2 summarizes the principal steps in the diagnosis of tuberculosis.

> **Objective 8–2. Treat a patient with pulmonary tuberculosis.**

Two major advances have been made in contemporary antituberculous therapy: the rate of cures now approaches 100%, and the duration of treatment has been shortened.

The wall of *Mycobacterium tuberculosis* is rich in lipids, and most common antibiotics are ineffective against it. The mean doubling time of *M. tuberculosis* is long, approximately 20 hours. Therefore, tuberculosis can be

Table 8–2. Diagnostic Examinations in Tuberculosis

	Comparison of Current with Previous Roentgenograms	Bacteriologic Study of the Sputum	Gastric Aspiration	Bronchoscopy	Transbronchial Biopsy	Transthoracic Needle Biopsy	Lumbar Puncture	Needle Biopsy of Liver	Bone Marrow Biopsy	Thoracocentesis	Pleural Biopsy
Abnormal roentgenogram of lung											
Infiltrations	+	±	±	±	0	0	0	0	0	0	0
Isolated nodule	+	±	0	±	+	+	0	0	0	0	0
Miliary tuberculosis	+	±	0	+	+	0	+	+	+	0	0
Tuberculous pleurisy	±	±	0	0	0	0	0	0	0	+	+
Classic reactivated tuberculosis	+	+	+	±	±	0	0	0	0	0	0

+ useful; ± of variable use; 0 not useful

treated by a single daily administration of antituberculous drugs, but the duration of the treatment has to be extensive. The frequency of mutations in a population of *M. tuberculosis* requires that treatment be undertaken with at least 2 antibacillary agents, to prevent the emergence of a resistant bacterial population. Tuberculous foci contain 2 populations of bacilli: extracellular, with a rapid growth, and intracellular, in macrophages, with a slower growth. Certain drugs are known to act preferentially on the extracellular forms. Moreover, some drugs are bactericidal, for example, isoniazid, rifampin, streptomycin, and pyrazinamide; others are bacteriostatic.

With the exception of patients with advanced cases, the duration of hospitalization can be brief (2 to 4 weeks). The patient should generally be removed from his home temporarily, to reduce the risk of contagion, to confirm the diagnosis, and to initiate the treatment. At the same time, hospitalization provides an opportunity to educate the patient and to make him aware of the importance of taking his medication as prescribed. After 3 to 4 weeks of treatment, the contagiousness of the illness is decreased.

DRUG THERAPY

Isoniazid is active against both intracellular and extracellular *M. tuberculosis* (Table 8–3). This drug is believed to act by blocking DNA synthesis. When taken on an empty stomach, isoniazid is absorbed completely from the intestinal tract. The adult dose is 5 mg/kg/day. The drug is metabolized by acetylation in the liver. According to the rate of acetylation, the population of patients falls into two phenotypes: rapid acetylators and slow acetylators. The proportion of these phenotypes varies among different races; for example, rapid acetylators are more frequent among Orientals. The serum level of isoniazid reveals the rate of acetylation. Because the hepatotoxicity of isoniazid is linked to the acetylated metabolites, this complication is more frequent in rapid acetylators. At current recommended doses, polyneuritis is a rare complication. The concomitant administration of vitamin B_6 (pyridoxine) is unnecessary, except in populations at high risk, such as patients receiving high doses of isoniazid and alcoholics.

Rifampin is active against extracellular and intracellular *M. tuberculosis*. It is absorbed completely from the intestinal tract. Its mechanism of action is probably by inhibiting RNA synthesis. The daily dose is 10 mg/kg (450 to 600 mg/day). Intolerance to rifampin is manifested by nausea and vomiting. Other side effects are seemingly allergic and are favored by the discontinuous administration or the reintroduction of the drug. These effects consist of febrile reactions, thrombocytopenia, hemolytic anemia, interstitial nephri-

Table 8–3. Dosages, Side Effects, and Activity of Major Antituberculous Agents

Drugs	Dosage	Side Effects	Activity
Bactericidal			
Isoniazid	5 mg/kg	Polyneuritis Hepatotoxicity Hypersensitivity	Extra- and intracellular bacilli
Rifampin	10 mg/kg (450–600 mg)	Hepatitis Nausea Vomiting Febrile reaction Thrombocytopenia Renal insufficiency	Extra- and intracellular bacilli
Streptomycin	15–25 mg/kg	Eighth cranial nerve involvement	Extracellular bacilli (neutral or slightly alkaline pH)
Pyrazinamide	30–35 mg/kg	Hyperuricemia Hepatotoxicity	Intracellular bacilli (acid pH)
Bacteriostatic			
Ethambutol	15–25 mg/kg	Optic neuritis Skin eruption	Extra- and intracellular bacilli

tis, and hepatitis. Rifampin also reduces the effectiveness of oral contraceptives.

Streptomycin is administered intramuscularly at a dose of 15 to 25 mg/kg/day. It is especially active against the extracellular population of *M. tuberculosis* and acts by inhibiting protein synthesis. Its toxicity for the eighth cranial nerve is related to sustained high serum levels, notably after renal insufficiency, and to the total dose administered.

Pyrazinamide, a bactericidal drug, is more active against the intracellular population of bacilli. It is administered orally at a dose of 30 to 35 mg/kg/day. Its principal side effects are hyperuricemia and hepatotoxicity.

Of the bacteriostatic antituberculous agents, only ethambutol is still used today. Its absorption is variable and incomplete following oral administration. Ethambutol is active against the intracellular and extracellular forms of *M. tuberculosis* and is believed to act by interfering with the metabolism of nucleic acids. The daily dose is 15 to 25 mg/kg. The therapeutic safety margin is narrow, however, and side effects, such as retrobulbar neuritis, are frequent at the highest doses, so ophthalmologic observation is necessary.

Most authors recommend, for minimal and moderately advanced pulmonary disease, a total treatment 9 months in duration, starting with a triple chemotherapeutic regimen, including isoniazid, rifampin, and streptomycin or ethambutol, for a period of 8 to 12 weeks, followed by a 2-drug treatment with isoniazid and rifampin for the remainder of the 9 months. With this regimen, the rates of failure and of recurrence are approximately 1% each. Some authors recommend treatment for 12 months, others a 2-drug treatment for 9 months, and some even recommend biweekly administration of the drugs.

Objective 8–3. Prevent tuberculosis.

The two goals in the prevention of tuberculosis are to reduce the incidence of the infection and to prevent a tuberculous infection from developing into active disease.

REDUCING THE INCIDENCE OF INFECTION

By the end of the 19th century, the incidence of tuberculosis was declining rapidly in both Europe and North America, even before the introduction of BCG vaccination and effective chemotherapies. Indeed, the improvement in socioeconomic conditions is considered to be the main factor in the regression of tuberculosis.

Because tuberculous infection is transmitted by a respiratory aerosol by a patient, it is important to isolate persons who harbor the bacillus for the duration of the contagious period; it is equally important to identify contacts. This screening process is initially limited to close contacts, such as family members and fellow workers. If cases of recent infection are found among these persons, the screening

Table 8–4. Evaluation of Annual Risk of Development of Tuberculous Disease

Clinical Situation	Annual Risk
Change in tuberculin skin test from negative to positive within one year	1/50
Positive PPD test in a young person	1/150–1/350
Sequelae of improperly treated tuberculosis	1/80
Close tuberculosis contact with positive PPD	1/50
Close tuberculosis contact with negative PPD	1/200

Table 8–5. Indications for Antituberculosis Chemoprophylaxis

1. Close contact with an individual with active tuberculosis.
2. Positive tuberculin skin test with nonprogressive radiologic anomalies; negative cultures for *M. tuberculosis*; no satisfactory previous treatment.
3. Recent tuberculin test conversion (<2 years).
4. Positive tuberculin skin tests associated with predisposing factors:
   Corticosteroid therapy
   Immunosuppressive treatment
   Immunosuppressive disease (lymphoma, leukemia)
   Diabetes
   Silicosis
   Gastrectomy
5. Positive tuberculin skin tests in an unvaccinated individual under 35 years of age.

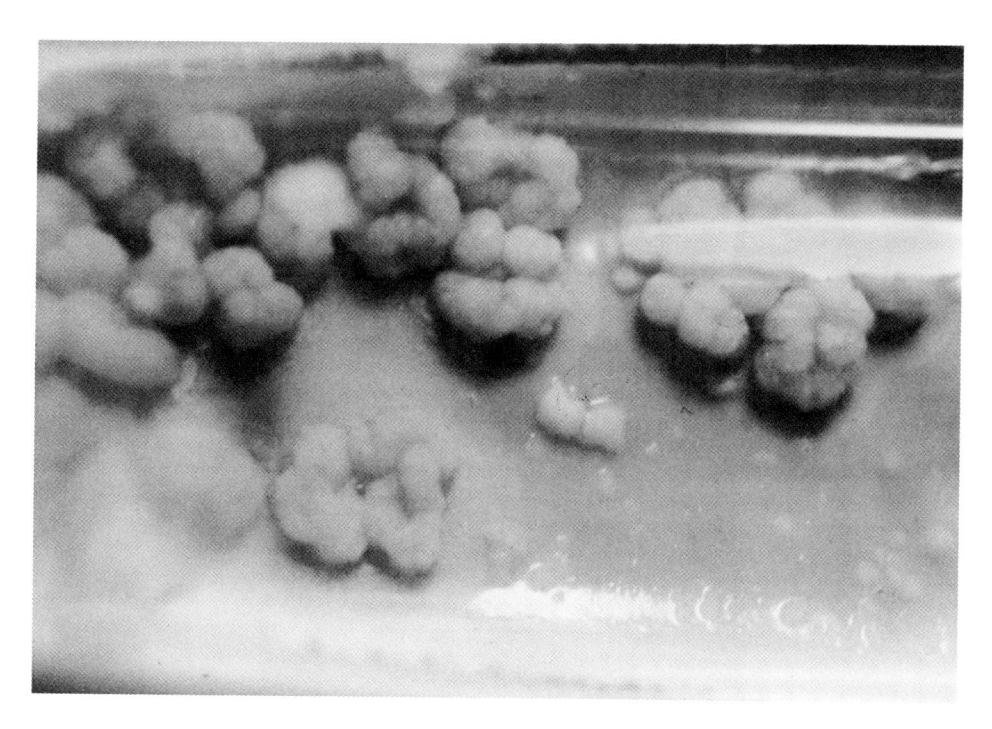

Fig. 8–5. Characteristic appearance of colonies of *Mycobacterium tuberculosis*.

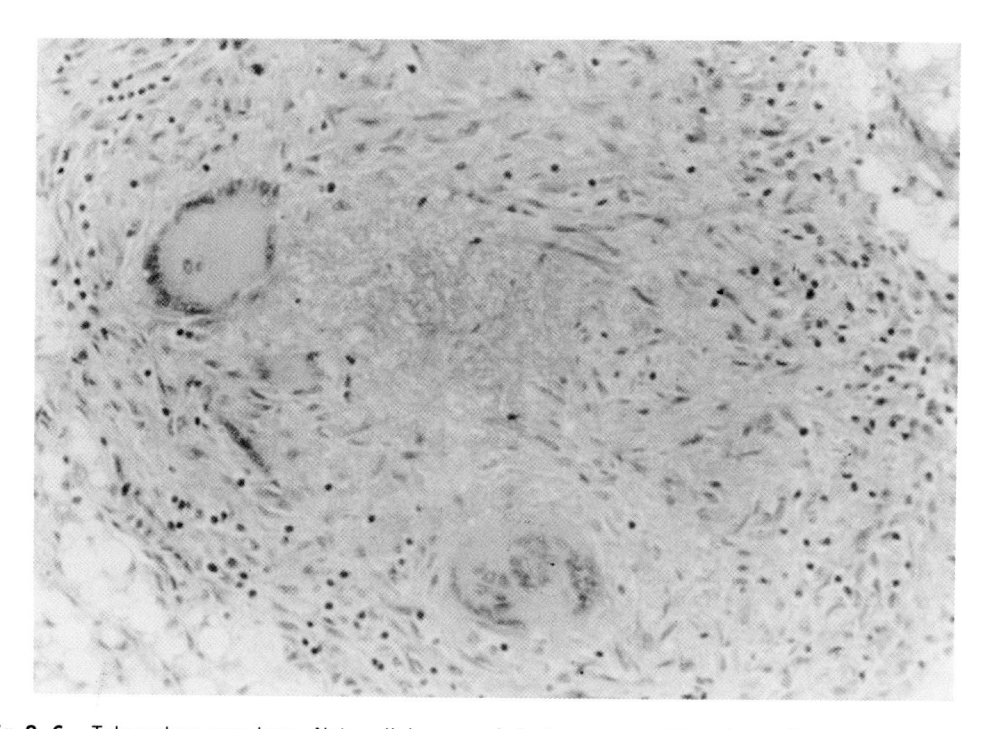

Fig. 8–6. Tuberculous granuloma. Note cellular necrosis in the center and two giant cells on the periphery; also note the infiltration of epithelioid, lymphocytic, and plasma cells.

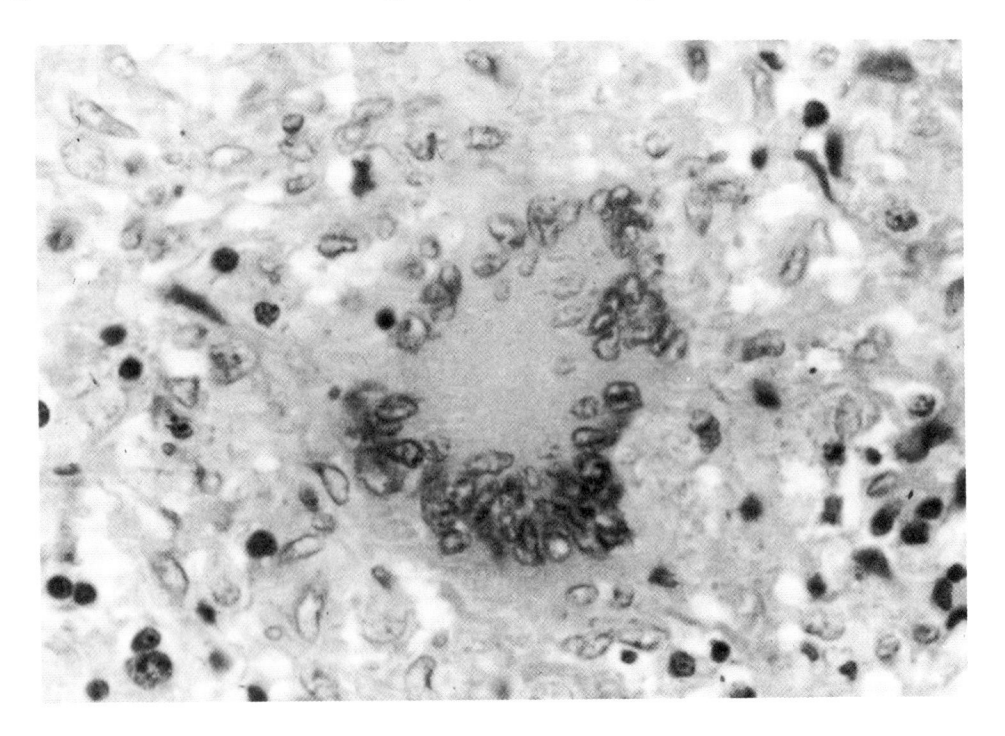

Fig. 8–7. Tubercle, a multinucleated giant cell.

is then extended to those at lower risk. Investigatory procedures include clinical history taking, tuberculin skin testing (PPD 5 U, or IP-48 10 U), and a chest roentgenogram. If the skin test is positive, as indicated by an induration of more than 10 mm, in the absence of a recent BCG vaccination, chemoprophylaxis should be proposed. The status of persons with a negative test result is re-evaluated 6 to 8 weeks later. During this period, chemoprophylaxis can be initiated in children who have been in close contact with the index case. If the test is still negative, BCG vaccination may be suggested, and chemoprophylaxis may be suspended. If the test has become positive, chemoprophylaxis is continued for a year, with appropriate medical surveillance. When chest roentgenograms and clinical findings indicate active tuberculosis, full therapy should be administered as described in Objective 8–2.

Vaccination is based on the bacille Calmette Guérin, a live strain of *Mycobacterium bovis* whose virulence has been attenuated while its immunogenic properties have been preserved. The efficacy of this vaccination has been established: approximately 70% of vaccinated individuals are protected after 10 years. The apparent failure of the vaccination has been traced to poor strains used in the vaccines and to an immunity conferred upon certain unvaccinated individuals by infections with atypical mycobacteria.

Prior to vaccination, the absence of tuberculous infection should be verified by means of a tuberculin skin test. The vaccination of tuberculin-positive individuals is unnecessary, although harmless. Vaccination consists of the intradermal injection of 0.1 ml lyophilized BCG in dilute suspension. Other vaccination methods should be avoided.

Complications of a well-performed vaccination include prolonged local ulcerations, adenitis, and osteomyelitis, but they are rare. Nonetheless, several cases of fatal dissemination have been observed in immunodepressed individuals. Approximately 6 weeks after vaccination, the PPD test becomes positive in 85% of patients. It has not been established whether the absence of a positive

BIOLOGIC PROPERTIES OF *MYCOBACTERIUM TUBERCULOSIS* AND THEIR MEDICAL CONSEQUENCES

Biologic Properties of *M. tuberculosis*

1. *M. tuberculosis* is resistant to acid and alcohol. It stains with difficulty, but once stained, for example by heating a slide covered with carbolfuchsin for 2 to 3 minutes or by using a detergent in the cold method, it retains its color, despite washing in 95% ethanol with 3% HCl (Ziehl-Neelsen). This property, no doubt connected to the abundance of lipid in the cell wall (60% of the dry weight of the cell), is shared only by a few bacteria pathogenic for man, that is, the other mycobacteria and nocardia.

2. The abundance of lipids probably explains the remarkable resistance of *M. tuberculosis* to acids and bases, as well as to various antiseptics and antibiotics.

3. *M. tuberculosis* multiplies slowly: division takes 10 to 20 hours; under similar conditions, only 20 minutes are necessary for *Escherichia coli* to divide.

4. *M. tuberculosis* is strictly aerobic.

5. *M. tuberculosis* does not possess well-identified *virulence factors,* such as toxins, extracellular enzymes, or capsule. As soon as it invades the host, it is quickly phagocytized by polymorphonuclear and monocytic cells. In addition, an affinity exists between the phagocytic cell membranes and the mycobacterial cell wall, both rich in lipid fractions.

6. Once it is intracellular, *M. tuberculosis* solidly resists digestion by phagocytes. It can survive within a macrophage for years and is capable of multiplying yet again after this long period of time.

7. Within host tissues, *M. tuberculosis* leads to the formation of *granulomas*. These are produced by the local proliferation of macrophages that constitute a specific diagnostic histologic syndrome (Fig. 8–6). Some macrophages undergo an epithelioid metaplasia or fuse to form multinucleated Langhans giant cells (Fig. 8–7). This property has been associated with a substance that contains trehalose and dimycolate and is located on the surface of the bacterium. In addition, this substance allows cell multiplication in an arrangement of parallel "ropes," an arrangement first noted by Robert Koch, who discovered the organism in 1882. In the center of the granuloma, caseation is often observed. Caseation is associated with a delayed cell-mediated hypersensitivity response against the organism and its products.

8. All populations of *M. tuberculosis,* without exception, contain mutant organisms resistant to antituberculous agents. In so-called wild strains, which have never been exposed to these agents, the frequency is 1 in 10^6 to 1 in 10^2, according to the nature and concentration of the substance. When the proportion of mutants reaches a certain threshold, the strain is called resistant because, in ordinary clinical conditions, therapy is likely to fail if the agent is prescribed by itself.

Medical Consequences

1. This staining property is useful in identifying the organism on smears of tissue secretions or drainage. Not all "acid-fast bacilli" are *M. tuberculosis,* however. The staining techniques used are the Ziehl-Neelsen, the Kenyon modification using polysorbate 80 (Tween-80) and fluorescent stain in which the stain (auramine) fluoresces.

2. *M. tuberculosis* survives even in such hostile environments as gastric acid and after exposure to the majority of ordinary disinfectants. Sputum can be "homogenized" with sodium hydroxide, which kills most bacteria, but leaves *M. tuberculosis* still viable. Few antituberculous agents are available.

3. The development of colonies (Fig. 8–5) on a selective solid medium, such as Löwenstein-Jensen, requires at least 2 to 3 weeks, usually up to 6 weeks. The former experimental diagnostic technique using live guinea pigs also required several weeks.

4. In the human host, *M. tuberculosis* particularly affects regions with high oxygen tension, such as the apices of the lungs, or well-vascularized areas, such as the vertebral bodies and the kidneys.

5. *M. tuberculosis* is a facultative intracellular parasite that shares several properties with other, similar organisms (see Table 25–2). It produces a delayed cellular hypersensitivity, which can be tested for by "tuberculin" intradermic inoculation, and a tendency to lymphatic spread probably by parasitized macrophages. Vaccination requires the use of a live vaccine.

6. Tuberculosis may manifest itself years after the primary infection by reactivation of quiescent organisms. Obviously, a lapse in cellular immunity favors this eventuality.

7. Whatever the localization of tuberculosis, the particular histologic structure of a characteristic granuloma helps the diagnosis. This granuloma is not entirely specific for tuberculosis however; similar lesions can be seen in sarcoidosis and in infections such as brucellosis, which causes caseation, contrary to widespread opinion.

8. All clinical isolates of *M. tuberculosis* should have their antimicrobial sensitivity tested. The testing consists of enumerating the colonies that form on agar containing antituberculous agents at concentrations chosen to correspond to those obtainable in patients (i.e., 0.2 and 1.0 μg/ml for isoniazid). It is also necessary to prescribe 2 or 3 drugs simultaneously, to limit the multiplication of resistant mutants.

PPD test indicates a failure of the vaccination. BCG vaccination is mandatory in certain countries. Other countries reserve it for children and young adults who have had contact with a tuberculous individual, for persons potentially exposed to repeated contact, such as hospital personnel, and for those in whom the risk of infection is high, such as immigrants to North America, Indians, and Eskimos.

PREVENTING TUBERCULOUS INFECTION FROM DEVELOPING INTO TUBERCULOUS DISEASE

Chemoprophylaxis is based on single-drug therapy with isoniazid at a dose of 300 mg/day in the adult and 10 mg/kg/day in children for a year. This regimen reduces the number and virulence of the bacilli present in small lesions. The indications for chemoprophylaxis take into account the risk of the patient's developing tuberculous disease in accordance with the clinical circumstances. This approximate risk is given in Table 8–4. The indications for chemoprophylaxis are listed in Table 8–5. The physician must also bear in mind the availability of supervision of the patient, the patient's compliance with the treatment, and the side effects of this chemoprophylaxis.

The hepatotoxicity of isoniazid is the only potentially serious complication of this regimen. This side effect is more frequent in older individuals: the rate of clinical hepatitis is 0.06% and the rate of isolated transaminase elevation is 5% in children under 15 years of age, whereas, in persons over 55 years of age, these rates are 4.3 and 19%, respectively. A few fatal cases have been reported. An isolated elevation of transaminase levels usually returns to normal even when treatment is continued. The patient should be observed clinically and should be evaluated at the onset of any symptoms compatible with hepatitis.

Contraindications to chemoprophylaxis include active tuberculosis, which should be treated with at least 2 agents, a history of allergy to isoniazid, active hepatic disease, pregnancy, and advanced alcoholism.

SUGGESTED READINGS

Addington, W.W.: The treatment of pulmonary tuberculosis: current options. Arch. Intern. Med., *139*:1391, 1979.

Banner, A.S.: Tuberculosis: clinical aspects and diagnosis. Arch. Intern. Med., *139*:1387, 1979.

Byrd, R.C., Horn, B.R., Salomon, D.A., and Griggs, G.A.: Toxic effects of isoniazid in tuberculosis chemoprophylaxis: role of biochemical monitoring in 1,000 patients. JAMA, *241*:1239, 1979.

Dash, L.A., Comstock, G.W., and Flynn, J.P.G.: Isoniazid preventive therapy. Retrospect and prospect. Am. Rev. Respir. Dis., *121*:1039, 1980.

Dutt, A.K., Jones, L., and Stead, W.W.: Short course chemotherapy for tuberculosis with largely twice weekly isoniazid-rifampin. Chest, 75:441, 1979.

Iseman, M.D., et al.: Guidelines for short-course tuberculosis chemotherapy. Am. Rev. Respir. Dis., *121*:611, 1980.

Iseman, M.D., et al.: Guidelines for the investigation and management of tuberculosis contacts. Am. Rev. Respir. Dis., *114*:459, 1976.

Jindani, A., Aber, V.R., Edwards, E.A., and Mitchison, D.A.: The early bactericidal activity of drugs in patients with pulmonary tuberculosis. Am. Rev. Respir. Dis., *121*:939, 1980.

Leff, A., and Geppert, E.F.: Public health and preventive aspects of pulmonary tuberculosis. Arch. Intern. Med., *139*:1405, 1979.

Mitchell, J.R., et al.: Isoniazid liver injury: clinical spectrum, pathology and probable pathogenesis. Ann. Intern. Med., *84*:181, 1976.

Mitchell, J.R., et al.: Increased incidence of isoniazid hepatitis in rapid acetylators: possible relation to hydrozine metabolites. Clin. Pharmacol. Ther., *18*:70, 1975.

Reichman, L.B. (ed.): International conference on tuberculosis. Chest, 76 (Suppl.):737, 1979.

Sahn, S.A., and Neff, T.A.: Miliary tuberculosis. Am. J. Med., 56:495, 1974.

Salvin, R.E., Walsh, T.J., and Pollack, A.D.: Late generalized tuberculosis: a clinical pathologic analysis and comparison of 100 cases in the pre-antibiotic and antibiotic eras. Medicine, 59:352, 1980.

Weg, J.G., et al.: Classification of tuberculosis. Am. Rev. Respir. Dis., *123*:356, 1981.

CHAPTER 9

Pulmonary Mycosis

D.H. Lederer and A.A. Medeiros

> **Objective 9–1.** Review the findings that lead one to suspect a fungal pulmonary infection.

The diagnosis of pulmonary mycosis usually requires consideration of a fungal origin in the differential diagnosis of a pulmonary lesion. Elements of the patient's medical history, physical examination, and laboratory data in pulmonary mycoses are often nonspecific and mimic other diseases. Therefore, one must be alert to clues that point to a possible fungal infection. This discussion considers factors that should raise the suspicion of a fungal infection as the cause of an acute respiratory illness, chronic pulmonary disease, or progressive, invasive, or disseminated illness.

Acute primary fungal infections of the lung are the result of spore inhalation. Mycotic disease is often considered only when a patient's acute respiratory infection fails to respond to broad-spectrum antibiotics, but a variety of findings may suggest a primary fungal infection earlier in the patient's illness.

First, the patient may reside in or may have recently visited an area that is endemic for a specific fungus. For example, in North America, *Histoplasma capsulatum*, the causative agent of histoplasmosis, is endemic in the valleys of the Mississippi and St. Lawrence Rivers and their tributaries, as well as in some of the river valleys of Central and South America, India, Africa, and Southeast Asia. The endemic area for *Blastomyces dermatitidis*, the agent causing blastomycosis, coincides in North America with that for histoplasmosis, although it extends further eastward and northward. *Coccidioides immitis*, which causes coccidioidomycosis, is endemic in a region that corresponds to the lower Sonoran life zone, which includes much of southern California, some of the Mexican states, and parts of Arizona, New Mexico, Texas, Utah, and Nevada; the organism is also endemic in parts of Argentina, Paraguay, and Venezuela. Although *Paracoccidioides brasiliensis*, which causes paracoccidioidomycosis, is endemic from southern Mexico to northern Argentina, most cases have been reported from Brazil.

Certain occupations or hobbies may predispose an individual to an acute fungal infection because of an increased exposure to spores. For example, disease may result from contact with bird droppings, especially from chickens, starlings, and black birds in histoplasmosis, and from pigeons in cryptococcosis. Bat droppings may contain histoplasma, and exploring caves may therefore carry an increased risk of infection. Digging in soil or using earth-moving machinery may, in endemic areas, give rise to coccidioidomycosis or, when the soil is contaminated by bird or bat droppings, histoplasmosis. Agricultural workers have a higher incidence of paracoccidioidomycosis because of their exposure to vegetation and soil. Similarly, small outbreaks of blastomycosis have occurred among persons exposed to decaying vegetation, particularly rotting timbers. The natural habitats of *Blastomyces dermatitidis* and *Paracoccidioides brasiliensis* have, however, not been firmly established. Horticulturists are at risk of contracting sporotrichosis, an illness due to *Sporothrix schenckii*, which is a ubiquitous dimorphic fungus that usually causes cutaneous-lymphatic disease, but it may also produce a pulmonary infection.

ACUTE INFECTION

Symptoms of an acute, primary fungal infection include fever, cough, shortness of breath, and chest pain and are similar to symptoms with infections by other agents and, therefore, rarely call attention to a fungal disease. On the other hand, the presence of erythema nodosum or erythema multiforme should suggest the possibility of histoplasmosis or coccidioidomycosis; the latter infection may also cause a transient erythematous maculopapular eruption. Hepatosplenomegaly may be a feature of acute histoplasmosis. When a chest roentgenogram shows patchy densities or regions of airspace consolidation, it is difficult to distinguish bacterial infection from the fungal illnesses that give a similar picture, such as histoplasmosis, coccidioidomycosis, and blastomycosis. Parenchymal nodules should suggest histoplasmosis or coccidioidomycosis, however; in coccidioidomycosis, excavation of nodules or regions of consolidation with resultant formation of thin-walled cavities may be seen. Histoplasmosis may cause a miliary radiographic pattern in someone previously infected who has cellular immunity. Histoplasmosis often produces hilar adenopathy, as does coccidioidomycosis on occasion. A pleural effusion is seen in approximately 10% of patients with acute coccidioidomycosis. Finally, lesions in the oral, nasal, or anorectal mucosa or in the lymphatic vessels that drain these areas should lead one to suspect paracoccidioidomycosis.

CHRONIC INFECTION

Chronic, stable pulmonary mycoses may follow acute infections and may not be recognized for years; it is therefore much more difficult to elicit a history of exposure. Most often, symptoms are absent or are nonspecific. An exception is the expectoration of mucous plugs that suggests allergic bronchopulmonary aspergillosis, a disorder in which the mucous plugs usually contain *Aspergillus fumigatus*.

Certain underlying diseases predispose patients to chronic fungal infections. For example, chronic histoplasmosis occurs almost invariably in the presence of abnormal underlying lung parenchyma, especially in emphysema. Cavitary disease may be complicated by an aspergilloma, which is a mass of fungal hyphae and fibrin that gives a characteristic roentgenographic pattern of a movable mass with a surrounding crescent of radiolucency. Less commonly, other fungi may manifest as a mycetoma. Allergic asthma is the usual setting for allergic bronchopulmonary aspergillosis.

Physical findings are rarely helpful in chronic fungal infection. On the other hand, these diseases most often are suspected because of distinctive radiographic findings. Bronchial casts in central bronchi are characteristic of allergic bronchopulmonary aspergillosis. Interstitial densities in upper lobes are seen in chronic histoplasmosis. Small single or multiple fibrotic subpleural nodules may be due to cryptococcosis. Nodules with central ("bull's-eye") or concentric calcifications are characteristic of histoplasmosis. A histoplasmoma may grow slowly and may mimic a neoplasm. In cryptococcosis and blastomycosis, one may also see mass-like lesions that occasionally cavitate. Cavitary disease can occur with histoplasmosis, coccidioidomycosis, paracoccidioidomycosis, or sporotrichosis and may easily be confused with tuberculosis, which on occasion coexists with these fungal infections.

Hilar calcifications suggest histoplasmosis, which may also produce mediastinal lymph node enlargement and perinodal fibrosis, with resultant obstruction of the trachea, esophagus, superior vena cava, pulmonary artery, or pulmonary veins. When these mediastinal nodes become calcified, broncholithiasis may result and may cause hemoptysis. Finally, splenic calcifications, resulting from a benign dissemination during primary infection, are characteristic of histoplasmosis.

DISSEMINATED INFECTION

Progressive, invasive, or disseminated fungal disease most frequently occurs in patients with undeveloped or altered immune mechanisms. Thus, infants, the elderly, and patients receiving corticosteroids, cytotoxic drugs, or long-term antibiotic therapy are particularly at risk, as are drug abusers, patients receiving hyperalimentation, and patients with prosthetic heart valves. Hodgkin's disease and other lymphomas predispose individuals to cryptococcosis. Invasive aspergillosis occurs in patients with acute leukemia or lymphoma, especially when they are neutropenic, as well as in renal transplant patients and in persons recovering from influenza. Mucormycosis, caused by organisms of the subclass Zygomycetes, such as absidia, rhizopus, mucor, and saksena, has a predilection for patients with diabetic ketoacidosis. Patients with indwelling urinary or intravenous catheters are predisposed to infection with *Candida albicans,* as are patients taking antibiotics on a long-term basis.

Symptoms of disseminated fungal disease are nonspecific and depend on the affected organs. Physical examination suggests systemic disease, often with persistent fever that is unresponsive to antibiotics. Blastomycosis may produce characteristic skin lesions, such as verrucous granulomas and subcutaneous nodules, that may cause chronic draining sinuses and ulcers. Ulcerating skin lesions also can occur in disseminated coccidioidomycosis and in paracoccidioidomycosis. In cryptococcosis, the lesions often appear gelatinous. The findings of a black nasal turbinate, thick, blood-tinged nasal discharge, or a necrotic palatal ulcer suggest mucormycosis. An oropharyngeal or laryngeal ulcer often appears in disseminated histoplasmosis when the course of the illness is not fulminant. Meningitis may be seen in cryptococcosis, coccidioidomycosis, mucormycosis, and candidiasis; it also occurs, rarely, in patients with histoplasmosis and sporotrichosis.

The chest roentgenogram may show minimal or no evidence of fungal infection, despite the occurrence of dissemination, or one may see regions of consolidation that are indistinguishable from the radiographic manifestations of bacterial pneumonia. On the other hand, certain patterns may suggest disseminated infection from specific fungi. A diffuse interstitial or miliary pattern can occur with coccidioidomycosis, paracoccidioidomycosis, cryptococcosis, histoplasmosis, or candidiasis. Invasive aspergillosis may cause necrotizing pneumonia characterized by airspace consolidation with cavitation, often in a segmental distribution consistent with lung infarction. This pattern is due to blood vessel occlusion, a phenomenon also seen in mucormycosis. Paratracheal adenopathy may occur in early infection with histoplasmosis, coccidioidomycosis, or blastomycosis, particularly in children. Dissemination of the infection may become manifest as adrenal insufficiency in histoplasmosis, in blastomycosis, or rarely, in coccidioidomycosis. These same organisms may also cause bone lesions.

> **Objective 9–2. Confirm the diagnosis of a specific pulmonary mycosis.**

The definitive diagnosis of a pulmonary fungal infection requires demonstration of organisms in tissue by direct examination or culture. Skin and serologic tests may be useful in certain well-defined clinical situations, but these methods provide only a presumptive diagnosis at best. In general, the diag-

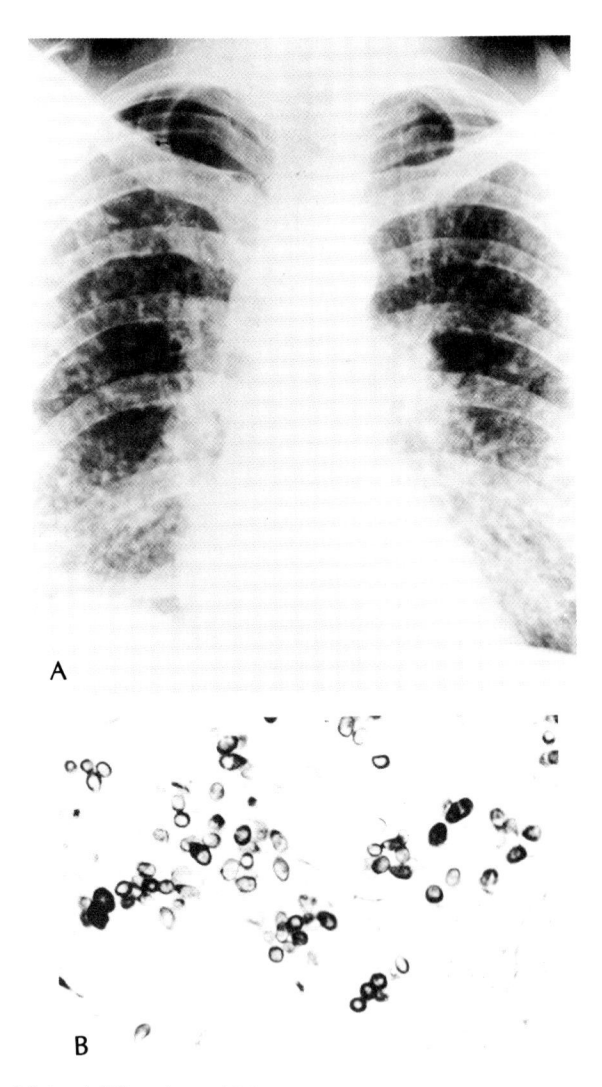

Fig. 9–1. Histoplasmosis. *A*, Bilateral diffuse interstitial and nodular infiltrates and hilar involvement. *B*, *Histoplasma capsulatum* in lung tissue.

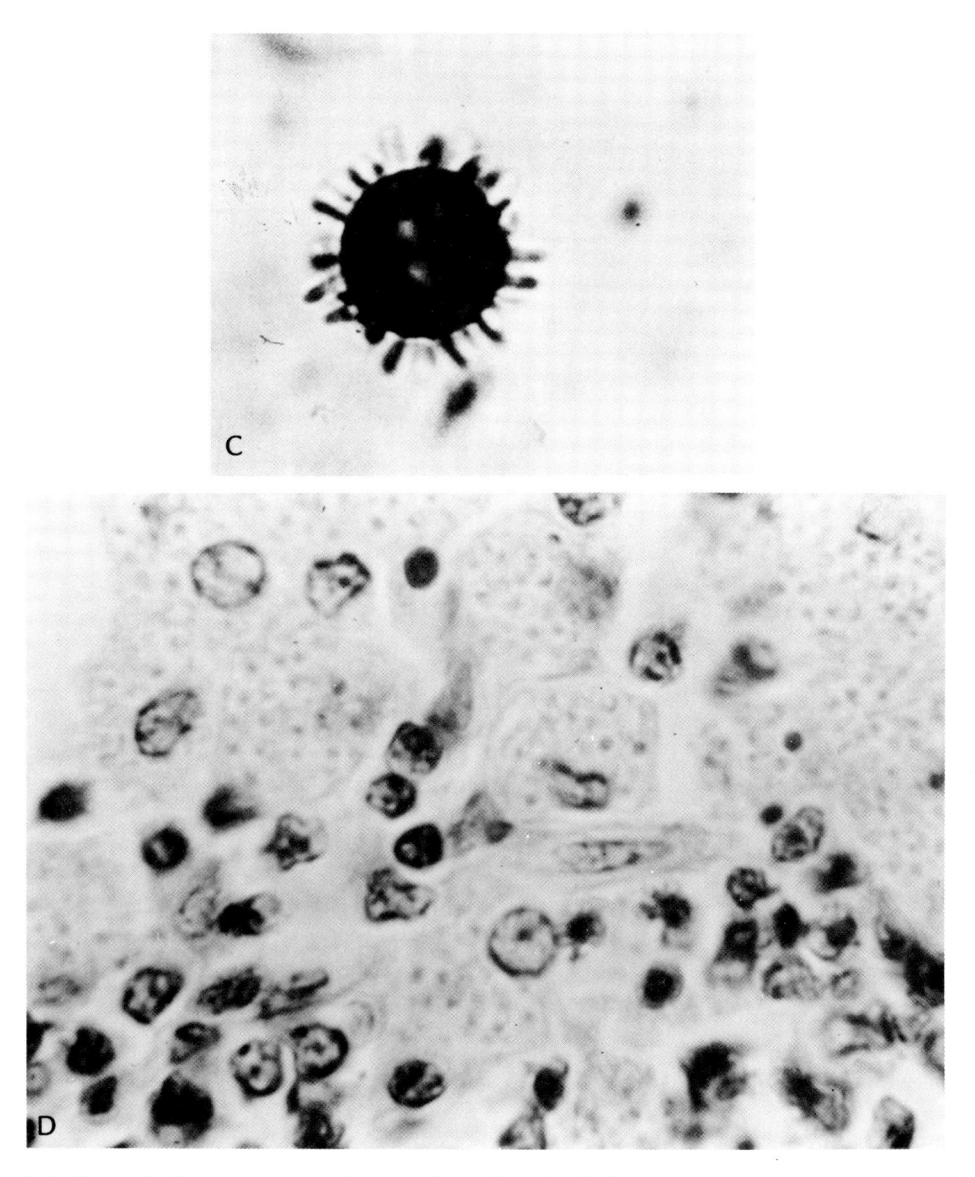

Fig. 9–1. Cont. C, *H. capsulatum* on Sabouraud's medium. *D,* Histiocytes containing numerous yeast cells. (*B* and *C* courtesy of the Pneumology Service, Laval Hospital, Québec, Canada.)

nostic approach should include culturing all available sites, especially sputum, or in the absence of sputum, bronchial washings and brushings. If these cultures are nondiagnostic, one should consider lung biopsy, using either the transbronchial technique or an open procedure. Rapid identification may be possible by examining fresh material with a Giemsa stain (histoplasmosis), an india ink preparation (cryptococcosis), or a potassium hydroxide preparation (most other fungal infections). Cultures on Sabouraud's medium should be incubated at both room temperature and at 37° C, to allow demonstration of the dimorphic character of some fungi, and should be retained for at least 3 weeks. This general approach may be modified, depending on which fungus is suspected and whether the disease is acute, chronic, or disseminated.

The following few sections review the diagnostic methods most appropriate for specific pathogenic fungi (Table 9–1).

HISTOPLASMA CAPSULATUM

Acute primary histoplasmosis (Fig. 9–1) is rarely severe, and invasive diagnostic procedures are therefore not usually indicated. The histoplasmin skin test converts to positive approximately 2 weeks after the patient inhales the fungal spores. In interpreting the skin test, however, one must remember up to 80% of the population in endemic areas will show dermal reactivity to histoplasmin. The skin test is most useful in patients with a previously negative reaction. Most patients with active pulmonary histoplasmosis react to the skin test antigen, but cross-reactivity with other fungi may occur. For this reason, a coccidioidin skin test should be applied simultaneously. A negative reaction may occur early in the course of acute pulmonary infection; however, a positive reaction develops in most patients when testing is repeated.

Skin testing should be done using an antigen derived from yeast cells (histoplasmin-CYL) because the antigen derived from mycelia may cause a rise in the complement fixation titer. It is still advisable to draw blood for serologic testing before applying the skin test, however. Agglutination, precipitation, and complement fixation tests are available. These tests become positive approximately 4 weeks after the primary infection. A titer of 1:4 for mycelial or 1:16 for yeast antigens is considered significant. The titer usually rises over time during or after the acute illness. Most patients with primary infection show elevations of titer, but patients with an acute illness resulting from reinfection have titer rises less often. Unlike in coccidioidomycosis, the height of the antibody titer in histoplasmosis does not correlate with the severity of the disease.

In chronic pulmonary histoplasmosis, the positivity of the histoplasmin skin test is no different from that of the general population in endemic areas and thus has limited usefulness. Complement fixation titers are positive about three-fourths of the time when one seeks both mycelial and yeast phase antibodies; a positive result suggests the possibility of chronic infection. Definitive diagnosis, however, depends on isolating the organism, which may be identifiable in sputum. An immunofluorescence technique that uses fluorescein-tagged antihistoplasma globulin may allow rapid identification of the organism. Colonies grow on Sabouraud's agar at room temperature. If tissue is obtained, one will see granulomas, occasionally with caseating necrosis, and the organism will stain with periodic acid-Schiff (PAS) or methenamine-silver stains.

In disseminated disease, skin and serologic testing are of limited usefulness because 50% of patients may have a negative skin test and 25% may have no detectable circulating antibodies. The organism may be isolated from sputum or from other sites such as blood or urine. Biopsy of an oropharyngeal ulcer, bone marrow, or liver may be diagnostic. Trephine biopsy of bone marrow is especially effective for diagnosing disseminated histoplasmosis; the organism is identified either by PAS or silver stains or by culture. The histologic features indicate the prognosis in that diffuse proliferation of macrophages in histoplasmo-

Table 9–1. Selected Features of Specific Pulmonary Mycoses

	Histoplasmosis	Coccidioidomycosis	Blastomycosis	Paracoccidioidomycosis	Sporotrichosis	Aspergillosis	Zygomycosis	Cryptococcosis	Candidiasis
Historical									
Endemic area	+	+	+	+					
Exposure to bird droppings	+							+	
Exposure to soil	+	+		+					
Exposure to decaying vegetation			+	+	+				
Physical									
Erythema nodosum or multiforme	+	+							
Skin ulcers		++	+	+	+			++	+
Meningitis		++			++		+	++	
Oropharyngeal ulcers	+			+					
Arthritis		+			+				+
Radiographic									
Hilar adenopathy	+	+		+					
Mass-like density			++					++	
Cavities	+	+	+	+	+	+		++	
Pulmonary infarction pattern						+	+		
Miliary pattern	+	+		+				+	+

sis has been associated with a fulminant course and a fatal outcome.

COCCIDIOIDES IMMITIS

Primary coccidioidomycosis (Fig. 9–2) can be diagnosed by a combination of skin and serologic tests. Skin testing with coccidioidin, which is a mycelial filtrate, or with spherulin, an antigen prepared from the sporangium of the organism, shows a positive reaction in virtually all patients by the third week of primary infection. Many patients with benign disease gradually lose this positivity over subsequent years, or much sooner if dissemination occurs. The usefulness of skin testing is limited by the skin test positivity of 50% of people in endemic areas. Only the conversion of a skin test from negative to positive is definite evidence of recent infection. The reaction is considered positive when an induration is 5 mm or more in diameter. A negative skin test does not rule out the diagnosis of active infection because patients may have defects in immune function. The coccidioidin skin test may affect the serologic tests for histoplasmosis. One must exercise caution when using either skin test antigen in any patient with erythema nodosum because the patient's reaction to the test may be severe. For this reason, the antigen should be diluted to 1:10,000 before use.

Agglutination and precipitation serologic tests become positive between 1 and 3 weeks after exposure, followed by complement fixation tests. A positive tube precipitin test almost always indicates recent infection; this test is frequently positive in symptomatic patients during the second and third weeks of infection. The test measures IgM antibody, as does the latex particle agglutination test, which is more sensitive and is simpler to perform. Because of the transient nature of IgM antibodies, a negative test does not rule out the diagnosis. In a patient with a well-established infection, one should check the IgG antibody by means of complement fixation testing. Immunodiffusion testing parallels the tube precipitin test if the coccidioidin is heated, and it parallels the complement fixation test if the coccidioidin is subjected to ultrafiltration. Complement fixation tests for coccidioidomycosis may be positive in patients with histoplasmosis.

Approximately two-thirds of patients with chronic infection continue to have one or more positive serologic tests. Definitive diagnosis requires isolation of the organism in culture or demonstration in tissue, however. Expectorated sputum samples show the organism in only 10 to 20% of patients with active coccidioidomycosis, whereas the yield is much greater from washings and brushings obtained by flexible fiberoptic bronchoscopy. If purulent material can be obtained, the organism may be seen with a potassium hydroxide preparation. The spherules may contain no endospores and then may be morphologically indistinguishable from blastomyces; it is therefore important to culture all biopsy material on Sabouraud's agar. The organism appears in tissue as a thin-walled spherule with multiple endospores and has the same appearance in cultures when grown on Sabouraud's glucose medium at 30° C. Mycelia can be seen in 2 to 8 days of culture; spherules may become apparent in liquid synthetic medium in 1 to 8 days. In tissue, spherules stain with PAS. A mycelial phase occasionally occurs in lung parenchymal cavities. As with other mycoses, the prominent pathologic feature is granuloma formation.

In disseminated disease, the patient may lose skin reactivity to coccidioidin and spherulin and may become anergic to other skin test antigens. A high or rapidly increasing complement fixation titer suggests extrapulmonary dissemination, with the titer higher in more severe extrapulmonary disease. A level of 1:16 or higher should raise the suspicion of dissemination, but the correlation of titers with disseminated disease must be determined by each individual laboratory. A lower complement fixation titer does not rule out dissemination of a fungal disease. The persistence of a positive precipitin reaction for longer than 6 months also suggests dissemination.

When pleural effusion is present, pleural

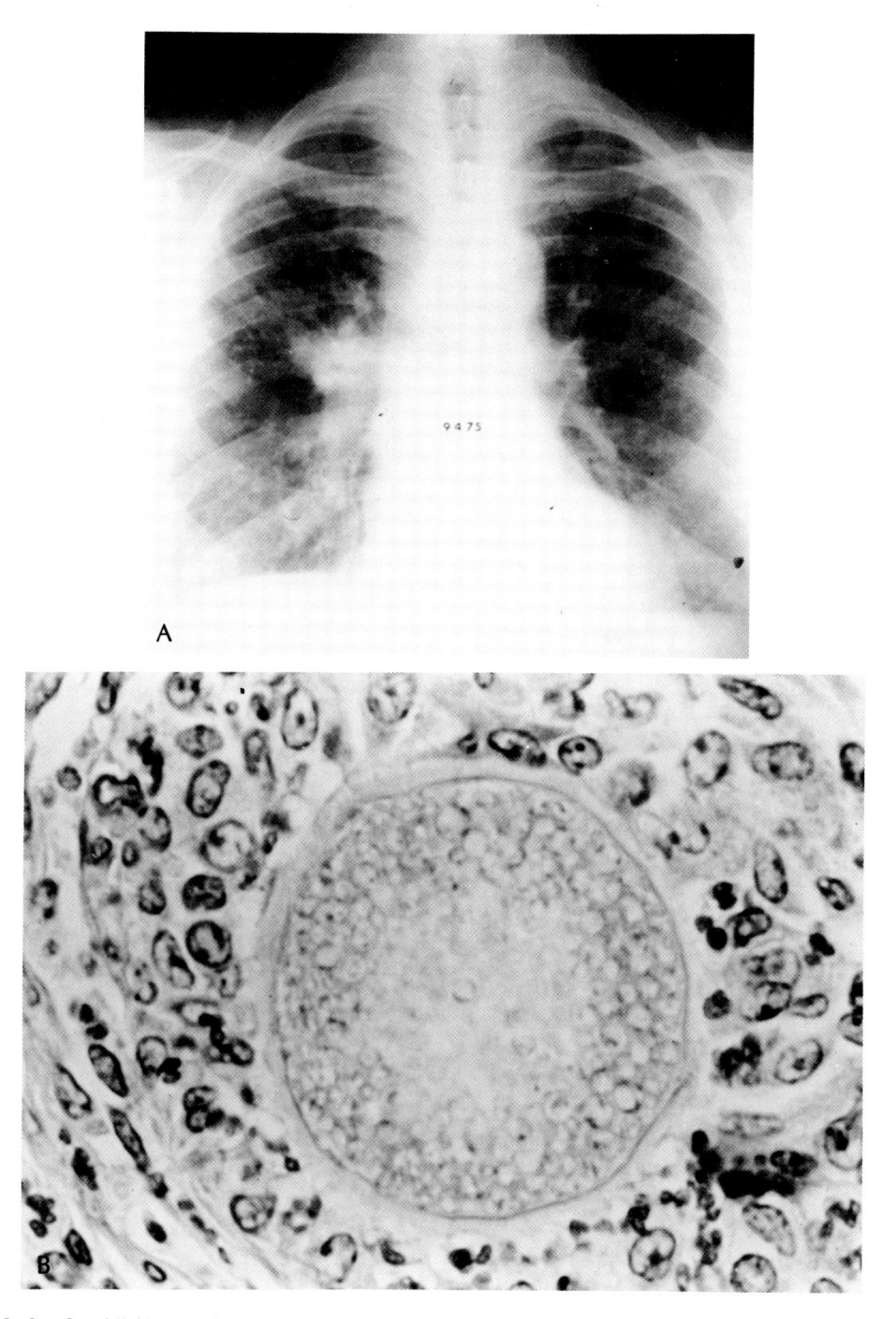

Fig. 9–2. Coccidioidomycosis. *A,* Right hilar lesion with a few radiating lesions in the medial region of the lung. *B,* Spherules and endospores. (*A* courtesy of the Pneumology Service, Laval Hospital, Québec, Canada.)

biopsy may demonstrate the organism. Meningitis may constitute the only site of extrapulmonary involvement. Complement fixation antibodies may be found in the spinal fluid in meningitis. A positive culture of cerebrospinal fluid is seen less often, but specific antigens may be detectable in spinal fluid. The presence of complement fixing antibody in spinal fluid can be considered diagnostic.

BLASTOMYCES DERMATITIDIS

Skin and serologic tests with blastomycin are of little value, partly because of cross-reactivity with histoplasmin and coccidioidin. One useful observation is that the presence of a strongly positive skin test, associated with lower serum titers of complement fixing antibody, points to a favorable prognosis, whereas the converse is associated with a poor prognosis. Sputum may be diagnostic in acute, chronic, or disseminated forms of the disease; organisms may be seen with a potassium hydroxide preparation. Culture on Sabouraud's glucose agar at 25° C yields growth in the mycelial phase of these fungi, and culture on blood agar at 37° C allows growth in the yeast form. If sputum is not readily available, bronchial washings or brushings obtained by the fiberoptic bronchoscope may be diagnostic. If tissue is obtained, a PAS or methenamine-silver stain demonstrates the organisms.

Diagnosis of disseminated disease is not difficult when skin lesions are present because the organism is easily seen on skin scrapings treated with potassium hydroxide. Sputum may show the organisms on smear or culture even in the absence of roentgenographic abnormalities of the chest. Prostatic fluid or aspirations from bone lesions may also contain organisms.

Figure 9–3 illustrates radiologic and clinical manifestations of blastomycosis.

PARACOCCIDIOIDES BRASILIENSIS

The diagnosis rests mainly on demonstrating the fungus in either sputum or tissue specimens. Direct examination of sputum, bronchial washings, or pus using potassium hydroxide may show yeast cells ranging in size from 2 to 60 µ, the large cells often having a doubly refractile wall. A cell may be surrounded by multiple smaller, "daughter" cells, attached by a narrow-necked base and giving the appearance of a "ship's wheel." As with other dimorphic fungi, specimens should be cultured on antibiotic-containing media at both 25° C and 37° C for several weeks. The paracoccidioidin skin test is not helpful because many patients with active disease are nonreactive. Conversely, cross-reactions occur in patients with histoplasmosis. An agar immunodiffusion serologic test is specific in 95% of patients, but this test does not indicate the activity of the infection. Although a high titer of complement fixing antibodies suggests an active process, cross-reactions may occur with histoplasmosis.

SPOROTHRIX SCHENCKII

In the chronic form of sporotrichosis, the organism can usually be isolated from sputum by culturing on Sabouraud's agar at room temperature or on cystine-containing blood agar at 37° C. The sporotrichin skin test does not distinguish between present or past infection, and serologic tests are unreliable.

ASPERGILLUS SPECIES

In allergic bronchopulmonary aspergillosis (Fig. 9–4), the expectorated brown sputum plugs may show mycelia microscopically or may yield the organism on culture. One sees eosinophilia, high IgE levels, elevated titers of precipitating antibodies, and a dual skin test reaction with both an immediate wheal and flare and a delayed, Arthus-like reaction. In addition to the typical chest roentgenogram showing mucoid impaction, the patient may have proximal bronchiectasis noted on bronchography. Patients with an aspergilloma do not have a positive skin test reaction but usually have elevated IgE and serum precipitins. The fungus is rarely found in expectorated sputum. The diagnosis of an aspergilloma can only be made definitively after resection and examination of the fungus ball

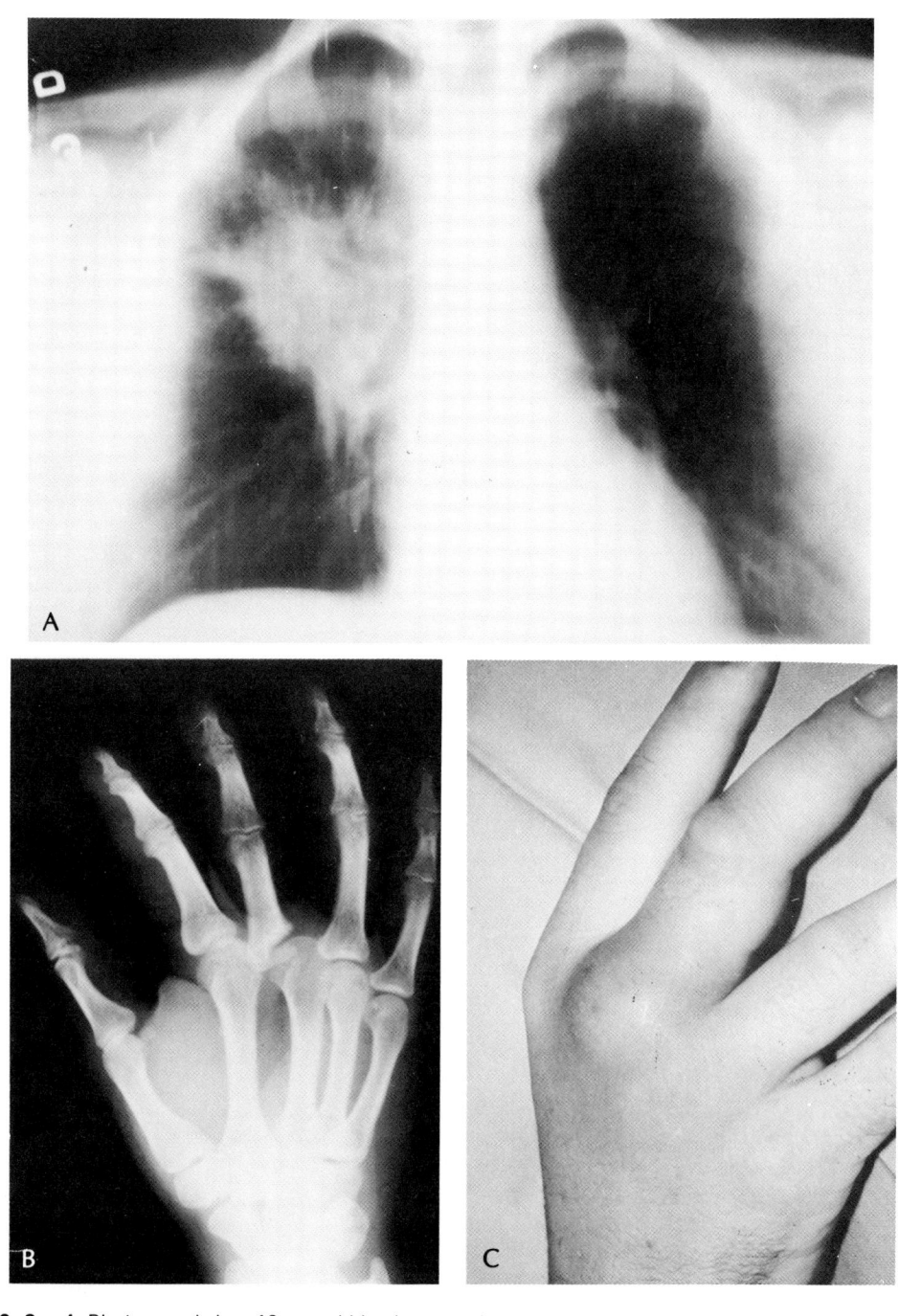

Fig. 9–3. *A,* Blastomycosis in a 42-year-old lumberman with an occasional fever and cough with whitish expectorations. The patient had lost over 20 pounds and complained of painful swelling at the base of the middle finger. Roentgenograms show an infiltration over the right small scissura. *B,* Roentgenograms show the destruction of the head of the first phalanx of the middle finger in blastomycosis. *C,* Clinical appearance of the patient's finger. (*B* and *C* courtesy of The Pneumology Service, Laval Hospital, Québec, Canada.)

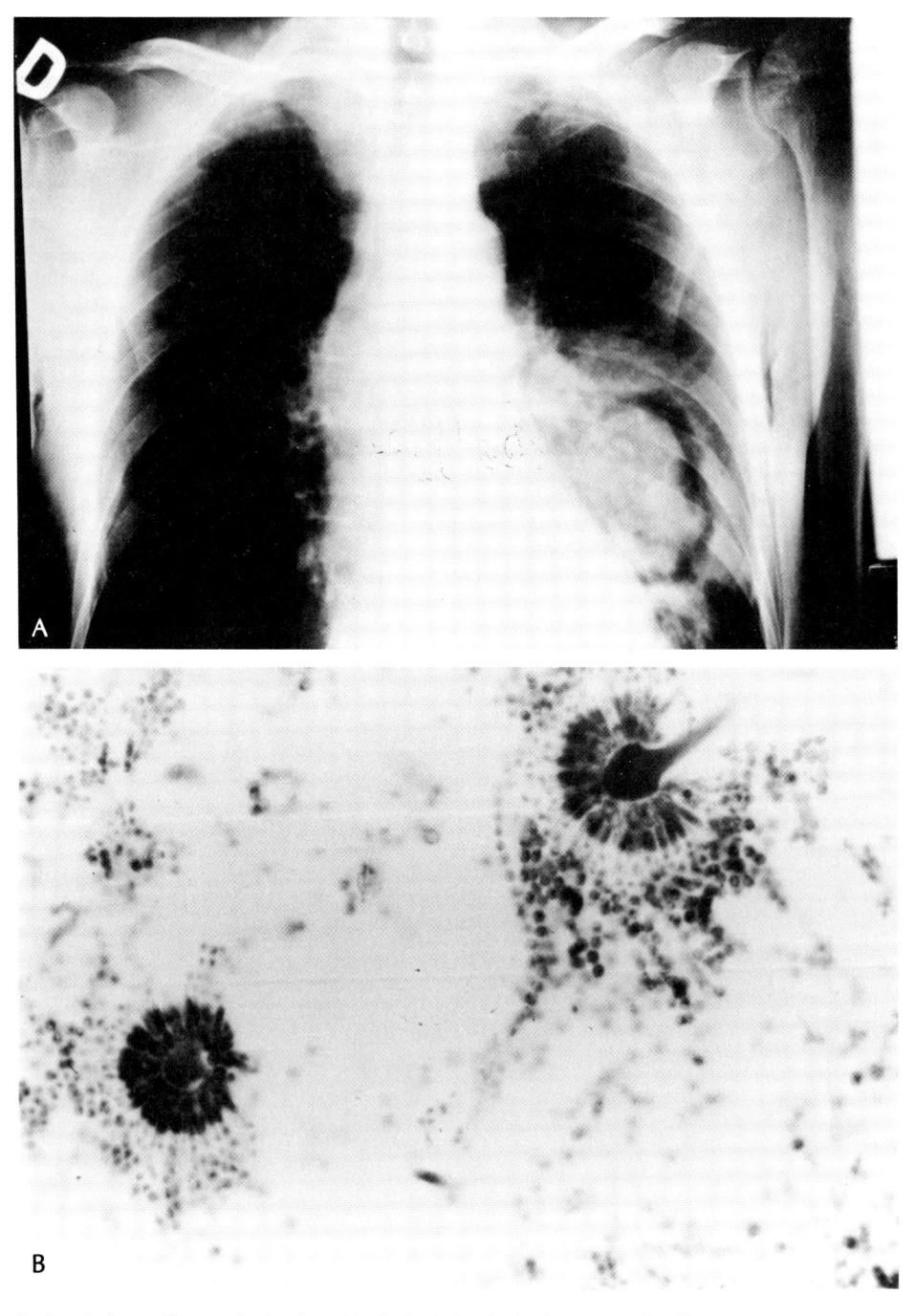

Fig. 9–4. A, *Aspergillus fumigatus* fungal ball. B, *A. fumigatus* in an expectoration.

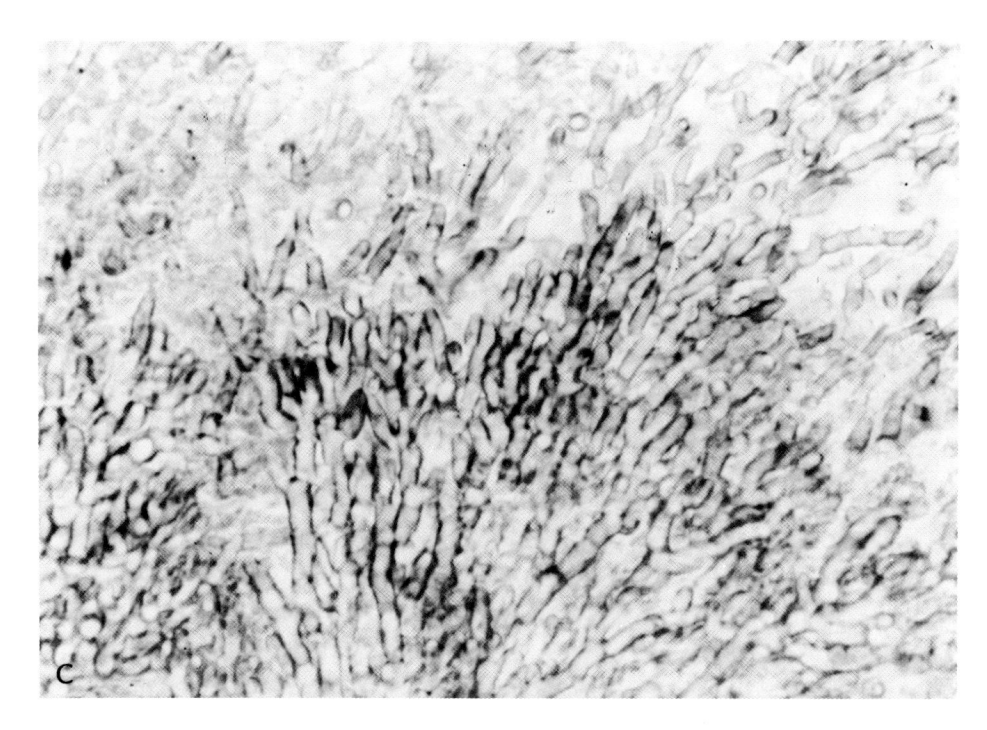

Fig. 9–4. Cont. *C,* Lung tissue biopsy in aspergillosis.

itself, because other fungi can also form mycetomas.

In invasive aspergillosis, the organism usually cannot be cultured from sputum. Although aspergillus may be present in the mouth and even in sputum cultures in the absence of actual infection, some consider the finding of organisms in any location, especially the nasopharynx, as adequate evidence for a presumptive diagnosis of invasive disease in the proper clinical setting, especially in an immunosuppressed patient. Invasive disease can only be established with certainty by identifying the organism in tissue. Biopsy specimens reveal hyphae invading pulmonary vessels with resultant hemorrhagic infarction of lung tissue. Either the transbronchial approach or an open procedure can be used, although an open operation is more likely to yield a diagnosis. Serologic testing is usually not helpful in diagnosing invasive aspergillosis.

ZYGOMYCETES

Definitive diagnosis depends on finding organisms of this subclass in biopsy material. A positive sputum culture, although unusual, is considered presumptive evidence of infection in high-risk patients. The organism can be grown on Sabouraud's agar.

CRYPTOCOCCUS NEOFORMANS

In chronic cryptococcosis, one occasionally is able to identify the yeast cells in sputum mixed with india ink and viewed under the microscope. Although it is difficult to culture the organism from the sputum, an attempt should be made on Sabouraud's agar at room temperature for 1 to 2 weeks. Bronchoscopic washings may yield the diagnosis; however, definitive diagnosis often requires lung tissue biopsy, which reveals granulomas with caseous necrosis and organisms that stain with silver chromate, PAS, or by means of fluorescent antibody. This organism does not evoke the active inflammation that one sees with other fungi, and the cellular reaction, which develops slowly, is rarely intense.

In disseminated cryptococcosis, pleural effusion is rarely present; when it is, cryptococcal antigen in the pleural fluid may be diagnostic. More commonly, the patient has meningitis, and the diagnosis is made by examination of the cerebrospinal fluid. Countercurrent immunoelectrophoresis (CIE) can detect cryptococcal polysaccharide antigen in cerebrospinal fluid as well as in urine, even when the organism cannot be seen or cultured. A latex agglutination test can detect circulating polysaccharide antigens in serum and urine. Serologic tests for antibodies are generally unrewarding.

CANDIDA SPECIES

Candida is a common saprophyte of the upper respiratory tract and is frequently present in sputum, urine, and even blood in the absence of invasive disease. It rarely causes primary pulmonary disease even in the immunosuppressed host. Diagnosis depends on demonstrating the organism in tissue, where it may be seen in both mycelial and yeast form. This organism stains with hematoxylin-eosin or with PAS. Serologic tests do not establish the diagnosis of invasive candidiasis.

> Objective 9–3. Present the indications for treatment of specific pulmonary mycoses.

HISTOPLASMOSIS

Acute histoplasmosis rarely requires treatment unless symptoms persist beyond 10 days. Even then, therapy of severely symptomatic or prolonged primary infection is controversial. On the other hand, in chronic disease, persistent cavities should be treated with amphotericin B. Occasionally, surgical resection of cavities is necessary. Intravenous amphotericin B is the treatment of choice for disseminated disease (Tables 9–2 and 9–3).

COCCIDIOIDOMYCOSIS

No specific treatment of the primary disease is necessary when it is self-limited. Stable nodules, regions of parenchymal consolidation, and small cavities can be safely observed without treatment. On the other hand, any of the following findings, suggestive of impending dissemination, constitute an indication for treatment: weight loss, cough, or hemoptysis; progression of pulmonary consolidation; persistence of adenopathy after clearing of parenchymal densities; a rising or persistently elevated complement fixation titer; or the appearance of mediastinal adenopathy. Patients who are immunocompromised, are pregnant, or are members of some racial groups, such as blacks and Filipinos, are especially prone to develop disseminated infection.

When extrapulmonary dissemination has definitely occurred, treatment is always indicated. A rapidly expanding cavity, bronchopleural fistula, and persistent, severe hemorrhage are indications for surgical resection. In all these instances, treatment consists of the administration of amphotericin B. When meningitis is present, the drug must also be given intrathecally. Transfer factor may have a role, especially when blood is obtained from a related donor.

BLASTOMYCOSIS

Treatment is indicated in all culture-proved disease. Amphotericin B is the therapy of choice. Hydroxystilbamidine isethionate has been used successfully, but cure and relapse rates are not as favorable as with amphotericin B.

SPOROTRICHOSIS

Chronic cavitary disease and disseminated disease require treatment with amphotericin B. Miconazole has been used successfully in a few patients.

ASPERGILLOSIS

Management of allergic bronchopulmonary aspergillosis usually requires a combination of corticosteroids, bronchodilators, and cromolyn sodium. Percutaneous instillation of intracavitary amphotericin B is an option for aspergilloma, but is usually not necessary. If associated hemoptysis is severe, surgical resection is indicated. Invasive aspergillosis always requires rapid treatment, although mortality rate is high even then. In the presence

Table 9–2. Therapy of Pulmonary Mycoses

Mycoses	Drug(s) of Choice	Alternatives	Comments
Histoplasmosis	Amphotericin B	? Ketoconazole, ? sulfonamides	Therapy is usually given only to patients with severe primary pulmonary infection, chronic cavitary disease, or disseminated infection. The usual primary pulmonary infection is self-limited. Surgical treatment may be necessary in patients with enlarging cavities and hemoptysis.
Coccidioidomycosis	Amphotericin B	Ketoconazole, ? miconazole	
Blastomycosis	Amphotericin B	Hydroxystilbamidine	
Paracoccidioidomycosis	Amphotericin B	Ketoconazole, ? miconazole, ? sulfonamides	
Sporotrichosis	Amphotericin B	? Miconazole, ? potassium iodide, ? hydroxystilbamidine	
Aspergillosis	Amphotericin B	? Amphotericin B plus rifampin	Pulmonary aspergilloma and allergic bronchopulmonary aspergillosis do not require amphotericin B therapy. Surgical resection of aspergilloma is necessary when life-threatening hemoptysis occurs. Allergic aspergillosis may respond to steroid therapy. Outcome of invasive pulmonary infection depends on prompt treatment and improvement in underlying disease.
Zygomycosis	Amphotericin B		Many patients improve without therapy. Those with progressive pulmonary infection or disseminated disease should be treated.
Cryptococcosis	Amphotericin B (? plus 5-fluorocytosine)		
Candidiasis	Amphotericin B	? 5-fluorocytosine, ? ketoconazole, ? miconazole	

Table 9–3. Major Characteristics of Antimycotic Drugs

Drugs	Fungi Likely to be Susceptible	Resistance Developing During Therapy	Dosages	Duration of Therapy	Precautions
Amphotericin B	Candida, aspergillus, and mucor species, Cryptococcus neoformans, Sporothrix schenkii, Coccidioides immitis, Blastomyces dermatitidis, Histoplasma capsulatum, Paracoccidioides brasiliensis	Rarely	Initial test dose: 1 mg in 100 ml 5% dextrose in water (D5W) given intravenously over 30 minutes. Then 0.25 mg/kg in 500 ml D5W given over about 4 hours. Dose is then increased 5–10 mg on each subsequent day to a maximum of 0.6 mg/kg/day	6–12 weeks	Fever and chills often develop 1–2 hours after the early infusions; may be helped by administering antipyretics, antihistamines, or hydrocortisone. Causes dose-dependent renal damage that is reversible early. Anemia due to suppression of red cell formation also occurs, but is reversible. Causes hypokalemia, which may require potassium supplementation. Hypotensive, hypertensive, and anaphylactic reactions have been reported.
5-Fluorocytosine	Candida species, Cryptococcus neoformans	Frequently	150 mg/kg/day in 4 divided doses given orally, often with 0.3 mg/kg/day amphotericin B IV for potential synergistic effect	2–6 weeks	May cause fatal dose-dependent bone marrow depression. Leukocyte and platelet counts should be done twice weekly. Dangerous to use in patients with diminished renal function. Also causes rash, hepatitis, and severe diarrhea. Adverse effects may occur more frequently in patients also receiving amphotericin B.

Ketoconazole	*Paracoccidioides brasiliensis, Blastomyces dermatitidis, Coccidioides immitis, Histoplasma capsulatum,* candida species, *Cryptococcus neoformans, Sporothrix schenkii,* dermatophytes	Rarely	200–1000 mg/day, given orally	6–12 months	Often causes nausea early in therapy. Taking half the daily dose twice a day may help. Rash, cholestatic hepatitis, and gynecomastia may occur. Antacids or H_2-blockers diminish absorption.
Miconazole	*Coccidioides immitis, Paracoccidioides brasiliensis,* candida species	Rarely	Initial test dose: 200 mg intravenously with physician in attendance. Then 20–40 mg/kg/day is given intravenously divided equally in 3 doses administered in 200 ml normal saline solution or D5W over 30–60 minutes	1–20 weeks	Acute cardiac arrest has occurred following an initial dose. May cause intense pruritus that may persist for weeks after stopping the drug. Hyperlipidemia, hypernatremia, and thrombocytosis also occur.
Griseofulvin	Dermatophytes	Rarely	500–1000 mg microsized crystals/day, given orally	6–12 months	Photosensitivity reactions may occur. Barbiturates interfere with absorption. Decreases activity of coumarin anticoagulants; dose of coumarin may have to be adjusted.

Table 9-4. Comparison of Yeasts and Molds with Dimorphic Fungi

Type of Fungi	Mycoses	Pathogenic Characteristics
Yeasts		Cause serious infection mainly in "immunocompromised hosts" (leukemia, lymphoma, or in transplant patients taking immunosuppressive drugs).
Candida	Candidiasis	
Cryptococcus neoformans	Cryptococcosis	
Molds		Invade through the gastrointestinal tract or lung.
Aspergillus	Aspergillosis	Cause a variety of clinical syndromes peculiar to each agent, but all can disseminate to many organs.
Rhizopus, mucor, absidia, saksena	Zygomycosis (phycomycosis, mucormycosis)	Usually evoke a suppurative rather than a granulomatous response in the host.
		Are widespread in nature.
		Colonization and mild localized infections are common even in otherwise healthy persons.
		Do not cause major epidemics.
		Have become increasingly more common as more patients are immunosuppressed.
		May be hospital-acquired.
		Are not contagious from person to person.
Dimorphic Fungi		Cause serious infection in otherwise healthy persons.
Histoplasma capsulatum	Histoplasmosis	Invade through the lungs.
Coccidioides immitis	Coccidioidomycosis	Cause acute pneumonia or chronic cavitation of lungs. Disseminate to many organs, as in tuberculosis.
Blastomyces dermatitidis	Blastomycosis (North American blastomycosis)	Evoke granulomatous response in the host, as in tuberculosis.
Paracoccidioides brasiliensis	Paracoccidioidomycosis (South American blastomycosis)	Exist in discrete foci in limited geographic (endemic) areas specific for each fungus.
Sporothrix schenkii	Sporotrichosis	Commonly cause mild (inapparent, subclinical) infection in lifelong residents of endemic areas.
		Cause major epidemics by airborne dissemination from point source.
		Have a stable overall incidence.
		Are not hospital-acquired.
		Are not contagious from person to person unlike *Mycobacterium tuberculosis*.

of a clinical picture compatible with invasive pulmonary infection, some consider isolating the organism from any site, especially the nasopharynx, as an adequate indication for treatment in an immunosuppressed patient.

MUCORMYCOSIS

In the appropriate clinical setting, a positive sputum culture, although unusual, is an indication for treatment. More often, the diagnosis is made by lung biopsy. Treatment involves the intravenous administration of amphotericin B and the surgical removal of necrotic tissue in the nasopharynx, paranasal sinuses, lung, or brain.

CRYPTOCOCCOSIS

The treatment of isolated pulmonary cryptococcal disease is controversial. Persistent or progressive pulmonary disease and disseminated disease, however, especially when associated with meningitis, always require treatment with intravenous amphotericin B and, usually, 5-fluorocytosine. Transfer factor therapy is occasionally effective in disseminated cryptococcosis. Successful therapy is usually accompanied by a drop in the titer of serum cryptococcal antigen, as measured by the latex agglutination test.

> **WHAT IS A FUNGUS?**
>
> Fungi are highly differentiated microorganisms. More complex structurally than bacteria, their DNA is surrounded by a nuclear membrane and segregates into chromosomes during cell division, like our own eukaryotic cells. Unlike bacteria, fungi have mitochondria and endoplasmic reticulum in their cytoplasm and sterols in their cell membrane. Their cell walls are made up of a tough polysaccharide polymer, which resists attack by antibiotics and even by heated alkali. A 10% solution of potassium hydroxide (KOH) is used for identifying fungi in direct smears. Fungi grow more slowly than bacteria, but they tolerate low pH and low temperature conditions better. Contaminated specimens are planted on a low-pH medium (Sabouraud's agar) incubated at 25° C to favor growth of fungi over bacteria. Fungi resemble plants because they are immotile and reproduce either by forming twig-like extensions (hyphae) and seed-like cells (spores) or by budding.
>
> Some fungi exist as single cells (yeast) and others as elongated filaments (molds). An important group of pathogens, dimorphic fungi, exists in both forms, that is, as molds in their natural habitats or at 25° C in the laboratory, and as yeasts in body tissues or at 37° C in the laboratory. See Table 9–4 for a comparison of yeasts and molds with dimorphic fungi. Many fungi flourish on vegetation, such as decaying grass, wood, and peat moss, all over the world, whereas others are limited to discrete geographic areas and are often prevalent in the soil of those regions, especially soil fertilized by bird or animal excreta. The commonest pathogen, candida, however, exists as part of our normal gastrointestinal flora and causes disease only when overgrowth occurs because of suppression of the bacterial flora by antibiotics. The other pathogenic mycoses usually enter the body by spore inhalation and, therefore, are the more frequent cause of pulmonary infections.

CANDIDIASIS

The presence of candida in sputum is not itself an indication for treatment. Conversely, organisms may be absent from sputum despite the presence of candidal pneumonia. Therefore, biopsy evidence of tissue invasion is mandatory before initiating treatment. Invasive candidiasis, documented by identification of the organism in tissue, is always an indication for treatment with amphotericin B, usually in combination with 5-fluorocytosine.

SUGGESTED READINGS

Davies, S.F., Khan, M., and Sarosi, G.A.: Disseminated histoplasmosis in immunologically suppressed patients. Am. J. Med., *64*:94, 1978.

Drutz, D.J., and Catanzaro, A.: Coccidioidomycosis. Part I. Am. Rev. Respir. Dis., *117*:559, 1978.

Drutz, D.J., and Catanzaro, A.: Coccidioidomycosis. Part II. Am. Rev. Respir. Dis., *117*:727, 1978.

Fraser, R.G., and Paré, J.A.P.: Diagnosis of Disease of the Chest. Philadelphia, W.B. Saunders, 1978.

Goodwin, R.A., and Des Prez, R.M.: Histoplasmosis. Am. Rev. Respir. Dis., *117*:929, 1978.

Masur, H., Rosen, P.P., and Armstrong, D.: Pulmonary disease caused by Candida species. Am. J. Med., 63:914, 1977.

Murray, H.W.: Pulmonary mucormycosis: one hundred years later. Chest., 72:1, 1977.

Sarosi, G.A., and Davies, S.F.: Blastomycosis. Am. Rev. Respir. Dis., *120*:911, 1979.

Sarosi, G.A., et al.: American Thoracic Society treatment of fungal diseases. Am. Rev. Respir. Dis., *120*:1393, 1979.

CHAPTER 10

Pleural Effusion

F. Waldvogel

Objective 10–1. Diagnose a pleural effusion using both clinical and radiographic findings.

Any disease process within the chest can reach the pleural space and provoke a localized inflammatory reaction, characterized at first by fibrin deposits followed by a serous exudate. The clinical evidence of such a development is the appearance of a pleural effusion on the side affected by the particular pathologic process. In situations involving hyperimmunity, the pleura and other serous membranes, such as the pericardium, react to an injury by forming, most commonly, a bilateral pleural effusion. In a polyserositis, the pleura is only one of many sites of the immunologic reaction. Finally, any hemodynamic or metabolic condition that leads to the development of peripheral edema can, for the same reasons, favor accumulation of fluid in the pleural space. Such transudates are seen most often in cardiac or renal failure and occasionally in portal hypertension and severe hypoalbuminemia.

Thus, pleural effusions can be caused by many pathologic processes and a host of etiologic agents. Successful clinical and radiologic diagnosis and etiologic and pathologic analysis of pleural effusions require a systematic approach and are of tremendous importance in the specialty of infectious diseases as well as in general medicine.

On a physiologic level, the equilibrium of Starling's forces, which act on intra- and extravascular fluid exchanges in the peripheral capillary bed, produces a small amount of plasma transudate from the parietal pleura because of the negative intrapleural pressure. This transudate, which has an estimated volume of 2 ml, is continually reabsorbed by the capillaries and lymphatic vessels of the visceral pleura. Any variation in the balance of forces, such as an increase in venous pressure, a decrease is plasma oncotic pressure, an alteration of capillary permeability, or lymphatic obstruction, can disturb the reabsorption of this small amount of pleural fluid and may lead to its accumulation. When a lesion of inflammatory origin involves a visceral pleural surface, which lacks sensory innervation, the disease becomes symptomatic only when pleural fluid is sufficient to cause dyspnea. If, on the other hand, the disease involves inflammation of the well-innervated parietal pleura, the fluid accumulation is usually preceded by severe pain: the warning symptoms in this case are pleuritic and include an excruciating pain exacerbated by coughing, breathing, or changes in position, and often a high fever.

CLINICAL FEATURES

Clinically, the effusion is manifested by a reduction or even an absence of diaphragmatic movement, a dullness to percussion with an attenuation of vocal fremitus, and the loss of vesicular breath sounds. The diagnosis is easily reached when the volume of fluid is greater than 500 ml, but becomes more difficult when an underlying disease process alters the auscultatory findings, as in a pneumonia, or when the effusion is of small size or has an unusual location, such as an interlobar or subpulmonary effusion. In such cases, one should turn the patient onto his stomach, with his head at the bottom of the bed, and demonstrate the displacement of fluid by percussion. Finally, a diaphragmatic paralysis or an extensive pleural fibrosis, such as secondary to a previous tuberculous pleuritis, or the long-term effects of a lobectomy, can occasionally be mistaken for a pleural effusion; this problem is solved by appropriate thoracic roentgenography.

RADIOGRAPHIC FEATURES

Pleural effusions greater than 500 ml in volume are easily detected on plain anteroposterior and lateral chest films. One should pay particular attention to the detection of bilateral effusions, which are most often secondary to a generalized disorder, such as the nephrotic syndrome or polyserositis, rather than to a localized condition. When conventional roentgenograms do not permit clear identification of the infiltrate, because of underlying pulmonary disease, pleural fibrosis, or subpulmonary or intrafissural effusion, one should first attempt radiographic visualization with the patient in a recumbent position, for example, lateral decubitus, before resorting to newer techniques such as ultrasonography. Decubitus films sometimes show fluid movement, even within loculated or encapsulated effusions; they may indeed reveal an underlying pneumonia or a tumor hidden on the plain films by a shifting of the fluid away from the underlying consolidation.

> **Objective 10–2. Distinguish an exudate from a transudate.**

Once the diagnosis of pleural effusion has been clearly established on the basis of the clinical or radiologic findings, it is necessary to determine whether the effusion is produced by an imbalance of hemodynamic forces in the capillary bed, as in congestive heart failure (transudate), or by a localized or general inflammatory process (exudate). The distinction between transudates and exudates can only be made with certainty by examining the pleural fluid obtained by thoracentesis. Thus, thoracentesis is the key to the differential diagnosis. Draining great quantities of fluid initially, unless the patient is severely dyspneic from a large effusion, using a wide-bore needle or trocar, or proceeding at once with a pleural biopsy are not recommended because risks inherent in these procedures are significant, particularly in an infected area.

LABORATORY VALUES IN PLEURAL EFFUSION

Which parameters are most reliable in making the distinction between a transudate and an exudate? The normal protein concentration of the pleural fluid varies from 1 to 2 g/100 ml; this value alone, however, does not suffice in distinguishing a transudate from an exudate. One must also take the patient's serum protein level into consideration. Probably, the most useful diagnostic criterion for an exudate is a pleural/serum protein ratio of 0.5 or more. Consequently, in a patient with normal serum protein concentration, the corresponding pleural protein would be greater than 3 g/100 ml. Another measurement equally useful in evaluating the degree of inflammation in pleural fluid is the determination of the lactose dehydrogenase activity (LDH). A value greater than 200 U/L, with a serum value of up to 280 U/L, and a pleural/serum ratio of greater than 0.5, suggest an exudate because these cytoplasmic enzymes are probably liberated into the effusion by the lysis of inflammatory cells. In contrast, neither the number of leukocytes nor the number of erythrocytes are reliable criteria in distinguishing between the two types of effusions. Parameters that permit specific identification of the origin of an exudate are discussed in Objective 10–4.

DIFFICULTIES IN DISTINGUISHING TRANSUDATES FROM EXUDATES

Two special clinical situations merit further discussion. First, the ratios of protein and LDH as defined previously are occasionally of borderline significance and do not allow one to distinguish clearly a transudate from an exudate. Although some chronic effusions, such as those of cardiac origin, may be rich in protein, clinical experience has shown that it is best to consider them as exudates while one is still investigating. Second, some effusions that are clinically or radiologically evident cannot be tapped using usual techniques. In such cases, when analysis of the pleural fluid is particularly important, it is advisable to use newer techniques for the localization of collections of fluid, by guiding the needle with the aid of sonography or CT scanning. This procedure has the additional advantage of providing densitometric information about the fluid that could be useful in determining the origin of the effusion.

> **Objective 10–3. Distinguishing among the major causes of exudates.**

The various disorders that cause pleural effusions can be classified into several large groups, according to their particular properties and symptoms. These groups are summarized in Table 10–1.

NEOPLASMS

Neoplastic effusions, whether primary, from mesothelioma, which is rare, or secondary (metastatic), are generally not painful and are often hemorrhagic. Cytologic examination of the pleural fluid usually yields both lymphocytes and neutrophils and reveals the presence of tumor cells in 65 to 96% of cases, depending on the number of times the patient's pleural fluid is examined. The finding of tumor cells is more valuable than the information yielded by biopsy of the pleura or immunologic testing of the fluid for carcinoembryonic antigen or alpha-fetoprotein. These tumor cells are usually pleural metastases arising from carcinomas of the lung, breast, ovary, or stomach. Polyserositis secondary to a carcinoma of the ovary is called Meigs's syndrome.

IMMUNE FACTORS

"Immune" effusions are encountered in the course of systemic lupus erythematosus (SLE) and rheumatoid arthritis (RA). Such effusions are also seen as part of the immunologic syndrome following myocardial infarction or cardiac surgery—Dressler's syndrome and postcardiotomy syndrome, respectively. Neither the cytologic examination nor the white blood cell count is diagnostic in this instance. Diagnosis of effusions related to SLE and RA can only be made upon discovery, in the blood or pleural fluid, of LE cells, anti-DNA antibodies, or high titers of rheumatoid factor. In addition, that the glucose levels are practically undetectable in a rheumatoid pleural effusion helps one to make the diagnosis. Circulating immune complexes are present in both diseases.

TUBERCULOSIS

Tuberculous pleural effusions generally have an insidious onset with little or no pleuritic pain and a fever that is often low-grade. The effusion is generally large and is easy to aspirate. The pleural fluid contains only a few mesothelial cells. Although at first the fluid may contain an equal quantity of polymorphonuclear cells and lymphocytes, the number of lymphocytes increases rapidly and usually represents 95 to 99% of all cells present in the pleural fluid. Patients with such effusions can sometimes be identified by their strikingly positive tuberculin skin reactions. Acid-fast organisms in a smear of the fluid sediment are rarely demonstrated, and the

Table 10–1. Major Types of Pleural Exudates

	Gross appearance	Microscopic appearance	Protein concentration	Glucose level	Most useful tests
Neoplastic	Amber, hemorrhagic	~2000 WBC/mm³ (lymphocytes and PMN); *malignant cells*; 50 to 5 × 10⁵ RBC/mm³	~4g/100ml	Normal	Cytologic examination
"Immunologic" (systemic lupus erythematosus, rheumatoid arthritis)	Clear, light-colored	Number of leukocytes variable	~4g/100ml	Low in rheumatoid arthritis	Tests for presence in serum and pleural fluid of abnormal immunoglobulins (Latex fixation, anti-DNA, immune complexes)
Tuberculous	Clear, light-colored	~1000–4000 WBC/mm³ (>90% lymphocytes); rare mesothelial cells	~4g/100ml	Normal	Pleural biopsy, for histologic study showing granuloma and for culture
Infectious metapneumonic	Usually cloudy	~2000–20,000 WBC/mm³ (>90% PMN); RBC rare; no organisms on Gram stain	~4g/100ml	Normal	Gram staining and culture of bronchial secretions or sputum and effusion
Infectious empyema	Cloudy to purulent thick fluid, difficult to aspirate	10⁴ to >10⁷ WBC/mm³ (>90% PMN), RBC rare; bacteria present on Gram stain	~4g/100ml	Normal, sometimes low	Gram staining and culture of the pleural fluid

WBC, white blood cells; PMN, polymorphonuclear leukocytes; RBC, red blood cells.

culture is positive in no more than 30% of cases. The pleural biopsy, provided it produces several fragments of pleural tissue, demonstrates typical caseating granulomas in 75% of cases. Thus, it is the examination of choice for making the diagnosis, although obtaining a technically adequate biopsy specimen may be difficult.

PULMONARY INFECTIONS

Finally, pleural effusions that accompany pulmonary infections due to pyogenic organisms can be of two types. Metapneumonic effusions occurring in the course of bacterial pneumonias manifest themselves by the development of pleuritic pain and fever. Auscultation often reveals a pleural friction rub, followed by a loss of vocal fremitus with the presence of local breath sounds just at the superior limit of the silent zone. The fluid is generally easy to obtain by aspiration: it contains a large number of white blood cells, more than half of which are neutrophils. Microscopic examination does not show any bacteria, and the culture is sterile. Generally, the effusion disappears with the resolution of the underlying pneumonia.

Occasionally, however, the effusion is of a totally different nature: the bacteria penetrate the pleural surface and produce a purulent infection within the pleural space, that is, an empyema. A smear reveals vast numbers of neutrophils, often in clumps. Microscopic examination reveals the causative organism, and the culture is usually positive. The conditions necessary for the culture and the microorganisms responsible are discussed in Objective 10–4. These infectious pleural effusions persist for long periods of time if they are not drained effectively because the host defense mechanisms seem to be incapable of controlling these space-occupying infections, even with the help of seemingly appropriate antibiotic therapy.

Pleural exudates can be secondary to an intra-abdominal process: both subdiaphragmatic and hepatic abscesses can manifest themselves either by the appearance of pleural effusions with "metapneumonic" characteristics or by a direct purulent extension across the diaphragm. Acute pancreatitis may also provoke a left-sided, right-sided, or bilateral pleural effusion with inflammatory characteristics and an elevated amylase level. Finally, eosinophils in the pleural fluid are seen with tumors as well as during the course of a pneumothorax.

> **Objective 10–4. Identify the microorganisms responsible for a pleural effusion.**

All effusions suspected of being exudates should be cultured without delay, immediately after aspiration of the pleural fluid.

CULTURE MEDIA

Blood and chocolate agar are the most suitable media for the isolation of the most frequently encountered bacteria,, such as pneumococci, staphylococci, and *Haemophilus influenzae*. In addition, a selective medium for gram-negative microorganisms should also be inoculated, particularly in patients with hospital-acquired pneumonias and effusions, which are often due to gram-negative bacteria. One should not omit a culture of the fluid for strict anaerobes as well. These organisms are responsible both for a majority of aspiration pneumonias and for the greater part of empyemas in patients hospitalized for bronchial aspiration. Obtaining an adequate anaerobic culture involves not only the immediate transport of the specimen to the laboratory and the use of an anaerobic transport tube or vial, but equally important, rapid inoculation of the specimen on a prereduced-deoxygenated solid medium and immediate incubation under strict anaerobic conditions. Finally, culture of the fluid on a Löwenstein or a liquid Dubos medium is also recommended for acid-fast bacilli, despite the low level of positive results.

"METAPNEUMONIC" EFFUSIONS VERSUS EMPYEMAS

Which microorganisms are responsible for metapneumonic effusions and which for em-

Table 10-2. Organisms Responsible for the Development of an Empyema

Organism responsible	Clinical characteristics	Population at high risk
Streptococcus pneumoniae	Bronchopneumonia or lobar pneumonia usually unilobar	Alcoholics
Staphylococcus aureus	Often multiple foci of bronchopneumonia	Infants, addicts, postoperative patients
Group A streptococci	Effusion minimally purulent, sometimes hemorrhagic	
Haemophilus influenzae	Tendency to rapid loculation	Children, older adults (alcoholics with chronic bronchitis)
Mixed anaerobic flora	Nauseating odor to fluid; often air-fluid level on chest roentgenogram	After aspiration (coma, convulsions, acute alcoholism)
Gram-negative bacilli	Effusion often minimally purulent; tendency to form bronchopleural fistula	Intensive care patients; patients undergoing endotracheal intubation
Mycoplasma pneumoniae	Large effusions rare, empyema exceptional	Primarily children and adolescents

pyemas, and what clinical findings point to one or the other of these bacteria? Table 10-2 partially answers these questions: In case of a metapneumonic serous effusion, the origin of the pneumonitis can be determined by means of a careful clinical examination and a smear and culture of the sputum or tracheobronchial secretions obtained under favorable conditions. Empyemas are most frequently due to such pyogenic organisms as pneumococci and staphylococci; the pus in these cases is often viscous and is consequently difficult to aspirate. Empyemas due to group A streptococci are, however, less tenacious and are often slightly hemorrhagic. Gram-negative bacteria, frequently the cause of empyemas in hospitalized, intubated patients, usually produce less of a pleural reaction than the usual pyogenic organisms previously mentioned. Finally, anaerobic organisms, often isolated from aspiration pneumonias, produce a thin, "dishwater" pus that is gray, black, or brown in color and usually has a nauseating odor. Usually these organisms are isolated in mixed culture.

"STERILE" EMPYEMAS

Occasionally, the physician is faced with the clinical paradox of a "sterile" empyema: the pleural exudate has the cytologic and other characteristics of an empyema, but the culture is sterile. Generally, this phenomenon can be explained by inadequate transport or improper culturing procedures of a fragile organism such as pneumococci or anaerobes. Sometimes, the empyema is loculated, and the encapsulated area with the active infection is not aspirated. In some rare cases, the effusions are caused by an organism for which no adequate routine medium exists, such as *Mycoplasma pneumoniae*, which should be considered in patients with persistent bronchitis, malaise, and atypical shifting pulmonary infiltrates, especially in patients with hemolytic anemia.

> Objective 10-5. Plan the treatment for a pleural effusion of infectious origin.

TUBERCULOUS EFFUSIONS

The treatment of tuberculous effusions is discussed here only briefly because this disorder is considered in detail in Chapter 8. The majority of these effusions are the result of dissemination from a primary infection with local reactivation, a situation in which conventional antituberculous treatment is generally adequate and in which major problems of bacterial resistance should not be found. Nevertheless, whenever *Mycobacterium tuberculosis* is isolated in culture, it is wise to submit the organism to sensitivity testing. Concomitant administration of corticosteroids has been recommended by some authors, but efficacy of these agents has not been demonstrated, although they at least have the advantage of rapidly improving the clinical symptoms. The pleural fluid should be removed by thoracentesis whenever possible because its high protein content often prevents its spontaneous and complete reabsorption.

METAPNEUMONIC EFFUSIONS

For metapneumonic effusions, treatment of the underlying pneumonia is all that is necessary. Some authors have proposed increasing the dose of penicillin to 10 million U/day or more when such an effusion is present, to treat or to avoid an incipient infection of the fluid collection. This recommendation is based more on theoretic considerations than on clinical data or solid experimental evidence, and I do not think it appropriate in all situations. On the other hand, some infected effusions are loculated; the pleural fluid sample obtained is not always representative of the whole of the effusion. When fever persists, a second aspiration may reveal a small, as yet undiagnosed, empyema; however, an uninfected, persistent pleural effusion can itself cause a lingering, low-grade fever.

EMPYEMAS

In patients diagnosed as having empyema, parenteral antibiotic therapy against the organism seen on smear or cultured from the pleural fluid should be started immediately. Pneumococci, as well as group A streptococci and nearly all respiratory anaerobes, can be treated with penicillin G at 12 to 24 million U/day. Ampicillin can be used against sensitive *Haemophilus influenzae*, and the penicillinase-resistant penicillins such as oxacillin and nafcillin are appropriate for *Staphylococcus aureus*. For ampicillin-resistant *H. influenzae*, chloramphenicol, cefotaxime, or other third-generation cephalosporins (see Table 13–7) are the agents of choice. Gram-negative nosocomial empyemas cannot be treated definitively without resorting to antibiotic sensitivity testing, although the newer cephalosporins may offer an initial, presumptive therapeutic approach. Use of the direct injection of antibiotics or proteolytic enzymes into the pleuritic space has lost its popularity because of its lack of effectiveness, the rapid transport of the drugs across the pleural surface, and the occasionally severe local or general febrile reactions to the injections of these products.

Surgical Treatment. This method of treating empyema is of major importance. Repeated aspiration or closed-tube drainage of the purulent material allows the pleural space to close and improves the efficacy of antibiotic therapy. The drainage tube should remain in place until the space closes, the fever abates, and the drainage is less than 100 ml/24 hours.

If these measures are not successful, recourse to open drainage of the pleural space will become necessary, to sever the adhesions and to evacuate the purulent material adequately. Such surgical intervention must not be delayed too long, particularly if the patient remains febrile and if the pH of the purulent pleural fluid stays below 7.25, a sign of unresolved infection.

SUGGESTED READINGS

Berger, H.W., and Mejia, E.: Tuberculous pleurisy. Chest, 63:88, 1973.

Black, L.F.: The pleural space and pleural fluid. Mayo Clin. Proc., 47:493, 1972.

Chernow, B., and Sahn, S.A.: Carcinomatous involvement of the pleura: an analysis of 96 patients. Am. J. Med., 63:695, 1977.

Lew, P.D., et al.: Decreased heat-labile opsonic activity and complement levels associated with evidence of C3 breakdown products in infected pleural effusions. J. Clin. Invest., 63:326, 1979.

Potts, D.E., Levin, D.C., and Sahn, S.A.: Pleural fluid pH in parapneumonic effusions. Chest, 70:328, 1976.

Storey, D.D., Dines, D.E., and Coles, D.T.: Pleural effusion: a diagnostic dilemma. JAMA, 236:2183, 1976.

Weese, W.C., Shindler, E.R., Smith, I.M., and Rabinovich, S.: Empyema of the thorax then and now: a study of 122 cases over four decades. Arch. Intern. Med., 131:516, 1973.

CHAPTER 11

How to Approach a Fever

M. Armengaud

> **Objective 11–1. Evaluate the severity of a fever.**

In most cases, fever in itself does not have serious implications; however, if severe it sometimes becomes a medical emergency.

FEVER IN INFANTS

In the young infant, major hyperpyrexia is potentially responsible for delirium, coma, convulsions, and dehydration. Biochemical evaluation demonstrates effects on the liver (elevated transpeptidases), the kidney (raised creatinine), and the muscles (increased creatinine phosphokinase). The consequences can be serious, if not fatal. Therefore, everything must be done to prevent a small infant from developing and maintaining an extremely high temperature.

MALIGNANT HYPERTHERMIA

A medical emergency can also arise during the administration of anesthesia, when a few rare individuals develop malignant hyperthermia, a condition that responds only if recognized early and treated with forced cooling. At any age, fever above 40° C (104° F) contributes to the discomfort of the patient and can play a role in the severity of septic shock. The patient usually becomes unconscious at 42° C (107.6° F) and rarely survives above 42.2° C (108° F). In addition, patients with particular problems, such as cardiac or pulmonary insufficiency, have difficulty tolerating even a small amount of hyperpyrexia because it decompensates their already fragile cardiopulmonary equilibrium.

OTHER CIRCUMSTANCES AND RESPONSE

A clinical appreciation of the patient's degree of fever tolerance can be obtained from the pulse, respiratory rate, blood pressure, and level of consciousness. These simple measures permit one to detect the first signs of a fever-related acid-base imbalance or diencephalic involvement without elaborate laboratory apparatus. Polypnea or rapid breathing is possibly the first and best sign that the fever is poorly tolerated. In such a case, the physician should attempt to reduce the fever without delay.

If common antipyretic agents are ineffective, or if action must be taken immediately, some "heroic" measures can be attempted. Small infants can be placed in a cool bath, with the water temperature at 36 to 38° C (97 to 101° F) for 5 minutes. For an older child, a wet sheet can be placed on top of the bare body, or alcohol sponges may be laid across the chest. In the adult, ice packs can be positioned over the major superficial vessels in

> **MECHANISMS OF A FEVER**
>
> A fever is a temperature above 37° C (98.6° F) in the morning and above 37.5° C (99.5° F) in the afternoon if taken rectally in an individual at rest; taken orally, a fever is above 36.7° C (98.1° F) in the morning and 37.2° C (99° F) in the afternoon. The determination of a patient's temperature is an essential part of every complete medical examination. Omission of this step may permit a low-grade febrile disorder, such as subacute endocarditis, to go undetected. The physician should take and should read the temperature himself in order to avoid errors of transmission. By this procedure, one often detects a number of otherwise unrecognized fevers, and one may thereby unmask factitious ones.
>
> In the course of infectious or inflammatory diseases, fever is produced by the action of substances called pyrogens, which are either endogenous, from the cells of the host, or exogenous, from sources other than the host, mostly bacterial. Whether the stimulus is exogenous or endogenous, an endogenous pyrogen represents the final common pathway. A molecule of 10,000 to 20,000 daltons is released by granulocytes, monocytes, and tissue macrophages. The lymphocytes play an indirect role by secreting a lymphokine, which, in turn, is capable of inducing the granulocytes to produce endogenous pyrogens. The main exogenous stimuli are the lipopolysaccharide endotoxins of gram-negative bacteria. Gram-positive cocci and viruses have no special pathway; their action is similar to that of inert particles of colloidal gold, iron oxide, kaolin, or dextran, which are capable of producing fever when they are injected into the blood. Their phagocytosis by granulocytes and the inflammation they induce are the steps usually necessary to produce a fever. Soluble antigen-antibody complexes help to produce fever in hypersensitivity reactions.
>
> In addition to its appearance in conjunction with infectious or inflammatory diseases, fever can also occur when the host is no longer able to control either heat production or heat loss. The body prevents overheating by sweating and by a vasodilation that directs the blood flow toward the skin. This control is more difficult when the ambient air is saturated with water vapor or when the patient's serum osmolarity is high. Therefore, sweating is less effective, and one's temperature increases under these conditions. The body's ability to regulate cold or "overcooling" involves shivering and increasing the metabolic rate, to raise the body temperature. The equilibrium between heat production and heat loss is controlled by centers located in the hypothalamus that are regulated at about 37° C (98.6° F). Raising the equilibrium point engenders shivering; lowering the point, sweating. This phenomenon occurs in a typical, high, intermittent fever. Dehydration, anticholinergic drugs that impede sweating and heat loss, and thyroid hormones or dinitrophenol, as well as similar drugs that uncouple oxidation-phosphorylation and produce accelerated glycolysis, either increase heat production or reduce heat loss to the point at which metabolic or toxic fever results.
>
> Major alterations in thermoregulation depend upon the secretion of epinephrine, norepinephrine, serotonin, and the prostaglandins. Acetyl-salicylic acid (aspirin) appears to act by suppressing the synthesis of some pyrogenic prostaglandins. This drug may also slow the release of endogenous pyrogen from granulocytes; its mechanism of action remains to be demonstrated.

the groin, axilla, neck, and occasionally, the chest and upper abdomen, or a cooling blanket can be applied either alone or in conjunction with wet sheets or alcohol sponging.

In malignant hyperthermia caused by halothane, succinylcholine, or methoxyflurane, or during the course of encephalitic syndromes, small doses of morphine may be used for vasodilation, in addition to the techniques already mentioned. In Europe, 3 to 6 ml Laborit's mixture (chlorpromazine, 50 mg; promethazine, 50 mg; meperidine, 100 mg; and 5% glucose solution, 10 ml) is usually recommended.

FEVER AS A SIGN OF SERIOUS ILLNESS

Fever may also be an essential element in the clinicopathologic picture of a serious illness because it is often the initial warning symptom of an underlying disease.

High fever preceded by initial shaking chills and followed by profuse sweating is an indication of malaria in individuals who have recently returned from areas where the disease is endemic. Severe headache and even minor disturbances of consciousness in these patients should immediately suggest the possibility of pernicious or malignant falciparum malaria. Once the blood smears have been taken, chloroquine or quinine-pyrimethamine therapy can be started, depending upon whether chloroquine-resistant plasmodial strains have been reported from the area visited.

A fever of the same abrupt onset in a patient who has *not* been to an area where malaria is endemic suggests a more mundane septicemia of urinary, biliary, or intestinal origin, usually caused by gram-negative bacilli. Such patients require immediate blood cul-

> **COMMON THERAPEUTIC MEASURES FOR FEBRILE PATIENTS**
>
> The following antipyretic agents are commonly administered:
>
> *Acetyl-salicylic acid* (aspirin): 0.3 to 0.9 g 4 to 6 times a day when the patient's temperature rises above 38.6° C (101.5° F). Injectable intramuscular or intravenous aspirin is seldom used.
>
> *Acetaminophen:* 0.3 to 0.6 g every 4 hours in adults and in older children; 0.1 g 3 to 4 times a day in younger children. The total dose in children is not to exceed 1.2 g/day. Larger doses cause hepatic damage; therefore, the drug should probably not be given to patients with severe liver disease.
>
> *Indomethacin, tolmetin, and the fenamate* derivatives such as *mefenamic acid** have, in addition to their other effects, antipyretic properties that are sometimes spectacular and may produce an apyrexia for 6 hours. It is said that these agents provide a prolonged antipyretic effect only when the causative disease is cancer, leukemia, or a collagen disorder, however, and not when the fever is due to an infection, although this opinion is not confirmed in the literature.
>
> *The corticosteroids* have a spectacular antipyretic activity in rheumatic fever, collagen diseases, vasculitis, and other hypersensitivity states, as well as in tuberculosis and typhoid fever.
>
> Corticosteroids are specifically indicated in severe cases of infectious mononucleosis and in cold hemagglutinin hemolysis accompanied by fever. In febrile patients with lymphomas and solid tumors, corticosteroids are prescribed only when the diagnosis is confirmed and an infectious cause is excluded. The use of these drugs in fevers due to bacterial infections, whether local or generalized, is advisable only when the febrile state is life-threatening. In typhoid fever, for example, even a small dose of a corticosteroid leads to a rapid lowering of the patient's temperature and sometimes to hypothermic levels with arterial hypotension. Similar hypothermic responses occur in tuberculous meningitis. The main indications for corticosteroids in infectious diseases occur in tuberculosis, either miliary or complicated by meningitis, and in pneumonitis with severe hypoxia in which a decrease in the inflammatory reaction may allow the patient to survive until the antimicrobial agents take effect.
>
> The measure most commonly recommended for fever is bedrest. Food should be easy to eat and to digest. In the first few days of the illness, when anorexia is a significant symptom, one must ensure adequate fluid intake. After 3 to 4 days, it may be necessary to coax patients to eat. Hydration by mouth is adequate when specified quantities are taken: in an adult, about 1500 ml basic fluid loss and 400 ml supplementary loss are necessary for every degree of fever. A variety of fluids are acceptable: water, fruit juices that contain both sugar and potassium, skimmed milk, foods without roughage, and of course, the traditional clear vegetable soups or bouillon to provide salt. Sometimes hydration by mouth is insufficient, most commonly in young infants and in the elderly. In such patients, parenteral fluid should be administered without delay. Nursing care takes on tremendous importance in the febrile and dehydrated patient because with proper care one can keep the patient from developing oral candidiasis or decubitus ulcers, to mention only two possible complications.
>
> When the patient is an infant, the following instructions should be given to the parents: dress the child lightly, keep the temperature in the bedroom cool (20° C [68° F]), provide fluids on a 24-hour basis, and maintain a constant surveillance, to prevent the child from struggling or crying, by predicting its needs.

*In the United States this drug is only used for analgesia.

ture and antibiotic therapy based on an informed guess about the nature of the bacteremia.

Fever accompanied by neurologic signs, disturbed consciousness, or a change in behavior strongly suggests a central nervous system infection, encephalitis, meningitis, or abscess and indicates the need for hospitalization and an immediate spinal tap (see Objective 29–1).

A high fever associated with petechiae or purpuric plaques on the trunk and limbs should make the physician suspect a meningococcemia and other infections (see Objective 27–1). If intestinal symptoms such as diarrhea or hemorrhage are present, typhoid or paratyphoid fever should be suspected.

Sometimes, fever is seen in a patient on the verge of shock, with a profound reduction in perfusion and hence hypo-oxygenation of tissues. In such a patient, the first signs of shock may be a peripheral vasoconstriction, and the patient's extremities will be cold and sweaty; mottling of the skin (livido reticularis) is sometimes seen. These signs appear before the patient's blood pressure falls (see Objective 13–4).

All fevers accompanied by acute distress of recent origin, whether respiratory, cardiac, renal, or metabolic (as in diabetic acidosis and adrenal or hepatic insufficiency), demand specific emergency therapy as well as a search for an inciting or accompanying infectious disease.

Fever in the last trimester of pregnancy is ominous and suggests a septicemia such as listeriosis. Immediate therapy is required in order to protect the fetus (see Objective 24–3).

All fevers in the newborn, up to 2 to 3 months of age, must be treated without delay. Hospitalization, blood culture, and lumbar puncture are essential because the two life-threatening problems in this age group are septicemia and meningitis (see Objective 24–4).

Any fever in a neutropenic patient (< 500 granulocytes/mm^3) requires hospitalization and immediate antibiotic therapy to cover the vast range of possible gram-positive and gram-negative bacterial pathogens (see Objective 33–5).

> **Objective 11–2.** Identify the most likely causes of a recent fever with clinical and simple laboratory or radiologic evidence.

Fever is a common symptom compatible with a broad spectrum of causes. Once the physician is sure that no emergency measures have to be taken, he must strive to discover the fever's origin, with the help of an extensive medical history, epidemiologic or seasonal evidence, a complete clinical examination, and subsequent, appropriate, first-line laboratory tests.

FEVER WITH LOCALIZED SIGNS AND SYMPTOMS

The diagnostic process is much easier when the patient has signs or symptoms of the malfunctioning of an organ or of a physiologic system. A cough, dysuria, or diarrhea usually indicates that the fever's origin is in the pulmonary, urinary, or gastrointestinal tract. Then, it is no longer a matter of diagnosing and treating a fever, but of evaluating, confirming, and treating an infection in these specific areas.

Some simple procedures can be useful in detecting overlooked infections: placing pressure over the patient's sinuses, examination of the teeth and gums, inspection for Koplik's spots (measles) and for a possible tumefaction of the parotid canal orifice (mumps), rectal and vaginal examination, inspection of intravenous and intramuscular injection sites, inspection of the scalp for tick bites or abscesses, and percussion of the costovertebral areas. Pressure or percussion over the dorsal processes of the vertebrae may provide the clue needed to detect a spondylitis or an epidural abscess. Careful palpation of different lymph node areas, including the epitrochlear, sometimes leads to the diagnosis of local infection or lymphoma. Visceral involvement may be minimal or slow in appearing, however, and daily examination of the febrile patient is therefore obligatory for early diagnosis of the condition.

Disseminated or diffuse infectious processes involve more than one organ system. Each organ is not necessarily affected by a separate process, and all such processes may have a single origin.

FEVER WITHOUT LOCALIZED SIGNS AND SYMPTOMS

Where no localization can be found, diagnostic clues may be obtained from the patient's medical history or from epidemiologic evidence, as illustrated in the following paragraphs.

Thrombophlebitis and Embolism. Fevers may be caused by thrombophlebitis and embolism, which may not be obvious on superficial inspection of the patient's arms or legs because these disorders may involve the deep veins of the legs or the pelvis. Such silent pulmonary emboli may be evident only by changes in the pulmonary scan or by linear opacities at the pulmonary base, sometimes visible only on lateral chest films. This possibility should be considered in aged or bedridden patients who have spent a prolonged convalescence immobilized. In this type of patient, the diagnosis may be particularly difficult. Heparin therapy has had a spectacular effect, and a trial of this therapy may confirm a diagnosis based on presumptions made from the patient's medical history or the unequal warmth or volume of the patient's legs.

Myocardial Infarction. In a patient who

has suffered a myocardial infarction, Dressler's syndrome may cause persistent fever.

Drug-Associated Fever. Such fevers are becoming more and more frequent, probably because of the increasing use and consumption of new pharmaceutic agents. A number of these products are known to cause prolonged fever in many patients; for example, penicillins and cephalosporins in high dose, sulfonamides, isoniazid, para-aminosalicylic acid, barbiturates, phenothiazines, minor tranquilizers, allopurinol, atropine and haloperidol by inhibition of sweating, quinidine, procainamides, and hydantoins. Fever has been observed in patients taking alpha-methyldopa and in those taking birth control pills. In fact, all drugs can be the potential source of fever, usually low-grade, but occasionally elevated. Because of this possibility, all previous medication should be discontinued when a physician is trying to discover the reason for a long-term fever.

Factitious Fever. Fevers may be factitious. These types of fevers are, unfortunately, not rare. The physician must consider the patient's psychologic motivation carefully and must handle the situation tactfully because the fever may be a means of attracting attention and perhaps of asking for help. Sometimes, other members of the family are part of the conspiracy. The physician should, therefore, use his own or the institution's thermometer and take the temperature personally, to prevent the substitution of a thermometer with a prearranged reading. A factitious fever can always be checked by taking the temperature of a freshly voided urine specimen, which is ordinarily about 1° C (1.8° F) lower than the rectal temperature.

Tropical Diseases. Fevers may be caused by tropical diseases, mostly malaria and hepatic amebiasis, which can be diagnosed without too much difficulty, provided one thinks about them. Malaria is confirmed by a blood smear, and hepatic amebiasis by amebic serologic study and liver scanning.

Occupational Exposure. The diagnosis of fever due to occupational exposure is suggested by specific items in the patient's medical history: factory workers may be exposed to zinc-cadmium metal fumes, polymers, dinitrocresol, and other organic nitrates, slaughterhouse workers may be exposed to brucella, and sewer workers may be exposed to leptospira.

Immunologic Status of Patient. Knowledge of the immunologic status of the patient allows the physician to anticipate abnormal host responses to infection and to foresee certain peculiarities in the clinical picture. Immunosuppression generally favors abnormal clinical presentations of infection, frequently nosocomial in origin, due to unusual organisms, often resistant to conventional therapy. The responses of the host to the organism in the course of an infection often form a special clinical picture for each type of patient. Patients with normal responses develop the typical or "classic" forms of the disease. Such signs may be abrupt and violent, such as in meningococcemia, or insidious and progressive, such as in pulmonary tuberculosis. Individuals with diminished responsiveness have attenuated reactions and symptoms that are barely recognizable, if present at all. It is, therefore, important to gauge the patient's whole condition ("terrain") by more than a cursory glance at general health, age, or color. Possible defects such as diabetes, cirrhosis, and respiratory, cardiac, or renal insufficiency, as well as the role of certain relevant medications, such as corticosteroids and cytotoxic and immunosuppressant drugs, must also be taken into consideration.

ISOLATED FEVERS

Some fevers appear to be isolated, with no other visible signs or symptoms. In such a case, the search for the origin of the fever is difficult. The diagnosis must then depend on the characteristics of the fever itself and on routine laboratory tests.

Clinical Features. The clinical characteristics of an isolated fever are simply the symptoms accompanying the elevated temperature. A rapidly rising fever produces shaking chills; when it falls rapidly, profuse sweating results. These pseudomalarial types of fevers are seen in pyelonephritis, ascending cholangitis, and septicemia. The opposite symptom, that is, the absence of chills and fever, is noted when the fever plateaus and when the daily fluctuations in temperature are less than 1° C (2° F).

The myalgias that almost always accompany a fever are particularly severe in leptospirosis, some enteroviral infections, and arboviruses (dengue), whereas arthralgias are seen in all rheumatic disorders, the preicteric phase of hepatitis B virus infections, septicemic brucellosis, Lyme arthritis, rubella (although usually accompanied by a rash), and gonococcal septicemia. Stiffness and aching, aside from muscle or joint tenderness, are found with nearly all fevers; however, they are sometimes totally absent. The symptoms are not characteristic of any particular disorder, but instead constitute the basis for the older terms "flu syndrome" or "the grippe."

Alteration in the patient's general condition, such as insomnia, loss of appetite, and loss of weight and energy, are also observed in nearly all high or prolonged fevers. Insomnia is common in typhoid fever, anorexia and changes in the taste of food and cigarettes in viral hepatitis, prostration and loss of energy in brucellosis and in polyarteritis nodosa, and rapid weight loss in malignant diseases. The patient may, however, retain his appetite in brucellosis and in early local forms of tuberculosis, little asthenia may be present in Q fever, and a moderate loss of weight (less than 10% of body weight) may occur in all the severe infectious diseases mentioned previously.

The form of the temperature curve itself may suggest (1) malaria (tertian or quartan fever); or (2) borreliosis, leptospirosis, or brucellosis (recurrent fever).

Laboratory and Radiologic Findings. On the other hand, the laboratory and radiologic findings are useful in emergencies when the fever is poorly tolerated. Laboratory tests should be performed systematically if the patient's fever is abnormally prolonged, for example, after the third or fifth day, depending on the severity of the fever. The following procedures are the first line of investigation recommended in the course of any unusually severe or abnormally prolonged fever:

1. Blood cultures may be used to detect the presence of septicemia. Negative results generally eliminate the diagnosis unless effective antibiotics were previously administered or unless the organism is fragile, fastidious in its growth requirements, or slow growing.
2. A white blood cell count may be useful, mainly to detect polymorphonuclear leukocytosis. Some viral infections, typhoid fever, and brucellosis can produce a polymorphonuclear leukopenia with reversal of the usual adult white blood cell ratio. A predominance of monocytes or atypical lymphocytes raises the possibility of viral hepatitis, cytomegalovirus, or infectious mononucleosis, eosinophilia, parenchymal parasitic infection, or an allergic reaction. AIDS shows a lymphopenia.
3. A sedimentation rate above 80 mm/hour, much higher than usually noted in fever, points to rheumatic fever, a collagen vascular disorder, a circulating immune complex disease, a hypersensitivity reaction, or, sometimes, a deep abscess.
4. A chest roentgenogram may disclose an unsuspected pulmonary infiltrate, often seen in mycoplasma, Q fever, and chlamydial infections.
5. Microscopic examination and culture of the urine, usually performed in the physician's office, may reveal bacteria in an otherwise poorly symptomatic pyelonephritis.

Objective 11–3. Approach a prolonged fever of undetermined origin (FUO).

A fever of unknown origin (FUO) is traditionally defined as a medically verified fever with no known cause after 21 days of well-conducted medical investigation.

FUOs can be classified as follows: infection

Table 11-1. Classification of Fevers of Undetermined Origin (FUO)

Cause of Fever	Recommended Treatment
Septicemia, such as from endocarditis, with fastidious or metabolically deficient organisms	
Various infections: salmonellosis, such as typhoid, osteomyelitis, or endarteritis, borreliosis, rat-bite fever (sodoku), rickettsiosis, such as recurrent or murine typhus, yersiniosis	
Osteomyelitis, chiefly vertebral	
Ascending cholangitis	
Miliary, hepatic, bone, peritoneal, or pelvic tuberculosis; pulmonary tuberculosis is too readily detectable by chest roentgenograms to constitute an FUO	Antimicrobial Chemotherapy (Antibiotic or Antiparasitic)
Hepatic granulomatosis	
Whipple's disease or Crohn's disease, granulomatous colitis	
Deep mycoses, such as cryptococcus, histoplasmosis, coccidioidomycosis, and paracoccidioidomycosis, and many other fungal and yeast infections in the immunosuppressed	
Trypanosomiasis	
Amebic and pyogenic liver abscesses	
Urinary infections in the male infant, nearly always associated with obstruction	
Deep abscess: hepatic, subphrenic, abdominal, retrocecal, retroperitoneal, appendiceal, pancreatic, pelvic, perinephric, prostatic, and cerebral	
Deep abscesses resulting from prior surgical or endoscopic procedures	Surgical Intervention
Foci of latent infection in the teeth, bone, or other otorhinolaryngeal localizations	
Malignant tumors of some organs, such as kidney, colon, pancreas, lung, stomach, brain, and thyroid; unfortunately, at present, this type of operation is performed primarily to confirm the diagnosis	
Leukemias, Hodgkin's and non-Hodgkin's lymphomas, hepatoma, and, in some cases, carcinomatosis	Cytotoxic Therapy
Collagenoses: lupus erythematosus, periarteritis nodosa, polymyositis	Anti-Inflammatory or Immunosuppressive Therapy
Acute rheumatic fever, sarcoidosis, thyroiditis, Still's disease, and Crohn's disease	

(40%), lymphoma and other malignant diseases (20%), and collagen, hypersensitivity, or autoimmune disorders (15%). This division accounts for most FUOs, but exact causes vary with the patient's age. Below the age of 6 years, generalized or respiratory viral infections or urinary infections associated with obstruction (in male infants) are the most frequent causes. Later on, through puberty, juvenile rheumatoid arthritis is a likely cause. In the adult, the percentage of fever with malignant diseases increases with age. In indigent adults, more than half the time the cause is tuberculosis, whereas in the affluent, it is usually a lymphoma or another malignant disorder.

When the fever persists for several months, infectious causes are less frequent, and the incidence of granulomatoses, such as of the liver, sarcoidosis, Crohn's disease, pulmonary angiitis, and vasculitis, juvenile rheumatoid arthritis, Still's disease, and malignant disorders rises.

The diagnosis must be clearly established before the physician should consider antimicrobial therapy with toxic agents such as amphotericin B, surgical intervention, and administration of corticosteroids or other potentially hazardous anti-inflammatory chemotherapeutic methods. Sonography and CT

Table 11-2. Chief Metabolic Causes of Fevers of Undetermined Origin (FUO)

Hyperthyroidism, principally thyroid storm
Pancreatitis
Familial periodic fever
Fabry's disease
Hyperglyceridemia and familial hypercholesterolemia
Cyclic neutropenia
Exaggeration of the normal circadian rhythm of temperature (neurologic fever?)

scanning are helpful in difficult cases; the classic laparotomy is seldom ordered nowadays (Tables 11–1 and 11–2).

INFECTIONS

The diagnosis and treatment of the FUO described in Table 11–1 vary according to the suspected category of the fever.

For infections, a logical approach is to identify the organism by culture or serologic study. Thus, abnormalities, clinical findings, or test results, once noted, should be pursued to verify the diagnosis; for example, biopsy should be performed on an enlarged liver with an elevated alkaline phosphatase level because it may reveal a granulomatous hepatitis. In some cases, it may be necessary to start therapy before definitive answers are available, either because of the urgent and serious nature of the illness or because of the slow growth of the organism in culture. For example, the *Mycobacterium tuberculosis* takes up to 6 weeks to grow on the Löwenstein-Jensen medium; therefore, it is usually necessary to begin therapy before the culture results are available.

In fact, the quality of the bacteriologic samples, the culturing on various specific media, and the use of modern serodiagnostic techniques, such as enzyme-linked immunosorbent assay (ELISA) and gas chromatography, provide the basic and essential knowledge required for many diagnoses. A systematic search for deep foci of infection in the head, neck, liver, and pelvis, best identified by nontraumatic diagnostic procedures, such as roentgenograms, isotope scans, sonographic examination, and CT scans, should also be conducted.

MALIGNANT DISEASE

For the diagnosis of malignant disease, further development of CT scans should eventually replace many other, less-useful procedures. The alpha-fetoprotein and carcinoembryonic antigen tests are useful, although nonspecific to the cell type or location. Radiographic studies of the particular organ suspected, such as the lung, colon, and bone, isotope scans of the liver, lung, and bone or whole-body gallium scans, and sonographic examination should constitute the first line of investigation. These procedures can be accompanied and extended by a variety of endoscopic tests, for example, of the stomach, lungs, and colon. Arteriography may also prove useful as a secondary procedure. For lymphomas, biopsies of the enlarged lymph nodes, and occasionally even lymphangiography, are the procedures of choice. For leukemias, bone marrow aspiration or biopsy are standard investigative techniques. More aggressive diagnostic procedures should be a last resort. In the absence of specific local findings, exploratory laparotomy is contraindicated because its usefulness is questionable.

INFLAMMATIONS

For inflammatory disorders, initial investigations should include the following tests: antistreptolysin O (ASLO), antinuclear antibody, serum iron, serum haptoglobins, protein electrophoresis, and biopsy of skin lesions or, if involved, the temporal artery. Skin, muscle, or liver biopsies, along with the Coombs test and tests for antimitochondrial or thyroid antibodies and immune complexes, are then indicated if the diagnosis is still in doubt. Treatment with corticosteroids constitutes too broad a therapeutic test to be diagnostic. When all signs indicate an inflammatory, noninfectious disorder, however, corticosteroids should be administered in large doses initially. The doses may then be progressively reduced.

At least 10% of FUO fail to reveal their origin, but they do spontaneously regress after several months. Most of the foregoing investigative procedures are best performed in a hospital. Many may be accomplished in extended-care facilities offering daytime hospitalization, thus permitting the patient to remain in contact with his family. For individuals who live far from outpatient diagnostic centers, hospitalization is suggested from the tenth day of such a fever.

SUGGESTED READINGS

Atkins, E., and Bodel, P.: Fever. N. Engl. J. Med., 286:27, 1972.

Dinarello, C.A., and Wolff, S.M.: Molecular basis of fever in humans. Am. J. Med., 72:799, 1982.

Dinarello, C.A., and Wolff, S.M.: Fever of unknown origin and approach to the patient with fever of unknown origin. *In* Principles and Practice of Infectious Diseases. Edited by G.L. Mandell, R.G. Douglas, Jr., and J.E. Bennett. New York, John Wiley and Sons, 1979.

Jacoby, G.A., and Swartz, M.N.: Fever of undetermined origin. N. Engl. J. Med., 289:1407, 1973.

Petersdorf, R.G., and Beeson, P.B.: Fever of unexplained origin: report of 100 cases. Medicine, 40:1, 1961.

Wolff, S.M., Fauci, A.S., and Dale, D.C.: Unusual etiologies of fever and their evaluation. Annu. Rev. Med., 26:227, 1975.

CHAPTER 12

Fever in the Drug User

C. Cherubin

Objective 12–1. Determine the site of the infection and specify the nature of the infecting organism in the drug addict with a fever.

Most recognized complications of narcotic drug abuse either have an infectious cause or are associated with common complications of infectious diseases. Thus, the differential diagnosis of fever in a narcotic addict encompasses virtually the entire list of the medical sequelae of drug use (Table 12–1). This chapter proceeds from the most frequent and best recognized of these disease entities and moves in order of their frequency, to those rare and uncertain disease associations that usually do not produce fever.

ABSCESSES AND CELLULITIS

The most common cause of emergency room visits and surgical hospitalization for addicts is superficial soft tissue infection. The infection sites cluster around those areas most often used for injection, that is, the forearms, thighs, and deltoid muscles, and the lesions are usually obvious on casual inspection and palpation. The associated thrombophlebitis may be missed unless the course of the neighboring veins is palpated.

At least half these infections are due to coagulase-positive staphylococci and are typical of lesions caused by these organisms in their similarity to an abscess or cellulitis in other patients. Occasionally, a group A streptococcus is found. Again, the infection is typical for this organism, with less swelling, heat, and tenderness locally than a staphylococcal cellulitis, but with more generalized toxicity and more frequent septicemia. A considerable number of these abscesses are caused not by a single pathogen, but instead by a mixed flora (Table 12–1). These abscesses are usually more indolent and chronic than those due to staphylococci alone. Surgical drainage is of primary importance, and it is not necessary to select an antibiotic directed against *all* bacteria isolated from the lesion.

In general, the temperature of patients with these superficial infections seldom rises above 38° C (102° F), and systemic toxicity and septicemia are unusual, except when group A streptococci are involved.

Unlike superficial infections, anaerobic cellulitis and necrotizing fasciitis, which usually occur on the lower half of the body, are deep, intensely painful infections of the soft tissues generally caused by a mixed flora (Table 12–1) and accompanied by high fever, toxicity, and leukocytosis. Necrotizing fasciitis, in particular, is characterized by hard, painful swelling of the deep facial planes and is unresponsive to antibiotics alone. This disorder

Table 12–1. Causes of Fever in Drug Addicts

Disorder	Organism(s) Responsible
Abscesses and cellulitis	*Staphylococcus aureus,* beta-hemolytic streptococci (rarely *Streptococcus pneumoniae* or *Haemophilus influenzae* B), or mixed infections, gram-negative aerobes, microaerophilic and anaerobic streptococci; *Streptococcus mullerii;* bacteroides; and *Eikenella corrodens* Anaerobic cellulitis with anaerobic streptococci, bacteroides, or clostridia species Necrotizing faciitis due to a mixture of aerobes and anaerobes
Septic phlebitis	Mainly *Staphylococcus aureus* and group A beta-hemolytic streptococci
Pneumonia	Mainly pneumococci, but aspiration pneumonia with a mixed flora occurs with overdoses or endotracheal intubation *Staphylococcus aureus,* mainly due to tricuspid endocarditis Klebsiella or proteus, usually upper-lobe, necrotizing pneumonias Beta-hemolytic streptococci, usually secondary to septic phlebitis
Tuberculosis	*Mycobacterium tuberculosis*
Solitary lung abscess	Usually mixed flora
Overdose with pulmonary edema	Unknown whether fever is transient in this syndrome or whether caused by bacterial superinfection
Endocarditis	50 to 60% due to *Staphylococcus aureus;* most hospitalized cases involve the tricuspid valve, but rapidly fulminating cases involve the aortic and mitral valves; 20% are due to various streptococcus (including viridans groups, microaerobes, and anaerobes) and enterococci 20% due to various gram-negative aerobes: *Pseudomonas aeruginosa* (rarely *P. cepasia*), serratia, and Klebsiella Fewer than 1% of cases are due to candida, and a fraction of 1% are polymicrobial, including bacteroides and haemophilus
Septic arthritis and osteomyelitis (usually of the spine)	*Staphylococcus aureus,* gram-negative bacteria (predominantly pseudomonas and serratia), and *Mycobacterium tuberculosis* (Pott's disease)
Tetanus	*Clostridium tetani;* does not produce fever initially, but aspiration pneumonia and hyperpyrexia during generalized convulsions are usually seen
Angiitis	Secondary to intravenous catecholamine (metamphetamine) abuse, which is fortunately out of fashion
Malaria	Plasmodium species; a disease of the past in drug addicts; the last addiction-transmitted cases were noted in California after the Vietnam War. Could be seen readily in countries with endemic malaria
Cytomegalovirus and hepatitis B virus	Cytomegalovirus infection is only suspected of being an addiction-transmitted disease; hepatitis B virus produces fever, generally only during the prodromal period, unless considerable hepatitic necrosis occurs during the acute phase
Traumatic injury with infections	Various organisms; fever seen in surgical abdomen, gunshot and stab wounds, ruptured viscera, perforated duodenum, appendicitis, ruptured spleen, and pelvic inflammatory disease
Acquired immune deficiency syndrome	Cause unknown; associated with infections caused by *Pneumocystis carinii,* cryptococcus (meningitis), *Toxoplasma gondii, cryptosporidiosis,* and with Kaposi's sarcoma (among others)

requires surgical tension-releasing incisions and drainage. Therapy directed against aerobic gram-negative rods and anaerobic streptococci seems rational.

PNEUMONIA

When a drug user has a fever in the presence of cough, chest pain, or shortness of breath, the diagnosis of pneumonia should be considered.

Even without the intervention of narcotic-induced stupor, vomiting, aspiration, and pulmonary edema, drug users suffer from a remarkable frequency of bacterial pneumonias, at least from the hospital physician's point of view. The majority of these pneumonias are single, lower lobe infiltrates that produce sputum in which pneumococci that respond to penicillin are the predominant organisms. In these patients, however, one also sees aspiration pneumonias, necrotizing pneumonias, solitary lung abscesses, pulmonary tuberculosis, and septic pulmonary embolization. Multilobar infiltrates with staphylococci in the sputum should not be considered as primary staphylococcal pneumonia, which is an unusual event except after an influenza epidemic, but rather should be treated as a staphylococcal tricuspid endocarditis under the classification of "worst possible treatable." The only way in which the diagnosis can be excluded is to stop therapy before 4 weeks have passed and to wait for a relapse—a risky procedure indeed.

DRUG OVERDOSE

If the addict is stuporous and has constricted pupils, then he may have taken an overdose of narcotics. The most common cause of death in narcotic addicts is pharmacologic overdosage, which has several distinctive features, pulmonary edema among them. Half the patients with overdoses seen in emergency rooms have this type of edema, which, incidentally, is not experimentally reproducible and is not due to congestive heart failure. Obviously, a great proportion of those admitted to the hospital mainly because of severe respiratory insufficiency have pulmonary edema. Some authors disagree as to whether an overdose with pulmonary edema can itself produce fever and leukocytosis. Because half the patients with pulmonary edema have one or both of these signs, this clinical problem is considerable. To complicate the situation, the physiologic effects of the narcotic, combined with pharyngeal stimulation during intubation, lead to vomiting and aspiration.

Because one does not definitely know, in an individual case, whether a bacterial pneumonitis is associated with the overdose, it is best to order bronchial aspirate cultures and gram-stained smears and to treat the patient for this condition if bacteria and pus cells are seen. Autopsy evidence suggests that pulmonary infection is universal in those who survive the first 12 hours. Chest films subsequent to clearing of the edema, in 36 to 48 hours, will show any residual consolidation; such a picture suggests a pneumonitis caused by aspiration or superinfection.

BONE AND JOINT INFECTIONS

If the patient has local pain and swelling over a bone or joint, then the possibility of bone and joint infections should be considered. Septic arthritis caused by staphylococci, candida, and gram-negative organisms, predominantly pseudomonas, is seen in drug addicts, even without obvious sources of infection such as a direct injection or endocarditis. One of the joints, the sternoclavicular joint, is seen more commonly in drug users than in others. Localized pain, tenderness, heat, and swelling are clearly more impressive diagnostic clues with staphylococcal infections than with other organisms. Aspiration of joint fluid is the most important diagnostic procedure.

The spine, mainly the lumbar spine, and the pelvis are the most common sites of osteomyelitis. Almost all cases are without known antecedent septicemia and are usually due to pseudomonas or to serratia. Although localized pain and tenderness over the lesion are usually present, fever may be low-grade or absent, and leukocytosis is unusual. Because they cross the vertebral disc and involve two adjacent vertebral bodies, these spinal lesions resemble tuberculous or salmonella spinal osteomyelitis both in this and the previously mentioned characteristics. The final diagnosis can only be made by bone biopsy.

ENDOCARDITIS

Because of the higher mortality rate and the longer duration of therapy needed to treat it, endocarditis must be given priority among the diagnostic possibilities, in line with the general operating principle of considering the worst possible treatable situation. Blood cultures should be taken in any drug addict with fever, myalgias, or malaise.

The acute, fulminant form of the disease is prevalent among drug addicts (Table 12–1), even though the milder, subacute form is usually seen in nonaddicts of the same age. As a consequence, a brief course of symptoms, including high fever and moderate-to-considerable toxicity, is common in addicts with endocarditis. The presence of Osler's nodes, Janeway lesions, or a palpable spleen and a history of pre-existing valvular disease are infrequent findings. Half or more of the cases are due to coagulase-positive staphylococci (Table 12–1); a quarter are caused by various streptococci, of which enterococci are the most important; a fifth or so are produced by a variety of gram-negative rods, especially pseudomonas and serratia; and a small percentage are due to several different species of candida. The last organism, the exception to the stated rule, produces an insidious onset of the disease, which consequently develops with a long symptomatic period, with little or no fever, and a normal leukocyte count. Candidal endocarditis develops only on valves with pre-existing damage and frequently comes to medical attention only when a major arterial embolization occurs.

When the lesion is on the left side of the heart (Table 12–2), the organisms just described, especially staphylococci, rapidly erode the valvular substance so that regur-

Table 12–2. Characteristics of Left- and Right-Sided Endocarditis

Characteristics	Left	Right
Incidence	For hospitalized patients diagnosed during life, usually 40–60%	In autopsied cases, half have tricuspid involvement alone, and half have tricuspid involvement in combination with left-sided lesions; in hospitalized patients diagnosed during life, tricuspid involvement is usually 50–60%
History of underlying heart disease	About 30–40%	Uncommon
Murmurs	Rapidly developing and changing "aortic" diastolic and "mitral" systolic murmurs in 90%	Faint left-sternal-border murmurs are found in about 67% of patients; these may sometimes have a noticeable inspiratory accentuation; in the remaining third, the physical findings have been misleading or even absent (about 10%)
Organism	Mainly *Staphylococcus aureus;* also gram-negative bacteria, various streptococci, and fungi	Virtually all due to *Staphylococcus aureus;* occasionally caused by pseudomonas, serratia, and rarely candida
Course	Fulminant, with frequent valve rupture, and with embolization to brain, heart, and kidney	More slowly progressive; always have septic emboli to lungs; condition may be misdiagnosed as staphylococcal pneumonia or septic pulmonary emboli from phlebitis
Valve	Aortic, mitral, or both	More than 95% are tricuspid; pulmonic valve is involved less than 10% of the time

gitant murmurs are usually present on admission or within a week; catastrophic embolization, congestive heart failure due to aortic valvular perforations, or rupture of the chordae tendineae are considerable hazards. So rapid is the course of this illness that many such patients die of cardiac decompensation or embolization either before hospitalization or immediately afterwards, and before a definitive diagnosis can be reached. Tricuspid valve involvement follows a slightly slower course, with similar fever and toxicity, but with less peripheral evidence of embolization and much less impressive murmurs. A systolic, left-sternal-border ejection murmur of grade 1 to 2/6 or less intensity, usually without clear inspiratory accentuation, is characteristically heard on admission of the patient to the hospital. In a majority of cases, the proper inspiratory accentuation never appears; therefore, little is gained by arguing about its presence. Echocardiography does not identify vegetations on the tricuspid valve with sufficient sensitivity or specificity to be depended upon for the diagnosis.

Because of the infrequency of early congestive heart failure or major systemic embolization in tricuspid endocarditis, such patients account for about half the hospitalized cases of this illness diagnosed during life. Septic pulmonary embolization, characteristic of the involvement of this valve, usually occurs by the second or third week of symptoms. Intense pleuritic pain of sudden onset and dense, irregularly shaped pulmonary infiltrates throughout the lung field, but concentrated towards the bases, which later cavitate, are the manifestations. The emboli may also originate from pelvic or peripheral septic thrombophlebitis. If these possibilities can be eliminated diagnostically, then the tricuspid valve is the only alternative. Severe right-flank pain may indicate splenic infarct or abscess, sometimes seen in endocarditis in addicts. Hematuria, pyuria, and proteinuria are common in staphylococcal endocarditis.

Staphylococcal as well as enterococcal and gram-negative endocarditis (Table 12–2), produces positive blood cultures, no matter what valve they affect. Negative cultures discredit the diagnosis for the specific cause. If the diagnostic possibilities, on hospital admission, lie between endocarditis and another diagnosis, then the rule of "worst possible treatable" indicates treatment for endocarditis initially. After lengthy evaluation, if the diagnosis is still equivocal, no other disease process is indicated, and the initial blood cultures were positive, then the rule requires a complete course of therapy.

Antibiotic therapy for staphylococcal endocarditis without cardiac decompensation is effective if started early, particularly in tricuspid disease (Table 12–3). With the enterococci, it may be difficult to find an antibiotic combination sufficiently active against the particular strain. With gram-negative bacteria, this situation occurs even more frequently, and unless the organism is adequately sensitive to a penicillin or cephalosporin derivative, with or without an aminoglycoside, a medical cure is impossible. Candidal endocarditis requires surgical treatment. When cultures are not positive, often in 48 to 72 hours, the diagnosis of endocarditis can be discarded, and one can start to search for another cause. An exception is candida that may require a week to become evident in blood culture.

TETANUS

The diagnosis of tetanus is not likely to be confused with anything else in the physician's experience because strychnine poisoning is not common these days. Fever is not one of the early features of this disease. Although hyperpyrexia has been noted, presumably from catecholamine excess, when the disease is fully developed, the majority of fevers accompanying tetanus are caused by pulmonary infections. Because drug addicts have a severe form of tetanus progressing to generalized spasms within 24 hours, the diagnosis rapidly becomes evident. These patients should have a tracheostomy before general seizures set in, and they should then be treated for the disease itself.

Table 12-3. Therapy for Endocarditis in Drug Addicts

Origin of Endocarditis	Recommended Drug	Dosage
Initial therapy* and *Staphylococcus aureus* endocarditis†	Semisynthetic penicillins	
	Oxacillin or nafcillin	12 g/day, IV, q4h for 4 weeks
	Cephalosporins	
	Cefazolin (some treatment failures at lower doses)	8–12 g/day; IM or IV doses may be given q6h
	Cefoxitin	12 g/day q4h for 4 weeks
	Ceforonide	2 g q12h
	Cefamandole and cefonicid (definitely not indicated for *S. aureus* endocarditis)	
	Other penicillins	
	Penicillin G	20 million U/day, q4h for nonpenicillinase producers
	Vancomycin‡	25 mg/kg/day q6–8h for 4 weeks
	Clindamycin (not for erythromycin- or, obviously, clindamycin-resistant strains)	3.6–4.8 g/day, IV or IM
	Dicloxicillin, oral not recommended (addict patients walk out of the hospital before treatment is completed, and bactericidal levels are mandatory)	4 g/day with probenecid, 1–2 g/day
Enterococcal endocarditis	Ampicillin and aminoglycoside (bactericidal levels are mandatory; vancomycin may also be used but gentamicin may have to be added)	12 g/day in divided doses with gentamicin, 80 g, IM tid
Pseudomonas	Ticarcillin or mezlocillin, or piperacillin in high doses with tobramycin (therapy is often unsuccessful, and surgical removal of the infected valve is often necessary)	
Serratia	Antibiotic therapy often unsuccessful, but trimethoprim sulfonamide, and gentamicin may be tried; and cefotaxime has had some success	
Candida	Neither amphotericin B nor 5-fluorocytosine nor ketoconazole has been successful (the valve must be removed while the patient is receiving these agents)	

*Initial therapy with a combination of antibiotics is not recommended because no combination adequately covers *Staphylococcus aureus*, enterococci, and the various gram-negative bacteria. Synergistic action against *S. aureus* is not evident, and combined therapy increases the risk of renal toxicity.
†*S. aureus* is the most common and most serious problem in initial therapy.
‡Bactericidal levels can be recommended as appropriate monitoring tests for endocarditis of any origin. In addition, vancomycin levels may be recommended for patients with renal insufficiency. Peak serum levels should be kept above 5.0 meq/ml, although this regimen does not ensure freedom from drug toxicity.

MALARIA AND CYTOMEGALOVIRUS INFECTION

As far as we know, malaria appeared as a complication of drug addiction as soon as the intravenous route of narcotic abuse was adopted. This complication is now uncommon. Some recent infections with *Plasmodium vivax* have been noted in California, but until now, malaria has not reappeared on the East Coast, where *P. falciparum* caused several hundred fatalities among drug users in the 1930s in New York City alone. Nevertheless, in countries where malaria is endemic or imported, a malaria smear is part of the diagnostic workup of a fever of unknown origin in an addict. Wright's stain is satisfactory, if Giemsa's stain is not available, and it usually is not. One must, however, have a competent reader for the slide. Hematologists, even those without any experience with malaria, are usually most helpful.

Occasionally, an addict with a low-grade fever, lymphocytosis, and lymphadenopathy with or without splenomegaly subsequently has high or rising titers of anticytomegalovirus antibody. Whether this disease is transmitted by a shared needle, as it could be, cannot be said with certainty. Yet, this viral agent does appear to be the rare cause of febrile disease in a drug user.

HEPATITIS

As an initial symptom of viral hepatitis, fever is seldom noted clinically in drug addicts. The reason, simply, is that addicts rarely seek medical advice for hepatitis until they have been symptomatic for 1 or 2 weeks. Occasionally, drug users are seen during the prodromal period with skin rash or arthritis, which may be accompanied by fever.

ACQUIRED IMMUNE DEFICIENCY SYNDROME

Just recently, drug users have been described as having the same constellation of infectious and neoplastic disorders as described in male homosexuals: *Pneumocystis carinii* infection, pneumonia, cryptococcal meningitis, disseminated herpes infection, hepatitis B, cytomegalovirus infections, non-Hodgkin's lymphoma, cryptosporidiosis, typical and atypical acid-fast infections, and Kaposi's sarcoma (see Chap. 33).

SUGGESTED READINGS

Abrams, B., Sklaver, A., Hoffman, T., and Greenman, R.: Single or combination therapy of staphylococcal endocarditis in intravenous drug abusers. Ann. Intern. Med., 90:789, 1979.

Pradhan, S., and Dutta, S.: Drug Abuse: Clinical and Basic Aspects. St. Louis, C.V. Mosby, 1977.

Sapico, R.L., and Montgomerie, J.Z.: Vertebral osteomyelitis in intravenous drug abusers: report of three cases and review of the literature. Rev. Infect. Dis., 2:196, 1980.

Sapira, J., and Cherubin, C.: Drug Addiction: A Guide for the Clinician. New York, Excerpta Medica/American Elsevier, 1975.

CHAPTER 13

Bacteremia and Septicemia

J.C. Pechère and M. Laverdiere

Objective 13–1. Recognize those cases in which blood cultures are useful.

Blood is normally sterile; therefore, the presence of bacteria in the blood indicates a bacteremia or a septicemia. These two terms are not synonymous. Septicemia implies a degree of severity and persistence that, theoretically, is not found in a more transient bacteremia. Because it is difficult to make such a distinction when an infection first appears clinically, however, the terms are usually used interchangeably.

The blood for a culture is drawn under strict aseptic conditions. Blood culture represents a simple, effective, and inexpensive means of identifying the bacteria responsible for a severe infection. It also expedites the initiation of appropriate antibiotic therapy.

In the following situations, blood cultures may be useful as a diagnostic tool for bacteremia and septicemia:

1. Direct intravascular infections, such as endocarditis or suppurative thrombophlebitis, which occur as a complication of intravenous catheterization.
2. Diseases, such as typhoid fever, brucellosis, leptospirosis, tularemia, and plaque, which can rapidly become systemic and pass through a septicemic phase.
3. A bacterial invasion, which may occur following tissue and vascular trauma. (Systematic blood cultures after dental extraction are positive in more than 50% of patients. They are also positive in 8% of patients immediately following simple bladder catheterization. Both these bacteremias are usually asymptomatic.)
4. A complication of a paravascular focus of infection, such as pneumonia, biliary tract infections, salpingitis, abdominal suppuration, and osteomyelitis. (When the focus is deep, obtaining a bacteriologic specimen may be difficult; blood culture can be the simplest means of establishing a microbiologic diagnosis.)

The clinical picture of a septicemia may be characteristic. The patient's fever is irregular, with several spikes per day on the temperature curve; it is preceded by chills and is followed by sweating. These episodes correspond to discharges of bacteria into the blood. The patient quickly develops a "toxic" appearance. From the initial focus, bacteria carried by the blood can establish metastatic foci

171

in any organ of the body, particularly the liver and lungs, because of the function of these organs as capillary "filters." Obviously, any patient suspected of having this complication is an immediate candidate for blood cultures. Other indications for a blood culture are outlined in Table 13–1.

> Objective 13–2. Indicate the optimum conditions for a blood culture.

NUMBER OF BLOOD CULTURES

Certain bacteremias are practically continuous, as in endovascular infections, such as endocarditis, but most are intermittent. The reason is that bacteria do not normally survive for long in the blood, except in individuals with absent or weakened immunologic defenses. The body has several mechanisms designed to ensure bacterial destruction. For example, bacteria are rapidly phagocytized by the cells of the reticuloendothelial system contiguous to the blood vessels. This phenomenon is particularly apparent in the spleen, which often becomes palpable in patients with septicemia.

Evidence indicates the polymorphonuclear neutrophils act as a supplement to bacterial destruction. Subjects with neutropenia, for example, are at high risk for gram-negative septicemia; in this situation, a transfusion of granulocytes improves the prognosis temporarily. In subjects with normal white blood cell counts, however, almost one-third of the *Escherichia coli* isolated by a blood culture will prove resistant to phagocytosis by polymorphonuclear neutrophils. Complement is also useful in destroying bacteria because, in addition to its chemotactic action on polymorphonuclear leukocytes and its role in immunologic adherence and opsonization, it can perforate the walls of gram-negative bacteria and may produce their lysis (fractions 8 and 9).

The existence of these defense mechanisms makes it more difficult to obtain a positive blood culture; therefore, several samples must be taken. If 3 or 4 specimens are secured in the first 24 hours, an answer can be expected in 90% of cases without an excessive number of punctures. Then, depending upon the clinical situation, the decision whether to obtain further blood cultures may be made the following day.

Taking several blood cultures also helps the physician to interpret results because, in case of contamination during collection, only one culture is affected.

TIMING OF BLOOD CULTURES

The timing of a blood culture is of the utmost importance. In the most severe cases of bacteremia and septicemia, bacterial discharges occur rapidly in succession. Taking 2

Table 13–1. Indications for Blood Culture

1. Fevers of unknown origin in all cases, but especially if one or more of the following conditions are associated:
    When the fever occurs after a surgical procedure, instrumentation, catheterization, or dental extraction.
    When the patient has received continuous intravenous infusion for several days; in such a case, the catheter should also be removed immediately, and the tip should be cultured.
    When the patient suffers from an immunologic deficiency.
    In any heroin addict.
    In the presence of shaking chills and sweating.
    When the patient's general state of health is impaired.
    When the physical examination reveals an enlarged spleen, signs of peripheral embolism (cutaneous or on the fundus), valvular disease, or cardiac malformation.
    In the presence of multiple metastatic foci of infection
2. Unexplained shock or intravascular coagulation syndromes.
3. Neonatal distress of any type.
4. Severe localized infections, such as meningitis, pneumonia, suppuration within the abdominal cavity, ascending cholangitis, cholecystitis, or pyelonephritis.
5. An unexplained worsening of the general health of an immunosuppressed patient.

or 3 specimens 20 or 30 minutes apart usually provides an accurate result. The samples should be taken immediately before starting therapy. Unfortunately, however, septicemic discharges occur in many patients at greater intervals. If such is the case, the discharges can sometimes be detected through the temperature spikes and chills that they induce. The most favorable timing appears to be at the beginning of a series of chills. Because there is not the same urgency to institute therapy, an interval of at least an hour between blood cultures is preferable. Insofar as possible, the blood must be cultured prior to administering any antibiotic treatment; otherwise, the chances of isolating a microorganism are diminished.

In continuous bacteremias, a blood culture can be taken even though the patient has no fever, as in endocarditis.

ASEPTIC PRECAUTIONS FOR BLOOD COLLECTION

Once the puncture site has been selected, the patient's skin should be disinfected by a vigorous, concentric cleansing with a 2% tincture of iodine or an equivalent preparation of povidone-iodine (in case of allergy to iodine, use 70% alcohol). One should wait a minute before the specimen is taken, and the area of the puncture must not be touched with the finger unless the operator is wearing sterile gloves.

The blood can be collected in a sterile syringe and inoculated immediately, but the use of Vacutainer or similar blood culture tubes is generally preferable because it reduces the possibility of contamination.

The quantity of blood taken from an adult should be approximately 10 ml, equally distributed between aerobic and anaerobic media. Several preparations are available, usually in liquid form. The proper proportion is 1 part blood to approximately 10 to 20 parts culture broth. A higher concentration of blood reduces the chances of isolating certain bacteria, particularly pseudomonas. For an aerobic culture, the type of broth most often used is trypticase soy, brain-heart, or brucella, with a 10% CO_2 atmosphere. After introducing 5 ml blood, sterile air is admitted to replace the residual vacuum. The same media are generally adequate for anaerobic culture, although, of course, no air is allowed to enter. The addition of 0.05% cysteine has the double advantage of maintaining a low pH and helping certain streptococci to grow, such as mutants requiring thiol. The bottles also contain an anticoagulant, generally polyanethosulfonate (0.025 to 0.05%). A final consideration might be to add commercial-grade penicillinase for those patients who are treated with a beta-lactam antibiotic, provided the product is sterile and is handled with perfect aseptic technique.

The clinician must communicate his diagnostic hypotheses to the microbiologist because certain organisms, such as brucella, pasteurella, leptospira, neisseria, haemophilus, L forms of bacteria, and fungi, require special culture techniques.

In the *laboratory*, the bottles are placed in the incubator and are read daily. Cloudiness, hemolysis, gas production, and the appearance of colonies indicate growth, but microscopic examination is much more accurate. If the result is negative, readings should be resumed daily for at least a week. Certain organisms take longer to appear; for example, brucella may require 10 to 15 days of latency before growing.

The following techniques have been proposed to accelerate the culture procedure:

1. Immediate microscopic examination of the buffy coat; in special cases, such as in immunodepressed individuals, the offending microorganism can be seen within minutes.
2. Early routine "blind" subculture on solid media, usually done on the second day.
3. Production of $^{14}CO_2$ by microbial catabolism of labeled amino acids placed in the medium (Bactec).
4. Gas chromatography of the metabolites.

> Objective 13–3. Predict, if possible, the organism responsible for bacteremia before the blood culture results are known.

Blood culture is the most reliable means of identifying the organism responsible for a septicemia, but it involves a delay that is often incompatible with the urgency of the clinical situation. Therefore, an informed guess about the identity of the causative organism must be made at the time of the initial examination so that some type of therapy may be begun. Definitive signs are rare; thus, the physician is compelled to arrive at a diagnosis using reasonable probabilities.

Useful indexes in this regard are age, such as in neonatal septicemia (see Objective 22–3); the condition of the host, particularly in immunodepression or if a possibility of hospital- or community-acquired bacteremia exists, the former primarily caused by gram-negative bacilli and staphylococci; the circumstances that may have precipitated the bacteremia; and the portal of entry (Table 13–2). Associated cutaneous signs may also be helpful (Table 13–3 and see Objective 27–1), provided they are interpreted within their clinical context. Note that dermatologic

Table 13–2. Etiologic Probabilities According to Portal of Entry of a Septicemia

Portal of Entry	Circumstances	Most Probable Causative Organism
Skin	Furuncle, abscess, or carbuncle	*Staphylococcus aureus*
	Infected wound	*Staphylococcus aureus*, *Streptococcus pyogenes*, gram-negative organisms, clostridium
	Cellulitis	
	Intravenous catheter	*Staphylococcus aureus*, *Staphylococcus epidermidis*, K-E-S*, acinetobacter, pseudomonas, candida
	Animal bite	See Table 1–8
Bronchi and Lungs	Pneumonia or bronchopneumonia acquired outside a hospital	*Streptococcus pneumoniae*, *Haemophilus influenzae*, *Klebsiella pneumoniae*, *Staphylococcus aureus*
	Aspiration pneumonia	Anaerobes, *Escherichia coli*, K-E-S*
	Tracheotomy or assisted ventilation	K-E-S*, *Pseudomonas aeruginosa*, *Escherichia coli*, acinetobacter, *Staphylococcus aureus*
Intestine	Obstruction, perforation, cancer, diverticula or surgical intervention	Bacteroides, *Escherichia coli*, K-E-S*, proteus, gram-positive anaerobes
	Diarrhea	Salmonella, campylobacter
Biliary tract	Cholecystitis, cholangitis, or obstruction	*Escherichia coli*, K-E-S*, proteus, bacteroides, clostridium
Urinary tract	Pyelonephritis, instrumentation, catheterization, surgical intervention, or obstruction	*Escherichia coli*, proteus, K-E-S, enterococcus, *Pseudomonas aeruginosa*
Female genitalia	Childbirth or abortion	*Escherichia coli*, streptococci (A, B, D, anaerobes), bacteroides, clostridium
	Salpingitis	*Neisseria gonorrhoeae*
None visible	Heroin addiction	*Staphylococcus aureus*, streptococci, gram-negative bacilli
	Leukemia, neutropenia, cancer, or immunosuppression	*Pseudomonas aeruginosa*, *Escherichia coli*, K-E-S, *Staphylococcus aureus*
	Valvular disease	Alpha-hemolytic streptococci, enterococci, *Streptococcus bovis*, other streptococci, *Staphylococcus aureus*
	Cardiac prosthesis	*Streptococcus epidermidis*, *Staphylococcus aureus*
	Occupation as farmer, veterinarian, or slaughterhouse worker	Brucella

*K-E-S, klebsiella-enterobacter-serratia group

Table 13-3. Cutaneous Signs of Septicemias

Lesions	Most Probable Causative Organisms
Ecthyma gangrenosum (Plate 3C)	*Pseudomonas aeruginosa*, but also other gram-negative bacilli, such as citrobacter, aeromonas, and klebsiella
2 to 20 papules, mainly on the extremities, sometimes pustular, vesicular, bullous, necrotic, or hemorrhagic (Plates 4A, 4B, and 4C)	*Neisseria gonorrhoeae*
Disseminated petechiae, sometimes with a vesicular, pustular, or necrotic appearance (Plates 5A and 5B)	*Neisseria meningitidis*, but also gram-negative bacilli and *Staphylococcus aureus*
Disseminated purpura	Causative agents of endocarditis, *Neisseria meningitidis*
Erythematous macules (Janeway's spots), painful papules of fingers and toes (Plates 5C and 5D)	Causative agents of endocarditis
Rose spots on trunk	*Salmonella typhi* and other salmonellae
Macules and maculopapules on extremities, including palms and soles, after a rat bite	*Spirillum minor* and *Streptobacillus moniliformis*
Disseminated pustules	*Staphylococcus aureus*
Small, disseminated macronodular lesions	Candida
Jaundice due to hemolysis	Clostridium
Jaundice without hemolysis	Gram-negative bacilli and leptospira
Marbling on lower limbs (livedo)	Gram-negative bacilli

Table 13-4. Localization and Complications of Septicemia that Suggest Etiology*

Localizations and Complications	Most Probable Germs
Septic shock (see Objective 13-4)	Gram-negative bacilli, *Neisseria meningitidis*, *Staphylococcus aureus*, clostridia, candida
Disseminated intravascular coagulation	Gram-negative bacilli, *Neisseria meningitidis*, *Staphylococcus aureus*, clostridia, candida
Acute hemolysis	*Clostridium perfringens*
Multiple pulmonary infiltrates with rapid cavitation	*Staphylococcus aureus*
Arthritis of limbs	*Neisseria gonorrhoeae*, *Staphylococcus aureus*, enteric bacteria, *Pseudomonas aeruginosa*, *Streptoccus pneumoniae*, *Haemophilus influenzae*, *Streptobacillus moniliformis*
Tenosynovitis	*Neisseria gonorrhoeae*
Osteomyelitis	See Table 28-1
Meningitis	*Neisseria meningitidis*, *Streptococcus pneumoniae*, *Haemophilus influenzae*, gram-negative bacilli
Orchiepididymitis	Brucella, *Neisseria meningitidis*, *Streptococcus pneumoniae*
Signs in ocular fundus	
Roth's spots (hemorrhage with clear center)	Causative agents of endocarditis
White spot ("cotton wool")	Candida

*For cutaneous signs, see Table 13-3.

appearance alone is rarely sufficient for an accurate, discriminating judgment, but some localizations or complications of septicemia may provide clues to its origin (Table 13-4).

GRAM-NEGATIVE BACTEREMIAS

The most common bacteremias today are caused by gram-negative bacilli. In the United States alone, 70,000 to 300,000 cases are seen annually. The number of cases per annum increased from the 1950s to the 1970s, probably because of the combined effect of new investigatory procedures and surgical instrumentation. The increased use of antibiotics encouraged the survival of the most resistant organisms, in addition to prolonging the lives of patients who would otherwise have died.

The etiologic role of gram-negative bacilli in bacteremias may be described as follows,

---

PRACTICAL MANAGEMENT OF CANDIDEMIA

RISK FACTORS

Isolation of *Candida albicans* from blood cultures is usually associated with a lowering of host defense mechanisms, with the use of certain medications, or with traumatic or iatrogenic breaks of natural barriers. A combination of these factors frequently occurs in the clinical entities commonly associated with candidemia: neonatal sepsis; neoplasia; immunosuppressive, corticosteroid, or antibiotic therapy; intravenous, intra-arterial, or Foley catheters; extensive surgical procedures; serious burns; and the intravenous use of illicit drugs.

MANIFESTATIONS

Although the clinical manifestations of candidemia can vary, fever is usually the only symptom. Occasionally, peripheral manifestations involve the eyes (chorioretinitis), the skin (subcutaneous hemorrhagic nodules), the bones (osteomyelitis), and the joints (arthritis). Infections of visceral organs involving the heart (myocarditis), the brain (meningitis), and the kidney (pyelonephritis) are also noted in *Candida albicans* sepsis.

DIAGNOSIS

Blood cultures are currently the only reliable method of detecting a candidemia. Media and atmosphere of incubation found in routine blood culture bottles support the growth of *Candida albicans*, although results are better if blood culture bottles are vented. The available serologic tests to detect candidal antigen and anticandidal antibodies are not reliable.

TREATMENT

The therapeutic approach to candidemia varies according to the clinical setting. Systemic antifungal therapy is not always indicated. A candidemia in a patient who is receiving central or peripheral hyperalimentation and who is not suffering from a deep organ involvement or an underlying debilitating disease can first be treated by the removal of all indwelling catheters, followed by a series of blood cultures. If the blood cultures are still positive for candida when the catheter has been removed, or if the course of the disease is worsening, systemic antifungal therapy is then indicated. Otherwise, only close observation of the patient is necessary. In the presence of peripheral embolic lesions or of visceral infections, antifungal therapy must be administered even if the candidemia is associated with catheterization. In immunosuppressed or severely compromised patients, systemic antifungal therapy is indicated.

The choice of systemic antifungal agents for the treatment of candidemia is limited. Amphotericin B is clearly the drug of choice for the treatment of *Candida albicans* sepsis.

Currently, few alternatives to this agent are available. Flucytosine is active against *Candida albicans*, but its use as a single antifungal drug in the treatment of candidemia is not recommended because resistant strains of candida often emerge during treatment. This agent can, however, be used in combination with amphotericin B in severe candidemia in which such a combination may be synergistic and may help to achieve therapeutic levels more rapidly.

The role of ketoconazole in the treatment of candidemia has not been clearly defined. Even though the efficacy of ketoconazole in chronic mucocutaneous candidiasis is remarkable, its role in single-drug therapy of candidemia does not look as promising and has not been established.

The optimal duration of systemic antifungal therapy for candidiasis is unknown. A dose of amphotericin B totaling 1.5 to 2 g has been proposed for deep-seated infection, whereas for catheter-associated candidemia with minor peripheral embolic lesions, a total dose of 0.5 to 1.0 g might be sufficient. The duration of therapy for candidemia must be based on the individual patient's overall clinical response, on the rapidity with which a favorable response is obtained, on the degree of involution of the clinical manifestations, and on the host factors.

---

in decreasing order of frequency: *Escherichia coli*, between one-fourth and half the cases; the klebsiella-enterobacter-serratia group; pseudomonas; hafnia; bacteroides; acinetobacter; alcaligenes; aeromonas; and achromobacter. In contrast, other gram-negative organisms, such as *Haemophilus influenzae*, salmonella, neisseria, francisella, and brucella, are considered as separate entities in determining the origin of a bacteremia.

Gram-negative bacteremias nearly always occur as a result of a precipitating cause that is usually diagnostic in itself. In approximately half the cases, these bacteremias are caused by the following conditions, in decreasing order of frequency: urogenital infections, instrumentation, gastrointestinal disease, such as postsurgical suppuration, colitis, perforations, Crohn's disease, cholecystitis, and cirrhosis of the liver, and pneumonia. Immunosuppressed individuals appear to be particularly at risk. Because these precipitating causes are so frequent, every physician must limit catheterization, such as of central venous pressure lines, and instrumentation as much as possible and must observe aseptic precautions scrupulously, to prevent the occurrence of bacteremia.

Septic shock (see Objective 13–4) occurs in more than 33% of these patients, often in the first hours of the illness, whereas clinically significant intravascular coagulation is observed in 5 to 10% of these patients (Plate 3B). These complications are also indications of the origin of the bacteremia. Because gram-negative bacteremias were so frequently associated with compromised host resistance, the mortality rate in several series has been in excess of 30%.

STAPHYLOCOCCAL BACTEREMIAS

Staphylococcal bacteremias often occur in hospital settings. They are habitually caused by *Staphylococcus aureus*; *S. epidermidis* often superinfects intravenous catheters and cardiac prostheses. The origin of staphylococcemias is varied. The disorder is usually cutaneous in origin, from infected wounds, furuncles, and carbuncles. Intravenous injections in drug addicts are increasingly seen as a cause. *S. aureus* may infect the shunt or fistula used for dialysis and is by far the most common bacterium in the septicemia of hemodialysis patients. The state of the host appears to play a major role in the production of this infection. Staphylococcal septicemias are rare in otherwise normal individuals, but they are often encouraged by various underlying conditions such as cardiovascular diseases, particularly those cardiovascular disorders related to arteriosclerosis, diabetes, renal insufficiency, leukemia, granulocytosis, dysproteinemia, cancer, immunosuppressive therapy, and hepatic insufficiency. The presence of a foreign body has been observed in most septicemias due to *S. epidermidis*.

Clinically, some forms of staphylococcemia are fulminating because the toxin-induced manifestations are rapidly complicated by fatal shock. The disease is usually less impressive, and in addition to the septicemic signs, one often sees various metastatic localizations (Plate 3D), such as multiple pulmonary abscesses, arthritis, and osteomyelitis, which generally affects the long bones of children and adolescents and the vertebrae in adults. The renal lesions cause cortical and perinephric abscesses, pyelonephritis, or more rarely, immune complex glomerulonephritis.

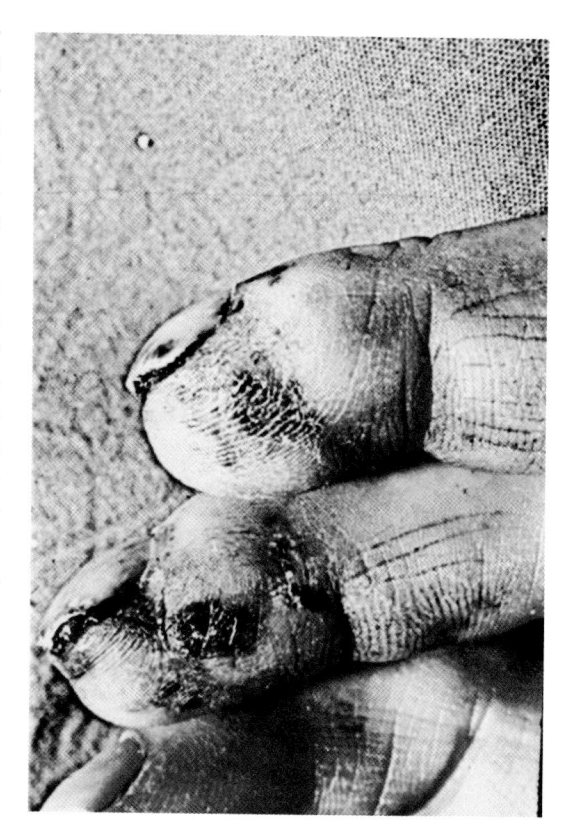

Fig. 13–1. Staphylococcemia: purpura of the fingertips.

The most dangerous localization is endocarditis, which worsens the patient's prognosis and requires a longer period of antibiotic therapy (4 to 6 weeks instead of 2). Endocardial involvement is not always easy to diagnose. Table 13–5 lists the principal elements of a differential diagnosis. On the whole, the prognosis is grave, with a mortality rate in excess of 30 or 40%, mainly when the

Table 13–5. Differentiation of Staphylococcemias Associated and Not Associated with Infective Endocarditis

Associated with Infective Endocarditis	Not Associated with Infective Endocarditis
Community-acquired illness	Hospital-acquired illness
Seen in illicit drug users	Obvious primary focus, such as intravenous catheter
No present or historical primary focus	No metastatic foci
Several metastatic foci, purpura (Fig. 13–1)	No cardiac murmur
Multiple septic pulmonary emboli, especially with rapidly cavitating infiltrates	Intermittent bacteremia
Pre-existing known endocardial lesions	Normal serum complement
Recent onset of regurgitant valvulitis, congestive heart failure, or systemic emboli	Normal rheumatoid factor
Classic peripheral signs of infective endocarditis, such as Osler's nodes	Normal echocardiogram
Hematuria	
All blood cultures positive (persistent bacteremia)	
Decreased serum complement	
Positive rheumatoid factor	
Positive anti-techoic acid antibodies*	
Echocardiogram shows valvulitis vegetation(s) (sensitivity 50–60%), underlying valvular lesion, and flail leaflet	
High level of circulating immune complexes	

*Positive in deep-seated staphylococcemias, such as originating from infective endocarditis, osteomyelitis, or pneumonias, and in staphylococcemias with metastatic foci; negative in superficial staphylococcemias, such as catheter-related illness without metastatic foci

underlying disease itself is severe. Septicemias due to *S. epidermidis* are clinically less severe and less acute than those due to *S. aureus*; their prognosis is also better, especially if the foreign body that led to the illness can be successfully removed.

ENTEROCOCCAL BACTEREMIA

Although enterococcus is frequently cultured in the clinical laboratory, the pathogenicity of this organism remains controversial, and hence ambivalence exists with respect to antibiotic therapy. Nonetheless, enterococcal bacteremias have been associated with a mortality rate higher than 50%. The main characteristics of these bacteremic events are as follows:

1. The primary sources of this illness are urinary tract, soft tissue (such as decubitus ulcers and burns), and intra-abdominal infections, but in some cases no primary focus can be found.
2. Many patients suffer from associated noninfectious diseases or injuries, such as central nervous system disease (for example, stroke), alcoholism, cancer, or multiple trauma. Failure of the host defenses is probably a critical predisposing factor in the pathogenicity of enterococcal infection. Concurrent administration of systemic antibiotics to which enterococcus is resistant, notably the cephalosporins (even the newer ones), may also be of pathologic significance.
3. Endocarditis should be suspected when the origin of the bacteremia remains unclear.
4. Bacteremias are often polymicrobial, the second organism being an organism belonging to the Enterobacteriaceae, candida, pseudomonas, clostridia, staphylococcus, or bacteroides, among others. Because of this phenomenon, a synergistic relationship may exist between enterococci and associated organisms at the primary site of infection.

Successful antimicrobial therapy requires a combination of penicillin G or ampicillin in addition to streptomycin or gentamicin. Vancomycin is an alternative when the patient is allergic to penicillins.

GONOCOCCEMIA—DISSEMINATED GONOCOCCAL INFECTION

Disseminated gonococcal infection (DGI) (Plate 4A to C) consists of a variety of clinical syndromes that are thought to be the hematogenous extension of local gonococcal infection. These syndromes occur in patients having a genital, rectal, or pharyngeal colonization of the organism. The primary site of infection is frequently asymptomatic. The incidence of DGI among individuals with symptomatic gonorrhea has been evaluated as 3% in females and 0.7% in males. The risk factors for gonococcemia include menstruation, pregnancy, the postpartum period, and genetic deficiency of the terminal components of complements C6 through C9.

Clinically, two stages, bacteremic and septic, have been recognized, but the practicing physician may find this distinction oversimplified.

The bacteremic stage is characterized by fever, chills, malaise, polyarthritis, and dermatitis. Polyarthritis has an inflammatory migratory pattern and usually involves the knees, followed by the wrist, hands, ankles, and feet. At this stage, gonococci can be cultured from the blood, but not from the joints. A characteristic feature of DGI is periarticular inflammation, especially tenosynovitis on the dorsum of the hand and wrist or the ankles. Typical dermatitis begins as small red macules or papules that may yield vesicular, pustular, hemorrhagic, or necrotic aspects. A patient generally has 2 to 20 skin lesions located on the extremities, including the palms and the soles, or near the joints. The bacteremic stage of DGI may also include transient electrocardiographic alterations and elevated hepatic transaminase levels. Classic complications, such as endocarditis and meningitis, are rare nowadays.

The septic joint stage involves 1 to 4 articulations. In about 40% of patients, only a single joint is involved. Oligoarthritis of 2 or 3 joints and polyarthritis represent 60% of the cases. Wrists, knees, hands, ankles, and elbows are most frequently involved, but any joint can be infected and may become painful and inflammatory. Joint fluid is usually purulent, and its culture on proper media yields gonococci in about half the cases. At this stage, however, systemic symptoms are minimal, and the blood cultures are negative.

The diagnosis of DGI is often suspected on clinical grounds in a young patient who has had a recent, unusual sexual exposure and, sometimes, who has symptoms of gonorrhea combined with the clinical features previously described. Confirmation is obtained by culturing gonococci from the patient's genitalia, rectum, or pharynx, and depending on the clinical stage, from the blood, the joint fluid, or the skin lesions. The forms of *Neisseria gonorrhoeae* responsible for DGI belong to particular biotypes that cannot synthesize certain nutrients, such as proline, arginine, hypoxanthine, or uracil (auxotrophic strains). Gonococci isolated from local symptomatic infections do not require these nutrients. Moreover, most DGI strains are sensitive to penicillin and resist killing by antibody and complement in normal human sera. Some strains of *N. gonorhoeae* resistant to penicillin have been found to be responsible for DGI, however.

Recommendations for the treatment of DGI are given in Table 22-6.

BRUCELLOSIS

Brucellosis is caused by a small, nonmotile gram-negative rod that grows slowly in vitro and requires an enriched culture medium. Four varieties are pathogenic for man: *Brucella melitensis*, *B. suis*, *B. abortus*, and *B. canis*. The disease is found mainly in domestic mammals, such as goats, cattle, pigs, sheep, dogs raised in kennels, and horses, in which it produces abortion as well as other disorders. Humans can become contaminated accidentally from the milk, placenta, or fetus of an infected animal. The portals of entry include the eyes, the nasopharynx, and the gastrointestinal or genital tract. In most cases, the human disease includes a septicemic phase that may be followed by a stubborn, recurrent, chronic infection.

The evidence that should lead the physician to suspect a brucella infection can vary. Occupational exposure often occurs in farmers, veterinarians, and employees in a slaughterhouse or a meat packing plant. The patient's medical history may also reveal consumption of unpasteurized dairy products. The illness begins progressively, and the principal symptoms are sweats, chills, headaches, myalgias, stiffness, and painful joints. The fever is often marked by undulations that occur over a period of several days; this classic temperature curve is not common, however.

The physical examination reveals small cervical and axillary nodes in 67% of patients, splenomegaly in 50%, and hepatomegaly in 25%. Certain focal findings, such as osteoarthritis (see Objective 26-8), orchiepididymitis, or abscess of the liver or spleen sometimes dominate the clinical picture. The patient's leukocyte count is normal or reduced, with relative lymphocytosis.

The diagnosis can be confirmed by isolating brucella through a blood culture, using a special medium and an atmosphere containing CO_2, or more rarely, from lymph nodes or by bone marrow culture. Serologic diagnosis with Wright's technique is also possible using agglutination of *B. abortus* antigen by serial dilutions of serum; the titer is more than 1/100, often > 1/1000, in 2 to 3 weeks. The melitin skin test, which is not available in North America, is less helpful because it is positive for life, and a negative reaction does not rule out the diagnosis.

Treatment during the acute phase of the illness should primarily consist of oral tetracycline, 2 loading doses of 1 g each at 4-hour intervals, then 500 mg every 6 hours for 21 days. In addition, in severe cases, 1 g streptomycin can be administered daily intramuscularly for 10 days. Rest is essential. Prednisone, an oral dose of 20 mg 2 or 3 times a day for up to 5 days, relieves patients who have high fever and marked toxicity; otherwise, salicylates can be used as supportive treatment. If, after this treatment, a relapse occurs within the following trimester, similar antibiotic treatment should be given.

> **Objective 13-4. Rapidly recognize shock and its cause in a septicemia, to initiate proper treatment.**

Shock is a major danger in septicemia from the first hours of the illness. Early diagnosis and treatment are the best guarantees of the patient's survival. To take the appropriate therapeutic measures, the physician must not only recognize the shock, but also must identify its causes and its possible consequences.

RECOGNIZING SHOCK

Recognizing shock is easy when the patient's arterial pressure has collapsed (systolic pressure < 80 mm Hg; diastolic pressure difficult to measure). Shock should be recognized earlier, however, before the blood pressure falls precipitously. An experienced physician is alert to a sudden fall of fever, an unexplained acceleration of the pulse and respiratory rate, a decrease in urine output, or an alteration of consciousness with confusion, agitation, or in contrast, a strange lucidity in which the patient appears too wide awake for his condition, all the while having lapses of memory or attention. The physician should also become alarmed when no evident disorder accounts for the development of sudden thrombocytopenia, respiratory alkalosis, metabolic acidosis, or arterial hypoxemia that is difficult to reduce.

IDENTIFYING THE CAUSE OF SHOCK

Some of the clinical possibilities that must be considered in a septicemia are found in Table 13-6. Interpretation of the physical signs can be difficult when several physiologic mechanisms are associated, but in the absence of involvement of a critical organ or in the case of a reduction in blood volume, one must always consider septic shock, in a differential diagnosis. In septic shock, the vascular space is normal in its volume, but abnormal in its distribution. The poor

Table 13-6. Causes of Shock with Septicemia

Type and Mechanism of Shock*	Examples	Signs Useful for Diagnosis
Cardiogenic shock due to cardiac lesion	Myocarditis in endocarditis Acute aortic insufficiency in endocarditis Associated myocardial infarction Cardiac abscess Tamponade in endocarditis	Auscultatory change, ECG abnormal, CVP and PAWP ↑
Cardiogenic shock due to pulmonary embolism	Multiple embolisms in endocarditis of right heart	Pulmonary clinical and radiologic signs, low Pa_{O_2}, scintiscan perfusion defects, CVP ↑, PAWP normal
Neurogenic shock	Central nervous system involvement in meningitis	Associated bulbar signs
Reduced blood volume due to dehydration	Typhoid with severe diarrhea	Weight loss, slow return to normal of pinched skin fold, dryness of mucous membranes
	Insufficient correction in febrile patient who refuses to drink and who may vomit and has diarrhea Uncontrolled diuresis in pyelonephritis with salt loss	Often blood electrolyte deficits, CVP ↓
Poor distribution of blood volume resulting from septic shock	Septicemia due to gram-negative bacilli, *Neisseria meningitidis*, *Staphylococcus aureus*, and clostridia	See text

CVP, central venous pressure; ECG, electrocardiogram; PAWP, pulmonary artery wedge pressure.
*In some patients, several mechanisms are involved simultaneously.

distribution of the blood is generally attributed to arteriovenous shunts, either truly anatomic, or functional in the sense that gas exchanges in the capillaries do not take place in a normal manner. The result is poor oxygenation of the tissues and, consequently, shock.

Clinically, two different entities can be distinguished. "Warm shock" is characterized by peripheral vasodilation; the patient's skin is warm and dry. This type of shock is particularly seen in septicemias due to gram-positive cocci and in the initial stages of a septicemia. In these patients, the cardiac output is increased, and peripheral vascular resistance is reduced.

In contrast, with "cold shock" peripheral vasoconstriction occurs. In this febrile patient, one finds cold, sweaty, and cyanotic extremities and sometimes marbling of the lower limbs. This condition may follow warm shock or may occur immediately by itself and is mainly observed in septicemias caused by gram-negative bacilli. In this instance, the cardiac output is reduced, and peripheral vascular resistance is increased. A portion of the blood is sequestered in the venous plexi and cannot be used for oxygenation of the tissues or for venous return to the heart. Therefore, a true, functional hypovolemia makes the shock similar to the one observed after hemorrhage.

IDENTIFYING THE CONSEQUENCES OF SEPTIC SHOCK

Many complications can appear during the course of septic shock. Renal insufficiency is common and usually follows tubular necrosis. Oliguria may supervene, but contrary to what is expected after simple dehydration, the excretion of urinary sodium remains high, at more than 40 meq/L. Secondarily, the patient's blood urea nitrogen and creatinine levels become elevated.

Another complication, "shock lung," often manifests itself by a stubborn arterial hypoxemia and by radiologic pulmonary infiltrates similar to those of pulmonary edema; however, this disorder occurs in the absence of heart failure. This syndrome has been attributed to increased pulmonary capillary permeability, which produces interstitial edema and alveolo-capillary block.

Disseminated intravascular coagulation can complicate any septic shock, but often takes on a particularly dramatic appearance in meningococcemia. In the small vessels, fibrin clots form and are lysed by the plasmin fibrinolytic system. On the one hand, this process results in a consumption of coagulation factors; besides thrombocytopenia, mentioned previously, prothrombin and thromboplastin times are prolonged and fibrinogen is reduced. On the other hand, the fibrin degradation products in the blood are increased. The clinical spectrum is variable. In some patients, the abnormalities remain purely biochemical; in others, cutaneous and visceral hemorrhages give an impressive appearance during life and at autopsy. In this context, the Waterhouse-Friderichsen syndrome includes adrenal hemorrhage, which is now generally considered to be the consequence rather than the cause of the shock.

Metabolic acidosis is another common finding. The poor tissue oxygenation shifts the cells toward anaerobic metabolism and causes organic acids, including lactic acid, to accumulate. Determinations of the serum electrolytes do not detect these acids, and the problem should be suspected when a deficit of anions of more than 10 meq is found, as compared to the cations (anion gap). Of course, the analysis is clearer if a blood gas analysis is used; this test indicates whether compensation exists. The possible sequelae of the ischemia should also be noted. Gangrene of toes, fingers, or limbs has been reported, particularly after meningococcemia. In the elderly, myocardial infarction and cerebral vascular accident are serious possibilities.

Overall, one ought not be surprised by the unfavorable prognosis in septic shock, especially when it is aggravated by the patient's advanced age or by an underlying disease, or when appropriate measures are undertaken too late in patients with collapsed blood pressure.

> **Objective 13–5. Plan the initial immediate therapy of a septicemic patient while awaiting the results of blood cultures.**

Initial treatment for septicemia should include the following:
1. Antibiotic therapy directed against the organism considered most likely to be responsible for the infection.
2. Measures to reverse possible septic shock.
3. Drainage of the original infection or metastatic foci if required.

ANTIBIOTIC TREATMENT

As soon as bacteriologic cultures have been taken, antibiotic treatment should be started. In the absence of precise bacteriologic identification, the physician's choice must be guided by the focus of infection that presumably produced the septicemia. (See specific chapters for treatment of various possible infections, such as cellulitis, pneumonias, and intra-abdominal suppurations.) When the organism is completely unknown and no initial infection serves as a guide, one should begin temporarily with broad-spectrum coverage, such as a combination of a cephalosporin and an aminoglycoside. Certain third-generation cephalosporins, such as cefotaxime, ceftazidime, and ceftriaxone, can be helpful and may be used for this purpose in the future. Naturally, once the organism has been identified, treatment must be adjusted on the basis of the results of the identification and sensitivity tests.

MEASURES AGAINST SHOCK

Several measures can be taken to limit the occurrence of severe shock. Delay in rehydration or in restoring the electrolyte balance must be avoided. Adequate oxygenation should be maintained, and the patient must be closely monitored. If septic shock should occur in spite of these precautions, the following procedures should be considered:

1. The first step is to refill the forward vascular bed by administering sufficient

> ### SEPTIC SHOCK AND ENDOTOXIN
>
> Most gram-negative bacteria possess complex molecules containing lipopolysaccharides (LPS) or endotoxins in their cell walls. When injected in animals, LPS produce a fatal disease seemingly related to septic shock, with hypotension, fever, and disseminated intravascular coagulation. The septic shock observed clinically seems more complex than this experimentally induced disease, however, and some microorganisms that have no LPS, such as *Staphylococcus aureus* or even influenza virus, can sometimes produce a clinical syndrome similar to septic shock. Thus, endotoxic shock and septic shock are not synonymous. Nevertheless, endotoxic shock is a useful animal model, and therapeutic deductions drawn from it may prove valuable.
>
> LPS are found at the surface of many species of gram-negative bacteria, for example, the Enterobacteriaceae, pseudomonas and various nonfermenting organisms, *Neisseria gonorrhoeae* and *N. meningitidis*, brucella, pasteurella, francisella, bacteroides, fusobacterium, and even the rickettsiae. The LPS molecule is composed of three parts. The deepest part, inserted in the cell wall, is lipid A, which appears responsible for the toxic properties. The central portion is closer to the surface and is attached to lipid A by a sugar, 2-keto-3-deoxy-octonate (KDO). This portion also contains a heptose, a phosphate, an ethanolamine, and three hexoses. Like lipid A, the central part of the molecule is the same in all bacterial species, and some have attempted to use it as an immunizing agent against endotoxin. The outer part of the molecule contains a series of repeated units of oligosaccharides that form the O antigen and permit serologic identification of various gram-negative bacteria including salmonella. The presence of O antigen gives the colonies a glossy, smooth appearance. These colonies, known as smooth (S) colonies, are missing in certain mutants. The colonies then have a rough (R) appearance, and their LPS core is bare.
>
> When labeled endotoxin is injected into an animal, it accumulates in the reticuloendothelial cells, notably those of the liver, spleen, and pulmonary alveoli, in the cells of the vascular endothelium, in the granulocytes, and in the platelets. Endotoxin has many biologic effects: hyperthermia due to the release of endogenous pyrogen by polymorphonuclear leukocytes; activation of the cascade sequence for coagulation; activation of the fibrinolytic system and complement; the release of vasoactive substances, such as catecholamines, histamine, serotonin, prostaglandins, and bradykinin; and the induction of hyperglycemia, followed by hypoglycemia. The sequence of these different events is still poorly known, however, as is the exact role, if any, of endotoxin in the production of septic shock in humans.

quantities of fluid. Saline solutions are used most frequently, but serum or even whole blood may be required, as in an associated anemia. To control the amount required, a central venous pressure (CVP) line is often used. Perfusions should be given rapidly until a CVP of 10 cm H_2O is obtained. One should not exceed 15 cm H_2O, to prevent an overload. Even in the absence of dehydration and diuresis, large quantities, such as several liters, may be necessary. If available, measurement of the patient's pulmonary artery wedge pressure (PAWP) is more reliable than that of the CVP for detecting the danger of pulmonary edema: the PAWP should rise to 15 mm Hg, but not over 20 mm Hg. Fluid replacement is often sufficient to restore an acceptable hemodynamic state. If this procedure fails, vasoactive drugs should be administered.

2. One should administer vasoactive agents to correct anomalies of blood distribution. Dopamine-type beta-adrenergic agents that reduce peripheral vascular resistance and increase cardiac output are most frequently used, but they are employed only *after* proper blood volume replacement. The patient must be kept under close observation for pulse, cardiac rhythm, urine volume, warmth of extremities, state of consciousness, arterial pressure, and CVP.
3. Any possible acidosis must be corrected by the usual measures, such as the administration of bicarbonate solutions.
4. Adequate oxygenation must be ensured. When arterial hypoxemia is irreducible, assisted ventilation may be indicated, either intermittent positive or positive end-expiratory pressure.
5. Digitalization must be done cautiously when the patient's CVP or PAWP rises to a dangerous level.
6. The use of corticosteroids is not universally recommended, particularly not by infectious disease specialists. Some

physicians, however, routinely use high doses of methylprednisolone or dexamethasone, for example, up to 30 mg/kg methylprednisolone for the initial dose.
7. The use of heparin for disseminated intravascular coagulation is even more controversial.

DRAINAGE OF INFECTION

In a septicemia, the physician must always ascertain whether an abscess or suppuration requires drainage or whether a catheter has become infected and needs to be removed.

> Objective 13–6. Interpret the results of a blood culture.

When blood culture results become available, after the required delay for bacterial growth, they must be carefully interpreted.

NEGATIVE BLOOD CULTURES

Negative blood cultures do not definitely rule out a diagnosis of bacteremia because the specimens may have been taken when no organisms were present in the blood, or previous or concurrent antibiotic therapy may have inhibited bacterial growth. Moreover, certain bacteria, such as haemophilus, leptospira, brucella, pasteurella, or an anaerobe, are difficult to grow and sometimes require special culture techniques. Therefore, these false-negative blood cultures deprive the physician of both a certain diagnosis and a reliable therapeutic guide.

POSITIVE BLOOD CULTURES

When blood cultures are positive, one must always make sure that the bacteria really came from the blood rather than from contamination by the skin, the air, or the physician's fingers. In the last case, contamination probably occurred because the specimen was difficult to collect. Often, the organism is in mixed cultures or is found in only one sample, or the bacteria belong to species of low pathogenicity, such as *Bacillus subtilis*, *Propionibacterium acnes*, other diphtheroids, or *Staphylococcus epidermidis*.

> Objective 13–7. Treat a septicemia due to gram-negative bacilli or to staphylococci according to the laboratory results.

Once the organism has been identified and sensitivity tests have been performed, a directed therapy may be chosen.

GRAM-NEGATIVE BACILLI

In bacteremias due to gram-negative bacilli, the choice is easily made by following the sensitivity test results. For Enterobacteriaceae, a beta-lactam antibiotic is generally used, preferably ampicillin or amoxycillin when these are in vitro, or an aminoglycoside, such as gentamicin, tobramycin or netilmicin, at a dose of 1.5 mg/kg every 8 hours intravenously, or amikacin, 7.5 mg/kg every 12 hours intravenously, or a cephalosporin such as cefoxitin or cefotaxime. In certain cases, such as neonatal septicemias, a combination of a beta-lactam antibiotic and an aminoglycoside is widely recommended, although a trend toward using the newer cephalosporins is likely.

Pseudomonas septicemias, particularly dangerous because they usually occur in immunodepressed individuals, require a combination of an aminoglycoside (same doses) with carbenicillin, 400 mg/kg/day intravenously, ticarcillin, 250 mg/kg/day intravenously, or, secondarily, mezlocillin or piperacillin. Ceftazidime is a possible future choice in such cases.

When the organism is *Bacteroides fragilis*, one may administer clindamycin, 30 mg/kg/day intravenously, cefoxitin, 100 mg/kg/day intravenously, or metronidazole, at 500 mg every 8 hours intravenously. With the other bacteroides and fusobacterium, penicillin G, 12 to 36 million U/day, is often preferred; clindamycin or chloramphenicol are alternatives.

On the whole, the site of infection determines the duration of treatment of gram-neg-

Table 13-7. Third-Generation Cephalosporins

I. Third-Generation versus First- and Second-Generation Cephalosporins	
Similarities among Cephalosporins	Peculiarities of Third-Generation Cephalosporins
Activity against gram-positive cocci and anaerobes other than *Bacteroides fragilis* Resistance of enterococci, listeria, legionella, mycoplasma, chlamydia, and rickettsia Relative safety	Low minimum inhibitory concentration for most susceptible gram-negative bacteria Longer half-lives for most Clinically significant meningeal penetration High cost

II. Comparison of 6 Different Third-Generation Cephalosporins

	Cefotaxime	Moxalactam	Cefoperazone	Ceftazidime	Ceftriaxone	Ceftizoxime
Antibacterial activity*						
Bacteroides fragilis†	○	◐	○	○	○	○
Escherichia coli	●	●	●	●	●	●
Haemophilus influenzae	●	●	●	●	●	●
Klebsiella	●	●	●	●	●	●
Pseudomonas aeruginosa	○	○	◐	●	○	○
Staphylococcus aureus‡	●	●	●	●	●	●
Streptococcus pneumoniae§	●	●	●	●	●	●
Serum half-life (hours)	1.3	2.5	2	2	6–9	1.4
Metabolization	yes (hepatic)	minimal	minimal	minimal	minimal	minimal
Main route of excretion	renal	renal	biliary	renal	renal and biliary	renal
Usual adult dose (grams)	1–2	1–2	1–2	1–2	1–2	1–2
Usual dosing interval (hours)	4–8	6–12	6–12	6–12	12–24	6–12
Dosage in severe renal failure (10% or less renal function)	unchanged	reduced	unchanged	reduced	reduced	reduced
Dosage in severe hepatic dysfunction	unchanged	unchanged	reduced	unchanged	reduced	unchanged

* ● More than 90% sensitive strains; ◐ 60–90% sensitive strains; ○ fewer than 60% sensitive strains
† Cefoxitin, a second-generation cephalosporin, is more often active
‡ Cephalotin is more active; moxalactam, cefoperazone, and ceftazidime are less active
§ Benzyl penicillin is equally or more active; activity of moxalactam in CSF is questionable.

ative septicemia; 10 to 14 days of treatment are often sufficient.

STAPHYLOCOCCUS AUREUS

In *Staphylococcus aureus* septicemias, the choice of antibiotics must take into account the bacterial resistance mechanisms, and the duration of treatment should depend on the presence of endocarditis.

The beta-lactam antibiotics are the most active against *S. aureus*, but their use is limited by three resistance mechanisms:

1. Many staphylococci (more than 90% in a hospital setting) have a plasmid that codes for a beta-lactamase active against penicillin G, but not against semisynthetic penicillins such as oxacillin.
2. A so-called intrinsic resistance is observed with certain bacterial strains with deficient cell walls. These bacteria then become resistant both to semisynthetic penicillins (methicillin resistance) and to the cephalosporins. These resistances may go unnoticed in disc tests performed by the conventional method, however. They are detected more readily by performing this sensitivity test at 30° C with a reading after 48 hours.
3. "Tolerant" *S. aureus* is characterized by a normal minimum inhibitory concentration (MIC), but a high minimum bactericidal concentration (MBC). The ratio of MBC to MIC is then more than 32, whereas the ratio is normally smaller.

Even though the question of the treatment of staphylococcal septicemias is not entirely clear, the following broad guidelines can be proposed.

1. If they are available, tests of bactericidal activity will be helpful in making a rational choice. Thus, the MIC, MBC, and, in the patient previously treated, the bactericidal activity of the serum (whose peak should be $\geq 1/8$) can be determined. These studies appear to be of special importance when endocarditis is present.
2. For the initial treatment before the sensitivity test results are known, a semisynthetic penicillin, such as oxacillin, cloxacillin, or nafcillin (1.5 to 2 g every 4 hours intravenously) is generally used. In patients allergic to penicillin, one should give cephalothin (2 to 2.5 g every 4 hours intravenously) or vancomycin (500 mg every 6 hours intravenously). Certain antibiotic combinations are synergistic in vitro, notably semisynthetic penicillins and aminoglycosides, cephalosporins and aminoglycosides, and nafcillin and rifampin. The addition of a second agent, often an aminoglycoside, is probably not necessary when endocarditis is not present or in cases of endocarditis of the right heart in drug addicts. A second drug may be useful in endocarditis of the left heart and in patients who have a prosthetic cardiac valve.
3. When sensitivity test results are available, one should follow these procedures: If the bacterial strain is susceptible to penicillin, this agent should be the antibiotic of choice (2×10^6 U every 4 hours intravenously). In case of intrinsic resistance or tolerance, one should administer vancomycin (500 mg every 6 hours intravenously) or vancomycin and rifampin (300 mg every 8 hours orally), although some question this combination.
4. The duration of treatment should be 10 to 14 days if endocarditis is not present; otherwise, it should be 4 weeks (Table 13–7).

SUGGESTED READINGS

Barth Beller, L., Murray, P.R., MacLowry, J.D., and Washington, II, J.A.: Blood Cultures. II. Cumitech, *1a*:1, 1982.

Bayer, A.: Staphylococcal bacteremia and endocarditis. State of the art. Arch. Intern. Med., *142*:1169, 1982.

Garrison, R.N., Fry, D.E., Berberich, S., and Polk, H.C., Jr.: Enterococcal bacteremia. Clinical implications and determinants of death. Ann. Surg., *196*:43, 1982.

Korzeniowski, O., Sande, M., and the National Collaborative Endocarditis Study Group: Combination antimicrobial therapy for Staphylococcus aureus endocarditis in patients addicted to parenteral drugs and in nonaddicts. Ann. Intern. Med., 97:496, 1982.

Kreger, B.E., Craven, D.E., and McCabe, W.R.: Gram-negative bacteremia. IV. Reevaluation of clinical features and treatment in 612 patients. Am. J. Med., 68:344, 1980.

Kreger, B.E., Craven, D.E., Carling, P.C., and McCabe, W.R.: Gram-negative bacteremia. III. Reassessment of etiology, epidemiology and ecology in 612 patients. Am. J. Med., 68:332, 1980.

Francioli, P., and Masur, H.: Complications of Staphylococcus aureus bacteremia occurrence in patients undergoing long-term hemodialysis. Arch. Intern. Med., 142:1655, 1982.

Lowder, J.N., Lazarus, H.M., and Herzig, R.H.: Bacteremias and fungemias in oncologic patients with central venous catheters—changing spectrum of infection. Arch. Intern. Med., 142:1456, 1982.

Mirimanoff, R.O., and Glauser, M.P.: Endocarditis during Staphylococcus aureus septicemia in a population of non-drug addicts. Arch. Intern. Med., 142:1311, 1982.

Roberts, F.J.: A review of positive blood cultures: identification and source of microorganisms and patterns of sensitivity to antibiotics. Rev. Infect. Dis., 2:329, 1980.

Stratton, J.R., Weiner, J.A., and Pearlman, A.S.: Bacteremia: echocardiographic findings in 80 patients with documental or suspected bacteremia. Am. J. Med., 73:851, 1982.

Weinstein, M.P., Reller, L.B., Murphy, J.R., and Lichtenstein, K.A.: The clinical significance of positive blood cultures: a comprehensive analysis of 500 episodes of bacteremia and fungemia in adults. I. Laboratory and epidemiologic observations. Rev. Infect. Dis., 5:35, 1983.

Weinstein, M.P., Murphy, J.R., Reller, L.B., and Lichtenstein, K.A.: The clinical significance of positive blood cultures: a comprehensive analysis of 500 episodes of bacteremia and fungemia in adults. II. Clinical observations, with special reference to factors influencing prognosis. Rev. Infect. Dis., 5:54, 1983.

Third-Generation Cephalosporins

Cherubin, C.E., Neu, H.C., Turck, M. (eds.): Current status of Cefotaxime sodium: a new cephalosporin. Rev. Infect. Dis., 4(Suppl.):281, 1982.

Cunha, B.A., and Ristuccia, A.M.: Third generation cephalosporins. Med. Clin. North Am., 66:283, 1982.

Moellering, R.C., and Young, L.S. (eds.): Moxalactam international symposium. Rev. Infect. Dis., 4(Suppl.):489, 1982.

Neu, H.C., Turck, M., and Phillips, I. (eds.): Ceftizoxime, a broad spectrum β-lactamase stable cephalosporin. J. Antimicrob. Chemother., 10(Suppl. C):1, 1982.

Williams, J.D., and Casewell, M.W. (eds.): Ceftazidime. J. Antimicrob. Chemother., 8(Suppl. B):1, 1981.

CHAPTER 14

Infective Endocarditis

H.F. Chambers and M.A. Sande

Objective 14–1. Prescribe antibiotics for the prophylaxis of infective endocarditis.

The use of antimicrobial prophylaxis to prevent infective endocarditis (IE) is standard medical practice and is justified mostly on theoretic grounds, based on our knowledge of the predisposing cardiac lesions, the pathogenesis of the disease, and the sources of bacteremias.

PREDISPOSING CARDIAC LESIONS

Pre-existing cardiac disorders are present in 50 to 80% of patients with IE. The variability in reported incidence is due to differences in age and etiologic agents among series. Elderly patients are less likely to report a predisposing cardiac condition, although one may be present, but are more likely to have a history of an antecedent heart murmur. Similarly, series composed of younger patients have proportionately higher numbers with congenital defects and rheumatic heart disease. Series of patients with IE caused by virulent organisms, such as *Staphylococcus aureus* or pneumococci, report a lower incidence of predisposing cardiac conditions. Presumably, most subacute cases are caused by bacteria unable to infect normal valves, a property reserved for the more virulent organisms.

The most common underlying disorder is still rheumatic heart disease, although the percentage of patients so affected has declined from 80 to 90% in older series to approximately 40%. This decline is associated with an increase in prosthetic valve endocarditis. Rheumatic heart disease is even less common in elderly patients, in whom other predisposing factors are more important. Patients with congenital heart disease account for 6 to 25% of cases, and the incidence may be increasing because of improved diagnostic methods and prolonged survival in this group of patients. Congenital valvular aortic stenosis, ventricular septal defect, coarctation of the aorta, arteriovenous fistula, patent ductus arteriosus, and tetralogy of Fallot constitute the highest risk categories. Isolated valvular disease of the right heart and idiopathic hypertrophic subaortic stenosis pose an intermediate risk. IE is uncommon in patients with atrial septal defect.

Patients who have undergone reparative or palliative cardiovascular surgical procedures constitute an increasing population at risk for IE. Most postoperative cases of IE occur in patients with prosthetic heart valves. The presence of a prosthetic valve is a predisposing condition in 13 to 33% of patients; the larger proportions are from referral centers that routinely perform cardiovascular opera-

DEFINITION AND EPIDEMIOLOGY OF INFECTIVE ENDOCARDITIS

Infective endocarditis (IE) is a bacterial, fungal, or viral infection of endocardial or valvular surfaces of the heart. Included within the definition are infections of patent ductus arteriosus, arteriovenous fistula, and coarctation of the aorta because of similar clinical manifestations.

Historically, IE was subdivided into acute and subacute syndromes, and the term "bacterial endocarditis" was used for both. The term "infective endocarditis" is now preferred because other organisms, such as fungi and rickettsiae, are known to cause the disease. Similarly, the distinctions between the acute and subacute varieties are not always clear. In the preantibiotic era, acute endocarditis was a fulminant disease with a rapid downhill course leading to the patient's death within a few days. The organisms most often implicated were virulent and included *Staphylococcus aureus, Streptococcus pneumoniae, Streptococcus pyogenes,* and *Neisseria gonorrhoeae.* The subacute form of the disease was of insidious onset, lasted for several weeks to several months, and typically occurred in patients with rheumatic heart disease. The responsible organisms were usually viridans streptococci.

As patients and treatment have changed, so has the disease. Repair of formerly lethal congenital defects and replacement of natural with prosthetic valves have become commonplace. Invasive monitoring techniques have brought with them attendant complications, one of which is IE. Clinical series now include a significant number of intravenous drug abusers. These patients make up an increasing proportion of cases in the face of a declining prevalence of rheumatic and luetic heart disease. It is now less common for endocarditis to go undiagnosed in a patient with a chronic illness characterized by weight loss, night sweats, low-grade fevers, fatigue, changing heart murmurs, and anemia. Intervention is generally earlier, the diagnosis is more easily made, and the treatment is more effective. Consequently, the distinctions between acute and subacute varieties are less clear, and the terms have lost much of their usefulness in predicting cause or outcome. An etiologic classification is now preferred and is more therapeutically relevant.

The true prevalence of IE is difficult to ascertain. Studies vary in criteria for diagnosis, and criteria may be omitted altogether. Data from 10 different hospitals in the United States indicate a prevalence of 0.16 to 5.4 per 1000 hospital admissions. Evidence from some hospitals of a decline in incidence since the advent of the antibiotic era suggests that infections of all types are treated earlier, chemoprophylaxis is more generally administered, and physicians are more aware of the disorder. Other series report a constant number of cases over the years. Recent reports all confirm that the character of the disease is changing.

The mean age of patients with IE has steadily increased during the antibiotic era. Series prior to 1940 reported an average age of 30 to 35 years, with 24 to 49% of patients over age 40. Studies from the late 1940s to the present report mean ages from 40 to 57 years, with 49 to 82% of patients over the age of 40. This change reflects the increasing age of the population in general, but it is also influenced by the improved survival rates of patients with congenital and acquired heart disease as surgical techniques improve. Because rheumatic heart disease has become less common, patients with degenerative valvular disorders make up an increasing proportion of patients with IE. The sex ratio has remained constant, males outnumbering females approximately 2:1 in most series. Women generally acquire IE at a younger age than men. Among elderly patients with endocarditis, males outnumber females by as much as 5:1.

---

tions. Of postoperative patients not requiring valvular replacement, those with cyanotic heart disease requiring shunting from a systemic artery to the pulmonary artery are at increased risk. Tetralogy of Fallot and transposition of the great vessels account for the majority of cases. Repair of ventricular septal defect carries a low risk of IE.

Other cardiac conditions have recently been recognized as predisposing a patient to IE. In one series, mitral valve prolapse was present in 11% of patients. More than a third of patients with isolated mitral valve infection had this syndrome. Mitral valve prolapse, however, occurs in up to 20% of college-age women, and the true significance of this observation remains unclear. Patients with syphilitic heart disease, Marfan's syndrome, hemodialysis shunts, intravenous lines, and central venous or pulmonary arterial catheters also are at an increased risk of IE.

Of the remaining 30% of patients without a specific predisposing cardiac disorder, most have degenerative heart disease with associated valvular, endovascular, and myocardial abnormalities. These disorders are more common in the elderly, but their exact contribution to the pathogenesis of IE is unknown. Over the past 20 years, the number of patients without detectable valvular or cardiovascular disease may have decreased.

Other specific conditions are commonly encountered in patients with IE. Intravenous drug abusers have an incidence of IE 30 times that of the general population and 7 times that of patients with known rheumatic heart disease. Prior episodes of infective endocarditis, cardiac operations, diabetes, immunosuppression, and possibly alcoholism are associated with an increased risk of IE.

PROCEDURES ASSOCIATED WITH BACTEREMIA

A predisposing event associated with bacteremia is identifiable in half the patients with IE. Dental disease or manipulation has been emphasized, but it probably accounts for fewer than 15% of cases of IE. Dental procedures that injure the mucous membranes and cause bleeding of the gingival surfaces are almost always accompanied by transient bacteremia; the incidence of bacteremia was up to 88% in one series. The greater the degree of gingival disease, the greater the degree of bacteremia. Endocarditis following such events is usually caused by the oral streptococci of the viridans group. Urologic manipulation or chronic urinary tract infection often precedes enterococcal endocarditis.

That *Streptococcus bovis* endocarditis is associated with a high incidence of colonic disease, especially carcinoma, suggests that this organism may spontaneously disseminate from the gastrointestinal tract. *Staphylococcus aureus* endocarditis can be traced to cutaneous staphylococcal infections, such as boils and infected intravenous catheter sites, in up to 50% of cases.

ANTIBIOTIC PROPHYLAXIS

Satisfactory prospective randomized studies of the efficacy of prophylactic therapy for IE do not exist and are unlikely to be conducted. The number of patients required for such a study would be excessive, and ethical

---

PATHOPHYSIOLOGY OF INFECTIVE ENDOCARDITIS

Despite a century of investigation, the exact mechanisms responsible for infection of cardiac valves remain elusive. Recent studies with animal models of IE have contributed much to the current understanding of the disease process. It appears that turbulence of blood flow, secondary to an abnormal or a damaged cardiac valve, produces endothelial damage leading to the formation of a fibrin-platelet thrombus. Circulating bacteria then adhere to these damaged cardiac surfaces. The lesions of IE occur at characteristic locations, such as the atrial side of the mitral valve in patients with mitral insufficiency, the ventricular surface in patients with aortic insufficiency, and the right ventricular orifice in those with ventricular septal defect. Three circulatory conditions help to explain these findings: (1) a regurgitant stream; (2) a high-pressure source directing this stream to a low-pressure sink, such as the left ventricle to the left atrium; and (3) the presence of a high diastolic pressure gradient.

The regurgitant stream traumatizes the endothelium and predisposes it to colonization by bacteria. Experiments using a venturi tube lined with sterile agar confirm the preferential deposition of bacteria at the expected sites, just beyond the orifice on the low-pressure side of the tube. Patients with valvular or congenital abnormalities having all three characteristics have the highest risk of IE. Conversely, patients with abnormalities lacking one or more conditions are at a lower risk. Thus, atrial septal defects that lack a high-pressure source and a high diastolic gradient are rarely complicated by IE.

Indirect evidence from pathologic studies in humans and data from animal experiments suggest that formation of sterile vegetation composed of platelets and fibrin follows endothelial injury. These vegetations, known as nonbacterial thrombotic endocarditis (NBTE), may be small and are occasionally seen on normal valves, but they are commonly associated with damaged valves. The NBTE thus appears to serve as a nidus for infection following chance bacteremia. The surface is most receptive early in the genesis of NBTE and before re-endothelization of the lesion. The exact mechanisms whereby organisms attach themselves to valves remain obscure. Gram-positive organisms, most often responsible for IE, adhere to heart valves or to fibrin and platelets more readily than gram-negative organisms. Dextran production by *Streptococcus sanguis* is directly correlated clinically with infectivity, and in vitro studies have demonstrated that dextran-producing strains adhere particularly well to damaged valves. These complex polysaccharides and other unknown cell-wall antigens enhance adherence to platelet-fibrin deposits on the cardiac valve.

After colonization of the sterile vegetation with bacteria, deposition of platelets and fibrin continues, and the organisms grow at a rate similar to that seen in broth cultures. A scaffolding effect of the platelet-fibrin mesh provides a milieu protected from the phagocytic defenses of the host. In animal models a fully mature vegetation may be seen in 24 to 48 hours. Thus, abnormal circulatory conditions associated with congenital and acquired valvular and nonvalvular heart disease cause mechanical stresses that damage endothelial surfaces, upon which platelet and fibrin deposition occurs. Bacteria, having gained access to the circulation, adhere to this lesion. Replication then begins, and a mature vegetation is formed.

considerations preclude such a randomized trial. Consequently, the current recommendations of the American Heart Association on antimicrobial prophylaxis are formulated from the best available epidemiologic, pathophysiologic, etiologic, and experimental data, as well as from clinical observations. These regimens were tested in animal models, and the experimental conditions were such that prevention was more difficult than in most clinical situations. The physician prescribing antimicrobial prophylaxis for IE makes five implicit assumptions:

1. The populations at risk for IE are known.
2. The situations likely to cause bacteremia and the species of bacteria present are defined.
3. Certain species of bacteria commonly cause IE, and therapy need only be directed against these organisms.
4. Prophylactic therapy effectively prevents infective endocarditis.
5. The risk of IE exceeds the risk of prophylaxis.

The patients at risk for developing IE are well characterized, although the magnitude of this risk is unknown. Risk may be categorized as high, intermediate, or negligible. High-risk lesions fulfill all the hemodynamic conditions outlined and include arteriovenous fistulas, patent ductus arteriosus, tetralogy of Fallot, coarctation of the aorta, ventricular septal defect, aortic or mitral valve disease, and Marfan's syndrome. Postcardiotomy patients and those with previous episodes of endocarditis, with hyperalimentation lines, and with prosthetic valves are in this high-risk category as well. Mitral valve prolapse, idiopathic hypertrophic subaortic stenosis, and tricuspid or pulmonary valve disease constitute an intermediate risk. Other conditions, most notably atrial septal defect and artificial cardiac pacemakers, are low risk factors, and prophylaxis is not indicated.

Numerous studies have examined the incidence of transient bacteremia after surgical, medical, and dental procedures. Although some differences exist, certain trends emerge. The association of bacteremia with dental manipulation has been mentioned, and prophylaxis is clearly indicated for patients at high and intermediate risk. Genitourinary surgical procedures and instrumentation including urinary catheterization are associated with a high incidence of bacteremia with enterococci. Operations involving infected soft tissues, gynecologic procedures in the presence of infection, drainage of abscesses, and upper respiratory tract operations are similarly high risk factors. All are indications for prophylaxis in patients at high and intermediate risk. Normal obstetric delivery and therapeutic abortion produce low degrees of bacteremia. Similarly, endoscopic procedures, endotracheal intubation, sterile surgical procedures, cardiac catheterization, and spontaneous loss of deciduous teeth are low risk factors, and prophylaxis is not indicated. Because prosthetic cardiac valves are particularly susceptible to colonization during bacteremia, and because endocarditis of a prosthetic valve causes substantial morbidity and mortality, prophylaxis even during low-risk procedures is advisable.

The bacteremia that follows diagnostic or therapeutic procedures is transient and polymicrobial. For example, aerobic enteric organisms rarely cause IE, but are commonly cultured from the blood after urologic procedures. Prophylaxis should be directed only against organisms likely to cause IE. In oral and upper respiratory tract procedures, viridans streptococci are of primary concern. After genitourinary procedures, enterococci are common offending organisms. Both coagulase-positive and coagulase-negative staphylococci predominate in postcardiotomy endocarditis and in endocarditis of prosthetic valves.

Prophylactic therapy is probably effective in preventing IE, provided certain conditions are met. Antibiotics must be administered so that maximal levels are present at the time of the procedure, that is, administered 30 to 60 minutes before the procedure. Low doses of antimicrobial agents are ineffective. Because gastrointestinal absorption may be erratic, parenteral therapy is preferred in high-risk situations and should be administered whenever feasible. Parenteral therapy is recommended in all patients with prosthetic cardiac valves. In other situations, oral therapy has the advantages of convenience and acceptance by both patient and physician. Because the bacteremia is transient, antibiotics should not be continued beyond 24 to 48 hours. Longer courses of treatment increase the risk of adverse effects without increasing the benefit. Only bactericidal agents have been thoroughly evaluated; bacteriostatic agents may not be as efficacious. Specific recommendations are listed in Table 14–1.

For dental procedures, penicillin is suggested, either alone or in combination with streptomycin. Oral penicillin may be used, provided a loading dose is given. Aqueous penicillin G and procaine penicillin G are given together to ensure an adequate peak level of antibiotic and a sustained level thereafter. Vancomycin or erythromycin is used in patients allergic to penicillin. For gastrointestinal and genitourinary tract procedures, we recommend penicillin, ampicillin, or vancomycin in addition to streptomycin or gentamicin. Patients undergoing cardiac surgical procedures should receive a penicillinase-resistant penicillin, a cephalosporin, or vancomycin. Patients with prosthetic cardiac valves should always receive parenteral penicillin or vancomycin in addition to streptomycin or gentamicin. Therapy is begun 30 to 60 minutes prior to the procedure and is continued for 24 to 48 hours.

> **Objective 14–2.** Find the clinical clues that suggest endocarditis in the febrile patient.

GENERAL CLINICAL MANIFESTATIONS

The signs and symptoms of IE are caused by cardiac dysfunction, systemic or pulmonary embolization, metastatic foci of infection, and immune complex disease. The verrucous valvular vegetation interferes with valvular function, serves as the source of continued bacteremia, and distributes septic emboli throughout the pulmonary or systemic circulation. The host response to the infection involves poorly understood immune mechanisms that may cause further injury, as in the case of glomerulopathy.

The symptoms of IE are often vague and nonspecific, reflecting the systemic nature of the disease. The mean duration of symptoms prior to diagnosis depends on the organism responsible. *Staphylococcus aureus* and pneumococcal infections are usually fulminant, and the diagnosis is made in a mean of 9 to 14 days. Patients with viridans streptococcal or enterococcal infections have a mean duration of symptoms ranging from 30 to 90 days. Longer durations of illness in streptococcal infections are associated with increased mortality rates because the incidence of complications progressively rises with a delay in therapy. In more recent series, the mean duration of symptoms before diagnosis appears to be shortening: 4 weeks for streptococcal disease and 9 days for *S. aureus* infection.

The most common symptom continues to be fever, a complaint in over 85% of patients. Apyrexia may occur in more chronic infections and in cases complicated by uremia or heart failure. Chills are a common accompaniment of infection with virulent organisms. Fatigue, sweats, malaise, and weight loss may be the predominant complaints, especially in chronic cases. Arthralgias, arthritis, and myalgias are presenting symptoms in up to 40% of patients. Headache, abdominal pain, and back pain are present in approximately a quarter of all patients. Chest pain, hemoptysis, and other pulmonary symptoms suggest right-sided infection and infection with *Staphylococcus aureus*. Complaints referable to involvement of the central nervous system (CNS), such as hemiparesis, visual field defects, lethargy, or obtundation, connote an unfavorable prognosis, whereas symptoms of congestive heart failure are elicited in 25 to 50% of patients. IE should always be considered when heart failure and fever

Table 14-1. Prophylaxis of Infective Endocarditis in Patients at Risk

Surgical Procedures	Risk Factors	Administration of Antibiotics — Adults	Administration of Antibiotics — Children
Dental and upper respiratory tract	Prosthetic heart valves	Aqueous penicillin 1 million U mixed with procaine penicillin 600,000 U IM *plus* streptomycin 1 g IM 30 min prior to the procedure, then penicillin VK 500 mg orally q6h for 8 doses or Vancomycin 1 g IV over 30 min, starting infusion 30–60 min prior to procedure, then erythromycin 500 mg orally q6h for 8 doses	Aqueous penicillin 30,000 U/kg mixed with procaine penicillin 600,000 U IM plus streptomycin 20 mg/kg IM 30 min prior to the procedure, then penicillin VK 500 mg q6h for 8 doses (250 mg for children under 25 kg) or Vancomycin 20 mg/kg IV as for adults, then erythromycin 10 mg/kg q6h for 8 doses
	Congenital or valvular heart disease, other factors	*Parenteral:* Same as adults with prosthetic valves; streptomycin may be omitted in situations associated with lower risk *Oral:* Penicillin VK 2.0 g 30 min prior to the procedure, then 500 mg orally q6h for 8 doses or	*Parenteral:* Same as children with prosthetic valves; streptomycin may be omitted in situations associated with lower risk *Oral:* For children under 25 kg, penicillin VK 1.0 g orally 30 min prior to the procedure, then 250 mg orally q6h for 8 doses; use adult regimen for children over 25 kg or

Infective Endocarditis

Procedure	Condition	Adults	Children
Genitourinary, gastrointestinal, incision and drainage of abscesses	Prosthetic heart valves, congenital or valvular heart disease, other factors	Erythromycin 1.0 g 2 hours prior to the procedure, then 500 mg orally q6h for 8 doses (1) Aqueous penicillin 2 million U IM or IV *or* Ampicillin 1.0 g IM or IV *plus* Gentamicin 1.5 mg/kg (up to 80 mg total) IM or IV *or* Streptomycin 1.0 g IM Give initial dose 30 min prior to procedure; repeat penicillin or ampicillin q8h for 3 doses; repeat gentamicin q8h for 2 doses; repeat streptomycin q12h for 2 doses (2) Vancomycin, 1 g IV *plus* streptomycin or gentamicin as above; repeat both drugs once in 12 hours	Erythromycin 20 mg/kg 2 hours prior to the procedure, then 10 mg/kg q6h for 8 doses (1) Aqueous penicillin 30,000 U/kg IM or IV *or* Ampicillin 50 mg/kg IM or IV *plus* Gentamicin 2.0 mg/kg IM or IV *or* Streptomycin 20 mg/kg IM Timing of doses is as for adults (2) Vancomycin 20 mg/kg administered as for adults *plus* streptomycin or gentamicin as above; repeat both drugs once in 12 hours
Cardiac, incision and drainage of staphylococcal abscesses	Prosthetic heart valves, congenital and valvular heart disease, other factors	Cefazolin 2.0 g IV or IM 30 min prior to procedure, repeated q8h for 5 doses *or* Vancomycin 0.5 g IV q8h for 5 doses	Cefazolin 30 mg/kg IV or IM administered as for adults *or* Vancomycin 20 mg/kg IV or IM administered as for adults

IM, Intramuscularly; IV, intravenously.

develop in patients with prosthetic cardiac valves.

The signs of endocarditis reflect the underlying cardiac infection, with dissemination of infected debris throughout the circulation. These signs must be specifically sought and may not be obvious when the patient is first examined. Fever is the single most common sign, and temperatures are only moderately elevated. In *Staphylococcus aureus* infections, however, the mean temperature is 39° C. The combination of fever and a heart murmur suggests cardiac infection, although murmurs may be absent or atypical initially. Up to 90% of all patients eventually develop an associated cardiac murmur, but murmurs may be absent in a third of patients with acute IE and in half the patients with tricuspid valve infection. Similarly, changing murmurs are observed in a minority of cases. The appearance of a new regurgitant murmur in the setting of positive blood cultures is diagnostic of infective endocarditis. The onset of heart failure with fever, with or without heart murmurs, also suggests the diagnosis.

In clinical series, isolated infection of the mitral valve is present in 35 to 45% of patients. The aortic valve is involved in up to 30% of patients, and some studies suggest that the proportion is increasing. Infection of both mitral and aortic valves occurs in approximately 20% of patients and has a worse prognosis. Aortic valve infection is more common in elderly males and is more often due to virulent organisms. Both factors are associated with increased mortality rates. Similarly, heart failure complicates aortic valve infection more often than mitral valve infection: 80 and 50% of cases, respectively. Once heart failure is present, it is more severe and is more poorly tolerated in aortic valve than in mitral valve infections.

In the general population, infection of the right side of the heart is uncommon and occurs only in 5 to 10% of cases, but the tricuspid valve is involved in up to 75% of cases of endocarditis in intravenous drug abusers. *Staphylococcus aureus*, other virulent gram positive cocci, gram-negative rods, and fungi are most often responsible. The clinical manifestations of tricuspid endocarditis are the signs and symptoms of septic pulmonary embolism. Congestive heart failure is rarely seen with this type of infection, but when present, it is due to occult left-heart failure with endocarditis, extensive pulmonary disease with cor pulmonale, or bacterial pericarditis with tamponade. Death is unusual in infections of the right heart chamber; if it occurs, it is generally secondary to uncontrolled infection in the lungs or to meningitis. Bilateral heart chamber infections are also uncommon, with an incidence of 1 to 2%.

Congestive heart failure is the most common cardiac consequence of left-sided IE. Other consequences include heart block, arrhythmias, valvular ring abscess, myocarditis and myocardial abscess, pericarditis with or without tamponade, myocardial infarction, aneurysms, and extension of infection with formation of fistulous tracts. Heart failure and cardiac complications are the most common cause of death in IE.

NEUROLOGIC SIGNS

Neurologic manifestations, septic and embolic in origin, are present during the course of IE in about a third of patients. Elderly patients, those infected with virulent organisms, and those with left-chamber involvement more commonly have neuropsychiatric complications. Three clinical syndromes are recognizable: (1) toxic encephalopathy, characterized by headache, inability to concentrate, irritability, confusion, disorientation, and psychosis; (2) meningoencephalitis, characterized by headache and meningismus, with or without acute organic brain syndrome; and (3) focal neurologic deficits with findings of a stroke, aphasia, cranial nerve deficits, ataxia, myelopathy, or peripheral neuropathy. Aseptic meningitis, cerebritis, and encephalopathy are most common. Lumbar puncture, especially in those with meningoencephalitis, typically reveals a mild pleocytosis, possibly a modest elevation in protein levels, normal glucose levels, and sterile cultures.

Clinical syndromes are not specific for pathologic entities. Pathologically, meningitis, infarction with or without abscess, mycotic aneurysm, or brain abscess may be present. All may have similar cerebrospinal fluid (CSF) findings. Mycotic aneurysms are usually clinically silent, with an unremarkable CSF formula until they rupture, sometimes months to years after cure of the infection. Focal neurologic deficits are unusual at first and generally occur shortly after the start of therapy. Fever in the presence of a stroke, however, especially in a younger patient, demands that IE be excluded by appropriate cultures.

Computed axial tomography and contrast angiography are useful in delineating the cause of a neurologic deficit. Angiographic examination is particularly helpful in evaluating subarachnoid hemorrhage, which may necessitate early surgical intervention. Medical therapy appropriate to IE usually treats neurologic manifestations, including unruptured aneurysm. Appropriate management of such an aneurysm is controversial. Rarely, brain abscesses require drainage after a course of antimicrobial therapy.

Central nervous system (CNS) complications are second only to cardiac complications as a cause of death in IE. Coma, meningitis, and brain abscess have been associated with up to 70% mortality rate. *Staphylococcus aureus*, in particular, is associated with a high incidence of CNS manifestations.

PERIPHERAL SIGNS

The peripheral manifestations of IE are caused by one of three possible mechanisms: embolism, immune complex deposition, or metastatic infection. The cutaneous stigmata classically described in patients with IE are subungual or splinter hemorrhages, subconjunctival and dermal petechiae, Osler's nodes, and Janeway lesions (Fig. 14–1). Roth's spots are similar hemorrhagic lesions of the optic fundus (Fig. 14–2). Splinter hemorrhages and petechiae, the most common signs, are found in a quarter to half of all patients. Although these findings are non-

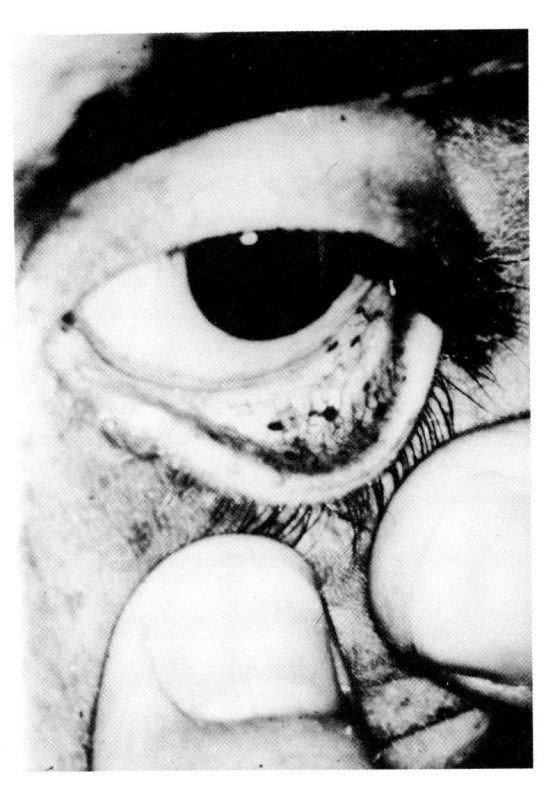

Fig. 14–1. Subconjunctival petechiae.

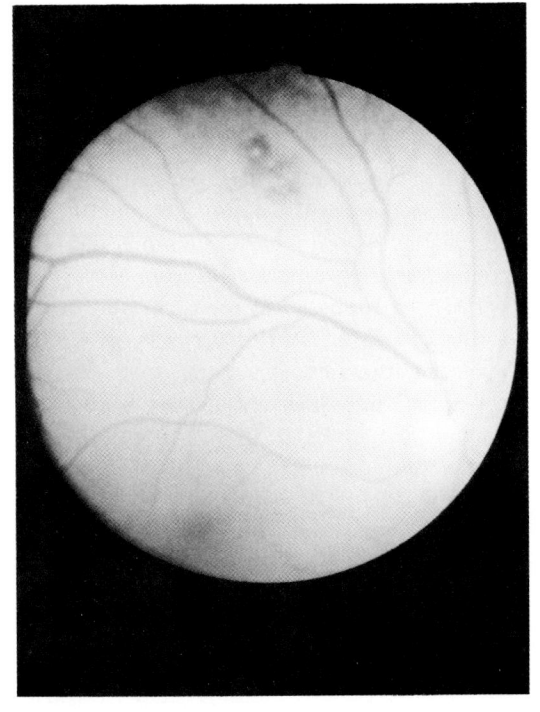

Fig. 14–2. Roth's spots.

specific, their presence in a febrile patient should prompt appropriate evaluation to exclude IE. Osler's nodes (Plate 5C and D) are tender, painful, erythematous or purplish, raised, pea-sized lesions generally localized to the pads of the toes or the fingers, although they are sometimes found on the palms of the hands or the soles of the feet; Janeway lesions are flat, painless, and nontender and are localized to the palms and soles, but they may otherwise resemble Osler's nodes in appearance. Osler's nodes, Janeway lesions, and Roth's spots are reported in 10 to 15% of patients with endocarditis, a much lower percentage than the 50 to 70% reported from the preantibiotic era. These lesions occur with about equal frequency in patients with acute or subacute left-sided disease.

The pathogenesis of these lesions remains controversial. Histopathologically, the lesions are described as a vasculitis with inflammation and central necrosis.

Other diseases characterized as immune complex mediated are rarely associated with these findings of IE. Some have attributed the phenomena to immune complex deposition and vasculitis. More recent data support Osler's original contention that these lesions are due to minute septic emboli lodging in the microvasculature.

Immune injury is important in other manifestations of endocarditis. Splenomegaly is probably the result of persistent antigenic stimulation. Assays for circulating immune complexes are frequently positive in patients with IE, rheumatoid factor is present in the serum of up to half the patients, and antinuclear antibodies have been reported. Occasionally, immune-mediated thrombocytopenia accompanies IE. Many musculoskeletal manifestations of IE, particularly culture-negative arthritis, likely involve immune complex deposition. The best-documented example of immune complex injury is acute glomerulonephritis, which occurs in up to 15% of patients. This disease is characterized by azotemia, hematuria, and sometimes, red blood cell casts and hypocomplementemia. Histopathologic studies reveal a typical lumpy-bumpy distribution of fluorescent antibody directed against complement and immunoglobulin along the basement membrane of the glomerulus. Electron micrographs disclose subepithelial electron-dense deposits common to other immune complex forms of nephritis.

Metastatic infection is encountered in IE of all origins, but it is more common in infection with virulent organisms, particularly *Staphylococcus aureus*. Virtually any organ or tissue may be involved. The myocardial and neurologic complications have already been described. Pneumonia, pulmonary abscess, and empyema are common in right-sided infection. Osteomyelitis, spinal epidural abscess, septic arthritis, splenic or hepatic abscess, pancreatitis, renal abscess, and systemic mycotic aneurysm may all be encountered.

Major artery embolism, other than to the CNS, is common in IE, but it is often clinically silent. Splenic infarcts may present as acute upper-left-quadrant pain. Renal infarction may be accompanied by flank pain and hematuria. Emboli may lodge in mesenteric arteries and may precipitate an acute abdomen. A cold extremity may be the first clue to an underlying endocarditis.

Although manifestations and complications may be viewed as primarily cardiac, septic, embolic, or immune mediated, in fact, a complex interaction among all these factors is more likely. Certain complications, such as empyema, are almost certainly infectious, but others, notably cerebral mycotic aneurysm, may be embolic and septic events modified by host immune responses.

> Objective 14–3. Select the tests that help to establish the diagnosis of endocarditis.

ROUTINE LABORATORY TESTS

Numerous laboratory abnormalities are encountered in patients with infective endocarditis, and most are nonspecific. Almost all patients have a normochromic, normocytic anemia. That the hematocrit is higher in patients with acute endocarditis reflects the shorter duration of illness. A mild leukocytosis occurs early in subacute infections, but it disappears as the disease becomes chronic. Leukocytosis is more marked in acute fulminant infection and is often associated with increased numbers of bands. White blood cell counts of 25,000 may be encountered in *Staphylococcus aureus* endocarditis. The patient's platelet count is normal or low; low counts are secondary to sepsis or immune mechanisms.

The erythrocyte sedimentation rate is elevated in over 90% of patients. A normal value calls the diagnosis into question. Associated abnormalities include hypergammaglobulinemia, positive rheumatoid factor (present in 25% of cases of acute endocarditis, increasing to 50% as the duration approaches 6 weeks), and circulating immune complexes. Values greater than 100 µg/ml by the Raji-cell radioimmunoassay are indicative of valvular infection, whereas undetectable levels are evidence against endocarditis.

Urinary abnormalities are common. Microscopic hematuria occurs in half the patients, and pyuria and positive urine cultures are also frequently seen. Azotemia occurs in fewer than 15% of patients, and frank renal failure is rare. Azotemia may be present because of prior renal disease, especially in the elderly, or because of heart failure with associated renal azotemia. In general, azotemia reflects an underlying glomerulonephritis documented by demonstrating hypocomplmentemia. Whether or not azotemia is present, 90% of patients have glomerulopathy demonstrable by renal biopsy.

CHEST ROENTGENOGRAM

The chest roentgenogram is particularly useful in patients with pulmonary complaints, in drug addicts, and in those with possible right-sided infections. In tricuspid infection with *Staphylococcus aureus*, the chest roentgenogram is abnormal in three-quarters of cases. Characteristic abnormalities are multiple peripheral, pleural-based defects, occasionally cavitating. Other findings include streaky pulmonary infiltrates, signs of pleural effusion or consolidation, and rarely, a picture compatible with adult respiratory distress syndrome. In patients with left chamber involvement, signs of heart failure predominate.

ELECTROCARDIOGRAM

The electrocardiogram is usually nonspecific, with sinus tachycardia the most common finding. Signs of myocardial infarction, pericarditis, or conducting defects are uncommon but ominous.

CULTURE OF BLOOD AND OTHER SUBSTANCES

Blood culture, by far the most useful test, identifies the responsible organism in approximately 90 to 95% of cases. Isolation and identification of the infecting agent is essential in planning rational therapy. Culture-negative cases occur, often because of previous antibiotic administration. The current decrease in incidence probably reflects improved culture techniques and strict case definition.

In cases destined to be culture-positive, at least 1 of the first 2 cultures is positive in 98% of cases. One can expect 95% of all cultures drawn to be positive. In the absence of previous antimicrobial agents, little is gained by obtaining more than 3 to 4 blood cultures. Cultures must be obtained prior to administration of antibiotics. Blood cultures of 5- to 10-ml samples, each obtained from multiple sites over a few hours, minimize delay if therapy must be initiated. This technique also maximizes the yield and obviates the problem of contamination. The venipuncture site must be prepared under sterile conditions, and the blood must be obtained by sterile technique. The bacteremia is on the order of 1 to 50 colony-forming units per milliliter, so the sample must be large enough to ensure an adequate inoculum.

In addition to blood, other valuable sources of culture material are urine, pleural fluid, cerebrospinal fluid, synovial fluid, abscesses, and embolic foci on the extremities. Gram staining of these specimens may provide early clues to the responsible organisms. Culture and microscopic evaluation of a major artery embolus may be the only source of positive culture material, especially in fungal and culture-negative endocarditis.

ECHOCARDIOGRAM

Echocardiography in the diagnosis and management of infective endocarditis continues to be investigated. Vegetations, detected in half of patients, are associated with an increased incidence of heart failure, cerebrovascular embolism, and death. The echocardiogram is useful in evaluating ventricular function and in detecting flail aortic or mitral valve leaflets. Mitral valve preclosure is an important sign of aortic regurgitation. Association of vegetations with any of these findings connotes a worse prognosis. Some investigators maintain that echocardiographic demonstration of valvular vegetations of the left heart constitutes an indication for early operation. Although the presence of valvular vegetations alerts the clinician to the increased likelihood of serious complications, this finding should be considered in light of the patient's hemodynamic status. Congestive heart failure, and not the presence or absence of vegetations, is the major indication for surgical intervention.

Echocardiography helps the clinician to categorize patients likely to be at increased risk, and if congestive heart failure supervenes, an echocardiogram is useful in selecting surgical patients and in directing treatment to the affected valve. Some centers proceed to operation without cardiac catheterization if valvular vegetations are demonstrated in a patient with serious hemodynamic compromise secondary to IE.

> Objective 14–4. Treat endocarditis properly.

The cornerstone of modern management of IE is antimicrobial therapy. Surgical treatment is reserved for special indications. Effective antibiotic therapy consists of prolonged courses of bactericidal agents in large doses. In general, bacteriostatic drugs have no role in the treatment of endocarditis. Because the infection is inaccessible to host phagocytic defenses, bacteriostatic agents, which depend on host responses for their efficacy, are unable to clear the infection, and the relapse rate is unacceptably high. The serum must be capable of rapid and complete killing without benefit of phagocytic cells; hence large doses may be needed. For similar reasons, prolonged therapy is recommended to ensure eradication of all organisms. Combinations of bactericidal antibiotics may be synergistic against certain organisms and may permit shorter courses of therapy in some patients.

GENERAL PRINCIPLES OF TREATMENT

General principles of management of IE include documentation of susceptibility of the organism to the antibiotics prescribed. Determination of minimum inhibitory and bactericidal concentrations (MIC and MBC) by broth dilution technique is recommended. Achievable serum antibiotic levels ideally must exceed the MBC severalfold to insure killing of the bacteria. What may seem adequate therapy in vitro may be inadequate in vivo. Determination of the serum bactericidal titers (SBT) attempts to circumvent this problem by demonstrating that a dilution of the patient's serum is bactericidal for the patient's infecting organism. A dilution of 1 to 8 or greater an hour after antibiotic administration is recommended.

Antibiotic failures occur, and these methods help to identify causes and to guide changes in therapy. Some organisms may be tolerant to single agents at achievable doses; that is, the MBC exceeds the MIC by a ratio greater than 32 to 1. Other organisms are insensitive to single agents; for example, the enterococcus resists killing by penicillin or vancomycin alone. Still others are sensitive by in vitro methods, but drugs fail to clear the bacteremia. A combination of agents demonstrating in vitro bactericidal synergy is indicated in patients who do not respond clinically or microbiologically to single-drug therapy.

INDICATIONS FOR ANTIMICROBIAL THERAPY

At times, antimicrobial therapy must be initiated prior to identification of the organism and its sensitivities. The clinical setting is a source of clues to the most likely responsible organism. Prosthetic cardiac valve infection within 3 months of operation is most likely due to *Staphylococcus aureus* or *S. epidermidis*. Late prosthetic valve infections are similar to natural valve infection in bacteriologic features, but *S. epidermidis* infection is still common. *S. aureus*, fungi, and gram-negative rods are more common in intravenous drug abusers. Endocarditis in patients with rheumatic heart disease is usually due to alpha-hemolytic streptococci. Infection with enterococci must be suspected in patients with endocarditis following genitourinary manipulation with prostatism, or with recurrent urinary tract infections. Administration of nafcillin, penicillin, and gentamicin is reasonable initial therapy, pending results of culture and sensitivity testing.

Recommendations for definite therapy for IE caused by the most common pathogens are outlined in Table 14–2. Certain situations merit special considerations. For example, endocarditis caused by viridans streptococci is cured by 4 weeks of penicillin alone. Combination therapy for a short course (2 weeks) is not advisable in complicated cases and when the risk of streptomycin toxicity is too high or is unacceptable at any level. Enterococci are not killed by single agents, and cephalosporins are totally ineffective against these organisms. Approximately 40% of strains are resistant to streptomycin, and gentamicin must be substituted.

Certain strains of staphylococci exhibit tolerance to various agents in that they are inhibited by low concentrations but are not killed by high concentrations of the antibiotic, and the clinical course is more complicated if these organisms are responsible for the illness. Most patients with staphylococcal endocarditis can be treated effectively with a semisynthetic beta-lactamase-resistant penicillin such as nafcillin at doses of 8 to 10 g daily for 4 weeks. Initial administration of an aminoglycoside such as gentamicin or tobramycin for the first 5 days may accelerate clearing of the bacteremia. The addition of either an aminoglycoside or rifampin, 300 mg bid orally, may be useful in the treatment of tolerant bacterial strains. Vancomycin or a cephalosporin may be given to patients allergic to penicillin.

Gram-negative rods, chlamydiae, rickettsiae, and fungi are notably resistant to antimicrobial therapy. Surgical intervention with extirpation of the infected valve is usually necessary, in addition to prolonged antibiotic therapy.

Anaerobic organisms are a rare cause of endocarditis, and little has been reported. Organisms resistant to penicillin, notably *Bacteroides fragilis*, are probably best treated with bactericidal antimicrobial agents such as metronidazole.

Endocarditis of prosthetic valves is a special problem often requiring both prolonged antimicrobial therapy and surgical intervention. Mortality rates are high, especially in the postoperative period. Possible mistakes in management are: failure to suspect the diagnosis in a febrile patient after operation; failure to anticipate complications once the diagnosis is made; and needless delays in early reoperation if the clinical course is complicated.

INDICATIONS FOR SURGICAL TREATMENT

Even the most appropriate antimicrobial therapy fails in some cases, and some complications of IE are not amenable to medical therapy alone. Clear-cut indications for early surgical intervention are rapid deterioration of the patient's condition and an inability to manage the patient's hemodynamic status medically. Persistence of infection despite antibiotic therapy, prosthetic valve dysfunction

Table 14–2. Definitive Therapy of Native-Valve Endocarditis*

Organism	Regiment	Duration of Therapy (weeks)
Viridans streptococci and *Streptococcus bovis* (MIC ≤ 0.2 μg/ml), penicillin-sensitive	(1) Penicillin G 2–3 million U IV q4h	4
	(2) Procaine penicillin G 1.2 million U IM q6h or penicillin G 2–3 million U IV q4h plus streptomycin 10 mg/kg (not to exceed 500 mg) q12h IM‡	2 2 2
	(3) Cephalothin 2 g IV q4h§	4
	(4) Vancomycin 1 g IV q12h§	4
Viridans streptococci and *Streptococcus bovis* (MIC > 0.2 μg/ml), relatively penicillin-resistant	Penicillin G 3 million U IV q4h plus streptomycin 10 mg/kg q12h IM (not to exceed 500 mg)	4 2–4‖
Enterococci, streptomycin-sensitive (MIC < 1500 μg/ml)	Penicillin G 3 million U IV q4h plus streptomycin 10 mg/kg q12h (not to exceed 500 mg)	4–6# 4–6#
Enterococci, streptomycin-resistant (MIC ≥ 1500 μg/ml)	Substitute gentamicin 1.0 mg/kg q8h IV or IM for streptomycin	4–6#
Staphylococcus aureus, methicillin-sensitive	(1) Nafcillin 1.5 mg IV q4h	4
	(2) Cephalothin 2 g IV q4h§	4
	(3) Vancomycin 1 g IV q12h§	4
Staphylococcus aureus, methicillin-resistant	Vancomycin 1 g IV q12h	4

*Dosages are for patients with normal renal function.
†For children the dosages are as follows: penicillin G, 150,000 U/kg/day; streptomycin, 15 mg/kg q12h (not to exceed 500 mg); cephalothin, 150 mg/kg/day; vancomycin, 20 mg/kg/day.
‡Not recommended for patients older than 65 years, with pre-existing renal or vesticular impairment, with prosthetic valve infection or extracardiac foci of infection, or with IE caused by nutritionally variant streptococci.
§For penicillin-allergic patients.
‖Two weeks of streptomycin may be sufficient if the MIC of the isolate is 0.5 g/ml.
#Six weeks of treatment are suggested if symptoms have been present for more than 2 months.

with associated infection, recurrent embolization, and possibly hemodynamic compromise caused by a large vegetation are other indications for surgical intervention. In a patient whose condition is stabilized with medical management, operation may be delayed until antimicrobial therapy is completed. Patients with moderate or severe congestive heart failure, especially when the aortic valve is involved, are best managed surgically. Most authorities agree that early operation is preferable in these patients, even before completion of antimicrobial therapy. Delays often result in further deterioration of the patient's condition. Concerns about implantation of a prosthetic valve in the presence of continued infection are, in general, outweighed by the increased risk and surgical mortality rates associated with delay.

Objective 14–5. Manage prosthetic valve endocarditis.

Prosthetic cardiac valve infections and postcardiotomy infections are serious complications of cardiovascular surgical procedures. Prosthetic valve infections may be characterized as either early or late. By definition, early infections occur within 2 months of operation, and late infections occur thereafter. These infections may be subtle, often manifesting only as a low-grade postoperative fever or insidious congestive heart failure, and peripheral stigmata of IE are usually absent. The risk of prosthetic valve infection is approximately 1% in the immediate postoperative period and falls to 0.5% per year thereafter. *Staphylococcus aureus* and *S. epidermidis* cause most early infections; the remainder are caused by streptococci, gram-negative rods, and candida. Late prosthetic valve infections, which make up two-thirds of all cases, resemble infection of a natural cardiac valve but staphylococcal species still are more common.

The mortality rate is up to 60% in some series and is worse in early infections. Prompt surgical intervention is often necessary to achieve a cure. A new heart murmur is the most reliable cardiac sign, and one should listen carefully for the regurgitant murmur of paraprosthetic valvular leak. Fluoroscopic examination is helpful in documenting suture disrupture by revealing a rocking motion of the valve. Arterial embolism may be a presenting sign. Proper therapy, which requires identification of the responsible organism, is discussed previously. In general, treatment should be continued for 6 weeks.

> **Objective 14–6.** Define a practical approach when blood cultures are negative, even though the clinical setting is consistent with endocarditis.

IE with negative blood cultures is diagnosed in the presence of fever, a pathologic heart murmur, and clinical manifestations of endocarditis such as cutaneous stigmata, major artery embolism, and congestive heart failure without other cause. Probably, the most common cause of culture-negative endocarditis is prior administration of antibiotics. Uremia has also been suggested as a possible cause. Almost any organism, including *Staphylococcus aureus*, has been reported to cause this syndrome. Whenever culture-negative IE is encountered, certain organisms should be suspected and excluded. Bacteria responsible for this syndrome are as mentioned previously if previous antimicrobial agents have been administered, but the list also includes anaerobes, nutritionally dependent streptococci, haemophilus and other fastidious organisms, L-forms, and brucella. Unusual causes are *Coxiella burnetti* (the agent of Q fever) and psittacosis. These organisms and fungi do not grow well on routine culture and also cause culture-negative IE. Serologic tests and careful examination of embolic debris may reveal the causative agent, but the organism is not always identified, even with surgical exploration or autopsy. In these patients, immune phenomena may play a role.

Once the diagnosis of culture-negative endocarditis is entertained, one should try to make a bacteriologic diagnosis. The procedure involves withholding or discontinuing antimicrobial therapy until sufficient and appropriate cultures are obtained, sometimes over several days. One should attempt to identify nonbacterial causes from laboratory, epidemiologic, or historical data. A therapeutic trial may be in order; most authorities feel that unless *Staphylococcus aureus* is the likely cause, treatment should be directed against enterococci. The clinical trial is followed by observing the patient for disappearance of fever, improved well-being, and resolution of symptoms.

SUGGESTED READINGS

Alpert, J.C., et al.: Pathogenesis of Osler's nodes. Ann. Intern. Med., 85:471, 1976.
American Heart Association Committee on Prevention of Bacterial Endocarditis: Prevention of bacterial endocarditis. Circulation, 56:139A, 1977.
American Heart Association Subcommittee on Treatment of Bacterial Endocarditis: Treatment of infective endocarditis due to viridans streptococci. Circulation, 63:730A, 1981.
Buchbinder, N.A., and Roberts, W.C.: Left-sided valvular active infective endocarditis. A study of forty-five necropsy patients. Am. J. Med., 53:20, 1972.
Cannady, P.B., and Sanford, J.P.: Negative blood cultures in infective endocarditis: a review. South. Med. J., 69:1420, 1976.
Cherubin, C.E., and Neu, H.C.: Infective endocarditis

at the Presbyterian Hospital in New York City from 1938–1967. Am. J. Med., 51:83, 1971.

Clemens, J.D., et al.: A controlled evaluation of the risk of bacterial endocarditis in persons with mitral valve prolapse. N. Engl. J. Med., 307:776, 1982.

Corrigall, D., Bolen, J., Hancock, E.W., and Popp, R.L.: Mitral valve prolapse and infective endocarditis. Am. J. Med., 63:215, 1977.

Dinubile, M.J.: Surgery in active endocarditis. Ann. Intern. Med., 96:650, 1982.

Durack, D.T.: Prophylaxis of infective endocarditis. In Principles and Practice of Infectious Diseases. Edited by G.L. Mandell, R.G. Douglas, Jr., and J.E. Bennett. New York, John Wiley and Sons, 1979.

Durack, D.T.: Experimental bacterial endocarditis. IV. Structure and evolution of very early lesions. J. Pathol., 115:81, 1975.

Everett, E.D., and Hirschmann, J.V.: Transient bacteremia and endocarditis prophylaxis: a review. Medicine, 56:61, 1977.

Kaplan, E.L., and Taranta, A.V.: Infective Endocarditis: An American Heart Association Symposium. Dallas, American Heart Association, 1977.

Kaplan, E.L., Rich, H., Gersony, W., and Manning, J.: A collaborative study of infective endocarditis in the 1970s. Circulation, 59:327, 1979.

Kaye, D.: Infective Endocarditis. Baltimore, University Park Press, 1976.

Lerner, P.I., and Weinstein, L.: Infective endocarditis in the antibiotic era. N. Engl. J. Med., 274:199, 259, 323, 388, 1966.

Mills, J., Utley, J., and Abbott, J.: Heart failure in infective endocarditis: predisposing factors, course and treatment. Chest, 66:151, 1974.

Pazin, G.J., Saul, S., and Thompson, M.E.: Blood cultures positivity. Suppression by outpatient antibiotic therapy in patients with bacterial endocarditis. Arch. Intern. Med., 142:263, 1982.

Pelletier, L.L., and Petersdorf, R.G.: Infective endocarditis: a review of 125 cases from the University of Washington Hospitals, 1963–1972. Medicine, 56:287, 1977.

Rahimtoola, S.H.: Infective Endocarditis. New York, Grune and Stratton, 1978.

Reisberg, B.E.: Infective endocarditis in the narcotic addict. Prog. Cardiovasc. Dis., 22:193, 1979.

Sabath, L.D., et al.: A new type of penicillin resistance of Staphylococcus aureus. Lancet, 1:443, 1977.

Sande, M.A., and Scheld, W.M.: Bacterial adherence in endocarditis: Interaction of bacterial dextran, platelets, fibrin, and antibody. Scand. J. Infec. Dis., 24(Suppl.):100, 1980.

Sande, M.A., and Scheld, W.M.: Combination antibiotic therapy of bacterial endocarditis. Ann. Intern. Med., 92:390, 1980.

Scheld, W.M., and Sande, M.E.: Endocarditis and intravascular infection. In Principles and Practice of Infectious Diseases. Edited by G.L. Mandell, R.G. Douglas, Jr., and J.E. Bennett. New York, John Wiley and Sons, 1979.

Stewart, J.A., et al.: Endocardiographic documentation of vegetative lesions in infective endocarditis: clinical implications. Circulation, 61:374, 1980.

Von Reyn, C.F., et al.: Infective endocarditis: an analysis based on strict case definitions. Ann. Intern. Med., 94:505, 1981.

Wilson, W.R., et al.: Valve replacement in patients with active infective endocarditis. Circulation, 58:585, 1978.

Ziment, I.: Nervous system complications in bacterial endocarditis. Am. J. Med., 47:593, 1969.

CHAPTER 15

Pericarditis and Myocarditis

Y. Morin

> Objective 15–1. Diagnose and treat pericarditis.

Pericarditis can be either dry, effusive, or fibrous. Pleuritis and myocarditis often coexist.

DRY PERICARDITIS

The initial symptoms of dry or fibrinous pericarditis are general and relate to the causal infection. The diagnosis of pericarditis should be suspected when the patient experiences characteristic chest pain. Usually sternal in location, this pain may be precordial or even epigastric and radiates widely, mainly to the neck and shoulders. The pain is increased by breathing, coughing, swallowing, and belching, and it is relieved by sitting up or by leaning forward. At times, the pain may be severe, but it may diminish when an effusion develops.

One specific physical sign of dry pericarditis is the pericardial friction rub, a rough, superficial sound, usually heard during both systole and diastole. The sound often increases during inspiration or when the patient leans forward.

The electrocardiogram is abnormal in 80% of patients with dry pericarditis. The first changes consist of generalized ST segment elevations without reciprocal ST depression. In approximately a week, the ST segment returns to the baseline, followed by a symmetric T-wave inversion that may persist for months. Atrial fibrillation or flutter is present in 10% of these patients.

Treatment of acute (usually viral) pericarditis consists of bed rest and pain relief. Aspirin or indomethacin should be prescribed. Corticosteroid administration is successful in severe cases, but the disease often recurs after cessation of steroid therapy.

PERICARDIAL EFFUSION

Although pericardial fluid accumulates, the pericardial friction rub does not usually disappear. The heart sounds may become faint and the cardiac apex difficult to palpate. The increasing pressure in the pericardial sac distends the jugular vein.

The electrocardiogram shows low voltage of the QRS complexes, and a chest roentgenogram reveals a global enlargement of the cardiac silhouette with clear lung fields. Serial examinations show enlargement of heart size. The echocardiogram (Figs. 15–1 and 15–2) is sensitive and specific in detecting

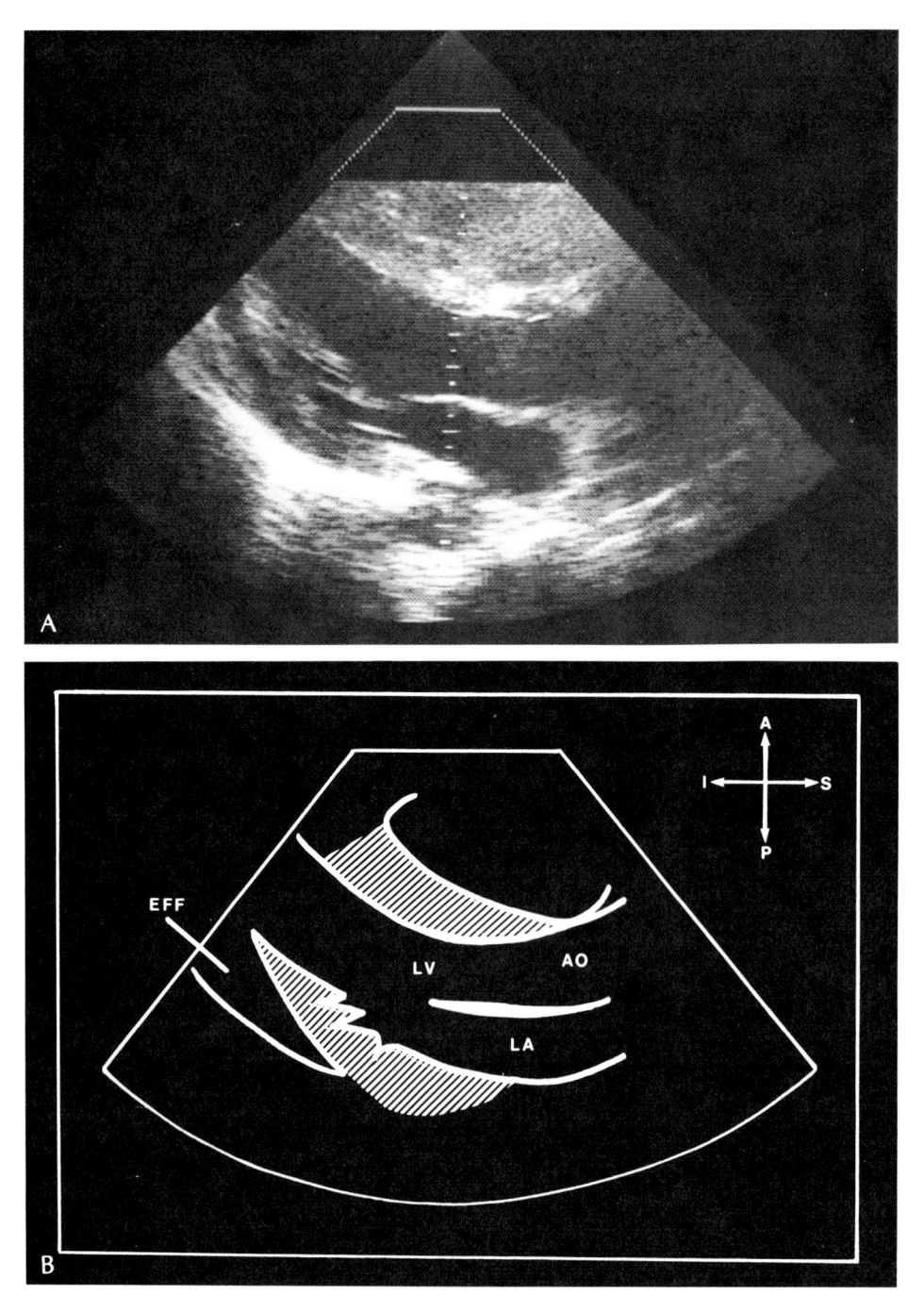

Fig. 15–1. *A* and *B,* Bidimensional echocardiogram showing a moderate posterior pericardial effusion (EFF). LV, Left ventricle; AO, aorta; LA, left auricle.

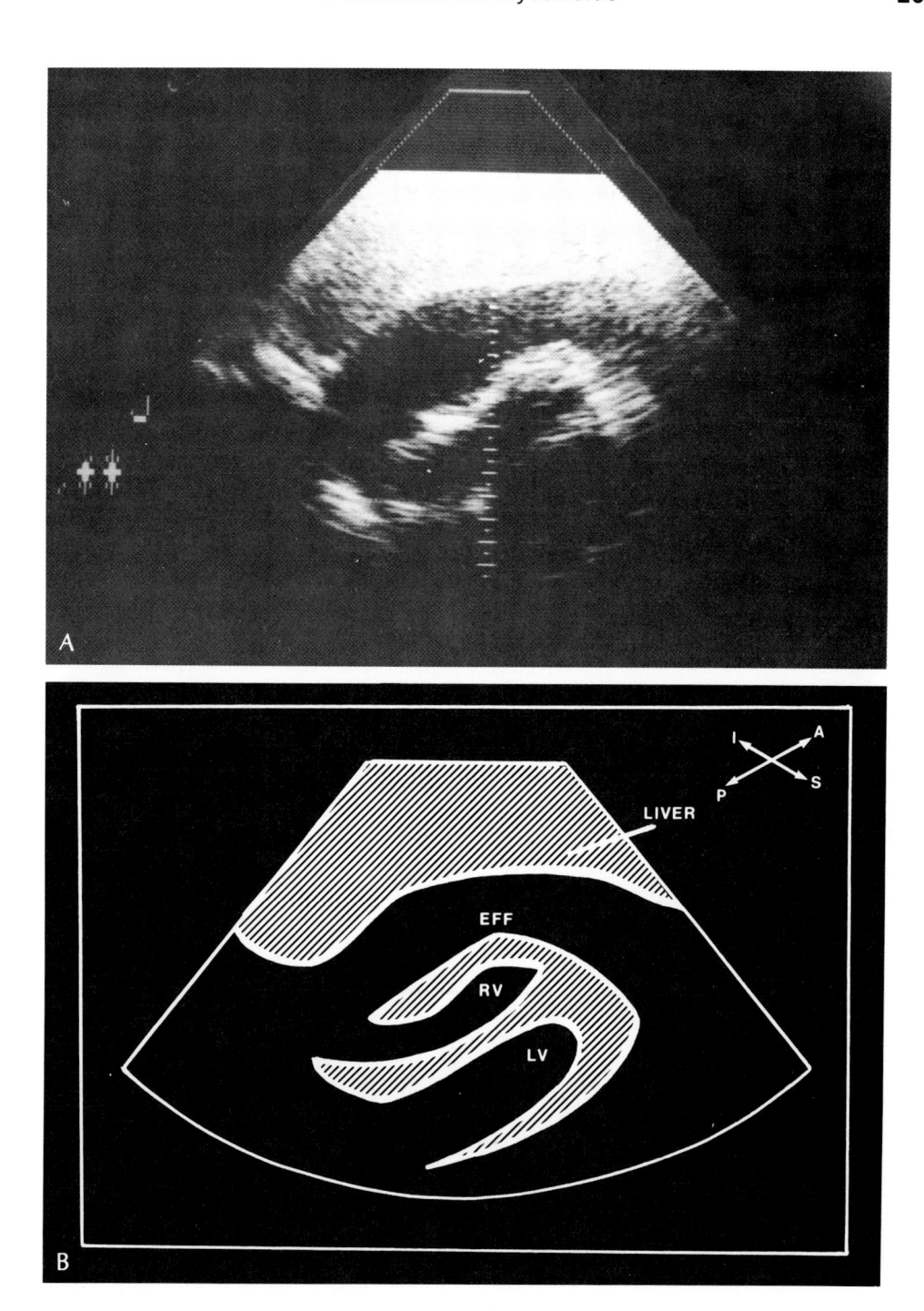

Fig. 15–2. *A* and *B,* Bidimensional echocardiogram. (subcostal view) showing a large pericardial effusion (EFF) and a pericardial thickening. RV, Right ventricle; LV, left ventricle.

pericardial effusion; it demonstrates as little as 30 ml excess fluid. Fluid usually accumulates posterior to the myocardium. When the effusion becomes moderate, it is detectable in the anterior space. At that point, the echocardiogram may show a swinging motion of the heart within the pericardial sac.

CARDIAC TAMPONADE

When fluid accumulates rapidly or when the pericardium is inflexible, the intrapericardial pressure will exceed normal diastolic pressure in both ventricles. As a result, cardiac filling is impaired, ventricular volumes are reduced, and cardiac output drops. Cardiac tamponade is a serious condition because it is often unrecognized and can be rapidly fatal.

Symptoms and signs of cardiac tamponade are related to increased venous pressure and to low cardiac output. Elevation of the jugular venous pressure is uniformly seen in this disorder, with a prominent systolic descent. The patient's heart rate is rapid, and pulsus paradoxus is found in 80% of cases. Defined as a fall of more than 10 mm Hg in systolic arterial pressure on inspiration, pulsus paradoxus is more easily recognized in intra-arterial pressure tracings. It is caused by the abnormal septal shift toward the left ventricle that occurs when the right ventricle is unable to accommodate the increased venous return during inspiration. Echocardiographic examination reveals the pericardial effusion, the marked changes of the right ventricular cavity with respiration, and the inspiratory shift of the septum to the left ventricle. Hypotension with narrowed pulse pressure is common, and frank shock occurs in severe cases.

The treatment of cardiac tamponade is pericardiocentesis.

FIBROUS PERICARDITIS

As pericardial inflammation becomes chronic, the pericardial cavity is progressively transformed into a sheath of fibrous tissue that may interfere with cardiac filling. As ventricular compliance is progressively reduced, diastolic filling generates abnormally high pressures in late diastole. Diastolic volumes drop as well as cardiac output. This syndrome is called pericardial constriction.

The onset of this disease is frequently insidious. Ascites, often the first sign, may be so severe that the physician confuses this disorder with cirrhosis. The patient's neck veins are distended and show an early diastolic dip caused by normal pressure in the ventricles during early diastole. This sign is not present in cardiac tamponade. On auscultation of the heart, a peculiar filling sound is heard in 50% of patients in early diastole; this sound is known as the pericardial knock. Atrial fibrillation or flutter is also common.

The chest roentgenogram shows a heart of normal size with, in half these patients, calcification of the pericardium. The echocardiogram is usually abnormal. The typical features are thickening of the pericardium, abnormal diastolic movement of the ventricular wall, and septal flattening. Cardiac catheterization should be performed to confirm the diagnosis; diastolic pressures in all chambers are uniformly elevated. In the ventricles, diastolic pressure is characterized by an early diastolic dip, that is, the square root sign.

The treatment of pericardial constriction is pericardectomy.

> Objective 15–2. Search for the cause of pericarditis of infectious origin.

Pericarditis can be infectious in origin, or it may be secondary to noninfectious systemic disorders. Only infectious pericarditis is considered in this section.

VIRAL PERICARDITIS

Viral pericarditis is often unrecognized and may be epidemic. Coxsackieviruses A and B are the most common causal agents and frequently affect the muscles and pleura, in addition to the myocardium. Other causative agents found in acute pericarditis are echoviruses, mumps virus, influenza viruses A and B, and Epstein-Barr virus. The virus can occasionally be identified by serial antibody titers during the acute and convalescent phase of the disease. In viral pericarditis, a small amount of exudate is usually found in the pericardium. The fluid is most often serous, but it can be purulent or hemorrhagic, especially in echoviral infections. Cardiac tamponade can occur suddenly and may even be the presenting syndrome. Constriction of the pericardium occurs in viral pericarditis, but its incidence is much lower than in other types of infectious pericarditis.

The first episode of viral pericarditis usually resolves in a few weeks. Half these patients have recurrences, however. In some patients frequent recurrences, immunologic in nature, become a serious clinical problem and even require pericardiectomy.

The place of corticosteroids in the treatment of viral pericarditis is controversial. They control symptoms quickly and are probably instrumental in reducing the amount of effusion that develops; however, no evidence suggests an improvement in the underlying pathologic process. Some patients with relapsing pericarditis become dependent upon corticosteroids. These agents are therefore contraindicated in bacterial pericarditis.

BACTERIAL PERICARDITIS

Nonpurulent pericarditis precedes bacterial pericarditis in approximately half the cases. The pericardium is rarely a primary site of bacterial infection; the source of the infecting organism is usually a pleuropulmonary infection. Bacterial pericarditis may develop from myocardial abscesses, from a perforating injury of the chest wall, or after a thoracic surgical procedure. Hematogenous spread occurs in debilated patients with chronic renal disease or diffuse carcinomatosis.

About a third of patients who died of purulent pericarditis had infections caused by gram-negative aerobic bacilli. In one-quarter of the patients, staphylococcus was the infecting organism, in the remaining cases, streptococci and pneumococci were responsible. Rarer causes included *Neisseria gonorrhoeae, N. meningitidis, Francisella tularensis*, and anaerobic bacteria. In an autopsy series of 55 patients with purulent pericarditis, the correct diagnosis had been made ante mortem in only 10 (18%).

Patients suffering from bacterial pericarditis are seriously ill. Cardiac tamponade may occur suddenly, and arrythmias are common.

The echocardiogram offers simple confirmatory evidence of effusion, and pericardiocentesis should be performed when fluid is demonstrated during the course of a febrile illness. This fluid shows a high leukocyte count ($> 50,000/mm^3$), a low glucose level (< 35 mg/dl), and a high protein content (> 3.0 g/dl). A Gram stain and smear should be done, as well as cultures (for acid-fast, aerobic, and anaerobic organisms) with antibiotic sensitivity testing. Antimicrobial therapy should begin promptly when the origin of the illness is unknown; oxacillin or a newer cephalosporin (cefotaxime, etc.), and an aminoglycoside are often combined as initial therapy. Local instillation of antibiotics into the pericardial sac does not seem indicated, but antibiotic treatment alone has a high mortality rate. Surgical drainage should be performed, followed immediately by pericardiectomy. Despite invasive management, the mortality rate for the condition remains high, at 30 to 40%.

TUBERCULOUS PERICARDITIS

Tuberculous pericarditis is now a rare condition (1% of pericardiocentesis) that occurs mainly in elderly patients, half of whom have pulmonary or disseminated tuberculosis. The course of the disease is insidious, often starting with mild chest pain. Tamponade is frequent, and the majority of those who survive develop pericardial constriction. On pericardiocentesis, the fluid is serous or, more often, serosanguinous, with the biologic characteristics described in Table 10–1. Culture results are positive in fewer than 15% of the cases. The effusion may reaccumulate despite repeated aspirations. Diagnosis depends on a high degree of suspicion. Tuberculous pericarditis should be considered in an elderly patient with an abnormal chest roentgenogram, a large intermediate or second-strength tuberculin skin test, and failure of the fluid to reduce after a week of corticosteroid therapy.

Echocardiograms should be performed regularly in patients with known tuberculosis. This routine procedure allows early detection of any pericardial involvement.

Treatment consists of antituberculous therapy, with corticosteroids reserved for severe cases with tamponade or persistent pericardial effusion. Pericardial drainage should be instituted early. In patients with pericardial constriction or repeated effusion, pericardiectomy should be performed after a course of antituberculous therapy.

OTHER TYPES OF INFECTIOUS PERICARDITIS

Fungal infection of the pericardium, such as candidiasis, coccidioidomycosis, histoplasmosis, and aspergillosis, occurs mainly in immunosuppressed and chronically ill patients. Cardiac tamponade is usually the presenting syndrome. Effusion is confirmed by echocardiography, and the etiologic diagnosis is made by pericardial biopsy.

Parasites such as *Entamoeba histolytica*, *Echinococcus granulosus*, *Toxoplasma gondii*, and *Trichinella spiralis* (see the boxed text on trichinosis later in this chapter) may also infect the pericardium.

> **Objective 15–3. Diagnose and treat an infectious myocarditis.**

Viruses are the most common causes of acute inflammation of the myocardium. In Latin America, however, Chagas myocarditis, caused by the protozoan *Trypanosoma cruzi*, is predominant. Although other infectious agents may produce cardiac inflammation, they do not present common clinical problems.

VIRAL MYOCARDITIS

Many viruses, such as echovirus, adenovirus, herpes varicella virus, poliovirus, mumps virus, and Epstein-Barr virus, may be associated with clinical evidence of myocarditis. Coxsackievirus B (6 types) is especially cardiotropic in humans and is the most common cause of myocarditis. Reports of epidemics of coxsackie viral infections have revealed that approximately one-third of the patients diagnosed develop myocardial disease as a result of the infection. Typically, patients suffering from coxsackie myocarditis also have clinical evidence of pericarditis and pleuritis.

In influenza, the incidence of myocarditis is approximately 10%, and the pericardium is not involved. Myocarditis is an important factor in fatal cases.

Clinical Manifestations. The clinical features of viral myocarditis vary widely. Patients may have tachycardia out of proportion to their fever, or they may have minor and evanescent electrocardiographic changes in the context of a known viral infection. In contrast to such minor clinical presentations, patients may also suffer from severe congestive heart failure, complex arrhythmias, or cardiogenic shock. Pulmonary and systemic emboli may be seen. Symptoms and signs are related to the severity of the disease and to the extent of cardiac involvement. In benign cases, dyspnea, atypical pain in the chest, and fatigue are the most common presenting symptoms. Physical examination reveals tachycardia, a third heart sound, and signs of cardiac enlargement. The electrocardiogram is abnormal (ST-T wave abnormalities), although the changes are nonspecific. Thus, a normal electrocardiogram prior to the illness is helpful in the diagnosis of viral myocarditis. Atrial arrhythmias and ventricular tachycardias are common. Conduction defects, bi- and trifascicular block, and complete atrioventricular block with Stokes-Adams attacks may dominate the clinical picture.

Myocardial enzymes, especially creatine phosphokinase isoenzymes, are elevated in the serum of patients with severe cases. The echocardiogram is most useful in assessing acute myocarditis because it helps to distinguish between patients in whom myocardial involvement is minor and those in whom contractility of the myocardium is depressed. The diagnosis is made on the diffuse character of hypokinesis. Echocardiograms should be repeated serially to evaluate heart chamber size and left ventricular function over the course of the disease. Gated cardiac blood pool imaging shows a drop in ejection fraction at rest in patients with severe myocardial damage. In patients who are asymptomatic or appear to have recovered, ejection fraction, although normal at rest, does not show the 15% increase normally found during exercise and usually falls below resting values.

The evolution of the disease is variable. In some patients, viral myocarditis is a fulminating often fatal, illness, as in nursery epidemics. It is not rare; 2.7% of sudden deaths in the population are caused by myocarditis. Generally, the prognosis for survival correlates well with the decrease in ejection fraction. The illness usually lasts 1 to 4 weeks. In 10% of patients, multiple recurrences are seen over a period of 2 to 3 years. In those patients, endomyocardial biopsy of the right ventricle should be considered. This procedure carries little risk if the surgeon is experienced, it shows the typical picture of a diffuse lymphocytic infiltrate with some plasma cells and histiocytes. Myocytolysis is also present. In severe cases, serial biopsies evaluate the treatment regimen. Biopsies repeated years after the initial episode have shown considerable fibrosis, but an absence of cell infiltrate. This finding suggests that chronic congestive cardiomyopathy is, in effect, a burnt-out acute viral myocarditis.

Treatment. Initially, the treatment of viral myocarditis should be directed to correction of the clinical consequences of myocardial involvement. Heart failure due to myocarditis responds to the usual treatment, although patients appear to be particularly sensitive to digitalis. Patients with severe cases require continuous hemodynamic monitoring and combinations of inotropic and vasodilating agents to maintain adequate cardiac output and satisfactory blood pressures.

Arrhythmias are treated in the usual way, and temporary or permanent artificial pacemakers are indicated for treatment of bradycardias. Anticoagulants should be prescribed, especially if ventricular thrombi are seen by echocardiography. Anticoagulant therapy is contraindicated if pericardial effusion is significant.

Bed rest is of the utmost importance because physical exercise has been shown to aggravate the disease in animal models. As a corollary, physical exertion should be avoided in patients with symptoms of a viral infection even if myocardial involvement is not apparent. Alcohol use is also contraindicated because it has been shown to aggravate the disease process. Physical exertion should be avoided in patients with convalescent myocarditis as long as the echocardiogram shows evidence of ventricular dilatation or hypokinesis.

Immunosuppression has been recommended for severe or relapsing cases of viral myocarditis. Therapy with prednisone and azathioprine has been shown, by serial endomyocardial biopsy, to eliminate the inflammatory infiltrate. Because of the serious side effects and the risks of superinfection, however, immunosuppressive therapy should be reserved for selected patients with intractable treatment failure or severe systemic toxicity.

CHAGAS MYOCARDITIS

Chagas myocarditis is the most common form of heart disease in Latin America; its geographic range is from Argentina to Central America. In affected areas, 50% of the population has been infected by the protozoan; 15% of these people have a chronic condition. Chagas myocarditis is caused by the protozoan *Trypanosoma cruzi*, which enters the human body through an insect bite, sometimes around the eyes. The triatomid insect vector, the vinchucha, is found on the thatched roofs of rural dwellings and typically attacks humans during the night.

Following inoculation of the host, the acute stage of the illness is usually asymptomatic. Occasionally, acute myocarditis is clinically evident, with tachycardia, gallop rhythm, and congestive heart failure. Other clinical manifestations include fever, asthenia, headache, diarrhea, lymphadenopathy, and hepatosplenomegaly. The site of the insect bite is sometimes visible, with unilateral periorbital edema and local adenopathy. Acute meningoencephalitis may complicate severe cases. At this acute stage, the diagnosis of Chagas' disease can be established by demonstrating the presence of *Trypanosoma cruzi* in the peripheral blood on microscopic examination or by xenodiagnosis. In xenodiagnosis, triatomid bugs are allowed to feed on the patient and are examined 30 and 60 days later for the presence of trypanosomes in their feces or gut. Several serologic tests are also available, including a promising enzyme-linked immunosorbent assay (ELISA).

The disease then enters a latent phase of 20 years, after which chronic Chagas myocarditis occurs. This chronic disease is clinically marked by cardiomegaly and congestive heart failure with mitral and tricuspid insufficiency, right bundle branch block, and complex arrhythmias. Echocardiographic examination shows congestive cardiomyopathy with apical akinesis and thrombus formation.

The diagnosis is established by serologic tests, such as complement fixation, hemagglutination inhibition, indirect immunofluorescence, and ELISA tests. Treatment for Chagas' disease is disappointing. In the acute stages, moderate successes have been reported with the administration nitrofurans, pyrimethamine, primaquine, nifurtimox, or metronidazole. No specific therapy exists for chronic Chagas myocarditis.

TRICHINOSIS

The presenting symptoms of trichinosis, a common helminthic disease, most often are periorbital edema and muscle tenderness. Rarely, signs and symptoms of acute myocarditis develop as the initial symptoms subside. Sudden death from acute myocarditis due to trichinosis has been reported.

The presence of eosinophilia and skeletal muscle biopsy confirm the diagnosis of trichinosis (Fig. 15-3). Management consists of

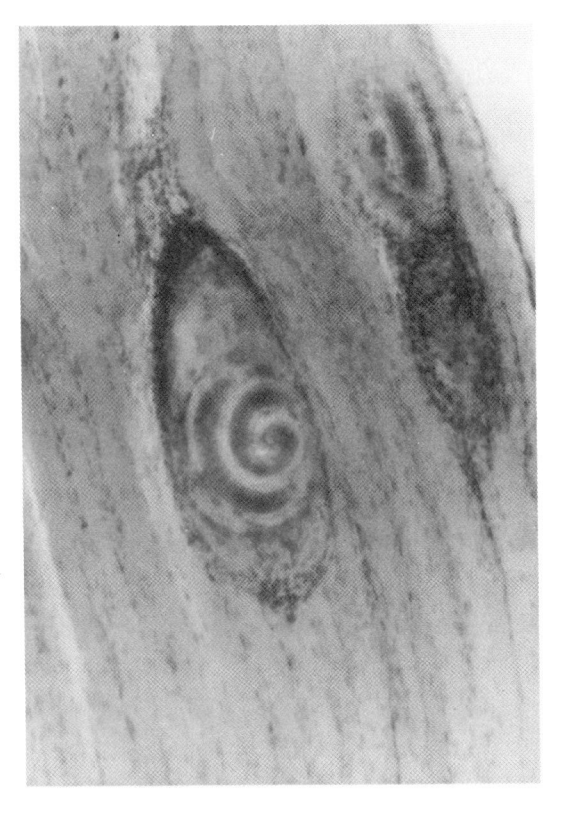

Fig. 15-3. Trichinosis.

corticosteroid therapy and thiabendazole administration.

DIPHTHERIC MYOCARDITIS

Myocarditis, the most serious complication of diphtheria, occurs in approximately 25% of patients. Symptoms and signs of congestive heart failure develop progressively during the second week of the illness. Death may suddenly occur from circulatory collapse or from complete heart block. Marked elevation of serum myocardial enzymes signals a poor prognosis. ST-T electrocardiographic changes are the rule. The development of bundle branch block or of atrioventricular conduction disturbances is characteristic and is associated with a 50 to 80% mortality rate. In addition to specific antitoxin and antibiotic therapy, treatment consists of respiratory and circulatory supportive measures and, if necessary, transvenous pacemakers. Digitalis is ineffective and may be contra-indicated if conduc-

> **TRICHINOSIS**
>
> *Trichinella spiralis* is the roundworm that causes trichinosis, also known as trichinellosis. Encysted larval forms of this worm can be found in the muscles of infected animals, notably swine or bear. The human disease is prevalent and sporadic wherever improperly cooked trichinous meat is eaten. Examples are homemade sausage and, in some American Indian communities, uncooked, smoked bear meat.
>
> When the trichinous meat is ingested, the cyst wall of the parasite is digested by the gastric juice of the host, and the parasitic larvae are released. Once liberated, the larvae develop to full sexual maturity in a few days. From 4 to 7 days after ingestion of the infected meat, fecund female trichinae, embedded in the intestinal mucosa of the host, produce embryos that penetrate into the host's lymphatic system, reach the blood through the thoracic duct, and gain access to the host's skeletal muscles. There, the larvae grow, become encased by a cyst wall made of connective tissue, and remain alive for many years. These cysts often become calcified.
>
> Clinically, the incubation period lasts from 2 to 30 days. The invasive stage, which begins with the release of larvae from cysts, is characterized by abdominal pain, nausea, and, in some patients, vomiting and diarrhea. About 7 to 10 days later, the stage of dissemination begins, marked by moderate fever, muscle pains, edema of the eyelids, urticarial rashes, itching, and, in severe cases, myocarditis and neuropsychiatric features. The blood cell count reveals leukocytic response with characteristic relative and absolute increases of eosinophils. A few weeks later, the stage of encystment occurs, and the clinical features disappear.
>
> Evidence confirming trichinosis includes the patient's medical history and presence of larvae in a biopsy specimen of the patient's muscle or in a sample of the suspected meat. Additional diagnostic aids are serodiagnosis studies such as complement fixation and ELISA and, to a lesser degree, skin tests. In patients with severe symptoms, one may attempt to control the disorder by administering thiabendazole, 20 to 25 mg/kg twice a day for 7 to 10 days. Corticosteroids are administered to critically ill patients, especially when symptoms indicate sensitivity phenomena.

tion disturbances are present. If the patient survives the acute episode, the long-term prognosis is good.

SUGGESTED READINGS

Burch, G.E., and Giles, T.D.: The role of viruses in the production of heart disease. Am. J. Cardiol., 29:231, 1972.

Das, S.K., Brady, T.J., Thrall, J., and Pitt, B.: Cardiac function in patients with prior myocarditis. J. Nucl. Med., 21:689, 1980.

Faubert, G.M., Pechère, J.C., and Delisle, R.: An outbreak of trichinellosis in Canada: the enzyme linked immunoabsorbent assay (ELISA) and clinical findings in trichinellosis. In Trichinellosis. Edited by C.W. Kimand. London, Reedbooks, 1981.

Fowler, N.O., and Manitsas, G.T.: Infectious pericarditis. Prog. Cardiovasc. Dis., 16:323, 1973.

Karjalainen, J., Niemenen, M.S., and Heikkilä, J.: Influenza A. 1 myocarditis in conscripts. Acta Med. Scand., 207:27, 1980.

Klacsmann, P.G., Bulkley, B.H., and Hutchins, G.M.: The changed spectrum of purulent pericarditis. Am. J. Med., 63:666, 1977.

Laurenceau, J.A., Cérèze, P.H., and Dumesnil, J.G.: Surveillance échocardiographique des myocardites. Coeur Med. Interne, 18:451, 1979.

Mason, J.W., Billingham, M.E., and Ricci, D.R.: Treatment of acute inflammatory myocarditis assisted by endomyocardial biopsy. Am. J. Cardiol., 45:1037, 1980.

Puigbó, J.J., et al.: Diagnosis of Chagas' cardiomyopathy. Non-invasive techniques. Postgrad. Med. J., 53:527, 1977.

Rooney, J.J., Crocco, J.A., and Lyons, H.A.: Tuberculous pericarditis. Ann. Intern. Med., 72:73, 1970.

Symmes, J.C., and Berman, N.D.: Early recognition of cardiac tamponade. Can. Med. Assoc. J., 116:863, 1977.

Tajik, A.J.: Echocardiography in pericardial effusion. Am. J. Med., 63:29, 1977.

Toala, P., Brown, A., and Russo, C.: Chagas' disease. In The Management of Infectious Diseases in Clinical Practice. Edited by P.K. Peterson, L.D. Sabath, E.C. Jaimes, and A.R. Ronald. New York, Academic Press, 1982.

Wentworth, P., Jentz, L.A., and Croal, A.E.: Analysis of sudden unexpected death in Southern Ontario with emphasis on myocarditis. Can. Med. Assoc. J., 120:676, 1979.

CHAPTER 16

Typhoid Fever

A.M. Geddes

> Objective 16–1. Recognize epidemiologic and clinical clues that suggest a typhoid fever in a febrile patient.

Typhoid and paratyphoid fevers, often referred to collectively as enteric fevers, are serious and sometimes fatal septicemic illnesses. *Salmonella typhi, S. paratyphi, S. schottmuelleri* (formerly paratyphi B), and *S. hirschfeldii* (formerly paratyphi C) only cause infection in humans, unlike the other salmonellae, which are also pathogens of animals and poultry. The source of infection in typhoid and paratyphoid fever is, therefore, always man and is frequently a symptomless carrier who excretes the organism in stool or urine. Transmission may be either direct, by contact with a carrier, or indirect, through food or water.

The vast increase in air travel over the past 20 years and the influx of immigrant workers from the Middle East, the Indian subcontinent, North Africa, the Mediterranean countries, and Latin America have led to the frequent importation of typhoid fever into more developed countries.

Infection almost invariably results from swallowing the organism, usually in contaminated food or drink. Experiments in volunteers have shown that many *Salmonella typhi* bacteria pass into the small intestine and invade the mucosa and Peyer's lymphatic patches. There the bacteria enter the blood and are disseminated throughout the reticuloendothelial system. Following a latent period of from 7 to 21 days, bacteremia recurs with the development of signs and symptoms of the disease. These signs and symptoms may originate in virtually any system or organ of the body, and therefore, the clinical features of the disease vary.

As an intracellular pathogen, *Salmonella typhi* is partially protected from humoral defense mechanisms as well as from antibiotics that penetrate poorly into human cells, such as penicillin G and the cephalosporins. The intracellular position of the organisms may have an immunosuppressive effect on host cells. The hypothesis might explain the slow response of patients with typhoid fever to antibiotic treatment, the frequent relapse after treatment, and the poor immunity against reinfection.

EPIDEMIOLOGY

Typhoid fever has a worldwide distribution, but it is most frequent in tropical and subtropical countries, where it is commonly contracted by travelers from temperate climates. The disease is not endemic in Northern Europe, North America, or Australia, but carriers of *Salmonella typhi*, especially food handlers, may be a source of infection anywhere in the world. Between January, 1978 and June, 1980, 615 cases of typhoid fever were diagnosed in England and Wales. Of these patients, 546 were considered to have contracted the infection during recent foreign travel, principally in the Indian subcontinent (68%), whereas the remaining 69 (11%) had not left the country. Fifteen of the 69 patients were contacts of known typhoid carriers; only 4 had been in contact with a patient suffering from the disease.

Sewer workers and those employed in bacteriology laboratories are particularly at risk of contracting typhoid fever.

Explosive outbreaks of typhoid fever, such as those in Zermatt, Switzerland in 1963 and in Aberdeen, Scotland in 1964, occasionally take medical authorities by surprise. In Aberdeen, over 500 people were eventually infected. The Aberdeen episode originated from a contaminated tin of corned beef imported from Argentina, and the Zermatt infection was due to contamination of the domestic water supply by sewage. Other commercial sources of typhoid fever have included shellfish and milk.

CLINICAL FEATURES

Early features of typhoid fever are frequently nonspecific. The patient often has a pyrexial illness associated with prostration and headache. Typhoid fever should be considered in any patient with undiagnosed fever, especially if the fever has been present for more than 3 days. If the patient has recently arrived from an area of the world where the disease is endemic, the diagnosis should be considered immediately. Early diagnosis and prompt institution of therapy lead to more rapid recovery and reduce the likelihood of complications. The frequency of symptoms and signs in typhoid fever is shown in Table 16–1. Of particular importance is the rarity of the "classic" signs of the disease, such as constipation, bradycardia, and "rose spots" on the anterior abdominal wall.

Atypical presentations of typhoid fever include respiratory symptoms, urinary tract symptoms, and signs of metastatic abscess formation, for example, osteomyelitis. I have recently seen a young woman with the classic features of acute schizophrenia whose urgent transfer to a psychiatric hospital was halted when *Salmonella typhi* was cultured from her blood. Blood culture had been performed principally because she had just returned from India. Treatment of the typhoid fever cured her psychiatric symptoms. Another atypical presentation occurred in a 3-month-old child who had acute septic arthritis of the hip. To the surprise of the orthopedic surgeon, culture of pus from the joint yielded *S. typhi*.

In the early stage of typhoid fever, pyrexia is often intermittent. As the disease progresses, however, fever becomes sustained.

Typhoid fever may sometimes be surprisingly mild, especially in children, and can be suppressed by "blind" antibiotic therapy for an undiagnosed febrile illness.

Objective 16–2. Confirm a suspected typhoid fever by the proper laboratory tests.

Confirmation can be achieved by direct or indirect laboratory methods.

DIRECT LABORATORY METHODS

The best way to confirm the diagnosis is to culture *Salmonella typhi* from the patient's blood. Blood culture is usually positive for at least the first 10 days of the illness and often longer. Indeed, *S. typhi* has been cultured from blood for up to 10 days *after* initial treatment with chloramphenicol. The organism may also be cultured from stool, urine, bone marrow, pus from an abscess, or rarely, cerebrospinal fluid. Culture of bone marrow is especially valuable in patients who received antibiotics before the diagnosis of typhoid fever was considered.

INDIRECT LABORATORY METHODS

The Widal reaction, which detects serum antibodies to *Salmonella typhi*, is the prin-

Table 16–1. Clinical Features of Typhoid Fever

Clinical Features	Geddes, Birmingham U.K. 1972–1978 %	Huckstep, Kenya 1954–1955 %	Stuart and Pullen, New Orleans 1939–1944 %
Systemic			
Pyrexia	96	94	Not given
Sweating	69	1	Rare
Rigors	31	23	Not given
Bradycardia	14	12	Not given
Gastrointestinal			
Anorexia	65	100	90
Vomiting	41	25	54
Abdominal pain	34	70	21
Diarrhea	31	37	43
Constipation	10	15	79
Other			
Cough	48	35	86
Splenomegaly	33	14	64
Dysuria	14	0.5	2.5
Meningism	10	1	10
Rose spots	10	5	14

cipal indirect method for supporting a diagnosis of typhoid fever. A rise in antibodies to the O antigen suggests active infection, whereas elevation of the H antigen points to previous infection or past immunization against the disease. The Widal reaction is of little value in the early stages of the disease, when the diagnosis of typhoid fever should be made by other methods. Its principal applications are to confirm the diagnosis of an atypical case, as well as to diagnose patients in whom the signs and symptoms may have been obscured by prior antibiotic therapy. The Vi antigen titer is increased in many carriers of *S. typhi*, but this method of screening can be unreliable for some typhoid excretors, such as food handlers or waterworks employees. A recently described counterimmunoelectrophoretic (CIE) technique for the detection of antibodies to the protein antigen of *S. typhi* is an alternative to the Vi antigen test for screening potential typhoid carriers.

Other indirect diagnostic aids are the white blood count, which is usually low, sometimes with relative monocytosis, and measurement of the liver transaminase levels, which are almost invariably elevated.

> **Objective 16–3.** Select and monitor the treatment of a typhoid fever.

In typhoid fever, as in any bacteremic illness, the earlier treatment is started, the better the outcome, especially with regard to duration of illness, incidence of complications, and mortality rates. Antibiotic therapy should therefore be commenced as soon as the diagnosis is considered likely on clinical grounds. It is not necessary, and it could be potentially hazardous, to wait until the results of laboratory investigations are available.

The response to treatment in typhoid fever differs from that of many other bacterial infections in a number of important respects, including slow defervescence, persistently positive blood cultures for up to 10 days after commencing antibiotic therapy, frequent relapses (10% of patients), usually occurring within 2 weeks of stopping treatment, and persistent excretion of *Salmonella typhi* in stools or urine following treatment in approximately 15% of patients. Some or all of these features may be due to the intracellular habitat of salmonellae that protects the organism from antibiotics and from host-resistance mechanisms.

SUPPORTIVE TREATMENT

Intravenous fluids are usually required for the first 2 or 3 days of treatment. The intravenous apparatus provides a convenient route for the parenteral administration of antibiotics. Food should be withheld from a sick patient at this stage and then gradually introduced as the patient improves.

SPECIFIC TREATMENT

Samonella typhi is sensitive to a number of antimicrobial agents, but few of these are therapeutically reliable. Chloramphenicol, co-trimoxazole, and amoxicillin-ampicillin are all effective.

The selection of antibiotic depends on individual preference, and little difference probably exists among the various agents, provided the infecting organism is sensitive. My personal choice is co-trimoxazole (trimethoprim and sulfamethoxazole), although chloramphenicol is most widely used. R-factor plasmid-mediated resistance to chloramphenicol was first recognized in the Eastern Mediterranean in 1967 and, since then, has appeared in Mexico, India, and Southeast Asia, especially Indochina. The same R factor codes for resistance to streptomycin, tetracycline, the sulfonamides, and sometimes amoxicillin and ampicillin as well. Chloramphenicol-resistant *Salmonella typhi* strains are increasingly isolated from European patients with imported typhoid fever.

It is preferable to administer the antibiotic by intravenous injection for at least the first 48 hours of treatment. Therapy should be continued for a total of 14 days. The dose recommendations for the various agents are shown in Table 16-2.

TREATMENT OF COMPLICATIONS

The complications of typhoid fever can be classified into three groups:

1. Local effects of infection in the mucous membrane of the small intestine that lead to perforation or hemorrhage.
2. Effects of toxemia, including myocarditis, encephalopathy, or intravascular coagulation.
3. Metastatic pyogenic lesions in bone, joints, liver, or meninges.

Gastrointestinal bleeding is treated by blood transfusion or, rarely, by surgical intervention, which is also indicated for perforation of the small bowel. If a trained surgeon and anesthetist are not available, however, treatment should consist of the administration of intravenous fluids and nasogastric suction. Metastatic collections of pus must be drained by needle aspiration or surgical incision.

Corticosteroids are indicated for the rare patient with profound toxemia. I have had to administer intravenous hydrocortisone to only 2 of almost 200 of my patients with typhoid fever. The dose is 100 mg every 6 hours for 48 hours.

PREVENTION OF CROSS-INFECTION

Stool and urine from patients with typhoid fever should be treated with disinfectant be-

Table 16-2. Chemotherapy of Typhoid Fever and Typhoid Carrier State

	Typhoid Fever	
	First 48–72 hours	To complete course
Chloramphenicol	750 mg q6h	500 mg q6h
Amoxicillin	1 g q6h	500 mg q6h
Co-trimoxazole	160 mg trimethoprim / 800 mg sulfamethoxazole } q12-h	160 mg trimethoprim / 800 mg sulfamethoxazole } q12-h
	Typhoid Carrier State	
Amoxicillin	500 mg q6h	To complete course
Co-trimoxazole	160 mg trimethoprim / 800 mg sulfamethoxazole } q12-h	For 4–6 weeks

> **Objective 16–4. Define the management required in a symptomatic *Salmonella typhi* carrier.**

Approximately 15% of patients temporarily excrete *Salmonella typhi* in stool and urine following clinical recovery from typhoid fever. These patients are referred to as convalescent excretors. Investigation or treatment is not indicated because most of these patients stop excreting the organism spontaneously; however, 1 to 2% continue to excrete the organism. If excretion persists for more than 3 months after treatment, the patient is classified as a carrier. The ineffectiveness of treatment in typhoid carriers may not be important if the patient is intelligent and is not involved in the preparation of food. Problems arise in patients who are food handlers or who fail to understand basic principles of personal hygiene.

Because short courses of antibiotics are ineffective, it is essential for patients to receive prolonged therapy lasting from 4 to 8 weeks or even longer in refractory cases. Co-trimoxazole or amoxicillin are recommended for typhoid carriers (Table 16–2).

One cannot be certain that a typhoid carrier has been "cured" by antibiotic therapy. For example, A. B. Christie of Liverpool, England obtained 196 negative stools in a typhoid carrier following a 12-week course of ampicillin, but culture of the 197th specimen yielded *Salmonella typhi*.

A proportion of typhoid carriers, especially middle-aged women, have chronic gallbladder disease, often associated with stone formation. It may not be possible to clear these patients of *Salmonella typhi* unless the gallbladder is removed; however, the patient may continue to excrete the organism in stools following cholecystectomy. Cholecystectomy should be recommended in typhoid carriers with gallstones only if (1) cholecystectomy is indicated in its own right or (2) patients are food handlers who have been forced to stop working because they excrete *S. typhi*.

> **Objective 16–5. Select individuals and population for whom antityphoid immunization is indicated.**

None of the available vaccines, all of which are inactivated preparations, give complete protection against typhoid fever. Of those currently available, however, the monovalent typhoid vaccine provides the best immunity with the lowest incidence of adverse reaction. Duration of immunity is limited, and immunization must therefore be repeated every 2 to 3 years.

TAB vaccine, which contains paratyphoid A and B as well as typhoid antigens, is less effective than the monovalent typhoid preparation and produces more local and systemic reactions. It remains popular, however, especially with travelers to the Middle East, to whom it is given in combination with cholera vaccine as one injection of TAB (C). It can also be combined with tetanus vaccine as TAB (T).

Type 21a strain for oral vaccination against typhoid, manufactured by the Swiss Serum and Vaccine Institute, appears promising and has recently been licensed in Switzerland. Field trials with single-dose administration are due to begin shortly in South Africa.

Immunization against typhoid fever should be offered to (1) travellers to tropical countries; (2) members of the armed forces; (3) microbiology laboratory staff; and (4) sewer workers.

SUGGESTED READINGS

Ball, A.P., et al.: Enteric fever in Birmingham: clinical features, laboratory investigation and comparison of treatment with pivmecillinam and co-trimoxazole. J. Infect. Dis., 1:353, 1979.

Christie, A.B.: Infectious Diseases: Epidemiology and Clinical Practice. 3rd Ed. Edinburgh, Churchill Livingstone, 1980.

Huckstep, R.L.: Typhoid fever and other salmonella infections. Edinburgh, E. & S. Livingstone, 1962.

Stuart, B.M., and Pullen, R.L.: Typhoid: clinical analysis of 360 cases. Arch. Intern. Med., 78:629, 1946.

CHAPTER 17

Acute Infectious Diarrhea

B. Grenier

> **Objective 17–1. Evaluate and correct the immediate consequences of diarrhea in an infant.**

Acute diarrhea, the passage of abnormally frequent and liquid stools for less than a week, is one of the most common pediatric complaints. Diarrhea is the clinical expression of an acute intestinal insufficiency with the following immediate consequences: (1) abnormal losses of water and electrolytes resulting in acute dehydration and ionic imbalance; (2) nutritional insufficiency, which, even though brief, may sometimes have severe repercussions; and (3) direct effects of the infectious agent on the patient (invasiveness and toxicity) and on members of the household (infectiousness).

The onset of diarrhea is sudden. In the space of a few hours, the child passes several soft or liquid stools; the volume is usually difficult to determine. It may be preceded or accompanied by vomiting, steady or colicky abdominal pains, fever, restlessness, irritability, and, at times, signs of upper respiratory infection.

EVALUATION OF VOLUME DEPLETION

The physician's immediate task is to assess the risks associated with dehydration and ion imbalance.

First, the frequency and appearance of the stools must be noted. The painless passage of 5 to 20 liquid, watery stools per day rapidly leads to severe volume depletion, especially when the diarrhea is accompanied by vomiting or the refusal to drink.

The immediate loss of weight is the most reliable gauge of water depletion. If it amounts to about 5% of body weight, it is clinically manifested by a sunken appearance of the eyes, a depressed anterior fontanelle, and oliguria. If the weight loss amounts to 10% of body weight, dehydration becomes clearly evident, with altered skin elasticity. When a fold of skin of the abdomen is pinched, it takes several seconds to regain its normal contour. Dryness of the mucous membranes and thirst reflect the hypertonic plasma. Profound hyperpnea reveals the existence of metabolic acidosis. If weight loss amounts to 15% or more of the patient's body weight, the volume depletion is serious and can be fatal as a result of circulatory collapse, shock, acidosis, or disseminated intravascular coagulation. The treatment is directed at urgent management of the shock, correction of the metabolic disorders, and palliation of the severe visceral insufficiencies that subsequently appear.

The approximate losses in acute diarrhea of moderate severity are indicated in Table

221

Table 17–1. Value and Mean Composition of Fecal Losses of Water and Electrolytes in Normal or Diarrheal Stools of an Infant

	Normal stools	Acute diarrhea
Water (ml/day)	20–30: 3 ml/kg	200–400: 5 to 20 ml/kg
Na (mmol/L)	1.3	50 to 100
K (mmol/L)	4	20 to 50
CL (mmol/L)	0.6	20 to 50
HCO_3 (mmol/L)	—	15 to 25

Table 17–2. Water and Electrolyte Depletion Caused by Severe Diarrhea

	Deficits (per kg body weight)
Water (ml/kg)	25 to 200
Na (mmol/kg)	4 to 20
K (mmol/kg)	3 to 15
CL (mmol/kg)	2 to 20
HCO_3 (mmol/kg)	2 to 20

17–1. Table 17–2 shows the approximate values of the water and electrolyte deficits produced by severe diarrhea. The loss of potassium is roughly equivalent to the loss of sodium. This information is useful in the determination of replacement therapy.

In any infant with acute diarrhea, fluid and electrolyte replacement must begin immediately. At the same time, etiologic investigations should be initiated.

Objective 17–2. Determine the cause of an acute infectious diarrhea.

Diarrhea may be produced by many infectious agents (Table 17–3). In an attempt to discover the cause, one begins by looking into the circumstances that preceded or accompanied the disease. Has the patient just returned from a trip? Have other diarrheas been reported in the patient's household? What foods were included in the meals eaten in the past few days? If a food is suspected, how much time elapsed between its ingestion and the onset of the first symptoms? Were

---

FLUID AND ELECTROLYTE REPLACEMENT IN AN INFANT WITH DIARRHEA

When the weight loss is not greater than 5% of the patient's body weight, oral replacement may be attempted by offering the following standard solution freely at an average dose of 15 ml/kg body weight/hour:

NaCl: 3 g (51 mmol)
KCl: 1.50 g (20 mmol)
$NaCO_3$: 1.50 g (18 mmol)
Glucose: 20 g (112 mmol)
Water: 1 L

Such a solution has a total osmolarity of 290 mOsm/L, of which 178 mOsm/L come from the electrolytes; 160 mOsm/L cannot be metabolized and contribute to restoring the osmolar concentration per liter absorbed.
Intravenous parenteral volume replacement is indicated if the loss amounts to 10% or more of body weight, or when oral therapy fails.
Several formulas exist for determining the volume and composition of the fluid to be infused. The composition may correspond to the formula 7:2:1:

7 parts 5.0 g/100 ml (5%) glucose solution
2 parts 0.9 g/100 ml NaCl solution
1 part 1.4 g/100 ml $NaHCO_3$ solution

The total volume to be infused in the first 24 hours must include the following:
1. The volume required to correct the initial deficit: 10% of body weight.
2. The normal daily intake: 1500 ml per m² body surface area or 120 ml/kg body weight.
3. The volume required to compensate for any additional losses through diarrhea: 5 to 10 ml/kg body weight.
Add 2 mmol/kg/day as soon as diuresis resumes.

Table 17–3. Principal Infectious Causes of Acute Diarrhea and their Mechanism of Action

	Invasion of the intestinal mucosa	Enterotoxin
BACTERIA		
Aeromonas hydrophila	0	+
Bacillus cereus	0	+
Campylobacter	+	?
Clostridium perfringens	0	+
Clostridium difficile and C. sordellii	?	+
Escherichia coli	certain strains	+
Salmonella	+	0
Shigella	+	+
Staphylococcus aureus types III and IV	0	+
Other Staphylococcus aureus	+	0
Vibrio cholerae	slight	+
Vibrio parahaemolyticus	+	+
Yersinia enterocolitica	+	+
PARASITES		
Balantidium coli	+	0
Entamoeba histolytica	+	0
Giardia lamblia	0	0
Isospora belli and I. hominis	+	0
VIRUSES		
Rotavirus	+	0
Norwalk virus	?	?
Coronavirus	?	?

there any associated signs and symptoms such as vomiting or fever? Did the patient take any antibiotic during the preceding weeks? The physician should look for evidence of skin rash, rhinopharyngitis, suppurative otitis, or bronchopulmonary infection. These diseases are sometimes accompanied by diarrhea and vomiting in infants, although no etiologic connection has been clearly established.

CLINICAL FEATURES OF DIARRHEA

According to the clinical picture and the microscopic examination of the stools, two distinct types of diarrhea can be identified. Cholera-like diarrhea is a profuse, liquid, watery diarrhea resembling rice water. It is preceded or frequently accompanied by vomiting and is essentially a gastroenteritis. The intestinal mucosa is not damaged, and few leukocytes are found in the patient's stools. This watery diarrhea, which carries a major risk of volume depletion, reflects a rapid and profuse fluid secretion by the epithelial cells of the mucosa of the proximal portion of the small intestine. This phenomenon of enterosorption is generally mediated by an enterotoxin elaborated by microbial organisms that adhere to the mucosal surface: *Vibrio cholerae* or, more commonly, enterotoxin-producing *Escherichia coli.*

In contrast, dysenteric diarrhea is expressed by violent colic, abdominal cramps, and tenesmus; the stools are glairy, mucosanguineous, and sometimes purulent. The diarrhea reflects a bacterial invasion of the ileocolic mucosa, with necrosis of the epithelium, ulceration of the mucosa, and intense inflammatory response of the submucosa. This disorder is mainly an enterocolitis. Erythrocytes and neutrophils are present in large numbers in the stools. This dysenteric syndrome is produced by "invasive" Enterobacteriaceae, essentially the shigellae and the non-typhi salmonellae, as well as by amebic infections. The major risk is the danger of suppurative foci around the colon, perforation, and dissemination as a result of spread of the intestinal infection.

DIAGNOSTIC TESTS

A rectocolonoscopy may help to diagnose a postantibiotic pseudomembranous colitis or an amebic colitis. The direct microscopic examination of the stools yields estimates of bacterial counts and permits one to recognize certain microbiologic morphologic features.

The next step is the stool culture, which must be interpreted in light of the information obtained from the stool smear and a knowledge of the normal flora (Table 17-4).

To increase the likelihood of isolating a bacterial pathogen, fecal specimens should be collected for 2 or 3 consecutive days. If a stool specimen is not available, a soiled diaper or a rectal swab may be sent to the laboratory. A routine stool culture is grown aerobically. The strictly anaerobic organisms, which constitute over 99% of the colonic flora, are thereby ignored. This deliberate neglect of an anaerobic pathogen is acceptable in most cases. *Clostridium difficile* is an exception, and its identification requires anaerobic culture or detection of the toxin (see Objective 17-5).

A possible source of error is the case of a carrier, principally of salmonella or shigella, who is suffering from diarrhea caused by an altogether different organism.

Viral diarrheas occur frequently. The most common agent, a rotavirus, cannot be cultured, but its morphologic identification can be established by electron-microscopic examination. More practically, the virus can be identified immunologically by a commercially available enzyme-linked immunosorbent assay (ELISA).

Serologic investigations may detect antibodies during infections with salmonella, *Vibrio fetus*, and rotavirus, but these antibody responses occur late and are not diagnostically reliable in the course of the illness.

Finally, the etiologic investigation of a diarrhea also extends to the bacteriologic study of suspected foods to demonstrate contamination, most often by *Staphylococcus aureus*, *Clostridium perfringens*, *Bacillus cereus*, or *Clostridium botulinum*.

> Objective 17-3. Determine the specific cause of an acute infectious diarrhea from among the principal causes on the basis of laboratory, epidemiologic, and clinical data, and implement appropriate therapy.

SHIGELLOSIS

Shigella infection produces a typical enterocolitis with a dysenteric diarrhea resulting from the invasion and destruction of the intestinal mucosa. The shigellae penetrate and multiply in epithelial cells. The bacterial invasion from cell to cell is limited to the superficial epithelial layer. Only rarely is the submucosa affected; therefore, the risk of bacteremic spread is low.

The inflammatory necrosis of the ileocolic

DIRECT MICROSCOPIC EXAMINATION OF THE STOOLS

This examination requires several steps, the first of which is a search for leukocytes in the stool smear. The technique is simple. First, take a fresh stool specimen the size of a pea—if possible, a sample that has been in contact with mucus or one that is blood-streaked. Then, mix the stool with an alkaline methylene blue stain (Loeffler's blue stain). Place it on a slide. Wait 2 to 3 minutes to allow adequate staining of the nuclei. Use a low-power objective to find clusters of leukocytes and examine them under high-power magnification. Blue staining can also be used on a thin smear of stool dried in air, but this technique is less reliable.

The presence of 20 to 50 granulocytes per high-power field reflects the inflammatory intrusion of so-called invasive bacteria in the ileocolic epithelium. This finding is particularly characteristic of the dysenteric diarrhea of shigellosis and salmonellosis.

The examination of a fresh specimen between slide and coverslip, preferably with a phase-contrast microscope, may show *Campylobacter* and vibrio organisms, which are motile, curved rods. In certain cases, some unicellular parasites, such as *Entamoeba histolytica*, *Giardia lamblia*, or *Balantidium coli*, may be present. On a dried smear, Gram staining makes it possible to recognize the gram-negative vibrios if their numbers are great. Parasitic cysts are more easily visualized using Lugol's iodine staining.

Table 17–4. Principal Bacterial Species Found in a Normal Stool

Always present	Usually present
Bacteroides fragilis	Lactobacillus
Bacteroides melaninogenicus	Clostridium (perfringens in particular)
Bacteroides oralis	Eubacterium limosum
Fusobacterium	Bifidobacterium bifidum
Group D streptococcus	Peptostreptococcus
Escherichia coli	Staphylococcus aureus
	Klebsiella and Enterobacter
	Proteus
	Pseudomonas
	Candida albicans

SHIGELLA

The genus shigella belongs to the family Enterobacteriaceae and is divided into four serologic groups.

Group A is the *Shigella dysenteriae* group. Uncommon in the United States, Canada, and Europe, these bacteria are occasionally responsible for severe cases of diarrhea in the Orient and Central America. This group contains 10 serotypes, of which only the first 2 cause diarrhea. Type I is the Shiga bacillus, which causes bacillary dysentery. It is unique in that it produces a heat-labile, cytotoxic, enterotoxic, and neurotoxic exotoxin, Shiga's neurotoxin. The exotoxin affects mainly the cells of the capillary endothelium. Its action on intestinal epithelial cells is believed to be similar to that of cholera enterotoxin, although it does not stimulate adenyl cyclase.

Group B is the *S. flexneri* group, which includes 6 serotypes and 9 subtypes. Group C is the *S. boydii* group, with 15 serotypes. Group D only has *S. sonnei*, the most common cause of shigellosis in children in the United States.

---

mucosa produces desquamation, ulceration, microabscesses, and hence the excretion in the stools of mucus, polymorphonuclear leukocytes, macrophages, blood, and cellular debris.

Clinical Features. The patient is feverish and suffers from abdominal pains for 1 to 2 days, after which the dysenteric diarrhea appears: 10 to 12 soft, foul-smelling, mucous, and often bloody stools per day. Vomiting may aggravate the volume depletion. Headaches, febrile convulsions, and a stiff neck may simulate a meningitis in young children. The course of the illness is brief. Diarrhea lasts for 2 to 5 days. It may be followed by severe constipation and, rarely, by thrombosis of the mesenteric artery.

Diagnosis. The diagnosis, which is based on the isolation and identification of shigella in the stools, may be initially suspected by observation in the stools of numerous clumps of cells, polymorphonuclear leukocytes, erythrocytes, and large mononuclear and epithelial cells. Although these organisms can survive for several months in a cold, dark, moist, alkaline environment, they are destroyed within a few hours of collecting the specimen if the pH of the stool is acidic. If the culturing of the stool specimen has to be delayed, it is advisable to use special transport media rather than relying on hope alone to keep the shigellae alive on the rectal swabs or stool specimen.

Because the bacterial invasion of the mucosa is superficial, the systemic immune response is weak, and serologic tests have no practical diagnostic value.

Treatment. Shigellosis responds clinically and bacteriologically to therapy. In practice, the specific indications for antibiotic treatment are as follows:

1. Severe dysenteric syndrome with volume depletion, related in particular to serotype 1 *Shigella dysenteriae* (Shiga's bacillus).
2. Dysentery affecting a young child, an individual suffering from malnutrition, or an old patient.
3. Shigellosis in a patient who has a high degree of contact with young children or whom elementary precautions of isolation and hygiene cannot be guaranteed.

Therapy today includes a trimethoprim-sulfamethoxazole combination or tetracycline in areas where the strains are likely to be susceptible. In most countries, *Shigella dysenteriae* and *S. sonnei* have become resistant to ampicillin, an antibiotic still usually effective against *S. flexneri* at a dose of 50 to 60 mg/kg body weight/day. Nonabsorbable, oral antimicrobial agents are not recommended. An adequate antibiotic treatment rapidly eliminates shigella from the feces; fever and diarrhea usually disappear within the first 24 hours of therapy. Short treatments of 3 to 5 days generally suffice, and single-dose regimens, for instance tetracycline, 2.5 g, have been proposed. Drugs that inhibit intestinal peristalsis should be avoided because they prolong the symptoms.

SALMONELLOSIS

Salmonellosis still ranks among the most important unsolved public health problems of the world, including the developed countries. These infections are most common in early childhood, although they are observed at any age. Disseminated salmonellosis is associated with certain underlying diseases such as sickle cell disease, systemic lupus erythematosus, lymphoma, and leukemia.

Salmonella. Salmonella is an immense genus with more than 1800 serologic types divided into 5 major groups, A to E, on the basis of their O somatic antigen characteristics. In practice, it is more useful to discuss these organisms on the basis of their host of predilection, whether man, animal, or both, and on the basis of their pathologic expression in humans after contamination of the digestive tract. Typhoid fever, bacteremic manifestations, and acute diarrhea with gastroenteritis ("food poisoning") comprise the three major groups of human salmonellosis.

The first group consists of a single species, *Salmonella typhi*, whose epidemiology is unique to man. This organism produces typhoid fever (see Chap. 16), which has become less prevalent in Europe and North America with the improvement of hygienic and sanitary conditions. *Salmonella cholerae-suis* forms a second group, characterized by early invasion of the blood after infection by the oral route and the absence of clinical involvement of the intestine. It produces bacteremia with metastatic suppurative foci in bones, meninges, endocardium, and lungs, especially in immunosuppressed patients. *Salmonella enteritidis* represents a third large group that includes close to 1800 different serologic types common to both humans and animals. These organisms represent a frequent cause of bacterial enteritis.

Clinical Features. The signs of salmonellosis appear from 8 to 48 hours after ingestion of contaminated food or liquid. Headaches, chills, and abdominal pains are soon accompanied by nausea, vomiting, diarrhea, and fever, which subside spontaneously in a few days. The patient's stools are foul-smelling, often stained with mucus and blood, and sometimes contain large numbers of polymorphonuclear leukocytes.

Blood cultures appear to be positive in about 5% of hospitalized patients. Stool culture generally makes it possible to isolate the organism, which must be serotyped to permit further epidemiologic investigations.

As with shigellae, the pathogenic action of salmonellae is related to their ability to adhere to the mucosa of the terminal intestine

---

EPIDEMIOLOGY OF SALMONELLOSIS

The epidemiology of gastrointestinal salmonellosis has two remarkable characteristics. Infection by these so-called minor salmonellae is common in man and many animals, and many animals are a source of human food through their meat or products. Some have suggested that better hygiene and supervision of food preparation would reduce the incidence of gastrointestinal salmonellosis. Actually, a sizable number of food-borne outbreaks have been related to the development of industrial techniques of stock farming and large-scale food processing. At the same time, an even greater number of hospital outbreaks have occurred; in these, transmission from person to person has played a major role.

The prolonged excretion of salmonellae in the stools of healthy individuals or of those convalescing from acute gastroenteritis represents another means of spreading the infection, notably through the use of food or water contaminated with feces. Minor salmonellae are present in stools more frequently than shigellae, but these salmonellae remain for a shorter time than *S. typhi*, rarely for more than a few weeks.

and to penetrate into the epithelium, where the bacteria multiply in the macrophages and polymorphonuclear leukocytes of the lamina propria. The mucosa of the terminal ileum and that of the colon are the sites of inflammatory foci and ulcerations. The deep penetration of salmonellae into the intestinal wall increases the risk of bacteremic spread.

Treatment. It appears that any antibiotic treatment of the acute gastrointestinal episode increases both the incidence and the duration of bacterial excretion of salmonellae during convalescence. In addition, the antibiotic treatment of gastrointestinal salmonellosis is particularly dangerous for the community because it rapidly promotes the acquisition of multiple plasmid resistance. Therefore, antibiotic treatment is indicated only when it is of definite, possibly vital advantage to the patient. Antibiotic therapy improves neither the intensity nor the duration of the gastrointestinal signs of this illness. Briefly, antibiotic therapy is indicated when a risk of bacteremic spread of the infection exists, as follows:

1. In patients at both extremes of age.
2. In patients with an immune deficiency, such as in leukemia, Hodgkin's disease, agranulocytosis, systemic lupus erythematosus, hypogammaglobulinemia, immunosuppressive treatment, severe alcoholic liver disease, advanced cancer, or malnutrition.
3. In patients with vascular disease, such as sickle cell anemia and vascular prosthesis or graft.
4. In highly febrile patients, notably when blood cultures are positive.

The treatment must be brief and should be administered either parenterally or using absorbable oral antibiotics selected on the basis of in vitro sensitivity tests whenever possible: ampicillin, chloramphenicol, or co-trimoxazole for 5 to 7 days. Throughout convalescence, it is useful to monitor the elimination of the bacteria in the stools and to make a periodic assessment of the antibiotic sensitivity profile. The persistence of bacteria in the stools does not in itself imply resistance.

DIARRHEA DUE TO *ESCHERICHIA COLI*

Pathogenesis. Escherichia coli, a normal host of the human intestine, has been linked to the pathogenesis of diarrhea in several ways. First, serologically agglutinable enteropathogenic *E. coli* have been implicated in some epidemics of acute diarrhea in children. These organisms have been recognized using the combination of certain somatic O antigen serotypes with capsular K or B antigen serotypes. The pathogenic role and mechanism of action of these bacteria have not yet been clearly established, however, and some observations seem inconsistent. It is not surprising that the same *E. coli* can be recovered from healthy children and 20 to 30% of carriers are asymptomatic, but it is more difficult to consider these *E. coli* as pathogens when, in some groups of children, their prevalence is higher in healthy subjects than in those with diarrhea.

More commonly, noninvasive, enterotoxin-producing *Escherichia coli* cause a generally mild illness known as traveler's diarrhea or "turista." These bacilli can also produce a severe, cholera-like syndrome that may be life-threatening in small children. The pathogenic mechanism of these bacteria reflects the combination of two properties conferred independently of one another by plasmids harbored within the bacteria. The first property is the ability of the bacteria to become attached to the initial portion of the small intestine during transit: this ability represents the colonization factor. The second property is the bacteria's ability to produce one or two exotoxins: a well-identified, heat-labile enterotoxin LT, which shares many properties with cholera exotoxin, and a heat-stable enterotoxin ST.

Less commonly, invasive *Escherichia coli* penetrate the intestinal mucosa and proliferate in the epithelial cells of the ileum and colon. Their pathogenic action is similar to that of shigellae. These *E. coli* produce an enterocolitis manifested by the presence of

> **ENTEROTOXINS FROM *ESCHERICHIA COLI***
>
> When it is fixed to the gangliosides of the intestinal epithelial cell membrane, *E. coli* toxin LT, like cholera toxin, stimulates the formation of membrane adenyl cyclase, which increases the concentration of intracellular cyclic adenosine monophosphate (cAMP). This change, in turn, results in the active secretion of Cl and HCO_3 ions and water into the intestinal lumen and leads to enterosorption. As soon as the enterotoxin has become fixed to the intestinal epithelial cell, the attachment is irreversible, although the effect does not last more than 20 to 24 hours. The toxin does not inhibit the absorption of water and sodium by the intestinal epithelial cell, particularly if glucose, at a concentration of 20 to 30 g/L, is added to the solution. This property is used for oral rehydratation with glucose-electrolyte solutions in cholera-like, bacterial, hypersecretory diarrheas. The "adhesiveness" of the bacteria is increased by a colonization factor antigen (CFA) and by pili that may be responsible for concentrations of bacteria as high as 10^5 to 10^7/ml. In vitro, this antigen can be demonstrated by agglutination of mannose-resistant, human group A erythrocytes in the presence of the bacteria. This agglutination response is directly attributable to the presence of the pericellular pili. A transmissible plasmid that may be lost during culture is the source of this antigenic property.
>
> Can other Enterobacteriaceae acquire colonization factor and the ability to produce an enterotoxin when exposed to the same plasmids? Such a potential has been ascribed to organisms belonging to the klebsiella, enterobacter, and citrobacter genera, but transformation probably only rarely occurs.

mucus and polymorphonuclear leukocytes in the diarrheal stools. The clinical picture includes abdominal pains, tenesmus, fever, and occasionally bacteremia, with its attendant risk of endotoxic shock or septic metastases. These bacteria generally belong to certain O group serotypes.

Overall, enterotoxigenic *E. coli* probably play a minor role in the origin of acute diarrhea in children living in developed nations. These bacteria may play a more important etiologic role in adults, particularly adults who travel to warm climates or who live in certain parts of the world, notably Southeast Asia.

Treatment. The clinical effectiveness of antibiotic treatment in enterotoxigenic *Escherichia coli* diarrhea is uncertain. The diarrheas produced by invasive *E. coli* can probably be treated as are diarrheas in shigellosis.

With regard to the treatment of diarrhea caused by enteropathogenic *Escherichia coli*, it is generally agreed that the administration of an oral antibiotic, even a nonabsorbable agent, eliminates the pathogenic bacteria in the stools. This effect probably reduces the risk of spread to those in close contact with the patient, but the benefit to the patient has not yet been clearly demonstrated. Either intravenous or oral electrolyte solutions may be used for fluid replacement when required.

DIARRHEA CAUSED BY CAMPYLOBACTER

Diarrheas caused by campylobacter mainly affect children, boys slightly more often than girls, and are unrelated to travel, the presence of household pets, or the parents' occupations. Asymptomatic carriers may play an important role in the transmission of this disorder. In addition to diarrhea, the clinical picture includes the presence of blood in the stools and fever in over 90% of the patients and abdominal cramps. Vomiting is minor, and volume depletion is moderate. Laboratory diagnosis of campylobacter diarrheas is aided by growth on selective media, Skirrow medium in particular. A filtration technique for separation of this organism from the other intestinal flora has also been proposed. Early in the investigations, it is sometimes possible

> ***CAMPYLOBACTER FETUS***
>
> *Campylobacter fetus* subspecies *jejuni* has now been isolated from close to 5% of the cases of diarrhea in many parts of the world. Campylobacter is a small, motile, gram-negative bacillus with a polar flagellum. The bacillus is usually curved, although it may be spiral. It was formerly classified as a vibrio, *Vibrio fetus*, but it is now considered to be related to the family Spirillaceae. The organism grows in enriched media and in CO_2 atmosphere or anaerobically, but not in room air. Its pathogenic role in humans, not suspected until 1947, has since been increasingly recognized in septicemia meningitis, in genital infections, and in acute diarrhea.
>
> The pathophysiology of this bacterium is still poorly understood.

to suspect campylobacter as the etiologic agent when the shape and the characteristic motility of the bacteria are observed using a phase-contrast microscope. Determination of IgG- and IgM-specific antibody titers rarely permits a serologic diagnosis.

Erythromycin, said to be effective, reduces the period of excretion of the bacteria in the stools; this excretion continues for 2 to 4 weeks in untreated individuals.

CHOLERA

Cholera, an ancient scourge that first penetrated Europe and America in the nineteenth century, is still with us.

It should be suspected in individuals with diarrhea who have returned from a stay in an endemic or epidemic zone, especially if the disease began abruptly and if the stools are abundant, watery, and painless. When volume depletion is not corrected rapidly, shock may supervene. The presence of *Vibrio cholerae* in the stools, the necessary criterion for diagnosis, is easy to demonstrate. The diagnosis is first suspected during the examination of a fresh stool specimen by dark-field microscopy if numerous small, actively motile, comma-shaped bacilli are seen. It can be further reinforced by direct immunofluorescence using a conjugated antiserum. The diagnosis can also be confirmed by bacterial growth on a number of selective media, including thiosulfate-citrate-bile salt-sucrose (TCBS) agar. Unlike most intestinal organisms, *V. cholerae* grows on this medium in 18 hours and produces yellow colonies.

Treatment. The treatment of cholera consists essentially of volume replacement according to the principles stated previously, with particular attention to the quantitative and qualitative compensation for water and electrolyte losses. Oral ingestion of a glucose solution increases the absorption of sodium by the small intestine. Antibiotic therapy is only an adjunct; oral tetracycline, 30 to 40 mg/kg/day in 4 equally divided doses for 2 days. A vaccine (see Objective 35–1), is required for travel in certain countries, but its effectiveness in a traveler from a Western country is doubtful. Better protection may be provided by taking proper hygienic precautions.

OTHER BACTERIAL DIARRHEAS

Other vibrios produce similar diarrheas. *Vibrio parahaemolyticus* is commonly responsible for food poisoning in Japan and is associated with the ingestion of raw shellfish. This infection has recently been observed in other countries, in North America in particular, after the ingestion of contaminated shellfish and shrimp.

Yersinia enterocolitica has been associated with diarrhea both in Europe and in North America. The epidemiologic features are poorly understood. This intestinal disease occurs primarily in young children. The organism is invasive, occasionally producing

---

PATHOPHYSIOLOGY AND EPIDEMIOLOGY OF CHOLERA

The causative organism is *Vibrio cholerae*, a small, curved, motile, gram-negative bacillus. The entire symptomatic picture derives from the tremendous loss of fluids and electrolytes through the intestine: the daily volume of stools may exceed 20 liters, and their composition is practically isotonic. This phenomenal loss is caused by an enterotoxin (Fig. 17–1) that becomes solidly fixed to the epithelial cells of the small intestine and produces effects similar to those of *Escherichia coli* enterotoxin LT: stimulation of adenyl cyclase, increase in the levels of intracellular cAMP, and leakage of chloride, bicarbonate, and water into the intestinal lumen. The bacterium itself does not invade the mucosa; therefore, blood cultures remain negative. No serologic reactions are helpful in the diagnosis.

Cholera is endemic in India and epidemic in the densely populated intertropical regions of Africa and Asia. Seven pandemics have occurred since 1817, the last of which, from 1961 to 1977, stopped at certain countries of the Mediterranean, apparently without reaching the American continent. The recent report of a series of cases in Louisiana, however, suggests that cholera may have established itself in North America during one of the pandemics. Man seems to be the only animal reservoir of the disease. Contaminated water and later food act as the principal vectors. The dissemination of *Vibrio cholerae* is promoted by the numerous asymptomatic carriers (one ill person for every four to ten carriers).

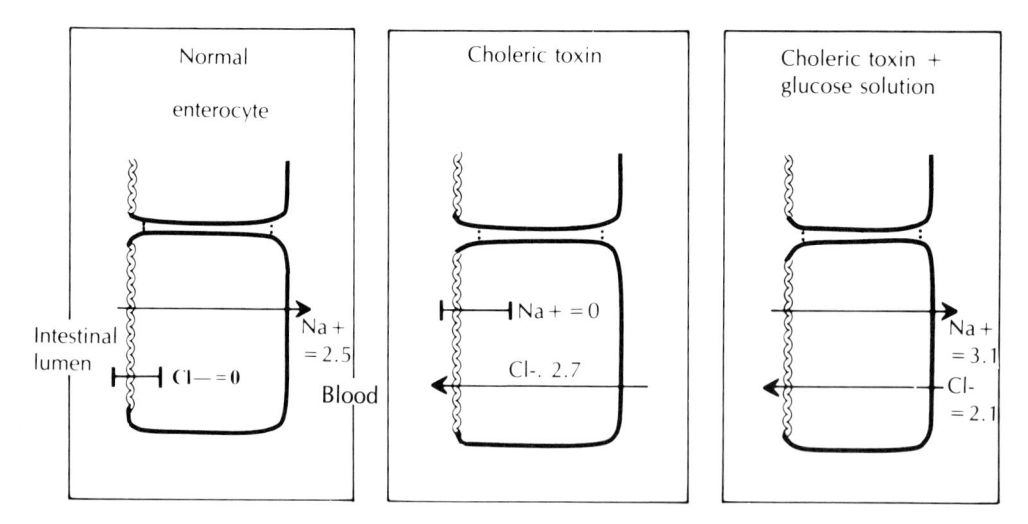

Fig. 17–1. Activity of choleric toxin and colibacillary enterotoxin on the hydroelectrolytic flow through the small intestinal epithelium. Flows are expressed in µeq/cm² per hour. The net flow of sodium becomes positive with the addition of glucose in the lumen and causes a simultaneous water resorption. (Modified from Hirschhorn, N., and Greenough, W.B.: Cholera. Sci. Am., 225:15, 1971.)

mesenteric adenitis and septicemia, and appears to produce an enterotoxin similar to those of *Escherichia coli* and *Vibrio cholerae*. In addition to diarrhea, the symptoms include fever and severe abdominal pains that may be mistaken for appendicitis. This infection may be accompanied by erythema nodosum (20% of the cases), polyarteritis, and Reiter's syndrome. The pathophysiologic features of these associations are unknown.

DIARRHEA CAUSED BY ENTEROPATHOGENIC VIRUSES

Rotaviruses. In 70 to 80% of the common diarrheas of early childhood, no bacterial cause is identified. The association of nonbacterial childhood diarrheas with the presence of rotaviruses in the stools has aroused much interest. Rotaviruses, which are similar to reoviruses, are virions without an envelope, with a diameter of approximately 70 nm, a nucleoprotein nucleus with a diameter of 45 mm, 2 superimposed capsid coats, and double-stranded RNA. They are ether-resistant. Human rotaviruses have not yet been cultivated. These viruses include 2 and possibly 3 different serotypes.

The infectious properties and pathogenic role of these rotaviruses are demonstrated by the following:

1. Their high concentration in the stools of children with diarrhea.
2. The specific serologic response in children who are infected.
3. The epidemic association of this intestinal infection with gastrointestinal disorders.
4. The presence of viral particles in damaged microvilli of the duodenal mucosa of children with diarrhea.

These acute rotaviral diarrheas generally affect children under 3 years of age, especially in the second year of life, nearly exclusively during the winter months in the temperate zones; that is, from November to May in the northern hemisphere. These disorders are occasionally preceded by a few signs of upper respiratory infection. The onset is abrupt and is marked mainly by vomiting. Sometimes, a slight nuchal rigidity prompts an examination of the spinal fluid, which is normal. The diarrhea, attended by moderate fever, is acute, with liquid stools that are neither fetid nor bloody and contain no mucus. The disease runs its course in 2 to 5 days. During the winter months, this virus may be related to

40 to 60% of diarrheas in children. Generally, diagnosis may be based on one or more of the following:

1. The morphologic identification of rotavirus in the stools by electron microscopic examination.
2. The existence of a serologic conversion by means of a complement fixation or an immunofluorescence reaction to either the human antigen extracted from positive stools or the bovine rotavirus antigen.
3. Identification of the virus in the stools by counterimmunoelectrophoresis or, more currently practical, by ELISA.

Norwalk-like Viruses. A second group of acute viral diarrheas is associated with the Norwalk-like viruses. These viruses are small, 27 nm in diameter, have no envelope, and are resistant to ether, acids, and heat, as are the RNA caliciviruses. Norwalk-like viruses are similar to parvoviruses and are closely related to many other strains of parvoviruses isolated in different parts of the world, such as Norwalk (Ohio), Hawaii, and Ditchling (England), and under different names such as W agent (Great Britain) and small round virus (Japan). This Norwalk-like virus includes at least 3 serotypes. After an incubation of 2 days, it produces, in about half the subjects infected, a gastroenteritis manifested by vomiting, liquid diarrhea, or both, with a moderate febrile reaction. The disease, which generally lasts for only a day, spreads as small explosive epidemics in the family or school and strikes older children and adults during any season of the year.

This disease is more difficult to identify than rotaviral infection because the concentration of Norwalk-like viruses in stool is much lower. Norwalk-like viruses can be identified in a stool sample by electron immunomicroscopic examination when the virus particles have been condensed and aggregated in contact with specific immune serum or convalescent patient serum, or more recently, by radioimmunoassay of a stool sample. These techniques are still limited to research laboratories. This virus cannot be cultivated in vitro. The presence of circulating serum antibodies demonstrates a previous infection, which apparently does not confer immunity. On the contrary, its presence indicates paradoxically a particular sensitivity to subsequent gastrointestinal infection.

GIARDIASIS

Giardia lamblia is a flagellated protozoan that may parasitize the initial portion of the small intestine and may produce abdominal pains, diarrhea, and sometimes a malabsorption syndrome. The diagnosis is based on the discovery of the parasite as a trophozoite in the duodenal aspirate or as a cyst in the stool. The most effective treatment is metronidazole or its derivatives, at a dose of 750 mg/day for 5 to 7 days in adults or 15 to 20 mg/kg/day in children. Quinacrine, 100 mg three times a day orally after meals for 5 days in adults and 2 mg/kg three times a day orally after meals for 5 days in children, and furazolidone, 100 mg 4 times daily for 7 days in adults and 1.25 mg/kg 4 times daily for 7 days in children, are also effective.

INTESTINAL AMEBIASIS

Symptomatic amebiasis has a worldwide distribution, with higher infection rates in tropical areas and where sanitary conditions are poor. The infection follows a fecal-oral contamination, and usual modes of transmission include contaminated fresh vegetables and water. Among the different amebas that inhabit the human intestine, only *Entamoeba histolytica* causes significant illness. *Entamoeba coli* and *E. hartmanni* are occasional intestinal saprophytes unable to provoke disease.

Pathogenesis. After being ingested, *Entamoeba histolytica* causes a variable range of symptomatic diseases reflecting the different pathogenicity of the strains and the differing susceptibilities of the hosts. For instance, a poor nutritional status favors a severe infection. Trophozoite forms of ameba can penetrate the intestinal epithelium and may spread laterally in the submucosa. This invasion can compromise the patient's blood supply to the overlying mucosa, which may undergo necrosis, with formation of ulcers. The trophozoites may then gain access to the patient's liver through the portal vein; they may also disseminate to other organs by rupture of a liver abscess into the pleural cavity, lung, or pericardium, or by the blood to the lungs or brain.

Clinical Features. The diarrhea, when present, typically reflects this invasive process and exemplifies the dysenteric syndrome with watery feces containing blood and mucus. The patient suffers from cramping abdominal pain, anorexia, nausea, and vomiting. A low-grade fever is often reported, but fluid depletion is uncommon because the volume of feces remains small. Many patients have only diarrhea, however. In some cases, the diarrhea is chronic, occurring several times a year with episodes lasting 1 to 4 weeks, alternating with periods of constipation.

Diagnosis. In addition to this clinical picture, other clues may lead to a presumptive diagnosis. For example, the patient lives in or has visited an infected area, although the disease can be caught in almost any part of the world. The rectosigmoidoscopy, which should be performed without preparation, to maintain the typical aspect of the mucosa, may reveal ulcers with punched out margins and covered by a whitish exudate; however, atypical or small ulcers and a nonspecific mucosal inflammation are not conclusively diagnostic.

The definitive diagnosis depends on identification of *Entamoeba histolytica* in the feces, in the scraping of a rectal ulcer, or in a rectal biopsy. Fresh specimens are required to enable one to observe the rapid and progressive motility of trophozoites, which characteristically engulf ingested red blood cells or starch granules. Stained trophozoites may also be recognized both by their size, 15 to 60 µm, and by their nuclei, which contain a central karyosome and a peripheral ring of chromatin. In some patients with chronic diarrhea, only cysts of *E. histolytica* can be seen. These cysts are 10 to 20 µm in size, with 1 to 4 nuclei; a large glycogen vacuole and rod-shaped chromatoidal bodies can be seen in the cytoplasm. This parasitologic diagnosis, however, is often hampered by many substances that destroy trophozoites and modify the morphologic features of the cyst. Interfering products include most antidiarrheal medications and antimicrobial agents, nonabsorbable antacids, and barium and a variety of other substances used for enemas.

Various serologic techniques can detect antibodies against *Entamoeba histolytica* when invasive disease occurs.

Treatment. A combination of 2 amebicidal drugs (Table 17–5) is often required because no product can act against *Entamoeba histolytica* at all sites, and most patients with amebic dysentery have parasites in the tissues as well as the intestinal lumen. Generally, metronidazole is used in combination with iodoquinol (diiodohydroxyquin). In all cases, at least one examination for amebas should be made 2 weeks after treatment, to assess the parasitologic cure. If the patient is not cured, another course of treatment must be prescribed.

Objective 17–4. Identify the main causes of bacterial food poisoning.

Certain bacteria multiply in food and secrete a toxin. When the food is later eaten, signs of intoxication appear. The importance of multiplication of the organism within the intestine is secondary, even if we grant that *Clostridium perfringens* and *C. botulinum* continue to secrete their toxins after the patient has swallowed these bacteria.

Clinically, some features help to characterize these forms of intoxication. The interval between ingestion of the contaminated food and the onset of the first symptoms is generally only a matter of hours. Usually, several persons who have shared the same meal are poisoned at the same time, but the degree of intoxication depends on the amount of the

Table 17–5. Drugs Active Against Amebiasis

Drug Category	Product Examples	Sites of Action in the Body	Dosages	Side Effects
Oxyquinolines	Iodoquinol	Intestinal lumen, intestinal wall	650 mg tid or 30–40 mg/kg body weight/day orally q8h for 20 days	Few; optic neuritis in prolonged therapy
Dichloroacetamides	Diloxanide furoate	Intestinal lumen, intestinal wall	500 mg tid or 20 mg/kg body weight/day orally for 10 days	Flatulence, loose stools
Imidazoles	Metronidazole	Intestinal wall and various tissues	750 mg tid or 20–40 mg/kg body weight/day orally q8h for 5–15 days	Few; digestive discomfort, Antabuse effect, rare paresthesia; not recommended during first trimester of pregnancy
Emetines	Emetine or Dihydroemetine	Different tissues; not used in amebiasis limited to the intestine	1 mg/kg body weight/day (not to exceed 60 mg) q12h IM or subcutaneously up to 5 days	Local pain, neuromuscular disability, cardiotoxic effects; ECG monitoring required
Chloroquine	Chloroquine phosphate	Different tissues; not used in amebiasis limited to the intestine	600 mg base (1 gm) or 15–17 mg/kg body weight/day, q6h for 2 days; then, 300 mg base (500 mg) or 7–8 mg/kg body weight/day q12h for 3–4 weeks	None with the recommended regimen

tainted food consumed (dose dependence) and the sensitivity of the individual to the toxin. Signs of infection such as fever are usually lacking. The patient appears seriously ill and often complains of violent abdominal cramps. The disease may progress to shock and may rapidly become fatal.

It may be difficult or impossible to demonstrate the organism in the stools, but the key to the diagnosis is often provided by a culture of the suspected food. Several distinctive characteristics of the four principal causes of food poisoning are given in Table 17–6.

With the important exception of botulism (see Objective 31–1), no specific therapy is available for bacterial food poisoning. Antibiotics are not indicated, and no known agents counteract the effects of the enterotoxin. Supportive therapy, such as administration of intravenous fluids, may be helpful if dehydration develops.

Objective 17–5. Determine the cause of diarrhea that appears during or at the end of antibiotic therapy and decide on appropriate therapy.

Most antibiotics, especially when administered orally, can accelerate gastrointestinal motility and may even cause true diarrhea. Several mechanisms are probably involved, such as a direct action on the mucosa (by neomycin, for example) or a disturbance in the "balance" of the intestinal flora by broad-spectrum antibiotics.

PSEUDOMEMBRANOUS ENTEROCOLITIS (PMEC)

Pseudomembranous enterocolitis (PMEC) is a more serious entity associated with the administration of many antibiotics. The direct cause of PMEC is not the antibiotic, but toxigenic *Clostridium difficile*.

The antimicrobial agents that carry the

Table 17–6. Principal Food Poisonings of Bacterial Origin

	Incidence	Foods usually involved	Time of onset after ingestion (hours)	Principal symptomatic features
Staphylococcus aureus phage groups III and IV	Frequent	Warmed-over food, pastry, whipped cream, canned foods, pork products, preserved meats, frozen foods	1–6	Vomiting, cramps, diarrhea, hypersalivation, headaches, sweating chills, possibility of shock (rare)
Clostridium perfringens	Frequent	Warmed-over food, sauces, insufficiently cooked pork (in New Guinea)	10–14	Diarrhea, abdominal cramps, possibility of shock
Bacillus cereus	Rare	Warmed-over sauces, Chinese food (in United States)	10–15	Profuse diarrhea, abdominal cramps, rectal tenesmus, nausea
Clostridium botulinum	Rare	Home-canned food, canned vegetables, preserved fish, canned fruit, warmed-over meat, Condiments, sometimes even honey	12–24 (up to 8 days)	Inconstant diarrhea (more commonly constipation), dry mouth, paralysis

---

CLOSTRIDIA

Clostridia are spore-forming, anaerobic, gram-positive bacilli that are widely distributed in the soil and in the fecal flora of humans and animals. When an antibiotic is administered either orally or parenterally, it suppress the growth of susceptible flora. *Clostridium difficile,* a resistant species, can then multiply and elaborate a cytotoxic toxin that produces postantibiotic pseudomembranous enterocolitis. This toxin is an antigenic protein. The exact causal relationship between the presence of the antibiotic and the production of the toxin is not clear. *C. difficile* is difficult to cultivate in vitro. The toxin can be more readily identified by its neutralization in a tissue culture with antiserum prepared against the toxin of antigenically similar *C. sordellii.* Thus, complete identification of the toxin in the stools can usually be accomplished in 2 days, but most microbiologic diagnostic laboratories are not equipped to perform this investigation.

---

greatest risk of PMEC are clindamycin, lincomycin, and the ampicillins; carrying a lesser risk are the other penicillins and the cephalosporins, co-trimoxazole, and metronidazole. PMEC has not been observed after treatment with erythromycin, parenteral aminoglycosides or antituberculosis, antifungal, or antiparasitic drugs. The frequency of PMEC following treatment varies from one study to another and with the age and sex of the population studied. The risk of PMEC is not directly related to the antibiotic dose.

Clinical Features. Although symptoms have been noted as early as a few hours after beginning antibiotic treatment, they more usually appear 4 to 10 days after the institution of the therapy, whereas a third of cases occur from several days to 2 weeks after discontinuance of the treatment. Usually, the enterocolitis is manifested by a watery diarrhea accompanied by abdominal pains or tenesmus. The patient may also have severe, bloody diarrhea, discharge of "false membranes," a fever of 40° C, and rapid deterioration of general health status.

Diagnosis. The diagnosis is based on proctocolonoscopy and the demonstration of *Clostridium difficile* toxin in the feces. Endoscopic examination reveals an inflammatory, edematous colorectal mucosa covered in some places by adherent, yellowish gray pseudomembranes. Barium enemas are contraindicated because they may increase the toxin absorption. The presence of *C. difficile* can be demonstrated by culture and by detection of the toxin. In a filtrate of stools, the presence of the toxin is demonstrated by its toxic action on a cell culture; it can be specifically identified by its neutralization with *C. sordellii* antitoxin. The presence of the toxin in the stools is not diagnostic in itself, however, because the toxin has been recovered from some asymptomatic patients.

Treatment. In all patients, the antibiotic should be discontinued as soon as the first signs of enterocolitis appear. Simple cessation is sometimes sufficient to control the iatrogenic diarrhea. Atropine and morphine preparations and, in general, all drugs that slow intestinal motility should be avoided.

Cholestyramine is an ion-exchange resin with the property of fixing *Clostridium difficile* toxin in vitro. In vivo, its therapeutic action can be dramatic, but it is inconsistent (approximately 50% of patients respond) and unpredictable.

If the diarrhea continues after cessation of the antibiotic therapy, oral vancomycin, in 4 daily doses of 500 mg each for 10 days, is prescribed for an adult. The therapeutic action of vancomycin is usually rapid, and it causes *Clostridium difficile* and the toxin to disappear from the patient's stools. Some patients may have a relapse after the cessation of vancomycin and may be cured by a second course of treatment. Vancomycin can be ototoxic and nephrotoxic, but because it does not cross the gastrointestinal barrier, no sign of toxicity is observed after oral administration. Metronidazole, a possible second choice, has itself been known to produce pseudomembranous enterocolitis.

Fortunately, fulminant hyperacute or incurable enterocolitis, for which an emergency colectomy may be necessary, is unusual.

Clostrial versus Staphylococcal Enterocolitis. In the 1950s and 1960s, *Staphylococcus aureus* was considered to be responsible for a severe enterocolitis, but this idea has been questioned since the discovery of the role of *Clostridium difficile* in the disorder.

Staphylococcus aureus can be isolated in the stools in 20% of normal infants or in those with diarrhea. This bacterium is not known to have any pathologic significance, except in the unusual staphylococcal enterocolitis in which staphylococci on smear predominate in the fecal flora. Some cases of staphylococcal enterocolitis have been reported in neonates subjected to tube feedings or intensive care units, or in those residing in institutions.

This rare enterocolitis should not be confused with staphylococcal food poisoning (Table 17–6).

Objective 17–6. Look for the cause of acute diarrhea in a neonate and determine appropriate management.

It is normal for a child to have 5 to 10 semiliquid stools per day in the first few weeks of life, particularly when the baby is breast fed. The baby's health is unaffected, and his growth after the first few days is rapid. In such a context, the diagnosis of pathologic diarrhea is not always easy, at least initially; pathologic diarrhea is manifested before long by pain and crying, abdominal distension, anorexia or vomiting, and, in particular, loss of weight.

Such a diarrhea may have a number of different infectious causes, all generally related to contamination in the home or the nursery; examples are salmonella, shigella, and enteropathogenic *Escherichia coli*. At this age, it is rare for a diarrhea of this type to be related to a rotaviral infection. Up to 40% of newborns in a hospital nursery may be carriers of

Clostridium difficile, in some cases with toxin production but without apparent pathologic consequences. The contamination is generally perinatal, via contact with the maternal vaginal flora.

ACUTE NECROTIZING ENTEROCOLITIS

The most alarming diarrhea or gastrointestinal disturbance in a neonate is that accompanying an acute necrotizing enterocolitis. The disease is rare, and its origin is obscure. The occurrence of limited epidemics suggests that this disorder may be infectious, related to clostridia, viruses, or other microorganisms. Preferentially affected are neonates of low birth weight who have suffered anoxia from any cause or who have undergone aggressive intervention or investigative procedures such as intubation or umbilical catheterization. Early hyperosmolar artificial alimentation is a contributing factor. After a symptom-free interval of a few days, the clinical picture includes the following:

1. A huge abdominal distension.
2. Presence of bile in the vomitus.
3. Bloody diarrhea.
4. Rapid and severe deterioration of the patient's general condition.

A plain roentgenogram of the abdomen confirms the diagnosis when it reveals gas-filled loops of bowel and the presence of air in the intestinal wall (parietal pneumatosis); sometimes, a pneumoperitoneum occurs as a result of perforation. The course of the disease is often rapidly fatal.

Treatment of acute necrotizing enterocolitis is based on the discontinuance of all oral intake and the implementation of parenteral alimentation and broad-spectrum antibiotic therapy with occasional recourse to bypass surgical procedures or colectomy.

SUGGESTED READINGS

Bartlett, J.G.: Antibiotic-associated pseudomembranous colitis. Rev. Infect. Dis., *1*:530, 1979.

Blacklow, N.R., and Cukor, G.: Viral gastroenteritis. N. Engl. J. Med., *304*:397, 1981.

Craig, J.P.: The enterotoxic enteropathies. Symp. Soc. General Microbiol., *22*:129, 1972.

Dupont, H., et al.: Treatment of traveller's diarrhea with trimetroprim/sulfamethoxazole and with trimethoprim alone. N. Engl. J. Med., *307*:841, 1982.

Echeverria, P.D., Chang, C.P., and Smith, D.: Enterotoxigenicity and invasive capacity of "enteropathogenic" serotypes of Escherichia coli. J. Pediatr., *89*:8, 1976.

Echeverria, P.D., et al.: Relative importance of viruses and bacteria in the etiology of pediatric diarrhea in Taiwan. J. Infect. Dis., *136*:383, 1977.

Evans, D.G., Evans, D.J., and Tjoa, W.: Hemagglutination of human group A erythrocytes by enterotoxigenic Escherichia coli isolated from adults with diarrhea: correlation with colonization factor. Infect. Immun., *18*:330, 1977.

Finberg, L.: The management of the critically ill child with dehydration secondary to diarrhea. Pediatrics, *45*:1029, 1970.

Finkelstein, R.A., Larue, M.K., and Johnston, D.W.: Isolation and properties of heat-labile enterotoxins from enterotoxigenic Escherichia coli. J. Infect. Dis., *133(Suppl.)*:120, 1976.

Fordtran, J.S.: Stimulation of active and passive sodium absorption by sugars in the human jejunum. J. Clin. Invest., *55*:728, 1975.

George, W.L., Rolfe, R.D., and Finegold, S.M.: Treatment and prevention of antimicrobial agent-induced colitis and diarrhea. Gastroenterology, *79*:366, 1980.

Kallings, L.O., Mollby, R., and Nord, C.E.: Antibiotic associated colitis and Clostridium difficile. Scand. J. Infect. Dis., *22(Suppl.)*:1, 1980.

Levine, M.M., and Edelman, R.: Acute diarrheal infections in infants. Hosp. Pract., *14*:89, 1979; *15*:97, 1980.

Sack, R.B.: Human diarrheal disease caused by enterotoxigenic Escherichia coli. Ann. Rev. Microbiol., *29*:333, 1975.

Santulli, T.V., et al.: Acute necrotizing enterocolitis in infancy: a review of 64 cases. Pediatrics, *55*:376, 1975.

Terranova, W., and Blake, P.A.: Bacillus cereus food poisoning. N. Engl. J. Med., *298*:143, 1978.

CHAPTER 18

Intestinal Helminthic Infections

J. Vincelette

> Objective 18–1. Suspect intestinal helminthic infections in a variety of clinical settings.

HIGHLY EXPOSED INDIVIDUALS

Intestinal helminthiasis is often asymptomatic, or the symptoms may be so discrete that the infection goes unnoticed. Nevertheless, the diagnosis is useful in preventing sequelae and transmission.

A careful history of recent or remote travel and a history of food consumption may give the physician the first diagnostic clue to intestinal helminthiasis. In a variety of clinical settings, a parasitic origin is not even considered unless a history of previous exposure is elicited. Patients at high risk who have been exposed to helminthiasis should be examined to detect asymptomatic carriers.

In large areas of underdeveloped countries, intestinal helminths are so common that only a small minority of the population is spared. Travel in those areas for an extended period or under poor conditions carries a significant risk of infection. Eating uncooked food certainly increases this risk; walking barefoot exposes a person to other helminths.

In short, it is difficult to share native life without sharing native parasites.

Similarly, intrafamilial transmission of pinworms is high, and it is usual for several members of one family to be infected, even though asymptomatically.

Even in the developed countries of Europe and North America, the consumption of raw or undercooked pork, beef, or fish may lead to infection by intestinal worms. Table 18–1 lists the characteristics of helminthiasis.

PASSING OF WORMS

Obviously, in a patient who reports passing a worm, the diagnosis of an intestinal helminthiasis is suggested. Two questions should be asked: is it really a worm, and if so, which worm? At times, poorly digested food or other small objects ingested by children can be mistaken for worms in the stools. Whenever possible, the physician should ask the patient to bring the worm to the physician's office, for expert identification. Otherwise, one should try to obtain a detailed description of the helminth.

Ascaris, pinworms, and tapeworm segments are most commonly seen. Ascaris may even be vomited, and occasionally the outline

Table 18-1. Characteristics of Helminthiasis

Helminths	Common Symptoms	Complications or Rare Symptoms
Roundworms		
Pinworm (*Enterobius vermicularis*)	Pruritis ani; pruritus vulvae; worm migration	Anal dermatitis or infection; perineal pain; vaginitis, endometritis, salpingitis (m̃), urinary tract infection (?) (in girls)
Whipworm (*Trichuris trichiura*)	—	Colitis; rectal prolapse (when severe)
Ascaris lumbricoides		
tissue-migration phase	Cough, bronchospasm; eosinophilia	—
enteric phase	Worm passed in stools or vomited; gastrointestinal disturbance	Intestinal obstruction; bile duct obstruction (m̃); appendicitis (m̃); m̃ at various sites
Hookworms (*Ancylostoma duodenale, Necator americanus*)	Epigastric malaise; hypochromic anemia (when severe)	Hypoproteinemia (when intense)
Strongyloides stercoralis	Epigastric pain; diarrhea	Cutaneous larva migrans at penetration site; cough (tissue-migration phase); vomiting; recurrent gram-negative bacteremia and other severe bacterial infection(s) (in hyperinfection syndrome and immunosuppression)
Tapeworms		
Diphyllobothrium latum	Gastrointestinal disturbance; pernicious anemia	Passing of segments of worm
Taenia saginata	Abdominal cramps	—
Taenia solium	Evacuation of worm segments	Cysticercosis (especially frequent in Latin America)
Hymenolepsis nana	Abdominal cramps; diarrhea	Dizziness, seizure
Flukes		
Faciolopsis buski	Abdominal pain; diarrhea	Vomiting, anorexia; ascites
Heterophyes heterophyes	Abdominal pain; diarrhea	Myocarditis; central nervous system symptoms
Metagonimus yokogawai	—	Gastrointestinal symptoms

*m̃, Migration of adult worm.

of an ascaris or tapeworm is visualized on a small bowel film of a gastrointestinal series.

PRURITUS ANI AND VULVAE

Intense nocturnal pruritus ani is typical of pinworm infection and may sometimes be complicated by perianal dermatitis, bacterial infection, or even abscess formation. Pruritus ani may produce a considerable sleep disturbance in children. The migration of pinworms occasionally causes an appendicitis-simulating peritonitis.

INTESTINAL SYMPTOMS

Most intestinal helminths can produce abdominal discomfort or pain, even if often ill defined. Epigastric pain is more characteristic of heavy infestation with hookworms (rare nowadays) or strongyloides. Intermittent loose stools or episodes of diarrhea are characteristic of amebiasis or giardiasis, but may be encountered with most of those infections. Whereas viral or bacterial diarrhea is usually acute and of short duration, parasitic diarrhea is intermittent and more persistent. In heavy strongyloides or whipworm infection, duodenitis or colitis may occur, accompanied by blood in the stools, especially with colitis when the patient is receiving corticosteroids or other forms of immunotherapy.

Intestinal obstruction may occur with

heavy ascaris infestation, notably in children. A rate of 2 per 1000 infected children, 1 to 5 years old, was calculated in rural areas of the southeastern United States some decades ago. Biliary colic has been noted following obstruction of the common bile duct by migrating ascaris. The adult worm may be visualized in the bile duct at cholangiography. Discharge of a hepatic echinococcus cyst through the biliary tree can also cause the same symptoms, with eosinophilia.

ANEMIA

Hypochromic anemia resulting from continuous blood loss is classically noted in heavy hookworm infections. Megaloblastic anemia, clinically similar to that seen in pernicious anemia, including glossitis, paresthesia, and numbness, occurs in some patients infected with the fish tapeworm *(Diphyllobothrium latum)*, owing to impaired absorption of vitamin B_{12} and folate.

PNEUMONITIS

Patients exposed to ascariasis in hyperendemic areas may have cough, mucoid sputum, dyspnea, wheezing, rales, and patchy pulmonary infiltration 5 to 14 days after the ingestion of ascaris eggs. The syndrome is due to the passage of larvae through the lungs during the tissue-migratory phase of the cycle. A parasitic origin should be suspected in a patient with a recent history of exposure and in the presence of a high eosinophilia (the last sign to occur in pulmonary ascariasis). Pulmonary symptoms may also occur in hyperinfective strongyloides infection and have been reported in experimental hookworm infections, again during the tissue-migratory phase.

CUTANEOUS LARVA MIGRANS (CREEPING ERUPTION)

An irregular linear papular skin eruption, which sometimes progresses in a few hours, is due to the penetration and migration under the skin of the infective (filariform) larvae of the dog and cat hookworm *Ancylostoma braziliense* or *A. asia*, of *Gnathostoma spinigerum*, or more rarely, of strongyloides. A rash caused by strongyloides is more frequently seen in the perianal area, usually within 30 cm of the anus. Infection is then due to autoreinfection from larva excreted in the stools. Ancylostoma and gnathostoma infections occur on exposed skin areas, mainly on the feet and legs.

EOSINOPHILIA

The eosinophil count is usually normal in presence of adult helminths in the lumen of the gastrointestinal tract. On the other hand, during the tissue-migratory phase of ascaris, strongyloides, or hookworms, a marked eosinophilic response may be elicited.

GASTROINTESTINAL SYMPTOMS AND PNEUMONIA IN AN IMMUNOCOMPROMISED HOST

As briefly mentioned, a lowered immune response in a carrier of *Strongyloides stercoralis* may allow internal autoinfection and dissemination of larvae throughout the patient's body. Gastrointestinal symptoms, including nausea, vomiting, anorexia, epigastric pain, and diarrhea, are usually present and may be severe. The diffuse pneumonitis often seen represents the migration and filariform larvae into the lung (larvae may be seen in the sputum) and can lead to respiratory insufficiency. Polymicrobial septicemia may result from the penetration of the intestinal mucosa by larvae. Peritonitis is also seen. Eosinophilia is present only in a minority of patients. A history of time spent in tropical areas of Africa, Asia, and South America, even decades before, should raise the possibility of this infection.

> **Objective 18–2.** Identify a helminthic infection of the gastrointestinal tract.

The diagnosis of intestinal helminthiasis can be made either by the identification of the ova (Fig. 18–2) or the larvae (Fig. 18–3) in the host's feces, by the identification of eggs in the perianal area, or by the identification of the evacuated adult worm or segments (Figs. 18–4, 18–5, and 18–6). Nonintestinal helminth eggs, such as from the liver

CHARACTERISTICS OF HELMINTHS

"Helminth" is derived from the Greek and means "worm." The term usually refers to several groups of parasitic worms with complex life cycles.

The host of the adult stage is called the definitive host; a host of developmental stages is an intermediate host. In human intestinal helminthiasis, the adult helminths live in the lumen of the host's gastrointestinal tract and usually attach themselves to the mucosa, or, as with strongyloides, penetrating the mucosa. For most helminth species, the biologic cycle is initiated when eggs are passed into the stools of the host. Exceptions are the pinworm, which lays eggs on the skin of the host's perianal area, and strongyloides, whose eggs hatch in the host's intestinal mucosa and whose larvae are passed in the stools. Even though the biologic cycle of each species has its own peculiarities, five general patterns can be traced (Fig. 18-1 and Table 18-2).

In the direct cycle (type I pattern), a mature ovum is ingested. It hatches in the host's gastrointestinal tract, and the parasite matures in the lumen or the wall of the gut up to the adult stage; ova are then laid in the stools or on the perianal skin. The next two patterns are characterized by a tissue-migration phase of the larva. The transmucosal pattern is peculiar to ascaris. After ingestion of the parasite by the host, the egg hatches in the duodenum, and the larva penetrates the mucosa to initiate the tissue-migration phase. The larva penetrates the lungs, is expectorated, and then is swallowed to mature in the lumen of the host's small bowel.

In the percutaneous pattern (type II), an infective (filariform) larva penetrates through the skin to initiate the tissue-migration phase. During this phase, larvae are brought to the lung capillaries by the host's circulation. Then, these larvae penetrate the pulmonary alveoli and follow the bronchial secretions up to the pharynx, where they are swallowed. The parasites mature to the adult stage in the host's gut. Thereafter, ova or larvae are evacuated in the stools.

Strongyloides follows the type III pattern, or it may have a complete cycle in the soil (broken line).

The last two patterns are characterized by one or two intermediate hosts during the larval stages of the helminth. In the ingested intermediate host pattern (type IV), the larva encysts in the intermediate host and infects the definitive host when the definitive host eats the uncooked flesh of the intermediate host (trichinosis, diphyllobothriasis, paragonimiasis). In the last pattern (type V), free larvae escape from the intermediate host and encyst on water plants, until these plants are eaten by the definitive host (*Fasciolopsis buski*).

Three main helminth phyla are found in humans: the nematodes or roundworms, the cestodes or tapeworms, and the trematodes or flukes.

The nematodes are unsegmented roundworms. Each worm is of one sex. Intestinal nematodes of man mate in the gastrointestinal tract. The larval stage requires no intermediate host, but occurs either in the gut (direct pattern), in the tissues of the definitive host (transmucosal and percutaneous patterns), or in the soil (percutaneous pattern). Pinworms (enterobius), whipworms (trichuris), ascaris, hookworms, and strongyloides are common intestinal nematodes in humans.

The cestodes or tapeworms are segmented flatworms. The cranial part is called the scolex or head and bears special organs, such as suckers or hooks, to anchor the helminth to the host's intestinal mucosa. Behind the scolex is a narrow neck, where the proglottids or segments are produced. These segments remain attached to one another while maturing and develop a long, tapelike shape. Cestodes have no digestive tract. Each segment has its own nervous system and musculature, male and female reproductive organs, and excretory canal. The caudal portion of the worm comprises gravid proglottids loaded with eggs. Cestodes have one or more intermediate hosts (type IV pattern), except for the dwarf tapeworm, which follows the direct cycle.

Trematodes or flukes are unsegmented flatworms. Intestinal trematodes are hermaphroditic. Eggs are passed in the host's feces and hatch in water, where the larva (miracidium) penetrates a specific species of snail and passes through several generations to produce free larvae (cercariae) that will encyst either in fish (type IV pattern) or on water plants (type V pattern). The cycle is completed when the cysts are ingested by the definitive host.

---

fluke, lung fluke, or schistosoma, can also be recovered from stools.

INTESTINAL ROUNDWORMS

Pinworms. Enterobius vermicularis (syn. *Oxyuris vermicularis*) is the most common helminth in United States, Canada, Europe, and other developed countries. The adult female is white, spindle-shaped, and 13 by 0.4 mm (Fig. 18-6). The male is smaller and is rarely seen. Adults live in the host's cecum. At night, the females migrate to the anus and lay embryonated eggs in the perianal area, where they become infectious in 6 hours. The oviposition often provokes an intense itching. Eggs may be taken up under the nails by scratching. Autoreinoculation occurs when fingers are put into the mouth or when food is contaminated by handling. The high intrafamilial transmission is due to person-to-person contact and to the ingestion or inhalation of dust from bed linen or clothes contaminated with pinworm eggs.

Anal itching may initiate a dermatitis that

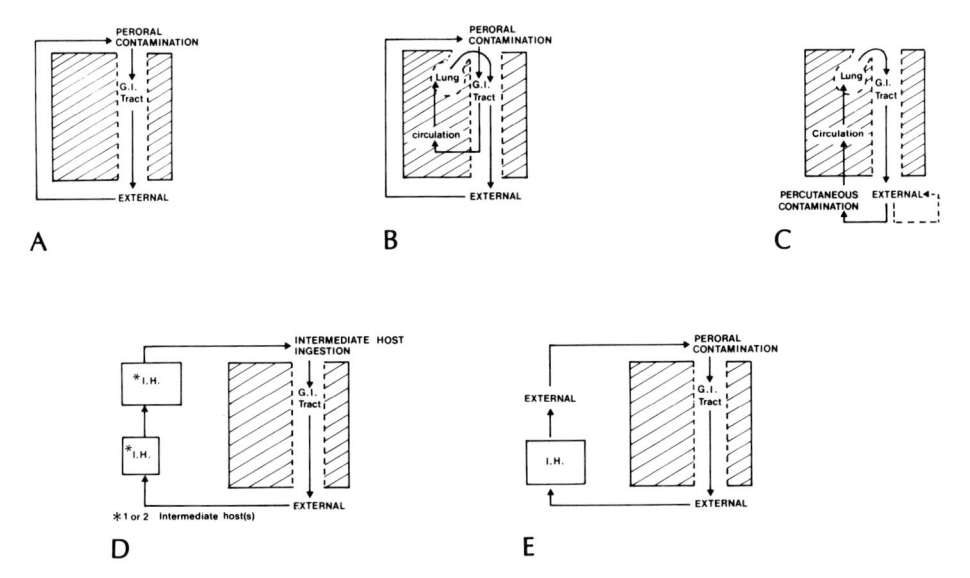

Fig. 18–1. Patterns of biologic cycle. *A,* Type I, direct; *B,* type II, transmucosal; *C,* type III, percutaneous; *D,* type IV, ingested intermediate host; *E,* type V, noningested intermediate host.

Table 18–2. Patterns of Biologic Cycles of Intestinal Helminths

Pattern Type	Nematodes	Cestodes	Trematodes
I: Direct	Pinworms Whipworms	Dwarf tapeworms	—
II: Transmucosal	Ascaris	—	—
III: Percutaneous	Hookworms Strongyloides	—	—
IV: Ingested intermediate host	—	Fish tapeworms Beef tapeworms Pork tapeworms	*Heterophyes heterophyes* *Metagonimus yokogawai*
V: Noningested intermediate host	—	—	*Fasciolopsis buski*

may be complicated by superinfection or, rarely, by an abscess. Female worms may be seen at the anus at night. It is not uncommon to see these worms on stools. Occasionally, migration of the worm may cause perianal pain, vaginitis, or deep genital tract infection.

The diagnosis of pinworm infection is made by the demonstration of eggs in the patient's perianal area with a cellophane tape swab (Fig. 18–7). This test is best done in the morning, before the patient takes a bath or has a bowel movement. The test has a 50% sensitivity when done once, 90% accuracy when performed 3 times, and 99% accuracy when done 5 times. Stool examination is rarely diagnostic.

Whipworms. *Trichuris trichiura*, when adult, is 30 to 50 mm long. These worms are rarely seen except during rectoscopy or on a prolapsed rectum. In the lumen of the bowel, females lay eggs that are passed in the stools. These eggs mature in about 3 weeks in the soil. Humans are infected by ingestion of the mature ova (direct cycle). *T. trichiura* is cosmopolitan and is common in warm and moist climates. It is one of the most common intestinal helminths seen in travelers returning from tropical areas. Trichuriasis is usually asymptomatic, although heavy infection may cause colitis with mucus and blood in stools and may be complicated by rectal prolapse. The diagnosis is made by the demonstration of typical ova in the patient's stools.

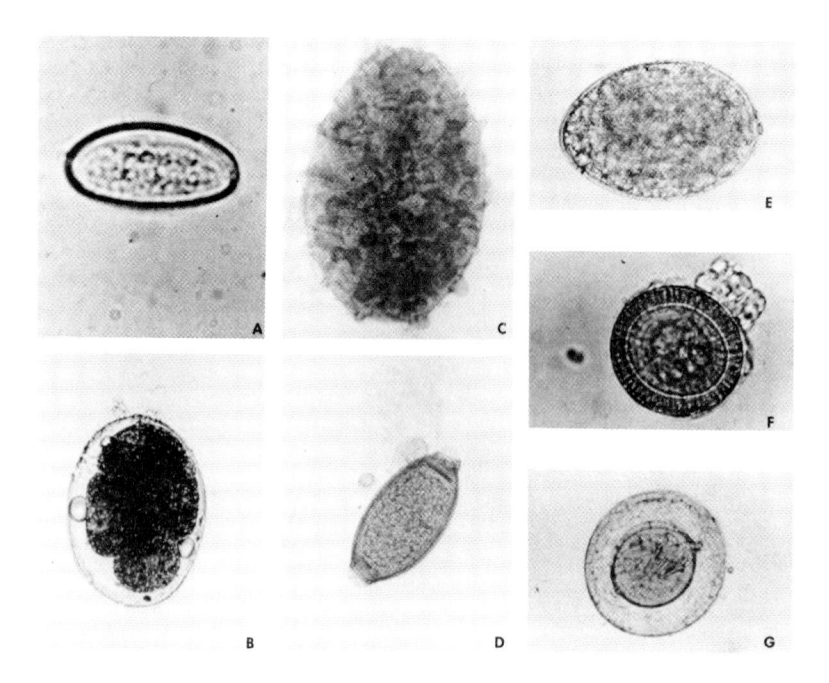

242　　Infections: Recognition, Understanding, Treatment

Fig. 18–2. A to G, Eggs of intestinal helminths. A, pinworm; B, hookworm; C, Ascaris; D, Trichuris; E, Diphyllobothrium latum; F, Taenia solium; G, Hymenolepis nana.

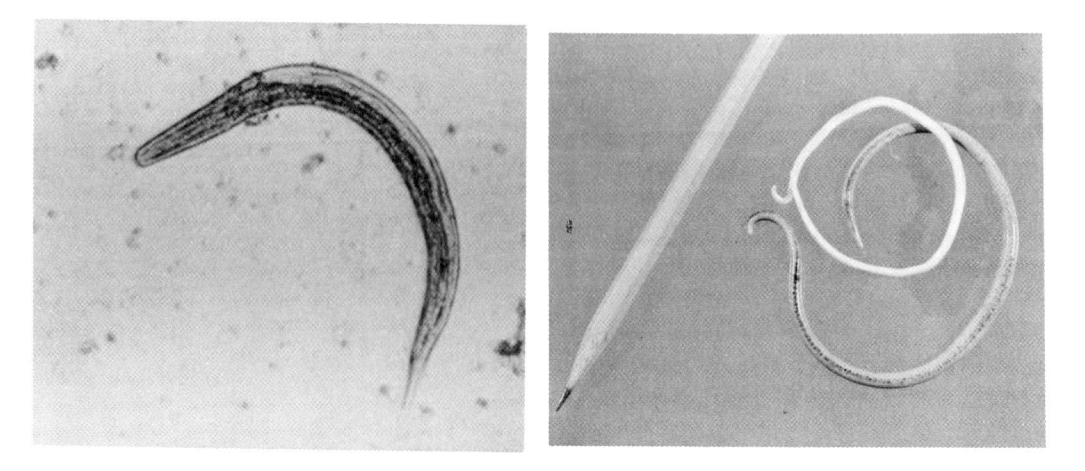

Fig. 18–3. Strongyloides stercoralis larva in feces (500 ×).

Fig. 18–4. Ascaris lumbricoides.

Intestinal Helminthic Infections

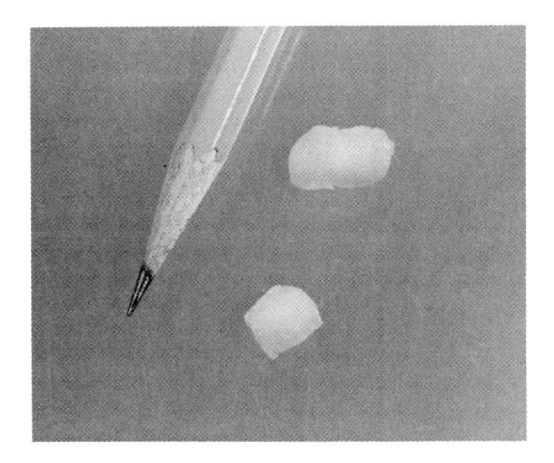

Fig. 18–5. Taenia proglottids.

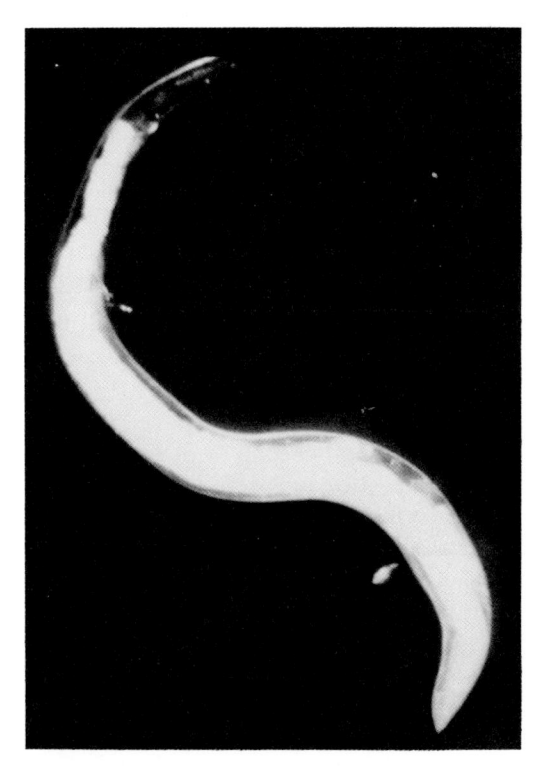

Fig. 18–6. Pinworm (15 ×).

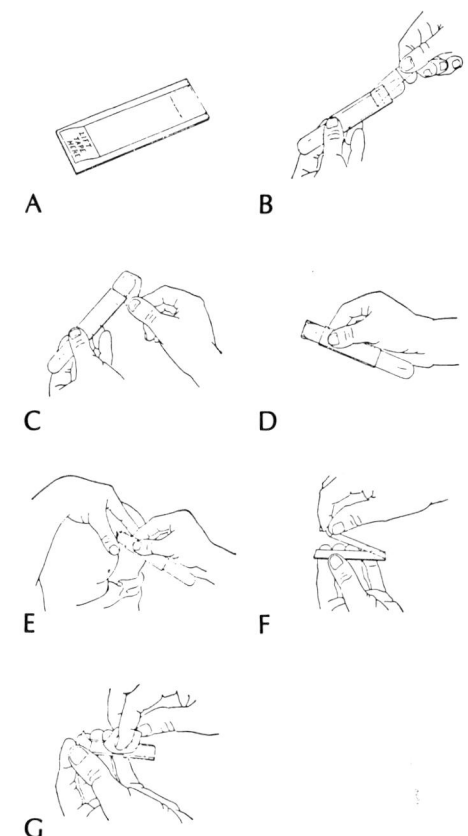

Fig. 18–7. Cellophane tape test. *A*, Slide preparation. *B*, Hold slide against tongue depressor one inch from end and lift long portion of tape from slide. *C*, Loop tape over end of depressor to expose gummed surface. *D*, Hold tape and slide against tongue depressor. *E*, Press gummed surfaces against several areas of perianal region. *F*, Replace tape on slide. *G*, Smooth tape with cotton or gauze. (From Henry, J.B. (ed.): Todd-Sanford-Davidsohn Clinical Diagnosis and Management by Laboratory Methods. 16th Ed. Philadelphia, W.B. Saunders, 1979.)

Ascaris lumbricoides. Cosmopolitan and common in tropical as well as temperate areas, this worm is by far the largest intestinal nematode of man. Its unique size (15 to 35 cm) among the roundworm parasites of man is pathognomonic, except for the rare case of human infection with an animal ascarid. A large, whitish or pink roundworm, 15 to 35 cm long, spontaneously expelled through the anus or by the mouth, is surely *Ascaris lumbricoides*. The biologic cycle is unique (transmucosal type): peroral infection and duodenal development of the ova are followed by a tissue phase in which the larva penetrates the host's intestinal mucosa and reaches the lung capillaries through the circulation. After maturation, the larva penetrates the alveolus, is expelled from the respiratory tract with the host's bronchial secretions, and is swallowed with sputum. When the larva again reaches the bowel lumen, it matures into its adult stage, mates, and lays eggs.

The tissue phase of infestation is characterized by respiratory symptoms such as cough, wheezing, dyspnea, mucoid sputum, and rales. Multiple small areas of infiltration may be seen on a chest roentgenogram. Eosinophilia is also present. The cause of the disorder is seldom suspected, and the specific diagnosis is rarely made. Larvae may be seen in the patient's sputum. Serologic tests are available in specialized reference laboratories. The diagnosis is more easily made detecting ova in stools, but only when maturation of the ascaris in the gut is complete, approximately 8 weeks later.

The enteric phase of ascariasis is diagnosed by the demonstration of ova in the patient's stools, but this test may be negative if only male worms parasitize the host. At times, the outline of ascaris may be seen on a small bowel film of a gastrointestinal series.

Hookworms. Two hookworms parasitize the human gut: *Necator americanus*, prevalent in central Africa, the Americas, eastern and southern India, Indonesia, and the South Pacific; and *Ancylostoma duodenale*, prevalent around the Mediterranean, in Pakistan, in northern India, and in the Far East. Both hookworms have a percutaneous biologic cycle. If ingested, filariform larvae penetrate the host's buccal mucosa. The tissue-migration phase usually goes unnoticed. *A. duodenale* larvae occasionally have a dormant phase in man, when development is arrested for up to 9 months. This dormant phase may explain apparent failures of treatment. Light hookworm infection is asymptomatic, but heavy infection may produce epigastric malaise and hypochromic anemia from chronic blood loss. *N. americanus* is estimated to cause its host to lose 0.03 ml blood per day, and *A. duodenale* 0.26 ml. Marked blood losses may produce hypoproteinemia. Diagnosis is made by the demonstration of eggs in the stools; the species of hookworms cannot be differentiated on this basis, however. Species identification requires the microscopic examination of adult worms recovered after purging, but this is rarely of clinical importance.

Stools should be either examined fresh or kept refrigerated if examination has to be delayed, because eggs may hatch in 24 to 48 hours under optimal conditions of warmth, and the larvae may be confused with strongyloides larvae by unexperienced microscopists.

Strongyloides stercoralis. This roundworm is endemic in tropical and subtropical areas. In addition to the percutaneous cycle, a complete biologic cycle may occur in the soil, including maturation and the laying of eggs without an animal host. Strongyloidiasis is usually benign or asymptomatic. Rarely, the penetration of the larvae produces a linear, papular rash with rapid progression known as cutaneous larva migrans. The tissue-migratory phase of the parasite's life cycle often goes unnoticed, but may produce respiratory symptoms and eosinophilia similar to those of ascariasis. The intestinal phase is asymptomatic in mild infection. Moderate infection produces abdominal pain, mainly epigastric, diarrhea, and sometimes vomiting. In some individuals, larvae mature in the intestine and produce autoinfection by penetrating the perianal skin. In a few patients, autoinfection increases the number of worms and causes the severe form of the disease, with bloody and mucous diarrhea, malabsorption, and hypoproteinemia. In immunocompromised hosts, internal autoinfection may occur. The larvae penetrate the mucosa, migrate to the tissues in large numbers, and cause shock and gram-negative bacteremia.

The diagnosis is generally made by the demonstration of larvae in the patient's stools on microscopic examination. Culture of a duodenal aspirate is a more sensitive means of detecting the parasite.

INTESTINAL TAPEWORMS

Fish Tapeworm. The fish tapeworm, *Diphyllobothrium latum*, is more common in Baltic Sea, in Scandinavia, and in the Great

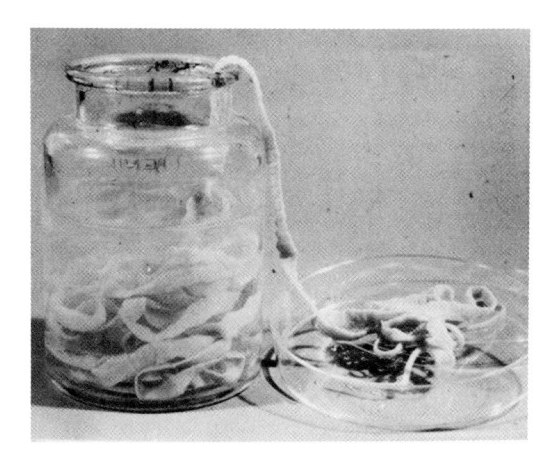

Fig. 18–8. Taenia saginata evacuated after treatment.

Lakes of North America. The intermediate hosts are copepods (minute crustaceans) and fish. The adult worm may measure 10 m in the human intestine. The infection may remain asymptomatic, or it may produce abdominal pain, loss of appetite, nausea, diarrhea, or weight loss. *D. latum* absorbs large quantities of B_{12} and interferes with the intestinal absorption of the vitamin by unbinding the B_{12}-intrinsic factor complex. Infection therefore may result in a pernicious anemia syndrome with megaloblastic anemia, glossitis, numbness, and other neurologic changes.

Beef and Pork Tapeworms. The beef tapeworm, *Taenia saginata* (Fig. 18–8), occurs frequently in Mexico, South America, West Africa, and Moslem countries. The pork tapeworm, *Taenia solium*, is common in Latin America, Western Europe, China, Pakistan, and India. Although these infections are not usually symptomatic, they may produce abdominal cramps or weight loss. The most common complaint is the passage of worm segments through the patient's anus.

Occasionally, man becomes an accidental intermediate host of *Taenia solium* when mature ova are ingested. The eggs hatch in the duodenum, and the larvae penetrate the intestinal wall and migrate into tissues in which an inflammatory reaction occurs. The larvae then encyst to become cysticerci. After about a decade, a cysticercus becomes calcified.

Clinical manifestations reflect the affected organ. When a cysticercus is present in the patient's brain, serious manifestations, such as seizures or symptoms of a space-occupying lesion, may occur.

A proglottid, or tapeworm segment, is a flat, motile worm, 0.5 cm wide by 1 or 2 cm long, roughly square, which passes through the host's anus (see Fig. 18–5). Sometimes, several segments are joined (up to 30 cm). Proglottid expulsion, common with *Taenia solium* and *T. saginata* infection, may also occur with *Diphyllobothrium latum* infection, especially after a purge. A *D. latum* proglottid is broader than long and has no lateral genital pore. Taenia proglottids have a genital pore on a lateral edge and are longer than larger. *T. saginata* has 15 to 20 uterine segments on each side, *T. solium* 7 to 13. These uterine segments are best seen when stained. If no segment is evacuated, diagnosis is made by microscopic stool examination, but the eggs of the species of taenia are similar.

Dwarf Tapeworm. *Hymenolepis nana* has a cosmopolitan distribution and requires no intermediate host. The ova hatch in the host's intestine, and the larva penetrates a villus and develops into a cyst that eventually breaks into the intestine, where the parasite matures into an adult 25 to 40 mm long.

Light infection is asymptomatic, whereas heavy infection can produce mucosal irritation with abdominal cramps and diarrhea. The diagnosis is made by the demonstration of typical ova in the patient's stool.

INTESTINAL FLUKES

Fasciolopsis buski. The large intestinal fluke, *Fasciolopsis buski*, is endemic in the Far East, particularly in China. The biologic cycle follows the type V pattern. Man becomes infected by eating raw, contaminated water chestnuts. The adult fluke, which measures 5 to 7.5 cm, attaches itself to the host's mucosa and produces local inflammation. The infection is either asymptomatic or is associated with abdominal pain and diarrhea. Heavy infection may lead to anorexia, nausea, malnutrition from vomiting, hypoproteinemia, edema, and even ascites. The diagnosis is made by stool examination, but ova may be mistaken for those of the liver fluke *Fasciola hepatica*.

Heterophyes heterophyes. This small intestinal fluke, 20 mm long, is endemic in Southeast Asia and in the Nile delta. Infection is acquired by the ingestion of raw, contaminated fish (type IV pattern with 2 intermediate hosts). Abdominal pain and diarrhea are common. Parasitic ova may be deposited in tissues and may be carried by the blood to the heart, the spinal cord, or the brain, to produce myocarditis or neurologic symptoms. Stool examination shows the characteristic eggs, which resemble those of the liver fluke *Opisthorchis (Clonorchis) sinensis*.

Metagonimus yokogawai. Infection with the smallest (0.7 mm) intestinal fluke, *Metagonimus yokogawai*, endemic in South East Asia, is usually asymptomatic. Heavy infection may produce diarrhea. Rarely, dissemination of eggs to various organs causes serious corresponding symptoms. The biologic cycle of this fluke is similar to that of *Heterophyes heterophyes*.

> **Objective 18–3.** Outline the treatment of intestinal helminthic infections.

Antihelminthic therapy is summarized in Table 18–3. Some of the drugs are still investigational or may not be readily available. In such instances, the practitioner should refer the patient to a tropical disease clinic for treatment or should communicate with either public health authorities* or the drug manufacturer.

On medical grounds, treatment of most asymptomatic cases of helminthiasis can be withheld, although people in western countries usually insist on treatment to relieve their psychologic stress.

---

*In the United States, one should contact the Parasitic Diseases Division, Center for Infectious Diseases, Center for Disease Control, Atlanta, Georgia 30333; telephone: (404) 329-3670

TREATMENT OF SPECIFIC INFECTIONS

Ascariasis. This disorder should be treated first in cases of multiple parasitic infections to avoid the migration of the worm and its possible complications. Asymptomatic ascaris infection may also require treatment to prevent such complications. Persons at high risk of ascaris infection and undergoing abdominal surgical procedures may be treated to prevent migration of worms into the surgical wound, even if the stool examination is negative; an infection with only male ascaris is possible and cannot be detected by stool examination. Biliary colic due to a wandering ascaris is treated by nasogastric suction and parenteral fluids or by endoscopic removal of the worm. Surgical intervention is indicated if medical treatment fails. Partial intestinal obstruction usually responds to conservative treatment, such as nasogastric suction, intravenous fluid administration, and repeated doses of piperazine citrate by nasogastric tube. Complete intestinal obstruction, however, requires prompt surgical intervention. The bolus of worms can often be dislodged by massage at laparotomy. If this maneuver is unsuccessful, then resection is preferred to enterostomy.

Pinworm Infection. The treatment of pinworm infection should include the patient's whole family and should be repeated in 2 to 4 weeks because of the prolonged viability of the ova, which are easily disseminated and may still be ingested after the initial dose of medication. Before the worms are fully mature, they are not as sensitive to therapy, and the rate of relapse is high; a second dose is usually needed. All members of the patient's family, even if asymptomatic, must be treated. The rate of transmission of the infection to parents and siblings is high. Even following treatment, enterobiasis may recur, mostly because of extrafamilial reinfection. When symptoms do recur, repeated treatments may be the only practical alternative. Various hygienic measures have been recommended to prevent reinfection, such as frequent hand washing, nail grooming, and a

Table 18–3. Treatment of Intestinal Helminthiasis

Recommended Treatment Regimens for Helminths

Roundworms	Mebendazole*	Pyrantel pamoate†	Others
Pinworm	100 mg (1 dose)	11 mg/kg, max. 1 g (1 dose)	Piperazine, 65 mg/kg (max. 2.5 g) for 7 days‡ Pyrivinium pamoate, 5 mg/kg (max. 250 mg)‡ N.B.: repeat in 2 weeks and treat all family members; take preventive measures
Ascaris lumbricoides	100 mg bid for 3 days	11 mg/kg, max. 1 g (1 dose)	Piperazine citrate, 75 mg/kg for 2 days
Hookworm	100 mg bid for 3 days	11 mg/kg, max. 1 g (1 dose)	Thiabendazole 25 mg/kg (max. 3 g/day) bid for 2 days for *Necator americanus*‡; treat anemia with iron
Trichuris	100 mg bid for 3 days	Not recommended	—
Strongyloides	Not recommended	Not recommended	Thiabendazole, 25 mg/kg bid for 2 days (max. 3 g/day)

Tapeworm	Niclosamide	Paromomycin	Other
Diphyllobothrium latum	4 tablets (2 g) 1 gm postoperatively then 1 gm in 1 hour	1g q15 min. for 4 doses	—
Taenia solium	1 gm postoperatively then 1 gm in 1 hour	1 g q15 min. for 4 doses	Quinacrine, 1 g orally or by nasoduodenal intubation, and a purgative given 3 to 4 hours after treatment
Taenia saginata	11–34 kg: 1 g; and > 34 kg: 1.5 g (child)	11 mg/kg (child)	—
Hymenolepsis nana	idem for 5 days	idem for 5–7 days‡	Praziquantel, 15–20 mg/kg (1 dose)

Flukes	Praziquantel	Tetrachloroethylene§	Other
Fasciolopsis buski *Heterophyes heterophyes* *Metagonimus yokogawai*	25 mg/kg tid for 1 day	0.1–0.12 ml/kg (max. 5 ml)	—

*Not recommended for children below 2 years of age, may produce diarrhea and abdominal cramps.
†Not recommended for children below 1 year of age.
‡Alternate treatment.
§Toxic drug, not recommended for children.

daily morning shower to dislodge parasitic eggs. The efficacy of these preventive measures, however, is uncertain.

Hookworm Infection. In well-nourished patients living in satisfactory sanitary conditions, light hookworm infection does not present any risk of transmission and does not require treatment. Heavy infection may require several courses of therapy to achieve a complete cure. That *Ancylostoma duodenale* larvae in their dormant state are not eradicated by treatment may explain apparent therapeutic failures. Patients with anemia require iron therapy.

Strongyloidiasis. This infection, even if asymptomatic, should always be treated in hospitalized patients and in those with underlying diseases because of potential autoinfection and hyperinfection in the event of impaired host resistance. Patients with moderate or severe forms of the disease should have weekly stool examinations for 4 weeks after treatment, to detect recurrence due to autoinfection. Patients with severe forms of the disease may require antibiotic treatment for concomitant bacteremia.

Tapeworm Infections. Niclosamide and paromomycin are currently preferred for the treatment of tapeworm infections. Although effective, quinacrine therapy is more cumbersome because it may require nasoduodenal intubation to instill the 1-g dose and to minimize nausea and vomiting. It also requires a purge to ensure rapid expulsion of the worm.

Treatment of *Taenia solium*, the pork tapeworm, should be followed in 3 to 4 hours by a purge because of the theoretic risk of cysticercosis, which is hatching of the eggs in the gut, penetration of larvae through the intestinal mucosa, and dissemination through the body.

In addition to the vermifuge, some patients with *Diphyllobothrium latum* infection need vitamin B_{12} and folic acid supplementation.

Dwarf tapeworm infection requires at least 5 days of treatment because the drug is ineffective against the larval stage (plerocercoid larva) of the worm, which develops for 4 days within the host's intestinal wall.

SUGGESTED READINGS

Anonymous: Drugs for parasitic infections. Med. Lett. Drugs Ther., 24:5, 1982.

Hunter, G.W., Swartzwelder, J.D., and Clyde, D.F. (eds.): Tropical Medicine. Philadelphia, W.B. Saunders, 1976.

Marsden, P.D.: Intestinal parasites. Clin. Gastroenterol., 7:1, 1978.

Schönfeld, H.: Antiparasitic chemotherapy. Antibiot. Chemother., 30:1, 1981.

Scowden, E.B., Schaffner, W., and Stone, W.J.: Overwhelming Strongyloidiasis. An unappreciated opportunistic infection. Medicine, 57:527, 1978.

Warren, R.E.: Intestinal nematodes. Med. Clin. North Am., 1:984, 1981.

Warren, K.S., and Mahmound, A.F. (eds.): Geographic Medicine for the Practitioner. Chicago, University of Chicago Press, 1978.

CHAPTER 19

Abdominal Infections

M.G. Bergeron

Intra-abdominal infections originate in the digestive or genital tract and are associated with certain specific illnesses and frequently follow trauma or surgical procedures. The vaginal and intestinal bacterial floras form a complex and diversified combination of anaerobic and aerobic bacteria that, together, induce the infectious process. This microbial synergy is selective and involves numerous bacteria such as *Escherichia coli, Streptococcus faecalis, Bacteroides fragilis,* and *Fusobacterium varium*. This complex flora is responsible for many clinical syndromes. Atypical clinical manifestations and the multiple possible localizations make the diagnosis difficult. Nevertheless, new diagnostic techniques, including isotope scanning, computerized tomography, and sonography, help one to localize visceral or intra-abdominal abscesses that would otherwise go undetected. The usual sites for these infections are the peritoneum, the retroperitoneum, and the abdominal viscera. Treatment consists of upsetting the microbial synergistic process by surgical intervention and appropriate antibiotic therapy.

> Objective 19–1. Recognize and locate intra-abdominal infection in a patient who has not undergone a surgical procedure.

A broad clinical spectrum of intra-abdominal infections exists in apparently normal persons who have not recently undergone a surgical procedure. Patients of all ages and with a widely variable picture of abdominal pains may call upon physicians, either for consultation or as an emergency. Furthermore, the same disorder can manifest itself in different guises. In general, the diagnosis of an intra-abdominal suppurative process should be considered in a patient in pain, with shaking chills accompanied by fever, and with a toxic appearance. Laboratory tests are of little use, except to detect leukocytosis or an elevated sedimentation rate. Locating the infection is an essential but often difficult step in formulating a precise therapeutic approach.

SECONDARY PERITONITIS

Secondary peritonitis, or inflammation of the peritoneum induced by the entrance of bacteria, intestinal fluids, such as gastric juice, pancreatic secretions, and bile, or blood into the peritoneal cavity, is characterized by fever, shaking chills, and abdominal pain, as well as by nausea and vomiting associated with an intense thirst. Peritoneal inflammation is responsible for the mobilization of fluids into the abdomen; this process leads to edema of the intestinal walls and paralytic ileus. During the physical examination, the absence of normal peristalsis is noted, along with abdominal distension and increased tympanic resonance. The abdominal wall is rigid and painful on palpation. Exquisite rebound tenderness is found on palpation and on rectal examination. The plain films of the abdomen may reveal free air in the peritoneal cavity and evidence of peritoneal fluid, extensive distension of the small bowel, and increased space between the loops of the bowel. The leukocyte count is usually more than 20,000/mm^3, with an increased percentage of polymorphonuclear leukocytes and band forms.

Patients suffering from bacterial peritonitis sometimes have a septicemia capable of inducing septic shock. The peritonitis is, generally, a consequence of the spread of a localized infection such as appendicitis, diverticulitis, or cholecystitis, but exceptions exist, such as "spontaneous peritonitis" or peritonitis associated with peritoneal dialysis.

SPONTANEOUS PERITONITIS

Also called "primary" because the original focus of infection usually cannot be demonstrated, spontaneous peritonitis is not an entirely specific entity and is rare. It occurs most frequently in children with the nephrotic syndrome or in adults with advanced cirrhosis and ascites, other hepatic diseases, or active systemic lupus erythematosus.

In the child, the onset of abdominal pain is dramatic and may simulate appendicitis. Pneumococcus, group A streptococci, enteric bacteria, and staphylococci appear to be, in order of importance, the most frequent organisms associated with this type of infection. The adult with cirrhosis and ascites often has modified, almost muted, symptoms, and fever may be the only clinical sign.

Escherichia coli, other enteric bacilli, group A and B streptococci, and some anaerobic bacteria are the most frequent pathogens. Where do these organisms come from, and how do they migrate into the peritoneum? In hepatic insufficiency, the antibacterial filtering functions of the liver and spleen may become less efficient. Once the reticuloendothelial system of the liver and spleen, responsible for eliminating portal and systemic microorganisms, is impaired, microorganisms, especially from the intestine, may disseminate throughout the body and may therefore be found in ascitic fluid. It seems equally probable that the hypertonicity of the ascites may enhance the passage of enteric bacteria across the intestinal mucosa and may thus favor the invasion of the peritoneum. Other organisms, such as *Neisseria gonorrhoeae* producing a perihepatitis, have as their portal of entry the female genital tract rendered more susceptible by menstruation or by localized infection. Tuberculosis can also produce spontaneous peritonitis both in alcoholics, in whom it seems to be the reactivation of a latent tubercule, and in women of child-bearing age, in whom it may spread from a tuberculous ovary, probably originally seeded years before by hematogenous spread.

APPENDICITIS

Appendicitis is the most frequent cause of acute intra-abdominal suppuration. Each year, more than 200,000 cases occur in the United States, 60,000 in England, and 20,000 in Canada. The population most affected is between 12 and 25 years of age.

Obstruction of the lumen of the appendix by a fecalith is thought to be responsible for distension and the resulting accumulation of intestinal contents. The patient complains first of umbilical or lower epigastric pain and later of pain localized two-thirds of the distance between the umbilicus and the right anterior iliac crest. Physical examination reveals tenderness and hyperesthesia, as well as guarding on palpation of the abdomen. The appendix becomes ischemic and can necrose, entirely or partially, leading to abscess formation. Anorexia, nausea, and vomiting complete the clinical picture. Rupture of the appendix may relieve the pain initially, but in the hours that follow, localized or even generalized peritonitis develops.

In individuals with a retrocecal appendix, the clinical diagnosis of appendicitis can be difficult. These patients may have a vague, unlocalized, abdominal pain, aggravated by hyperextension of the right leg, probably following inflammation of the right psoas muscle sheath. Palpation of right pararectal area provokes intense pain. This area may bulge inward eventually, and the abscess may seek to drain through the rectum. Signs of peritonitis are usually lacking.

Laboratory tests and routine roentgenograms are generally of little use, except for the infrequent detection of a lateral compression of the sigmoid colon by the appendiceal abscess. Even though the clinical manifestations of acute appendicitis are well characterized, several pathologic studies have demonstrated that 25% of surgically removed appendices are normal. It is therefore necessary to consider each case carefully, to rule out the following, for example: in a woman, pelvic inflammatory disease; in a child, mesenteric adenitis; and in patients over 50 years of age, diverticulitis.

DIVERTICULITIS

Diverticulitis usually occurs in the left colon and the sigmoid colon in Europeans and in patients of European descent and in the ascending colon in Orientals; in older patients, it causes intermittent abdominal pain accentuated by defecation. In general, patients with diverticulitis complain of constipation. An increase in interdiverticular pressure can produce local necrosis and perforation of the intestinal lining and may give rise to numerous small abscesses limited to the paradiverticular area. The erosion of blood vessels in the mucosa is responsible for intestinal bleeding. To avoid perforation of the colon, the diagnostic barium enema should be performed under low pressure. This procedure makes it possible to visualize the fistulas and pericolonic abscesses. A lack of intestinal motility and a narrowing of the lumen or sacculations of the intestinal wall may be demonstrated by sigmoidoscopy or colonoscopy. Sonography and gallium scanning are occasionally useful in detecting these paracolonic abscesses.

ACUTE CHOLECYSTITIS

One should always consider acute cholecystitis in the differential diagnosis of intraabdominal infections. In more than 90% of cases, a stone is responsible for an obstruction of the cystic duct. The gallbladder is dilated, and local circulation is compromised. The stagnation of bile leads to a proliferation of bacteria normally absent in the bladder. To relieve the obstruction, which could lead to empyema or necrosis of the bladder wall, more than 25% of these patients must undergo emergency operations. If the common duct is obstructed, the infection may produce an ascending cholangitis. Rarely, cholecystitis is complicated by pylephlebitis, which is phlebitis of the portal vein that may also be secondary to appendicitis, diverticulitis, or other types of intestinal diseases such as granulomatous or ulcerative colitis.

The physician should suspect the diagnosis of acute cholecystitis when a patient has severe pain, localized to the right upper quadrant and radiating to the tip of the right shoulder, accompanied by nausea, vomiting, fever, and a mild jaundice, as well as guarding over the gallbladder. The gallbladder may be palpable. The localization of pain to the epigastrium and the presence of jaundice suggest a common duct obstruction. In older patients, it is necessary to maintain a high degree of clinical suspicion because fever may be the only symptom of acute cholecystitis. Laboratory tests most often show variable leukocytosis, mild hyperbilirubinemia, and an elevation of the patient's alkaline phosphatase level. If the obstruction persists, or if the infection spreads through the biliary tree, transaminase and hepatic enzyme levels may become elevated.

Oral cholecystography is of little value in the investigation of acute cholecystitis. Occasionally, intravenous cholangiography is helpful, but it does not usually permit adequate visualization of the bile ducts. Sonography of the gallbladder, a useful noninvasive procedure, is increasingly employed to confirm the presence of gallstones, abscesses of the bladder, or dilation of the biliary tree following an obstruction. Blood cultures are positive in more than 50% of patients with cholangitis. The clinical signs of pylephlebitis are identical to those of cholangitis; however, the results of hepatic biochemical tests, such as that for transaminase levels, are generally normal. Portal venograms can help to confirm the diagnosis. Pylephlebitis may be complicated by an intrahepatic abscess.

HEPATIC ABSCESSES

These abscesses can be either bacterial, amebic, or hydatid. The absence of systemic manifestations in a proper epidemiologic context (endemic area) can suggest the diagnosis of echinococcosis. The serologic study, the Casoni skin test, and the presence of a slight eosinophilia should suggest the diagnosis of a hydatid cyst. Roentgenograms of the abdomen may show calcification of the cyst wall.

It is, however, more difficult to differentiate bacterial from amebic infection of the liver, inasmuch as, on rare occasions, an amebic abscess is complicated by an aerobic or anaerobic bacterial infection. The evolution of an amebic abscess often occurs over several months, and the patient's presenting symptoms are night sweats, fever, and loss of weight. Sometimes, the clinical manifestations are more acute and imitate cholecystitis or acute pancreatitis. The diagnosis is all the more difficult because, in more than a third of patients, diarrhea is absent, and examination of the stools does not reveal *Entamoeba histolytica*. The physical examination is usually normal, but intercostal pain in the lower thoracic area can be a useful clinical sign. A history of a recent trip to areas where amebiasis is endemic is sometimes helpful. Amebiasis, however, can be acquired in almost all parts of the world. The patient's alkaline phosphatase level may be slightly elevated, and the liver scan (Fig. 19–1) or the hepatic sonogram confirms the presence of a large, solitary abscess, often localized to the posterior portion of the right lobe of the liver. The serologic test for amebas is positive in more than 90% of patients. Amebic trophozoites or cysts are rarely found in the pus aspirated by needle or drained on operation. This pus is, typically, odorless, thick, and brownish in color. It may resemble anchovy paste in color and consistency, but it is sometimes a clear yellow color. The amebas can usually be found within the wall of the abscess (for more details on amebiasis, see Objective 20–6).

Bacterial liver abscesses can either be single or multiple. Although multiple abscesses are accompanied by fever, they are generally less symptomatic and are microscopic in size. These abscesses occur in the course of septicemias with staphylococci and streptococci or are associated with biliary obstruction. Most solitary hepatic abscesses are associated with intra-abdominal or biliary infections. Blunt trauma with hematoma or penetrating trauma can also be associated with hepatic abscesses. The clinical manifestations of a sol-

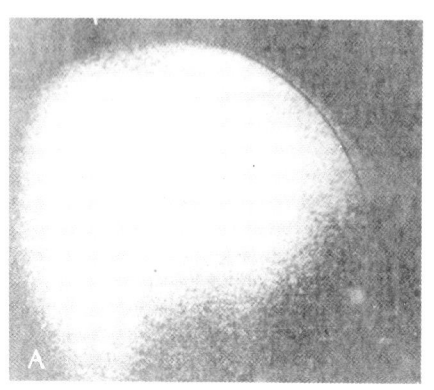

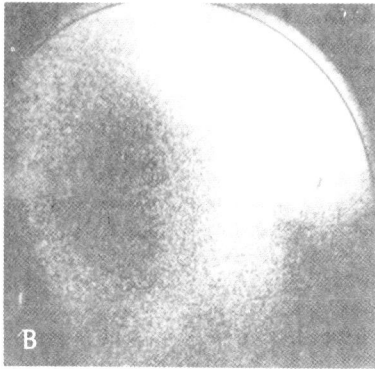

Fig. 19–1. *A*, Normal liver scan; *B*, hepatic abscess.

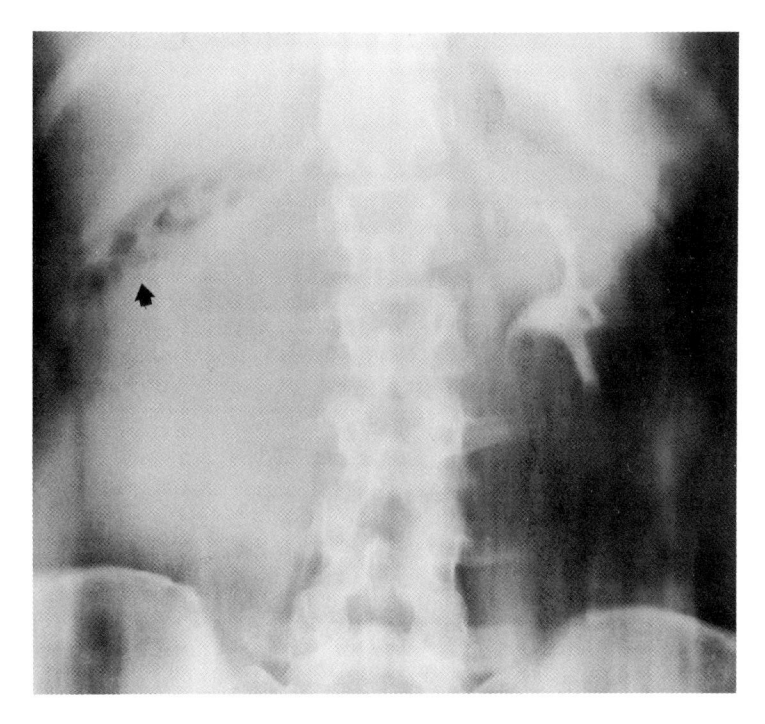

Fig. 19–2. Subhepatic abscess; note the gas bullae (arrow).

itary bacterial abscess are, as a rule, more acute than those of amebiasis. Fever is nearly always present and is accompanied by nausea, vomiting, systemic symptoms, hepatomegaly, and pain on hepatic percussion. A right pleural effusion is classically said to be present, but localizing signs are not always seen. Leukocytosis often occurs, and the alkaline phosphatase level is elevated. The sonogram, the hepatic isotope scan, and the abdominal CT scan are most useful in confirming the diagnosis of bacterial hepatic abscess. Angiographic studies may also be helpful.

PERIRECTAL ABSCESSES

Perirectal abscesses may be either superficial or deep. Superficial abscesses are diagnosed easily, both by severe anal pain on defecation and by a palpable and visible mass. Such an abscess is commonly seen with an anal fissure, perianal folliculitis, and sclerosing hemorrhoids.

Deep ischiorectal abscesses are usually more difficult to detect and are seen in diabetics, alcoholics, and in patients with leukemia. The abscess may precede or may accompany such diseases as ulcerative colitis or regional enteritis. Fever is often the only initial manifestation of the disease. The local signs may include severe rectal pain, diarrhea, perirectal swelling noted on palpation of the rectal mucosa, and much later, swelling of the perineum or groin. Occasionally, the presence of a localized abscess on the upper portion of the rectum is accompanied by symptoms of urinary bladder compression or of urinary retention and may suggest a urinary tract infection.

Excruciating pain can be elicited sometimes on rectal examination by pressing the examiner's finger toward the coccyx. On proctoscopy, a swelling or a narrowing of the rectal ampulla may be observed. In patients with a relapsing rectal abscess, the investigation should include colonoscopy, barium enema, and tests of intestinal transit time, to rule out an underlying intestinal disorder.

PELVIC INFECTIONS

In contrast to intra-abdominal infections that nearly always necessitate surgical intervention, many pelvic infections will respond to medical treatment and do not require surgical treatment. It is sometimes difficult, however, to separate these infections completely from upper abdominal infections, and the gynecologic exam should be an integral part of the general examination of a woman with abdominal pain. Culdoscopy and peritoneoscopy are sometimes necessary to confirm the localization of an abscess in the female genital tract, particularly because some infections are complicated by extrapelvic spread in the form of peritonitis or perihepatitis. As in other intra-abdominal infections, mixed aerobic and anaerobic floras, both gram-negative and gram-positive, can produce the disease, especially in patients with a history of chronic infection. Nevertheless, these infections are also frequently associated with sexually transmitted organisms, in particular, gonococci and chlamydia. Indeed, gonococci and chlamydia are probably the microbial initiators of damage to the fallopian tubes, damage that later permits progressive implantation of a normal flora from the vagina into an environment whose natural defenses have been neutralized by previous infection; thus, the development of recurrent salpingitis is favored.

> Objective 19–2. Recognize and locate intra-abdominal sepsis following a surgical procedure.

In contrast to the clear clinical picture discussed previously, the symptoms and signs of postoperative abdominal infections may be nonspecific and thereby difficult to evaluate. Fever is sometimes the only symptom. If this fever occurs 24 to 48 hours after a surgical procedure, it is necessary first to rule out a hematoma or an infection of the wound site, atelectasia, transfusion reactions, or anesthesia reactions. If a local wound infection cannot be found, the persistence of a spiking fever should lead one to search for a possible abscess of the abdominal wall or abdomen.

INTRA-ABDOMINAL ABSCESSES

Superficial abscesses are generally easy to detect because they can drain spontaneously or may produce telltale erythema around the surgical wound. Deep intra-abdominal abscesses are more difficult to detect. They may localize in the peritoneum, in the retroperitoneum, or in the viscera.

The majority of patients with postoperative intra-abdominal abscesses have spiking fevers, abdominal or back pain, general debilitation, and weight loss. Some laboratory tests (discussed later in this chapter) can be of assistance, but indeed, the patient's medical history and repeated physical examinations are often the only criteria by which the clinician arrives at a precise diagnosis.

Intra-abdominal and retroperitoneal abscesses are not necessarily found close to the source of the infection (Table 19–1). Their clinical manifestations are often perplexing. The history of a recent abdominal operation and the appearance of fever and chills several days after the procedure should cause the physician to suspect the diagnosis. A palpable mass on examination of the abdomen, with a tender mass felt on rectal or pelvic examination, should make one suspect a cecal, sigmoid, or pelvic abscess. By contrast, subdiaphragmatic and retroperitoneal abscesses are nearly impossible to identify on physical examination. Tenderness to percussion over the hepatic or renal area should suggest the presence of an abscess, but these findings are nonspecific.

Even in the absence of these signs, isotope scanning, computerized tomography, and sonography in these areas are more useful than the physical examination in locating an abscess. In addition, the following findings on the chest roentgenogram indicate a right subdiaphragmatic infection: abnormal elevation of the right diaphragm and less mobility on fluoroscopy, pleural effusion, widening of the costochondral angle, and obliteration of the costophrenic angle. This location can be further suggested by an abnormally large space between the liver and the lung on a

Table 19–1. Intra-Abdominal Abscesses

Localization	Most Frequent Source
Intraperitoneal	
Right lower quadrant	Appendicitis
Left lower quadrant	Diverticulitis
Pelvic area	Gynecologic infections and surgical procedures
Subdiaphragmatic	Perforated peptic ulcer
Subhepatic	Cholecystitis, pancreatitis
Middle abdominal	Surgical procedures of the stomach, duodenum, and biliary tract
Morison's pouch	
Peri-intestinal	Generalized peritonitis
Generalized ("horseshoe" distribution)	Fusion of several abscesses
Retroperitoneal	
Anterior	Pancreatitis, renal operations, trauma
Paravertebral	Osteomyelitis of vertebral bodies
Visceral	
Splenic	Extraintestinal septicemia
Renal and perirenal	Pyelonephritis or staphylococcal septicemia
Hepatic	Biliary surgical procedures, septicemias, intra-abdominal infections
Pancreatic	Acute pancreatitis and surgical manipulation
Ovarian	Salpingitis and pelvic surgical procedures

liver and lung scan. A simple roentgenogram of the abdomen may show the presence of gas under the diaphragm (evidence of perforation of hollow viscera) or, rarely, an air-fluid level within the abscess. Roentgenographic evidence of displacement of the liver, spleen, or intestines suggests their compression by a collection of pus. A gallium scan as well as a sonogram can help to outline an intra- or retroperitoneal abscess; however, the interpretation of these studies is difficult following surgical manipulation, and a CT scan is often the procedure of choice.

A pelvic or other abscess may obstruct the colon by compression. Such masses impinging upon the colon are detectable by barium enema (Fig. 19–3). If these abscesses descend inferiorly into the pelvis, a needle puncture, anterior from the rectum or posterior from the vagina, will permit localization as well as culture of the abscess.

Most visceral abscesses, with the exception of splenic abscesses, are secondary to intra-abdominal suppurative processes. Fever is nearly always present, and more than half these patients experience pain on percussion over the affected organ, whether liver, spleen, or kidney. A hepatic friction rub is sometimes heard on auscultation when a liver abscess is present. Pain of hepatic or splenic origin radiates superiorly to the patient's shoulders, whereas pain from renal abscesses radiates inferiorly to the hip, thigh, or even the knee. Two-thirds of patients with renal abscess do not have symptoms of a urinary tract infection, despite the presence of pyuria or concentrations of more than 10^5 bacteria/ml in the urine. Lower abdominal and pelvic abscesses are often palpable.

Perinephric and pancreatic abscesses are occasionally perceived on physical examination, but those of the liver and spleen are seldom felt. An epigastric mass in an afebrile patient suggests a pancreatic cyst. With an intra-abdominal abscess, the patient's white blood cell count is elevated to 15,000/ml, and blood cultures are positive in about 30% of cases. The alkaline phosphatase level is elevated in the presence of a hepatic abscess, whereas the amylase level is usually normal in patients with a pancreatic abscess. Gas bubbles, with or without an air-fluid level (Fig. 19–2), are more characteristic of pancreatic or hepatic abscess than of abscesses of other viscera. The isotope scan and the computerized tomograph are useful in detecting interhepatic and splenic abscesses; sonography is used increasingly to visualize those in

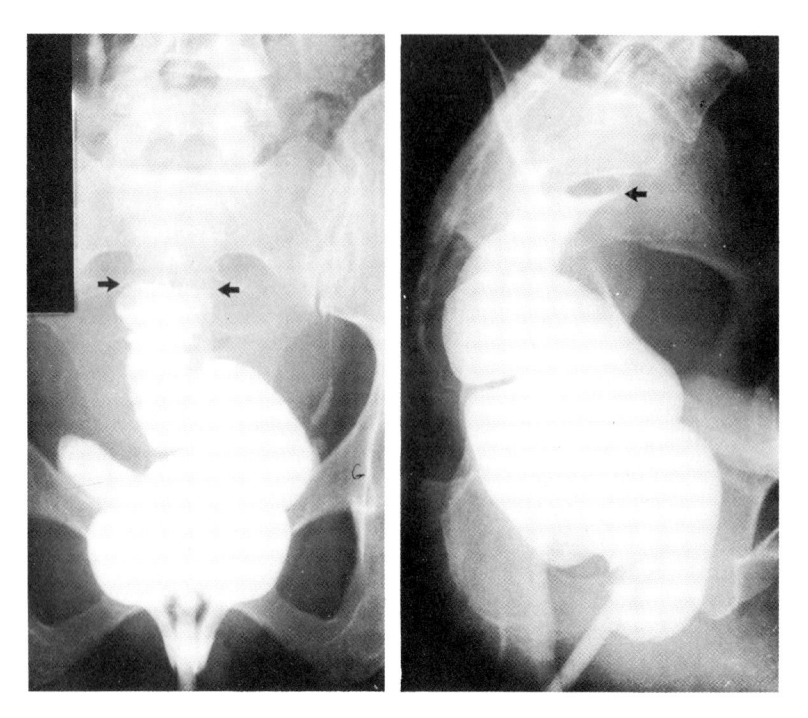

Fig. 19-3. Obstruction of the left colon (arrows) by an abscess; barium enema.

the pancreas and kidney. Arteriography is rarely used now to locate a hepatic abscess that has escaped detection by other techniques.

WOUND INFECTIONS

About 7% of individuals undergoing a surgical procedure develop infections of the wound site. The incidence is about 10% after clean-contaminated surgical procedures, such as excision of a tumor of the colon, and higher than 20% after dirty-contaminated procedures, such as traumatic perforation of the colon. The age of the patient, the duration of the surgical procedure, and the consecutive use of common operating rooms increase the frequency of wound infections. These infections prolong the patient's hospital stay threefold and have a high cost, both in terms of pain and suffering as well as in monetary terms. Of all postoperative infections, for example, peritonitis, abscess, septicemia, and urinary infections, wound infections are by far the most frequent.

Wound abscesses must be distinguished from superficial and deep cellulitis. Fever and drainage from suture sites suggest a wound abscess. Superficial cellulitis due to group A streptococci is distinguishable from that due to staphylococci by its raised erythematous area with a clearly defined border. In the absence of pus, a culture can be taken by aspirating the wound site after injection of 1 ml sterile saline solution without preservative into the advancing edge of the lesion. The different types of deep cellulitis are described in Table 19-2. These serious infections, often insidious in onset, are characterized by local edema without marked superficial inflammation, the presence of gas in the tissues, a putrid odor, and fistula formation because anaerobes are frequently present.

In contrast to the superficial infections that respond to appropriate antibiotics, infections involving mixed aerobes and anaerobes must be drained surgically. These severe infections, requiring an immediate response by the physician, occur mainly after penetrating trauma or abdominal surgical procedures,

Table 19–2. **Deep Cellulitis**

	Necrotizing Fasciitis (acute streptococcal gangrene)	Myositis due to Anaerobic Streptococci	Anaerobic Gas Producing Cellulitis	Myonecrosis due to Clostridium (Gas Gangrene)	Synergistic Necrotizing Cellulitis	Synergistic Progressive Bacterial Gangrene (of Meleney)	Chronic Necrotizing Ulceration
Origin	Aerobes: streptococci, *Staphylococcus aureus*, coliforms; anaerobes: peptostreptococci, bacteroides, fusobacteria	Peptostreptococci	Bacteroides; peptostreptococci; clostridium and similar coliforms (in hyperglycemia)	*Clostridium perfringens; C. novyi; C. septicum*	Coliforms; peptostreptococci; bacteroides	Microaerophilic streptococci; *Staphylococcus aureus*	Anaerobic streptococci; *Staphylococcus aureus*
Clinical Signs							
Toxicity	High	High	Low	Extremely high	Extremely high	High	None
Pain	Moderate	Intense	Moderate	Extremely intense	Extremely intense	Moderate	None
Skin appearance	Edematous, Erythematous	Edematous, copper-colored	Normal	Edematous, taut	Edematous, erythematous	Ulcerated, erythematous	Chronically ulcerated
Exudate	Serosanguineous	Seropurulent	None	Blackish serosanguineous	Purulent (dishwater appearance)	Seropurulent	Purulent
Gas	Little or none	Little	Much	Much if extension	Little (25%)	None	None
Tissues invaded	Fascial sheaths, skin	Muscles, skin	Skin, subcutaneous tissues	Muscle, fascia, skin	Muscle, skin	Skin, fascia	Skin
Mortality Rate	High	High	High	High	Very high	High	None
Treatment							
Surgical	Tension release of fascial spaces, drainage (primary)	Excision of necrotic tissue, drainage	Excision and exposure of tissue, drainage	Excision, amputation (Hyperbaric O₂ ?)	Excision of tissues, amputation	Excision, grafting	Excision, grafting
Antibiotic	Penicillin plus clindamycin plus chloramphenicol plus or cefoxitin	Penicillin G (first choice); clindamycin (second choice); cefoxitin	Penicillin G (first choice); clindamycin (second choice); cefoxitin (if coliforms present, choose cefoxitin)	Penicillin G (first choice); chloramphenicol	Clindamycin and aminoglycosides or cefoxitin	Penicillinase-resistant penicillin or clindamycin	Penicillin or cephalosporin

particularly in individuals suffering from diabetes or vascular insufficiency.

> **Objective 19–3. Confirm the presence of anaerobic bacteria in an abdominal abscess.**

Two groups of anaerobic bacteria are recognized: toxigenic anaerobes, represented by the genus clostridium, of which different species produce botulism, tetanus, and pseudomembranous colitis, and nontoxigenic anaerobes, which are more relevant to this discussion. Nontoxigenic anaerobes produce local or systemic infections involving one or more organisms. *Bacteroides fragilis, B. melaninogenicus,* the fusobacteria, and the anaerobic cocci are anaerobes most often implicated in abdominal suppurative infections.

Whichever type of infection is involved, the clinician can anticipate the presence of anaerobes by evidence of pus with a fetid odor and a dirty brown, black, or gray color, the appearance of gas within the tissues (although this can also be due to aerobic or facultative gram-negative bacilli), or the formation of abscesses (Table 19–5).

IDENTIFICATION OF ANAEROBIC BACTERIA

To identify these anaerobes, specialized culture techniques must be used. The simplest method is to use sterile glass tubes devoid of oxygen and containing carbon dioxide or nitrogen for the transport of swabs from wound specimens to the microbiology laboratory. These tubes may contain prereduced peptone broth with an indicator that turns red in the presence of oxygen. Small rubber-stoppered vials containing a nitrogen atmosphere and a solid agar, for instance Anaport, are available commercially.

In the absence of proper transport containers, the pus from an abscess can be aspirated directly into a syringe, from which all air bubbles are expelled. Further contact with oxygen is avoided by sealing the needle with a rubber stopper for transport to the laboratory. Some bacteria, such as the Bacteroides and the fusobacteria, can tolerate up to 6% oxygen, but *Clostridium haemolyticum* is killed on contact with even 0.5% oxygen.

The microscopic examination of a Gram stain of a sample of the exudate is an essential element in the bacteriologic diagnosis. Gram-

---

MICROBIAL ECOLOGY OF INTRA-ABDOMINAL ABSCESSES

With the exception of peritonitis due to *Streptococcus pneumoniae, Streptococcus pyogenes,* or *Escherichia coli,* which occur "spontaneously" in cases of cirrhosis or the nephrotic syndrome with ascites, and streptococci or *Staphylococcus aureus* invading the peritoneum from postoperative wound infections, abdominal suppuration is generally due to a mixed flora infection (Table 19–3). This flora consists of aerobic and anaerobic bacteria originating in the intestine or the female genital tract. Unless stasis and obstruction are present in the gastrointestinal tract, the stomach, duodenum, jejunum, and proximal ileum do not contain anaerobes in any great number.

The vagina and colon hold 10 and 1000 times more anaerobes than aerobes. At least 120 different species of bacteria are found in the colon, and 10 to 15 in the vagina. In spite of the imposing number of organisms, few bacteria are responsible for intra-abdominal infections (Table 19–4). *Escherichia coli* and *Bacteroides fragilis* seem particularly important because they are nearly always present, but they represent no more than 0.06 and 0.6%, respectively, of all bacteria found in stool.

More than 50% of splenic and pancreatic abscesses are caused by aerobic bacteria. In contrast, the other abdominal suppurations combine aerobic and anaerobic elements in more than 75% of cases. This rate is probably underestimated because recent studies suggest that, with better anaerobic techniques, these organisms would be isolated in nearly all such infections. Klebsiella, proteus, various clostridia, *Bacteroides melaninogenicus, Streptococcus faecalis,* peptococci, and peptostreptococci are the bacteria most often found, along with *Escherichia coli* and the encapsulated form of *Bacteroides fragilis.* Up to 12 species of bacteria can be found in intraperitoneal abscesses, whereas in perirenal abscesses, it is unusual to identify more than 2 or 3. One does not often find anaerobes in pure culture without an aerobic counterpart. Finally, acid-fast bacilli are, of course, responsible for renal and paraspinal infections and an occasional peritonitis or pelvic infection, and actinomycosis can produce abdominal symptoms, especially in the pelvis, where it is associated with intrauterine devices.

Table 19-3. Normal Flora of the Digestive Tract Below the Diaphragm

Sources	Number of Bacteria	Number of Species	Ratio between Anaerobes and Aerobes
Stomach	10^{3}*	0–5	No anaerobes present
Duodenum	10^3	1–5	No anaerobes present
Jejunum	10^4	1–5	No anaerobes present
Ileum	10^5	1–5	No anaerobes present
Terminal Ileum	10^8	25	1:1
Colon	10^{11}	110–120	1000:1
Vagina	10^9	10–15	10:1
Normal biliary tract	0	0	No bacteria present
Abnormal biliary tract (with stones)	10^1	2–5	1:3

*Number of bacteria per ml/g tissue.

Table 19-4. Bacteria Most Often Associated with Abdominal Infections

Aerobes (in order of importance)	Anaerobes (in order of importance)
Escherichia coli	Bacteroides fragilis
Streptococcus faecalis	Clostridia
Proteus	Bacteroides melaninogenicus
Klebsiella pneumoniae	
Staphylococcus aureus	Fusobacteria
Pseudomonas aeruginosa	Peptostreptococci
Alpha- and beta-hemolytic streptococci	Peptococci
Other streptococci	

MECHANISMS OF MICROBIAL SYNERGY

Several mechanisms are responsible for the induction of synergistic infections:

Mechanisms	Examples
1. Injury to the normal anatomic features of the host	Rheumatic valvular damage secondary to group A streptococcal infection leads to a risk that other organisms will engraft themselves on the valve and induce endocarditis
2. Change in flora	Colonization of the upper respiratory tract by pathogens (*Haemophilus influenzae*, staphylococci, group A streptococci) following a viral infection
3. Acquisition of pathogenicity by the merging of two microorganisms	Production of toxin by *Corynebacterium diphtheriae* when parasitized by a bacteriophage
4. Production of a favorable environment for the growth of pathogens	Reduction of oxygen tension and oxidation-reduction potential by aerobes, thus favoring the growth of anaerobes (intra-abdominal abscesses)

In mixed infections involving a limited number of microorganisms, some factors that permit potentiation of the pathogenicity of one organism by another are easily identifiable. For example, in Meleney's synergistic gangrene, the production of hyaluronidase by the staphylococcus allows the anaerobic streptococcus to invade the tissues. In necrotizing oral infections, the diphtheroids can furnish the vitamin K necessary for the growth of *Bacteroides melaninogenicus*, which plays an essential role in this type of infection.

In intra-abdominal infections, the mechanisms of synergy are most difficult to clarify, given the diversity and abundance of microbial partners. To understand better the relative roles of these different microbes in such infections, an animal model of intra-abdominal abscess has been created by implanting in the peritoneum of rats capsules containing stool with a mixed flora similar to that occurring in man. These investigations have demonstrated that the combination of *Bacteroides fragilis* or *Fusobacterium varium* with *Escherichia coli* or *Streptococcus faecalis* can produce intra-abdominal abscesses in this model. On the contrary, the two anaerobes alone never induced abscess formation. The mechanism of this synergy may be related to the reduction of oxygen tension and the oxidation-reduction potential by the aerobic component (*E. coli, S. faecalis*), creating an appropriate environment for the anaerobes (bacteroides, fusobacterium), which then grow to produce the abscess.

Table 19–5. Clues for Recognizing Anaerobic Infections

Predisposing factors
  Necrosis of tissue
  Underlying injury, such as cancer, irradiation, surgical manipulation, presence of foreign body, leakage of fecal material
  Contamination by material containing anaerobes
Clinical features
  Fetid odor
  Presence of gas in tissues (not pathognomonic, however; can be produced by *Escherichia coli,* klebsiella, or microaerophilic streptococci)
  Pelvic thrombophlebitis and emboli
  Multiple visceral abscesses
  Fever persisting despite antibiotic therapy
Microbiologic features
  Specific morphologic features on Gram stain
  Negative aerobic routine cultures, even when bacteria are seen on Gram stain

negative bacilli that have round ends, are pleomorphic, and are irregularly staining (Fig. 19–4) suggest the presence of bacteroides whereas bacilli with pointed ends may be fusobacteria. Thick, gram-positive rods suggest clostridia, and long chains of variably staining, sometimes indistinct cocci may be anaerobic streptococci.

Gram staining permits the physician to choose immediate therapy appropriate for the organism presumed to be present, and it serves as a method of quality control for the microbiologist; if the cultures remain sterile despite the presence of bacteria on the smear, then it is obvious that a problem exists in the method of taking cultures or of transporting them, or with the anaerobic culturing process itself. On arrival in the laboratory, the pus should be immediately seeded on blood agar, preferably deoxygenated, and on a gram-negative-selective medium such as MacConkey or eosin-methylene blue agar. In looking for anaerobic bacilli, a selective blood agar plate containing kanamycin, or gentamicin and vancomycin, which inhibits the other intestinal flora, can be used, as well as nonselective blood agar and a prereduced enrichment broth of cooked meat or thioglycolate. The previously deoxygenated plates should be seeded under carbon dioxide or nitrous at-

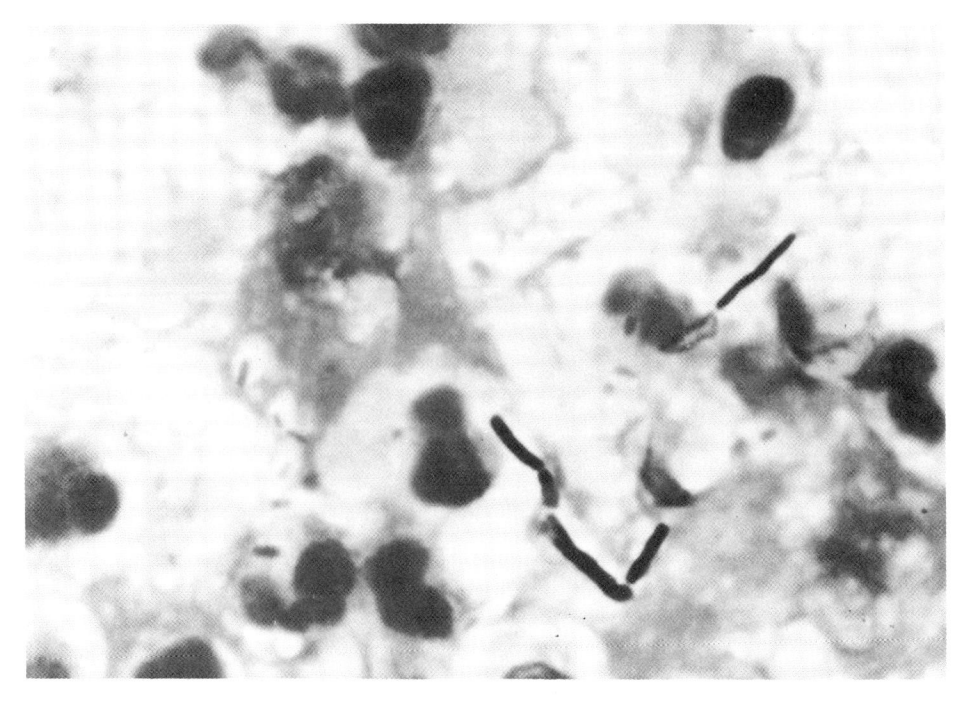

Fig. 19–4. Gram stain of bacterial pus showing *Bacteroides fragilis, Escherichia coli,* and clostridium. (Courtesy of Dr. J.C. Pechère.)

mosphere. If an anaerobic chamber is not available, the streaked plates must be placed as rapidly as possible into an anaerobic jar or incubator. The most common apparatus is the GasPak, which employs a cold catalyst to remove oxygen from the incubating jar and provides a source of carbon dioxide and water vapor.

After incubation under anaerobic conditions for 48 hours, colonies of bacteroides and fusobacteria, the morphologic features of which are given in Table 19–6, should be visible. If no growth is visible on the plates, the enrichment broth should be observed. If the Gram stain shows characteristic bacteria (Fig. 19–5), the positive broth should be reseeded on agar plates. Table 19–6 also indicates the biochemical reactions, the antibiotic susceptibility, and the properties on gas chromatography that permit the identification of anaerobic bacteria and their subspecies. A rapid fluorescent staining technique currently available for the identification of *Bacteroides fragilis* and *B. melaninogenicus* may become the most convenient method for identifying these organisms in a sample of pus, no matter how collected.

The antibiotic disc susceptibility test (Kirby-Bauer) is inadequate in this context and is not recommended for anaerobic isolates. Determination of the minimal inhibitory and bactericidal concentrations (MIC and MBC) is recommended to evaluate the antibiotic sensitivities of anaerobic bacteria.

Objective 19–4. Define appropriate therapy for patients with intra-abdominal infections.

With the exception of uncomplicated pelvic infections or primary or spontaneous peritonitis, which respond well to adequate antibiotic therapy, most patients with abscesses or suppurations of the abdomen, whether or not these persons have undergone a recent surgical procedure, require surgical or percutaneous catheter drainage, along with administration of the appropriate antibiotics. A surgical approach has the double advantage

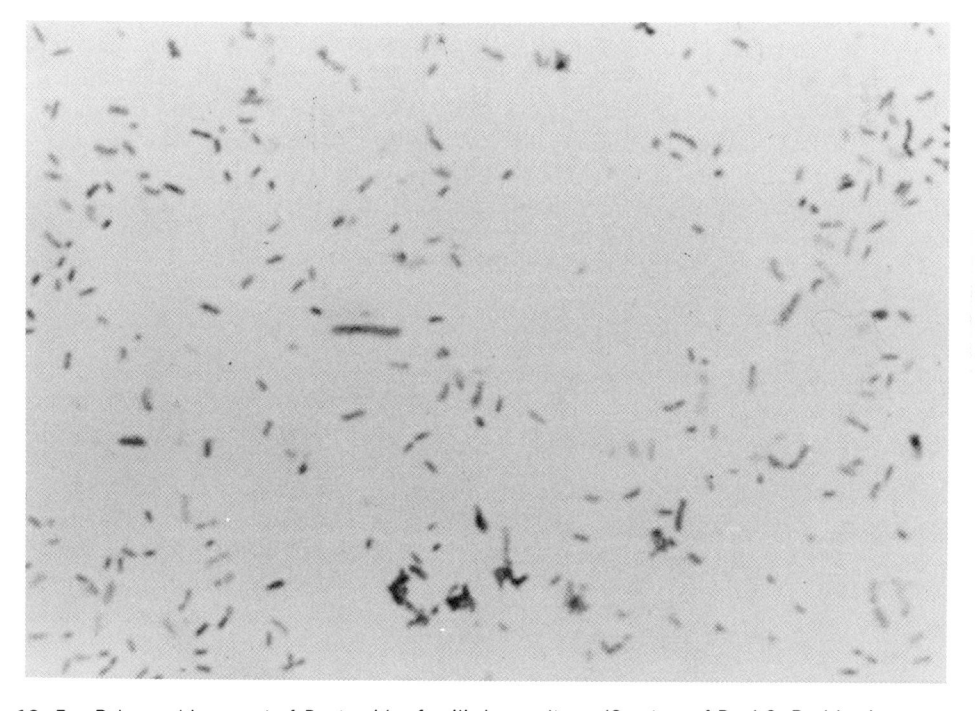

Fig. 19–5. Polymorphic aspect of *Bacteroides fragilis* in a culture. (Courtesy of Dr. J.C. Pechère.)

Table 19-6. Characteristic Features of Gram-Negative Anaerobic Bacilli

Features	Bacteroides fragilis	Bacteroides melaninogenicus	Fusobacteria
Morphologic and staining characteristics	Rods with rounded ends, pleomorphic; staining irregular	Bacillary and coccobacillary forms with rounded ends	Bacilli with pointed ends, pleomorphic
Colonial characteristics on blood agar	Grayish, transparent and convex	Black pigmented or with red fluorescence	Resembling fried eggs
Biochemical reaction	Indole-positive; catalase-positive	Indole-negative	Indole-positive; catalase-negative
Antibiotic susceptibility	Resistant to penicillin, to first-generation cephalosporins, and to aminoglycosides	Resistant to aminoglycosides; some produce beta lactamase	Resistant to aminoglycosides
Production of volatile acids (detected by gas chromatography)	Acetic, propionic, and succinic acids	Lactic and succinic acids	Acetic, propionic, and butyric acids

of localizing the site or sites of infection that might have been missed otherwise, of draining walled-off pockets of pus, and of eliminating devitalized tissue that favors the extension of these mixed infections.

ANTIBIOTIC THERAPY

Antibiotic therapy should, therefore, be aimed at neutralizing the mixed aerobic and anaerobic flora. Of all the aerobes in intra-abdominal infections, *Escherichia coli* seems most often responsible for septicemia and associated septic shock. In many areas, a significant number of *E. coli* are resistant to ampicillin and to the first-generation cephalosporins. In such a setting, the physician may wish to use a second- or third-generation cephalosporin or an aminoglycoside to treat *E. coli* and the facultative gram-negative bacilli adequately. The aminoglycosides, such as gentamicin, tobramycin, netilmicin, or amikacin, may be useful in patients who develop abdominal suppuration, especially during hospitalization, because an increased incidence of resistant gram-negative bacilli, including *Pseudomonas aeruginosa*, has been demonstrated in these patients. An agent effective against anaerobic organisms must be added to the aminoglycoside.

Table 19-7 compares the activity of several antibiotics against anaerobes. With *Bacteroides fragilis* infections, the mortality rate is about 50% if the antibiotic therapy is less than adequate, and it is less than 15% if clindamycin, chloramphenicol, cefoxitin, or metronidazole is administered. Carbenicillin, ticarcillin, mezlocillin, and piperacillin can also be considered, but some doubts exist about

Table 19-7. Antibiotics Effective Against Anaerobes

Bacteria	First Choice	Alternatives
Bacteroides fragilis	Metronidazole or clindamycin	Cefoxitin, chloramphenicol, or carbenicillin
Bacteroides melaninogenicus	Metronidazole or clindamycin	Penicillin G (some strains now resistant to penicillin) Cefoxitin, carbenicillin, or chloramphenicol
Clostridia	Penicillin G	Clindamycin, metronidazole, carbenicillin, or chloramphenicol
Fusobacteria	Penicillin G	Clindamycin, metronidazole, carbenicillin, or chloramphenicol
Anaerobic cocci	Penicillin G	Clindamycin, carbenicillin, or chloramphenicol

their efficacy against this type of infection. If the infection is due to clostridia, fusobacteria, peptococci, or peptostreptococci, penicillin G is the drug of choice.

The threat of aplastic anemia with chloramphenicol and the pseudomembranous colitis seen with clindamycin have limited the use of these products. Most antibiotics, however, except vancomycin, can induce a pseudomembranous colitis. In spite of this side effect, the combination of clindamycin and an aminoglycoside remains excellent and is widely used for intra-abdominal infections.

Cefoxitin, is effective against both gram-negative aerobes and anaerobes as well as against anaerobic gram-positive cocci. It may be a valuable alternative to combination therapy in the treatment of abdominal infections, in patients both with and without a history of prior surgical intervention. This monotherapy, which avoids the nephrotoxic potential of aminoglycosides, may be expanded even further in the future with the use of newer cephalosporins that have extended activity, such as cefotaxime, moxalactam, and others still under investigation.

For biliary tract infections, one should choose an antibiotic concentrated in the bile. See Table 36-5 for antimicrobial agents that concentrate in the bile. This concept may not be entirely valid, however, because concentrations of all antibiotics are much lower in inflamed and obstructed (and infected) bile ducts. At present, ampicillin with an added aminoglycoside is frequently employed for treating infections of the biliary tree because this combination is also effective against the enterococcus. Some newer cephalosporins, may prove promising.

If the general condition of the patient deteriorates, and if the fever persists after several days of what is considered adequate therapy, then it is necessary to rule out the possibility either of an underlying undrained abscess or of resistance to the antibiotic such as occurs infrequently with *Bacteroides fragilis* when clindamycin or cefoxitin is administered.

The approach to the treatment of primary or "spontaneous" peritonitis is different from that of secondary peritonitis. Because it is sometimes difficult to distinguish primary from secondary peritonitis in the child, many surgeons recommend surgical exploration. If paracentesis demonstrates gram-positive diplococci on a smear of the ascitic fluid in children with the nephrotic syndrome, then antibiotic therapy with penicillin alone can eliminate the infection. Cirrhotics tolerate surgical procedures poorly, and medical therapy based on the Gram stain or culture of the ascitic fluid obtained by paracentesis is recommended. When the pathogen is a pneumococcus or a group A streptococcus, penicillin is the drug of choice. When enteric bacteria are present, aminoglycosides are usually adequate, and clindamycin should be added if anaerobes are suspected; alternatively, cefoxitin may replace both aminoglycosides and clindamycin.

Objective 19-5. Make the proper choice of prophylaxis in abdominal surgical procedures.

Antibiotic prophylaxis today is mainly employed in abdominal surgical procedures (Table 19-8). Indeed, prophylactic indications account for only 10% of the antibiotics prescribed in internal medicine, whereas in a surgical context, 70% of antibiotics are now prescribed to prevent infection.

Chemoprophylaxis is defined as the prevention of infection by the administration of antimicrobial agents before, during, or just after exposure of the individual to a specific pathogen or group of pathogens. It is necessary to distinguish this form of preventive prophylaxis from the use of antimicrobial agents to prevent the eventual development of clinically evident disease in a patient already infected, for example, in penetrating bowel trauma and intestinal leakage, or following intraoperative slippage of a colonic clamp and subsequent contamination of the peritoneum with fecal contents.

Although controversy persists, it is now

Table 19–8. Prophylaxis in Abdominal Surgical Procedures

Type of Operation	Likely Pathogens	Antibiotics	Doses and Routes of Administration	Observations
Clean-contaminated Gastroduodenal	Enterobacteriaceae, gram-positive cocci	Cephalothin or Cefazolin	1 g IM or IV, 1 h preoperatively	Only in patients with special risks (achlorhydria, obstruction, cancer)
Biliary tract	Enterobacteriaceae, group D streptococci, clostridia	Cephalothin or Cefazolin	1 g IM or IV, 1 h preoperatively	Only in patients at high risk (age over 70 years, acute cholecystitis with jaundice or with stones in the bile duct)
Colorectal	Enterobacteriaceae, anaerobes including *Bacteroides fragilis*, group D streptococci	(1) *Oral* Neomycin AND Erythromycin	1 g each, at 1 P.M., 2 P.M., and 11 P.M. the day before the operation	For elective surgical patients
		(2) *Parenteral* Cefoxitin OR Clindamycin AND Gentamicin, Tobramycin, or Netilimicin OR Metronidazole AND Gentamicin, Tobramycin, or Netilimicin	1 g IV 600 mg IV 1.5 mg/kg IM or IV 500 mg IV 1.5 mg/kg IM or IV	To be given 1 hour preoperatively and repeated every 4–6 hours (depending on the drug used), during the operation until the end of the procedure

Vaginal hysterectomy	Enterobacteriaceae, anaerobes, groups B and D streptococci	Cefazolin or Cefoxitin	1 g IV or IM, 1 h preoperatively
Cesarian section	Enterobacteriaceae, anaerobes, groups B and D streptococci, *Staphylococcus aureus*	Cefazolin, Cefoxitin, or Cefotaxime	1 g IV or IM	Only in patients at risk (prolonged labor or rupture of membranes); the dose is given just after clamping of the umbilical cord
Dirty-contaminated			
Repair of ruptured viscera	Enterobacteriaceae, anaerobic bacteria including *Bacteroides fragilis*, group D streptococci	Clindamycin AND Gentamicin, Tobramycin, or Netilmicin	600 mg IV q6h 1.5 mg/kg IM or IV q8h	Because highly colonized material has contaminated the area, this represents actual treatment rather than prophylaxis; therapy should be continued for 5 to 10 days
		OR	
		Cefoxitin	1g IV q4–6h	
		OR	
		Cefoxitin AND Gentamicin, Tobramycin, or Netilmicin	1g IV q4–6h 1.5 mg/kg IM or IV q8h	
		OR	
		Metronidazole AND Gentamicin, Tobramycin, or Netilmicin	500 mg IV q8h 1.5 mg/kg IM or IV q8h	

IV, Intravenously; IM intramuscularly.

generally conceded that prophylactic antibiotics can decrease the frequency of both wound infections and intra-abdominal postoperative abscesses in abdominal surgical procedures, specifically of the colon and rectum, in vaginal hysterectomy, in primary cesarian section, and in some biliary operations. The choice of antibiotics in these situations (Table 19–8) depends upon the varieties of bacteria likely to be present in the operative field. For lower abdominal or pelvic procedures, prophylaxis should selectively aim to eliminate a mixed flora of aerobes and anaerobes. If infection or contamination is already present at operation, however, it is no longer a question of brief prophylaxis, but of an extended course of therapy. Moreover, this flora can be modified by prior antibiotic therapy, and resistant gram-negative bacilli and methicillin-resistant staphylococci, for example, may be selected and may evade the prophylactic regimen.

The antibiotic chosen should ideally be easy to administer, not too costly, and nontoxic, both for the patient and, in pregnancy, for the fetus. The agent should, in general, be administered intravenously 1 to 2 hours before the surgical procedure, to ensure high tissue levels at the time of the operation. The antibiotic should not be continued for more than 24 hours because prolonged administration adds nothing to its effectiveness, but rather alters the normal protective intestinal flora and increases the possibility of selecting resistant organisms and of developing gastrointestinal side effects such as pseudomembranous colitis. Oral prophylaxis, or bowel "sterilization," with neomycin and erythromycin or metronidazole is given 18 to 24 hours before bowel operations to suppress the patient's endogenous flora.

Prophylaxis is indicated only when the risk of serious infection is sufficiently great and when this risk can be reduced by such mode of therapy. In a clean surgical procedure, in which contaminated areas are not crossed by the scalpel, such as in thyroidectomies, herniorrhaphies, and removal of ovarian cysts, the risk of infection is low, and prophylaxis is not necessary.

SUGGESTED READINGS

Altemeier, W.A., Culbertson, W.R., Fuller, W.D., and Shook, C.D.: Intra-abdominal abscesses. Am. J. Surg., 125:70, 1973.

Anonymous: Antimicrobial prophylaxis for surgery. Med. Lett. Drugs. Ther., 23:77, 1981.

Berger, M., Smith, E., Holm, H.H., and Mascatello, V.: Utility of ultrasound in the differential diagnosis of acute cholecystis. Arch. Surg., 112:273, 1977.

Caffee, H.H., Watts, G., and Mena, I.: Gallium 67 citrate scanning in the diagnosis of intra-abdominal abscess. Am. J. Surg., 133:665, 1977.

Camer, S.J., Tan, E.G.C., Warren, K.W., and Braasch, J.W.: Pancreatic abscess. A critical analysis of 113 cases. Am. J. Surg., 129:426, 1975.

Chow, A.M., and Guze, L.B.: Bacteroidaceae bacteremia: clinical experience with 112 patients. Medicine, 53:93, 1974.

Chulay, J.D., and Lankerani, M.R.: Splenic abscess. Report of 10 cases and review of the literature. Am. J. Med., 61:513, 1976.

Finegold, S.M., Shepherd, W.E., and Spaulding, E.H.: Practical anaerobic bacteriology. Cumitech, 5:1, 1977.

Finegold, S.M., et al.: Management of anaerobic infections. Ann. Intern. Med., 83:375, 1975.

Gilmore, O.J.A., et al.: Appendicitis and mimicking conditions. A prospective study. Lancet, 2:421, 1975.

Gorbach, S.L.: Intestinal microflora. Gastroenterology, 60:1110, 1971.

Gorbach, S.L., and Bartlett, J.G.: Anaerobic infections. N. Engl. J. Med., 290:1177, 1237, 1289, 1974.

Harding, G.K.M., et al.: Prospective, randomized comparative study of clindamycin, chloramphenicol and ticarcillin, each in combination with gentamicin, in therapy for intra-abdominal and female genital tract sepsis. J. Infect. Dis., 142:384, 1980.

Mackowiak, P.A.: Microbial synergism in human infections. N. Engl. J. Med., 298:21, 83, 1978.

Onderdonk, A.B., et al.: Microbial synergy in experimental intra-abdominal abscess. Infect. Immun., 13:33, 1976.

Polk, H.C., and Stone, H.H.: Hospital Acquired Infections in Surgery. Baltimore, University Park Press, 1977.

Schimpff, S.C., Wiernik, P.H., and Block, J.B.: Rectal abscesses in cancer patients. Lancet, 2:844, 1972.

Sommers, H.M.: Anaerobic bacterial disease: general considerations. In The Biologic and Clinical Basis of Infectious Disease. Edited by G.P. Youmans, P.Y. Patterson, and H.M. Sommers. Philadelphia, W.B. Saunders, 1980.

CHAPTER 20

Liver Infections

F.A. Waldvogel

Objective 20–1. Gather clinical evidence of an infectious process involving the liver.

As a result both of its unique anatomic location at the junction of the veins that drain the abdominal cavity and of its close topographic relations with the biliary tree and digestive tract, the liver is subjected to a variety of repeated microbial challenges of viral, bacterial, or parasitic origin. In light of the many functions of this organ, such as the synthesis and secretion of bile salts and pigments, the synthesis of various proteins and their release into the circulation, a primary role in intermediary metabolism, and the detoxification of various exogenous and endogenous substances, the clinical manifestations of a hepatic infectious process naturally vary according to the causative microorganism and to the hepatic functions primarily affected. Furthermore, the position of the liver beneath the diaphragm sets a limit to its direct clinical examination. To sum up, the liver is subjected to various types of infections whose clinical manifestations, while often specific, are for detailed exploration dependent primarily on laboratory procedures.

CLINICAL MANIFESTATIONS OF LIVER INFECTION

Of all the clinical symptoms and signs of hepatic infection, four are of particular importance: *fever, jaundice, hepatomegaly,* and *pain in the right flank*. These are found individually or in combination in various hepatic diseases. By a thorough search for these four clinical signs and symptoms, one can, in general, orient the laboratory tests toward establishing an accurate etiologic diagnosis. Other symptoms, such as nausea, vomiting, and loss of appetite, are not specific enough to be of great help in the initial evaluation.

Fever. An elevated temperature is rarely absent in acute infections of the liver. The patient's fever curve and the accompanying symptoms are often a source of important information; thus, a febrile episode of insidious onset accompanied by joint pains and urticarial lesions is characteristic of viral hepatitis, particularly hepatitis B. In hepatic involvement induced by cytomegalovirus (CMV), Epstein-Barr virus (EBV), or even hepatitis A virus, fever may be the only early clinical manifestation.

In liver involvement due to *Leptospira icterohaemorrhagiae*, fever often occurs in two successive phases of a few days, the first phase accompanied by nonspecific systemic signs, and the second combined with hepatic, renal, or meningeal involvement. In brucellosis, the fever curve is undulant and is accompanied by recurrent chills, sweats, intense myalgias, hepatomegaly, and splenomegaly. Fever with hepatic involvement secondary to typhoid fever is continuous and is characterized by a dissociation of pulse rate and temperature. In focal pyogenic infection (abscess) of the liver or of the gallbladder, the patient has a high fever spiking to 40° C (104° F); the fever falls rapidly with antipyretic agents, but rises to even higher levels in the following hours, together with shaking chills and even mental confusion. In patients with biliary tract obstruction, these irregular febrile spikes are superimposed on an already elevated basal temperature, fulfilling the criteria of a Charcot's fever.

Jaundice. In general, jaundice is easy to recognize. One must remember that it cannot be detected until the serum bilirubin level rises to more than 25 mg/L, and skin discoloration due to jaundice is difficult to evaluate under artificial light. Provided a chemistry laboratory is at the clinician's disposal, determinations of serum bilirubin, serum glutamic-oxaloacetic and serum glutamic pyruvic transaminases (SGOT and SGPT), and alkaline phosphatase levels are of diagnostic help. Otherwise, urinalysis (bile pigments) or a rapid hematocrit determination (yellow color of supernatant plasma) may be helpful. Finally, extrahepatic or intrahepatic biliary obstruction is often heralded by persistent pruritus, preceding jaundice by several days or weeks and leading to excoriated skin lesions; such is the case, for example, in cholestatic hepatitis or in primary biliary cirrhosis. Not every case of jaundice, even when accompanied by fever, is necessarily of infectious origin; toxic agents such as alcohol or drugs, or the presence of a primary or secondary tumor of the liver, can reproduce all the clinical signs and symptoms of liver infection.

Hepatomegaly. The size of the liver is often difficult to evaluate. Hepatomegaly is measured by the span of the organ at the level of the midclavicular line (right lobe) and over the midsternum (left lobe). Normal values vary as a function of the height and sex of the patient, but they average 10 cm for the right lobe and 7 cm for the left lobe. A diffuse hepatomegaly, affecting both lobes, is preferentially found in diffuse hepatic infections (hepatitis), whereas an expanding lesion is suggested by localized hepatomegaly. An enlarged left hepatic lobe may be confused with splenomegaly: on deep respiration, the enlarged left lobe moves along the axis of the body, whereas the enlarged spleen moves along an oblique axis toward the umbilicus. Occasionally, careful palpation may demonstrate a gallbladder under tension, or may reveal a local inflammatory induration, as when cholecystitis is complicated by adhesions to the omentum.

Flank Pain. Spontaneous right subchondral pains are frequent, but can also be elicited by palpation. They are essentially of three different types. A pain localized to the right subcostal region, exacerbated by palpation during inspiration, constitutes Murphy's sign, a reliable finding in cholecystitis. This localized sign must be distinguished from pain produced by palpation of the entire free edge of the liver, a frequent finding in hepatitis with significant cellular necrosis and edema. Moreover, this diffuse tenderness is readily elicited by effort or by fist percussion. Finally, a sharper pain, accentuated by breathing, with almost a pleural characteristic, usually indicates an expanding process involving the fibrous capsule of the liver; careful auscultation occasionally reveals a friction rub indicating the presence of an abscess or a liver tumor or discloses a continuous systolodiastolic murmur suggestive of a tumor.

TYPES OF HEPATIC INVOLVEMENT

We have previously seen that the clinical symptoms and signs of liver disease help one to select the proper laboratory tests for an accurate etiologic diagnosis. This diagnosis presupposes correct interpretation of the many liver function tests and roentgenographic and radioisotope studies available to the physician. Because none of these tests are sufficiently specific to permit an unequivocal diagnosis, one must first consider the major impact of each of the toxic or bacterial etiologic agents.

Thus, one can usually distinguish four

major types of hepatic involvement: microbial and toxic agents can (1) localize preferentially to the gallbladder and the biliary tract; (2) produce diffuse hepatic involvement; (3) occasionally produce a cellular infiltration of the hepatic lobule or portal spaces; and (4) involve a circumscribed area of the liver, to produce one or more localized lesions of variable size. Each of these different types of involvement is discussed in this chapter.

> **Objective 20–2. Plan the investigation and treatment of an infection of the gallbladder and biliary tract.**

Infections of the gallbladder and biliary tract are nearly always secondary to an obstruction, whether by a stone or, more rarely, a parasite or a tumor. The fever is generally of sudden onset, often accompanied by repeated chills. Nausea and vomiting start at the onset of the first fever spike. Then, jaundice develops; it may be progressive and intense in case of complete obstruction or transient and slight if the stone is passed rapidly. Examination of the patient shows the abdominal wall overlying the gallbladder to be tender, with a positive Murphy's sign. The gallbladder may be surrounded by a palpable, inflammatory mass. In such a case, abdominal sounds are absent in the right hypochondrium.

DIAGNOSTIC PROCEDURES

The laboratory tests that help to confirm the diagnosis are microbiologic, radiologic, and biochemical. Blood cultures are occasionally useful in determining the bacterial origin of a biliary tract infection. A plain roentgenogram of the abdomen is always indicated; it may allow one to visualize the cholelithiasis responsible for the jaundice, to rule out the presence of air in the biliary ducts, and to eliminate the diagnosis of a gallstone ileus; nonfilling of the gallbladder on cholecystography is the rule at this stage of the disease. These studies have been superseded, however, by abdominal ultrasonography, which can determine the presence of stones and dilation of the bile ducts in a short time. Finally, conjugated bilirubin and alkaline phosphatase levels are generally disproportionately elevated in relation to tests for hepatic cell necrosis, such as the determination of SGOT, SGPT, and gamma glutamic transaminase (γGT) enzyme activity.

What microorganisms are responsible for this clinical picture? They are, primarily, the Enterobacteriacea (*Escherichia coli* and klebsiella) and anaerobic organisms, less commonly enterococci. Rarely, certain parasites (ascarides, flukes, echinococci) uncommon in temperate climates penetrate and obstruct the biliary tract and produce the inflammatory state.

PRINCIPLES OF TREATMENT

The management of a patient with acute biliary tract infection depends on his age and on the complications of the disease. The usual approach is to let the crisis abate by administering appropriate antibiotics and then to operate in the weeks that follow; however, the almost inescapable surgical intervention in an obstructed patient carries a certain operative risk in aged patients and in those with cardiovascular or pulmonary problems. This sometimes considerable risk must be weighed against the seriousness of the biliary infection. The manifestations and complications can be alarming in a patient in a highly septic state, or in one with localized peritonitis or renal failure. In such patients, the surgical intervention must be scheduled earlier and must be performed even under unfavorable circumstances.

I shall simply outline the broad principles of antibiotic therapy. A chemotherapeutic agent both effective against the Enterobacteriaceae and anaerobes that may be present and able to penetrate into the biliary ducts is indicated. The antibiotics most often prescribed are second- or third-generation cephalosporins, such as cefoxitin or cefotaxime, 4 to 6 g/day; ampicillin, 4 to 8 g/day; chloramphenicol, 2 to 3 g/day, or in Europe, thiamphenicol, 3 g/day. Therapy must be administered parenterally and continued for 2 weeks, to control these infectious episodes.

> Objective 20–3. Look for the cause of hepatocellular necrosis, to establish etiologic treatment and preventive measures.

DIAGNOSIS OF HEPATOCELLULAR NECROSIS

Diffuse involvement of the hepatic parenchyma poses no real diagnostic problem. Jaundice is progressive, fever is moderate, although it may exceptionally reach 40° C (104° F) in cases of sudden and massive hepatic necrosis such as caused by alcohol, viral hepatitis A and B, or drugs. The intensity of the initial systemic symptoms (nausea, vomiting, anorexia) and of the local signs (painful hepatomegaly) are proportional to the degree of hepatocellular involvement. Generally, the liver is diffusely enlarged, tender, and has a smooth edge. If the hepatocellular involvement is massive, rapid diminution of liver dullness may be seen, and the free border of the liver may disappear beneath the rib cage. Finally, other clinical findings that may provide important information regarding the origin of the disease are spider nevi suggestive of acute or chronic alcoholism, a morbilliform eruption as a sign of drug toxicity, a transient urticaria bringing viral hepatitis B to mind, and a collateral circulation revealing pre-existing portal hypertension.

In hepatocellular involvement, the transaminase levels are elevated, whereas the tests reflecting the synthetic activities of the liver, such as the tests for the albumin level, the prothrombin level, and even urea, are disturbed commensurately with the degree of hepatic disease. Occasionally, the hepatocellular involvement is preceded by a phase of intrahepatic cholestasis that is still incompletely understood. Biochemically, this cholestasis is manifested by a considerable elevation in alkaline phosphatase and leucine aminopeptidase levels; the transaminases show only a slight increase. In such conditions, provided extrahepatic biliary obstruction has been excluded by retrograde cholangiography or ultrasonography, the diagnosis can often be clarified by needle biopsy of the liver.

Although the diagnosis of hepatocellular involvement is usually easy to make, the determination of its cause may be difficult. Extensive destruction of the hepatocytes may have any of the following causes: hemodynamic collapse as in cardiogenic or septic shock; ingestion of toxic substances such as carbon tetrachloride, phosphorus, toxin from the mushroom *Amanita phalloides*, and viruses such as the ones responsible for viral hepatitis; other microorganisms such as *Leptospira icterohaemorrhagiae;* or, presumably, immunologic mechanisms, as suspected after the repeated use of halothane, anticonvulsants, or diuretics.

VIRAL HEPATITIS

Various laboratory tests, such as electron microscopy and immunofluorescence, have contributed to the demonstration of different biologic markers of the disease. These markers, which include DNA polymerase, HBs antigen (HBsAg) and HBc antigen (HBcAg) and their corresponding antibodies, e antigen and its corresponding antibody, and antibody to virus A, have helped to expand knowledge of viral hepatitis A and B, in recent years (Table 20–1). The discovery of animal models (chimpanzee, marmoset) and the establishment of tissue cultures permissive to the hepatitis virus B (hepatoma cells) have also enabled one to obtain more accurate information regarding these infections. These data, important both clinically and epidemiologically, are summarized in Table 25–1. In this respect, hepatitis A virus produces neither prolonged viremia nor long-lasting infection.

The demonstration of antibodies to hepatitis A virus by various techniques, such as the rise and fall of IgM during the disease and the persistence of IgG during convalescence, makes diagnosis possible at an early active stage as well as after infection and has

Table 20-1. Three Principal Hepatitis Viruses

Characteristics	Hepatitis A (epidemic, infectious)	Hepatitis B (serum, inoculation)	Non-A, non-B hepatitis
Virologic features	RNA virus, 27 nm	DNA virus, 42 nm (Dane particle)	DNA virus (?)
Virologic identification	By electron microscopy; anti-HAV antibodies (RIA, hemagglutination, CF); IgG, IgM (acute)	By electron microscopy; HBsAg, HBcAg and corresponding antibodies; DNA polymerase	By exclusion of other forms of hepatitis
Transmission	Stool, urine: second part of the intubation period (until 14 days after jaundice); blood: probably not infectious	Patient's blood, commercial blood, blood products; sexual activities; vertical (maternal-fetal)	Patient's blood, commercial blood, blood products, probably in 20 to 50% of patients with post-transfusional hepatitis
Portal of entry	Oral (parenteral)	Parenteral, transcutaneous, mucous, sexual	Parenteral
Incubation period	< 6 weeks (15-45 days)	> 6 weeks (60-180 days)	6-9 weeks
Clinical manifestations before jaundice	Headaches, myalgias, nausea	Few or none	Few or none
Chronic forms	None	About 10%	About 10%
Mortality rate	Low	High	High
Chronic carriers	No	Yes	Yes

helped to establish its epidemiologic profile. Although 80% of the children under 10 years of age in subtropical countries already have antibodies to this virus, the percentage is much lower in industrialized nations, where such figures are not even found in older adults. Moreover, in adults, the immunized subpopulation may vary by geographic region and by socioeconomic circumstances.

Hepatitis A virus is shed essentially by the fecal route during the latter part of the incubation period and during the icteric phase of the disease. This property explains the high transmission rate of the virus by the fecal-oral route in crowded environments or under poor sanitary conditions. A transient hematogenous transmission probably accounts for some cases of contamination by blood, blood products, or blood-contaminated biologic fluids. Finally, many point-source epidemics have been observed, usually ascribed to contaminated water or food. The disease generally has an acute clinical course, but these cases represent the tip of the iceberg: for every clinical case, probably close to nine anicteric cases occur and result in active, permanent immunization.

The immunologic profile of hepatitis B virus is far more complex than that of hepatitis A virus, and its epidemiology is complicated by the presence of a large human reservoir of virus carriers, estimated at more than 100 million individuals. Schematically, an electron microscopic study of the blood of an infected individual shows complete viral particles, called Dane particles (Fig. 20-1), containing the nucleocapsid, or HBc antigen,

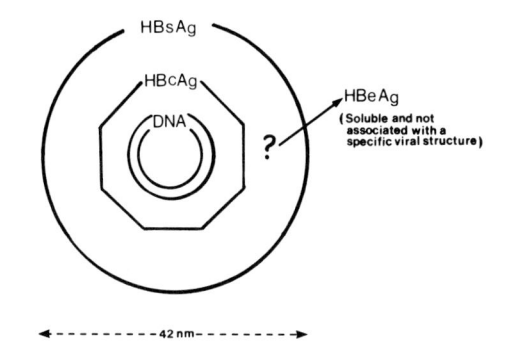

Fig. 20-1. Diagram of the Dane particle.

covered by a viral coat with its surface HBs antigen(s). In addition, the intact viral particle has an e antigen whose nature is still poorly understood, but whose presence is associated with the infectious-contagious character of the patient as well as with the progression to chronic disease. Furthermore, this infectious serum also contains an excess of spherical and filamentous structures without nucleic acid, composed essentially of material from the viral coat containing the HBs antigen, which is not infectious as such.

These three antigens, HBs, HBc, and e, induce the production of corresponding antibodies at the end of acute hepatitis, following a well-defined sequence. HBsAg and e antigen appear in the serum prior to the elevation of the transaminase levels. Anti-HBc antibodies make their appearance during the initial phase of the clinical illness and persist, although at reduced levels, during the convalescent phase. These antibodies are followed briefly by anti-e antibodies, and then by anti-HBs antibodies during the convalescent phase, protective antibodies that herald recovery. This immune response is modified when the infection becomes chronic (Fig. 20–2) (see Objective 20–4).

The possible persistence of hepatitis B virus in the blood as a fully infectious particle, its high pathogenicity, and the complex immune response all help to explain the complicated epidemiologic features of hepatitis B. Infection is essentially transmitted by blood or blood products from infected carriers; moreover, close mucosal contact is probably responsible for high transmission rates during sexual activity, particularly among male homosexuals.

Other "hepatitis" viruses now seem to be responsible for most cases of post-transfusion hepatitis. For lack of a better definition, these viruses are currently called "non-A, non-B hepatitis viruses." They possess certain biologic characteristics of hepatitis B virus, such as parenteral transmission by blood or blood products, a tendency to cause chronic infection, and the presence of an asymptomatic carrier stage. They differ, however, from hepatitis B virus immunologically by the absence of cross-reactivity. At this time, the inability to detect these viruses in the serum of blood donors prevents their elimination from blood banks.

The etiologic picture of hepatocellular involvement would not be complete without mentioning the rare and poorly understood causes of hepatic cell destruction. Thus, in the field of infections, leptospirae, particularly *Leptospira icterohaemorrhagiae* can cause severe hepatocellular involvement often associated with renal impairment. Yel-

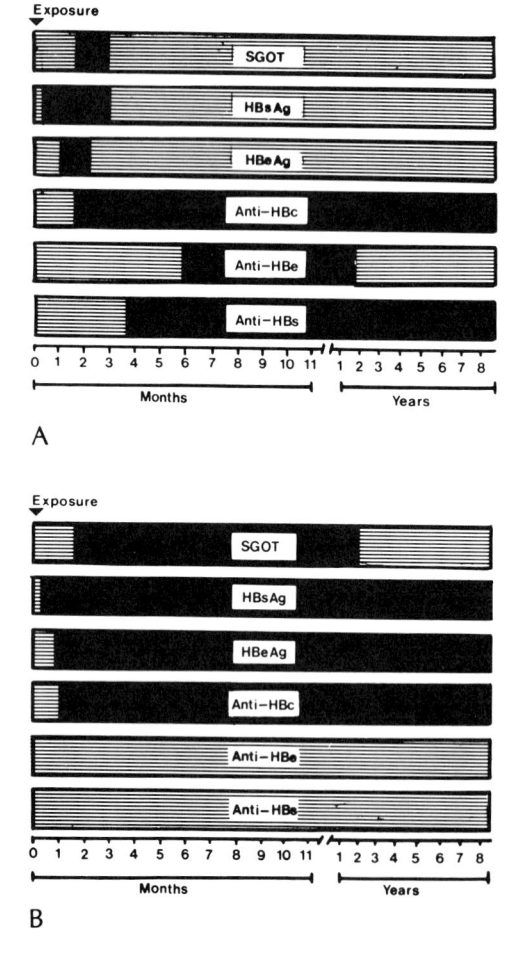

Fig. 20–2. Biologic and serologic events associated with acute viral hepatitis type B followed by recovery (A) and followed by chronic hepatitis (B). (Modified from Krugman, S., et al.: Viral hepatitis type B. Studies on natural history and prevention reexamined. N. Engl. J. Med., 300:101, 1979. Reprinted by permission.)

low fever can also be responsible for severe hepatitis in certain geographic areas. Cases of Reye's syndrome, fortunately still rare in children and exceptional in young adults, have been reported throughout the world. Clinical features of this disorder consist of fever, hypoglycemia, and severe hepatocellular damage without jaundice; the syndrome usually follows an episode of common influenza. Finally, the liver may be affected indirectly by various infectious processes, including acute pyelonephritis, gram-negative sepsis, and septic shock in the presence of severe neutropenia. In such cases, the hepatic injury is reflected by severe hepatocellular damage with jaundice. It is only through a complete clinical examination and careful microbiologic cultures, such as blood and urine cultures, that such complex manifestations can be understood. Finally, many toxic agents for example, *Amanita phalloides*, carbon tetrachloride, and isoniazid, or immunologic reactions, such as to halothane, can be manifested clinically and biologically by hepatotoxic damage.

Once the diagnosis of viral involvement of the liver parenchyma has been established, three problems remain to be solved: treatment of the disease, clinical and laboratory surveillance of the hepatitis, and reduction of the risk of transmission.

TREATMENT OF ACUTE HEPATITIS

At the present time, we are forced to admit that no chemotherapy is effective in acute hepatitis. Even in fulminant hepatitis, the administration of corticosteroids seems to be contraindicated because it increases the risk of gastrointestinal hemorrhage. Treatment of chronic hepatitis is discussed later in this chapter.

CLINICAL AND BIOCHEMICAL SURVEILLANCE OF HEPATITIS

Because many factors can affect the severity and prognosis of hepatic injury, the physician must try to determine their relative importance by means of repeated, careful clinical examinations and hepatic function tests. The various prognostic factors can be classified into three groups:

First, the previous condition of the patient's liver plays an important role in the course of the infectious episode; thus, alcoholism, previous toxic damage, and the administration of hepatotoxic drugs, reduce the liver's residual functional capacity and predispose it to hepatocellular insufficiency. Second, the infection itself helps to determine the course of the disease. At the present time, however, we still do not know whether fulminant hepatitis is due to a high number of infecting viral particles or to an abnormal immunologic response of the host. Recent studies favor the immunologic explanation. Although the severity of the acute illness cannot be gauged by its virologic and immunologic evaluation, it does not match with a unique biologic profile either. Certain patients lapsing rapidly into endogenous coma, and who have pathologic liver function tests, may improve spectacularly within a few days. In my experience, it takes a longitudinal evaluation of the hepatic function tests for a correct assessment of the risks of an imminent hepatocellular collapse or, on the contrary, of a progressive recovery.

The third prognostic factor, hepatocellular insufficiency, is heralded primarily by neurologic signs such as agitation, tremor, uncontrollable extrapyramidal movements (flapping tremor). Then, progressive coma occurs, sometimes accompanied by papilledema. At this stage, the patient is generally jaundiced and has the other stigmata of hepatic injury such as spider angioma and ascites. The clinical course of the illness, rather than the size of the patient's liver, confirms the suspicion of hepatocellular insufficiency; the zone of hepatic percussion shrinks within a few days by several centimeters.

The biochemical changes in hepatocellular insufficiency are characteristic: increased signs of liver cell necrosis (SGOT, SGPT), a precipitous decrease in the protein levels synthesized by the liver (prothrombin, albumin), hypoglycemia, and a decrease in urea concentration. In addition, such a patient may have pancytopenia, probably as a result of hypersplenism. Gastrointestinal hemorrhage nearly always occurs at this stage. It aggravates hepatocellular insufficiency and often leads to a fatal outcome.

All hope, however, is not necessarily lost at that stage. If the hepatocellular injury was a single, sudden event, for example, induced by drugs, involving an otherwise healthy liver, therapy to correct the various protein deficiencies, to control the blood sugar level, and to minimize gastrointestinal bleeding may save the life of a desperately ill patient. In view of the many medical measures used to support such patients, it is difficult to determine whether aggressive maneuvers such as exchange transfusion, charcoal hemoperfusion, and cross-circulation have an additional beneficial effect.

IMMUNIZATION AND PREVENTIVE MEASURES

Although chemotherapy is of no avail in acute viral hepatitis, many prophylactic techniques have been developed in recent years, and new active immunizations for viral hepatitis B have been marketed. The present status of passive immunization against hepatitis is summarized in Table 20-2. As to active immunization, the new hepatitis B vaccine offers a novel way to immunize a large segment of the population. Obtained from otherwise healthy carriers by purification and inactivation of HBsAg, the active vaccine offers protection against disease for several years. Indications for vaccination have not been fully delineated, but they include health professionals, patients receiving repeated blood transfusions or products, patients in dialysis centers, sexual partners of homosexuals, and drug addicts. We do not yet know the duration of the immunity conferred by the vaccine, however, and this factor is of concern in light of possible reinfection evolving into chronic hepatitis.

Objective 20-4. Distinguish between acute and chronic hepatitis.

As mentioned earlier, both hepatitis B and non-A, non-B hepatitis can become chronic. Moreover, the apparently benign course of such an illness can be complicated by alcohol abuse or drugs. In the absence of any viral damage, alcohol and drug ingestion can maintain the hepatocellular necrosis accompanied by hepatocellular regeneration and suggest the clinical and biochemical picture of chronic hepatitis.

The question of the diagnosis of chronic hepatitis arises primarily in two distinct clinical situations: first, when acute type B hepatitis follows an unfavorable course in which the liver function tests fail to return to normal after several months; second, when the results of liver function tests are found to be abnormal in a patient with vague symptoms

Table 20-2. Possible Protection against the Three Principal Hepatitis Viruses

	Viruses		
	Hepatitis A	Hepatitis B	Non-A, non-B hepatitis
Immunologic protection	Standard immunoglobulins administered within 1-2 weeks after contact to: intimate contacts (household, school, institutions); those exposed to a common source; persons traveling in endemic regions	Specific immunoglobulins: hepatitis B immune globulins* administered to†: intimate contacts with significant HBsAg and inoculum; infants at risk of maternal-neonatal transmission; patients in hemodialysis units	Nonspecific immunoglobulins; indications not clearly delineated
Prophylaxis	Improved social and hygienic conditions	Detection of carriers; active vaccination	Unknown at present

*Antibody titer > 1:100,000 by passive hemagglutination.
†Indications limited since the introduction of HB vaccine.

such as loss of appetite, unexplained asthenia, and abdominal pain.

CLINICAL FEATURES

Even though the solution to this diagnostic problem often requires a histologic study of the liver by needle biopsy, many clinical and biochemical findings are indicative of chronic hepatitis. Clinically, one must look for any signs of chronicity such as lichenified scratch marks, clubbing of the fingers, patent collateral circulation, and ascites. In certain forms of chronic hepatitis, remote clinical signs are noted, such as polyarteritis (lupoid hepatitis), Kayser-Fleischer ring (Wilson's disease), pulmonary disorders (α_1-antitrypsin deficiency). By means of a thorough history-taking, one must search for possible contributing factors, for example alcohol abuse, and repeated exposure to anesthetic agents such as halothane or to various other drugs including contraceptives and laxatives.

BIOCHEMICAL FEATURES

Biochemically, the degree of hepatic dysfunction does not allow one to distinguish between acute and chronic hepatitis. A record of the changing laboratory values over the course of the illness is useful, but it takes a long time to collect. On the other hand, certain immunologic parameters are often helpful to establish the diagnosis of chronic hepatitis: the search for LE cells or the determination of anti-DNA antibodies (lupoid hepatitis), the determination of anti-smooth-muscle antibodies (chronic active hepatitis), the presence of a rheumatoid factor (chronic active hepatitis), and the determination of the histocompatibility antigen B8 (chronic active hepatitis).

When a liver biopsy is performed, the pathologist should be questioned with regard to the histologic signs of active disease. In chronic persistent hepatitis, these inflammatory signs are minimal, and the course of the illness is usually benign. In chronic active hepatitis, on the contrary, signs of necrosis and regeneration are present, and the outlook is much less favorable. The prognosis may be bleak when the causative agent is clearly hepatitis B virus. Such patients present an immunologic profile of "nonhealing" hepatitis, as if the host defense mechanisms had been partially inhibited during the disease. HBsAg and e antigen are present in large quantities, as are intact viral particles (Dane particles); the patient is therefore highly infectious. Although the mechanisms leading to the production of anti-HBc antibodies are intact, no free anti-e and anti-HBs antibodies can usually be demonstrated.

Some patients with chronic active hepatitis have no immunologic sign of hepatitis B virus infection. They frequently are women who have both clinical and laboratory findings of systemic lupus erythematosus (lupoid hepatitis). Others are patients of either sex who are taking hepatotoxic drugs such as oxyphenisatin, aspirin, acetaminophen, methylcarbamate, and mefenamic acid. In this group, discontinuance of the drug may radically improve the clinical course of the disease.

TREATMENT OF CHRONIC HEPATITIS

What are the therapeutic possibilities in chronic hepatitis? In persistent disease, total abstinence from any toxic product and a conservative approach are usually sufficient. In chronic active hepatitis caused by hepatitis B virus, temporary success has been achieved with a combination of interferon and adenine arabinoside. In hepatitis without signs of B virus involvement, most investigators have reported success with prolonged prednisone treatment.

Objective 20–5. Determine the origin of infiltrative lesions of the liver.

Infiltrative lesions of the liver have few symptoms. When these lesions are infectious, they produce a nontender hepatomegaly accompanied by fever, which is usually well tolerated by the patient. In most cases, no jaundice is present. Hepatic function tests are only slightly disturbed, with a moderate elevation of the alkaline phosphatase level. Because of the infiltrative nature of the process, hepatocellular tests are usually normal.

Histologically, a great variety of infiltrative lesions may be found. These are sometimes due to tumor and may be discovered before the primary lesion is clinically detectable; they are found in acute and chronic leukemia; and they may reflect the progression of Hodgkin's disease or other lymphomas to stage IV. Finally, these infiltrates may be of infectious origin and may correspond to granulomas on occasion, containing giant cells in various stages of organization. The causative agent may be determined by the appearance of the granuloma's location, its degree of necrosis, and by special staining techniques for various types of microorganisms, such as *Mycobacterium tuberculosis*, rickettsiae, yeasts, and fungi.

The principal causes of granulomatous infiltrates of the liver are summarized in Table 20–3. Of all the tests available to the clinician, needle biopsy of the liver provides the most information at this early stage of investigation (Figs. 20–3 and 20–4).

The microscopic appearance of the granuloma may be helpful to the clinician, and such biopsies are always a fruitful topic for discussion at clinicopathologic conferences. Thus, the presence of polymorphonuclear leukocytes in the granuloma is evidence against a diagnosis of tuberculosis and suggests instead a diagnosis of rickettsia or coxiella infection; the presence of eosinophils suggests a hypersensitivity reaction, either drug-induced or parasitic. Occasionally, argentaffine staining reveals that a systemic infection is caused by yeasts or other fungi.

The laboratory studies should not be limited to a biopsy, however. Blood cultures are required for the diagnosis of brucella or salmonella infection. A radiographic examination of the chest may reveal undiagnosed miliary tuberculosis, and a rise in the levels of antibodies to EBV (infectious mononucleosis) or CMV has considerable diagnostic value. Finally, based on the patient's medical history or on epidemiologic considerations, one

Table 20–3. Causes of Granulomatous Hepatitis and Diagnostic Tests

Type of Infection or other Cause	Causative Agent	Diagnostic Tests
Viral	Cytomegalovirus	Serologic tests (specific IgM), isolation of virus (urine, saliva), blood smear
	Epstein-Barr virus	Serologic tests, heterophil antibodies, blood smear
Coxiella	*Coxiella burnetti* (Q fever)	Serologic tests: agglutination, complement fixation
Spirochetal	*Treponema pallidum* (syphilis)	Serologic tests
Other Bacterial	Salmonella, brucella, *Listeria monocytogenes*	Blood cultures
	Mycobacterium tuberculosis	Ziehl-Neelsen staining on biopsy specimen
Yeast or fungal	*Candida albicans*	Blood cultures, argentaffin staining of biopsy specimen
	Aspergillus, blastomyces nocardia, histoplasma	Culture, skin tests
Parasitic	Schistosoma	Search for eggs in biopsy of liver, serologic tests
	Toxocara, ascaris	Serologic tests
	Leishmania	Serologic tests
Hypersensitivity reactions	Sulfonamides, phenylbutazone	Medical history, provocative tests
	Sarcoidosis	Lung roentgenogram, Kveim test
	Collagen diseases	Biopsies of other tissues
	Hodgkin's disease (?)	Lymph node biopsy

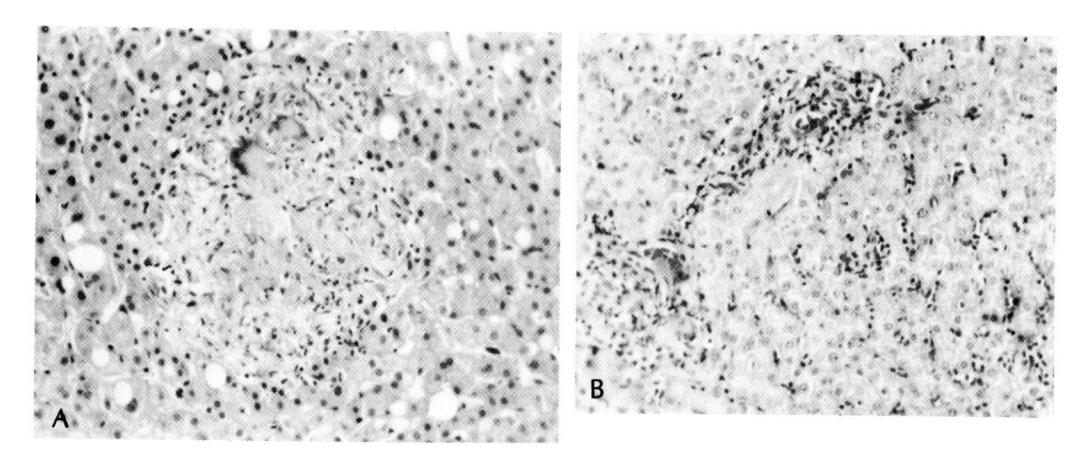

Fig. 20-3. *A*, Granulomatous hepatitis in a case of tuberculosis; note the two giant cells and the central caseous necrosis. *B*, Granulomatous hepatitis in a case of brucellosis; note the well-demarcated granulomas and the diffuse hyperplasia of the sinusoids.

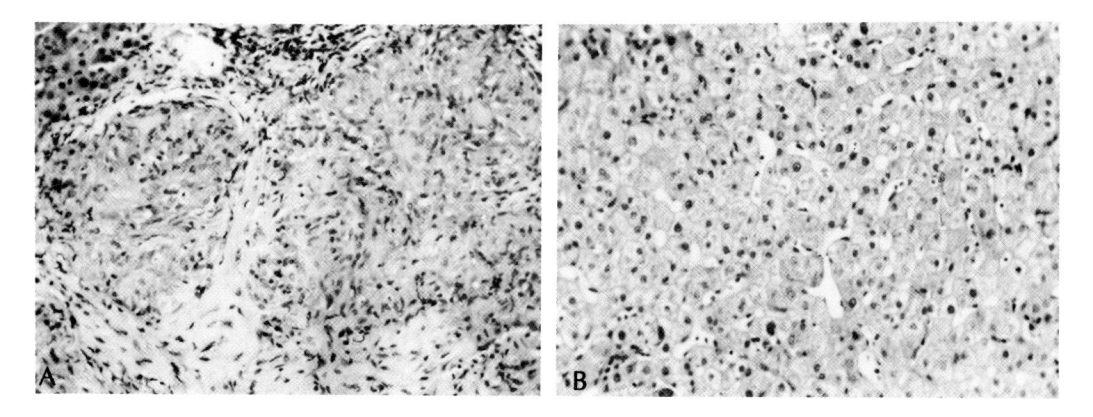

Fig. 20-4. *A*, Granulomatous hepatitis in a case of sarcoidosis; note the absence of caseous necrosis and the intense fibrosis. *B*, Reactive hepatitis occurring after salmonellosis; note the hepatocellular anisocytosis, the absence of necrosis, and the mild focal infiltration of the sinusoids by mononuclear cells. (Courtesy of J.J. Widmann, Pathology Institute, Cantonal University Hospital, Geneva.)

must search carefully for parasites; repeated collections of stool samples, rectal biopsy, and appropriate serologic tests sometimes show such infiltrative lesions to have a parasitic origin, as in schistosomiasis.

Infiltrative lesions, cytotoxicity, or even a cholestatic picture can be caused by drugs. In the case of infiltration, the microscopic lesion is characterized by focal changes that become organized in granulomas. With regard to cytotoxicity, these drugs produce hepatocellular necrosis. In view of the vast quantities of drugs used nowadays, it is not surprising that the list of hepatotoxic products keeps growing and ranges from antituberculous drugs, such as isoniazid and rifampin, to anti-inflammatory agents, such as aspirin, acetaminophen and phenylbutazone, to antipsychotic compounds, such as the phenothiazines. Therefore, such factors must always be considered in the presence of diffuse hepatic disease of unknown origin.

> **Objective 20-6. Differentiate between an abscess and a tumor in space-occupying lesions of the liver.**

Localized infectious lesions of the liver take the form of abscesses and have to be differentiated from primary or secondary tumors. Both abscesses and tumors can cause fever accompanied by a variable leukocytosis, an irregular hepatomegaly tender to palpation and percussion, an elevation of the right hemidiaphragm, and finally, a hepatic friction rub heard over the right upper quadrant. Neither a liver scan, which is indispensable for locating the lesions, nor a selective arteriogram provides decisive evidence in favor of an infection or a tumor. The same is true of hepatic function tests, which are often normal and show only a slight elevation of the transaminase level and a more significant increase in alkaline phosphatase levels. Ultrasonography and computed axial tomography are useful for estimating the density of the mass and sometimes for detecting other intra-abdominal metastatic lesions.

How can a firm diagnosis be established and adequate treatment be undertaken in the presence of such a lesion? Histologic confirmation of the diagnosis could be obtained by a simple, blind hepatic biopsy. If the lesion is a tumor, the risk of hemorrhage is high; if it is a focus of infection, a risk of dissemination exists. The pragmatic approach to such a diagnostic problem consists, first of all, in listing the infectious agents responsible for such abscesses: Enterobacteriaceae when the present episode is preceded by a biliary disorder, anaerobic organisms when it follows an appendicular or colonic infection. Sometimes, these abscesses are mixed and contain both the aforementioned flora, or *Staphylococcus aureus*. Abscesses of mixed origin are seen particularly following surgical intervention or abdominal trauma.

The other main causes of hepatic abscess are parasitic. At first sight, an amebic abscess is clinically, radiologically, and, in terms of laboratory findings, biochemically indistinguishable from a suppurative lesion. Only a particularly suggestive medical history and a positive amebic serologic test allow one to make this diagnosis without resorting to a direct puncture, which is felt to be a dangerous procedure without appropriate chemotherapeutic coverage. Indirect hemagglutination, complement fixation, and gel diffusion precipitation techniques are currently available. The first technique is perhaps the most sensitive and the most likely to turn negative within 6 months of adequate treatment. Finally, the last cause to rule out is a hydatid cyst, a diagnosis also confirmable by appropriate serologic tests.

If the various clinical and laboratory data fail to provide an unequivocal diagnosis, a histologic examination of the lesion will become mandatory, either through direct puncture or by laparoscopy. In such cases, the procedure should be preceded by a few days of chemotherapy, the choice of which depends on the probable infectious agent. Cephalosporins such as cefoxitin 6 to 8 g/day or cefotaxime 4 to 6 g/day (or similar third generation agents) can be used for Enterobacteriaceae or mixed flora infections. Metronidazole (2 g/day) or clindamycin (2.4 g/day) is indicated in infections specifically caused by anaerobic bacteria; a penicillinase-resistant penicillin, for example, nafcillin, the only one in this group that provides effective biliary levels, should be administered when the infection is thought to be due to *Staphylococcus aureus*. When the abscess is suspected to be of amebic origin, treatment with metronidazole (2 to 2.5 g/day for 5 to 10 days) is required; certain authors have observed relapses following the single-drug treatment of these abscesses and advocate the addition of a second amebicide of the chloroquine type (0.6 g/day for 10 days). The abscess is slow to clear under this treatment, and a liver scan may show a residual area of reduced uptake even at the end of the regimen. In contrast, fever responds to the therapy within a few days and is a reliable index of the effectiveness of the treatment. Because amebas residing in the intestinal tract are unaffected by this treatment, local adjuvant therapy with nonabsorbable iodoquinol or diloxanide furoate has been advocated by some authors to prevent reinfection of the liver.

Finally, it is possible to drain hepatic abscesses surgically. Such a procedure is mandatory in large abscesses caused by pyogenic organisms, yeasts, or fungi. The indication for surgical drainage is much more limited in amebic abscess, although the patient's recovery is faster and rupture of the abscess through the diaphragm may thereby be prevented. Surgical drainage also removes the last doubt concerning the origin of a solitary lesion of the liver.

SUGGESTED READINGS

Biological Laboratories of the State Laboratory Institute, Massachusetts Department of Public Health: Hepatitis B immune globulin—prevention of hepatitis from accidental exposure among medical personnel. N. Engl. J. Med., 293:1067, 1975.

Careoda, F., et al.: Persistence of circulating HBs AG/IgM complexes in acute viral hepatitis, type B: an early marker of chronic evolution. Lancet, 2:358, 1982.

Castell, D.O., O'Brien, K.D., Muench, H., and Chalmers, T.C.: Estimation of liver size by percussion in normal individuals. Ann. Intern. Med., 70:1183, 1969.

Coury, C., et al.: Résultats de 79 biopsies hépatiques chez le tuberculeux pleuropulmonaire bacillifère non traité. Sem. Hôp. Paris, 51:169, 1975.

Fischer, J.E., and Baldessarini, R.J.: Pathogenesis and therapy of hepatic coma. Prog. Liver Dis., 5:363, 1976.

Flemma, R.J., Flint, L.M., Osterhout, S., and Shingleton, W.W.: Bacteriologic studies of biliary tract infections. Ann. Surg., 166:563, 1967.

Gazzard, B.G., et al.: Charcoal haemoperfusion in the treatment of fulminant hepatic failure. Lancet, 1:1301, 1974.

Gregory, P.B., et al.: Steroid therapy in severe viral hepatitis. A double-blind randomized trial of methylprednisolone versus placebo. N. Engl. J. Med., 294:681, 1976.

Guckian, J.C., and Perry, J.E.: Granulomatous hepatitis: an analysis of 63 cases and review of the literature. Ann. Intern. Med., 65:1081, 1966.

Hoofnagle, J.H.: Serologic markers of hepatitis B virus infection. Annu. Rev. Med., 32:1, 1981.

Krugman, S.: The newly licensed hepatitis B vaccine. JAMA, 247:2012, 1982.

Linnenmann, C.C., et al.: Association of Reye's syndrome with viral infection. Lancet, 2:179, 1974.

Losowsky, M.S., and Scott, B.B.: Hepatic encephalopathy. Br. Med. J., 3:279, 1973.

Markoff, N., and Kaiser, E.: Krankheiten der Leber und der Gallenwege in der Praxis. Methodik Diagnostik, Therapie. Georg Thieme, Stuttgart, 1962.

Muller, R.: Liver flukes. In Infectious Diseases. 2nd Ed. Edited by P.D. Hoeprich. Hagerstown, MD, Harper & Row, 1977.

Prince, A.M., et al.: Hepatitis B "immune" globulin: effectiveness in prevention of dialysis-associated hepatitis. N. Engl. J. Med., 293:1063, 1975.

Redeker, A.G., et al.: Hepatitis B immune globulin as a prophylactic measure for spouses exposed to acute type B hepatitis. N. Engl. J. Med., 293:1055, 1975.

Remmer, H.: The role of the liver in drug metabolism. Am. J. Med., 49:617, 1970.

Sherlock, S.: Diseases of the Liver and Biliary System. 5th Ed. Oxford, Blackwell Scientific Publications, 1975.

Spiro, H.M.: Clinical Gastroenterology. 2nd Ed. London, Collier-Macmillan, 1977.

Walter Reed Institute of Research, United States Army Medical Research and Development Command: Prophylactic gamma globulin for prevention of endemic hepatitis: effects of US gamma globulin upon the incidence of viral hepatitis and other infectious diseases in US soldiers abroad. A cooperative study. Arch. Intern. Med., 128:723, 1971.

Zuckerman, A.J.: Specific serological diagnosis of viral hepatitis. Br. Med. J., 2:84, 1979.

CHAPTER 21

Urinary Tract Infections

J.F. Acar and F. Goldstein

> **Objective 21-1. Describe the clinical situations that call for a urinalysis and culture.**

SIGNS AND SYMPTOMS OF URINARY TRACT INFECTION

The symptoms of urinary tract infection may be grouped together into several syndromes.

Pain, when present, is generally felt in the area around the urinary tract. It is either suprapubic or retropubic, experienced during or immediately after urination, and is accompanied by burning on urination. The patient may also have continuous discomfort characterized by pelvic heaviness, unilateral lumbar pains with strain, or heaviness increased by palpation between both hands, or a paroxysmal type of pain such as occurs in renal colic.

Symptoms of disorders of micturition in particular include urgency and frequency of urination. Urinary incontinence may also be observed in children and in the aged, or acute urinary retention may occur, especially when an obstructive element exists, as in prostatitis.

Fever, which is inconstant, usually reflects an involvement of the upper urinary system or the prostate and is uncommon in pure cystitis. Generally, one or more fever spikes are accompanied by chills, malaise, and a deterioration of the patient's general health.

The patient may also complain about the appearance of the urine, which is cloudy or bloody, malodorous, and contains mucous filaments. In this case, examination of urine is a matter of course.

Despite the range of symptoms, however, urinary tract infections are clinically asymptomatic in approximately 30% of patients. Thus, in certain patients at high risk, urinalysis and culture may be necessary even in the absence of symptoms.

URINARY TRACT INFECTION IN DIFFERENT GROUPS OF PATIENTS

Children. The incidence of urinary tract infection is well below 1% in infants, and it generally occurs in males. These infections usually are complications of urinary system malformations. In preschool and school age children, the incidence of urinary tract infections reaches 1 to 2%, with a definite female preponderance. More minor anatomic malformations may be discovered at this stage, particularly vesicoureteral reflux, but most patients simply have asymptomatic bacteriuria.

Microscopic examination of urinary sediment should be performed routinely in any patient with a fever of undetermined origin, especially in children.

Women. In adults, the female preponderance of urinary tract infection is accentuated still further, and the incidence increases with age: 1% before age 20, 6% at age 60, and over 10% at age 70, with socioeconomic variation. Symptomatic urinary tract infection is also frequent during pregnancy. It occurs in 5 to 6% of pregnant women, but reaches 25 to 50% in those who had pre-existing bacteriuria. A systematic examination of the urine is justified in this high-risk group (see Objective 24–1).

Older Men. Beginning at age 50, urinary tract infection becomes more common in men, when obstructive prostatic hypertrophy first appears. This frequency further increases with age and reaches 4% in men over 60.

Aged Individuals. In the aged, confinement to bed and other age-related changes of habit increase urinary tract infection. Based on hospital statistics, up to 40% of elderly men and women may have an asymptomatic bacteriuria.

Diabetics. Even though not all studies agree on this point, urinary tract infection may be more frequent in diabetic women than in other women; the majority of these cases are asymptomatic, although symptomatic infections are generally more severe in the diabetic.

Individuals Who Have Undergone Invasive Examination. Patients who have had a cystoscopic examination, those who have had an operation of the urinary tract, and those who have an indwelling catheter are obviously at risk of infection. The same is true when the flow of urine is obstructed, whether by hypertrophy of the prostate, renal lithiasis, malformations, neurogenic bladder, or tumors. All such patients should have their urine examined.

> **Objective 21–2.** Ensure that an adequate urine specimen is collected and is properly delivered to the laboratory.

Urine from the bladder is normally sterile, but during urination it becomes contaminated while passing through the urethra. To obtain an adequate specimen for the diagnosis of urinary tract infection, this contamination must be limited, and the multiplication of bacteria in the voided specimen must be prevented.

CLEAN-CATCH METHOD OF URINE COLLECTION

Generally, the optimal specimen is morning midstream urine collected from an individual who has not urinated for some hours. After cleaning the external genitalia with a pad soaked with nonfoaming antiseptic, followed by a careful rinsing with physiologic saline solution, the patient is instructed to allow the initial urine flow (10 to 20 ml) to escape and then to fill three-fourths full a 50- to 100-ml sterile container. In some cases, the first part of the urine stream is collected and is compared to the second portion, for example in the diagnosis of urethritis.

Suprapubic Puncture. This method is certainly the most reliable for collecting urine without contamination. It carries no major risk. Fewer than 1% of patients develop a slight hematuria, which disappears within 24 hours. This procedure is not recommended for routine office patients, however, but rather is used in the presence of unusual organisms or an abnormally low bacterial count.

The sample is taken from the recumbent patient who has not urinated for at least 4 hours. The urinary bladder must be palpable as a spherical mass. After local disinfection of the skin with an alcohol-iodine solution, the bladder is punctured from 1.5 to 2 cm superior to the symphysis pubis over the midline with a 20-ml syringe and a long intravenous or lumbar puncture needle.

Collecting Urine Specimens in Infants. The simplest method is placement of an adhesive collection bag, following a thorough cleansing of the patient's skin. Keep checking the patient to see whether he has voided, so the bag may be removed without delay. The same method may be applied in an older patient with urinary incontinence.

Collecting Urine Specimens in Patients

with Urinary Catheters. This method applies to patients with urethral or suprapubic catheters, as well as to those with a ureterostomy or a nephrostomy. The specimen is taken by puncture of the catheter, after disinfecting its surface. It is a gross error to collect the urine in the drainage bag, where bacteria have been multiplying freely for hours or days.

DELIVERY OF THE URINE SAMPLE TO THE LABORATORY

Urine constitutes an excellent culture medium for bacteria. Because the diagnosis of urinary tract infection is based on a quantitative study of the number of bacteria in the urine, the count will be overestimated if the urine has been left for several hours at room temperature. The urine must be delivered rapidly to the laboratory. Failing that, it may be kept for 2 to 4 hours at $+4°$ C without altering its bacterial count. Another alternative is to use glass slides covered with agar (Uricult system) or to halt the growth of bacteria with boric acid.

The examination provides proof of urinary tract infection and guides the physician in the choice of an antibiotic.

> **Objective 21–3. Interpret the results of the urinalysis culture.**

The urine of a normal individual contains only the bacteria cleared during passage through the urethra, generally fewer than 10^3 bacteria/ml. In most cases of urinary tract infection, the bacteria multiply within the urinary tract and produce bacteriuria of 10^5 to 10^9 bacteria/ml. Thus, a count of 10^5 bacteria/ml or more generally indicates true bacteriuria. With properly obtained specimens, the probability of a urinary tract infection is 85%

URINALYSIS

1. Direct examination is the first step of the investigation. In a matter of minutes, the physician can obtain valuable data. This method allows one to determine the presence of significant numbers of bacteria in the urine. The white blood cells can be approximated by counting the number per microscopic field or by counting them in a hemacytometer. Hematuria can be estimated by counting the number of red blood cells per microscopic field. One may determine the presence of granular, hyaline, leukocytic, or epithelial casts, not always easy to distinguish, and the presence of epithelial cells, of round cells probably of renal origin, or of abnormal cells such as multinucleated giant cells in cytomegalovirus. The existence of urate, phosphate, and other crystals can be established by direct examination of the urine.
2. Certain screening tests have been proposed for a rapid diagnosis of infection, but they are open to considerable criticism. The nitrite test (Griess's test) is only valid for bacteria that convert nitrates into nitrites, mainly the Enterobacteriaceae, not enterococci or pseudomonas; the glucose oxidase activity in the urine specimen has a low specificity.
3. Urine culture and colony count involve the isolation and approximation of the number of bacteria in the urine sample. Several techniques can be used:
    a. The reference method is the direct dilution method in which the urine is diluted repeatedly by factors of 10. This technique makes it possible to count the number of bacteria per milliliter accurately, although the procedure is time-consuming.
    b. In the semiquantitative method, a small, exact volume of urine is spread on a Petri dish with a graduated platinum loop or a graduated pipette. The urine deposited is then spread with a glass rod. After 18 hours of incubation at 37° C, each bacterium in the urine produces a colony visible to the naked eye. The initial number of bacteria in the urine is calculated by counting the number of colonies and multiplying by the dilution factor (10,000). This method is the simplest and is most commonly used.
    c. Other methods involve a dip stick or paddle or slide covered with agar (Uricult type) immersed in the urine. The paddle is incubated, and the bacteria are identified from the growth on the device. This technique eliminates growth within the urine sample that causes false results. Special media must always be used for the culture of anaerobes, mycoplasma, and chlamydia.
4. In identification and susceptibility testing, plates can be examined for growth and presumptive identification 18 hours after inoculation of the slide with bacteria. From the primary culture, the antibiotic disc sensitivity test and the biochemical identification tests are prepared. These tests can be read after 8 hours or on the following morning, that is, no more than 48 hours after the culture plates are inoculated in the laboratory.
5. For other tests, refer to Objectives 21–6 and 21–8.

with a single examination of 10^5 bacteria/ml or greater and 95% with 2 successive examinations.

Under the proper conditions of collection and delivery to the laboratory, a count of 10^5 bacteria/ml is rarely due to contamination. On the other hand, authentic infection may be accompanied by a bacteriuria of under 10^5 bacteria/ml, as in the following situations:

1. When the infection is caused by certain organisms such as enterococci, which habitually produce low bacterial concentrations in the urine.
2. When the patient has a high urine volume (due to fluids or diuretics), which reduces the concentration of bacteria, especially in lower urinary tract infections.
3. In the presence of antibiotics or urinary antiseptics, which can reduce bacteriuria to nearly zero within a few hours.
4. When a low pH inhibits multiplication of the bacteria.
5. When two urine specimens have colony counts of between 10^4 and 10^5 bacteria/ml with the same organism; this finding is as indicative of true bacteriuria as one count over 10^5 bacteria/ml.

The inflammatory response of the urinary tract mucosa or the renal parenchyma to the microbial insult is responsible for an influx of leukocytes into the urine. A urine white cell count of 10,000/ml or 2 leukocytes per high-power field (centrifuged urine) can be considered abnormal. The results are often semiquantitated as $1+$, $2+$, and $3+$; however, counting the actual number of leukocytes per high-power field is usually preferred.

Pyuria does not occur in 10 to 15% of urinary tract infections. On the other hand, pyuria may be seen even when no bacteria is detectable by conventional means, as in urethritis, prostitis, urogenital tuberculosis, tumors of the genitourinary system, migrating renal calculi, and in certain cases of nephritis. This phenomenon may also be observed during analgesic nephrotoxicity, Legionnaires' disease, or in severely dehydrated patients.

> **Objective 21-4.** Identify the cause of a symptomatic urinary tract infection when no significant bacteriuria is present.

Some individuals have a symptomatic urinary tract infection without a significant urine bacterial colony count. Various possibilities must be considered.

Urethral Syndrome. A urethral syndrome generally occurs in a young woman without a history of urinary infection. Some consider the disorder to be the female equivalent of nongonococcic urethritis in men. The patient consults the physician because of frequent and burning urination as though she had cystitis. Fewer than 10^5 organisms/ml urine are found, and the patient's urine white cell count is often $\leq 10^4$ WBC/ml. The clinical examination must exclude vaginitis, vulval irritation, and genital herpes. The urethral syndrome is felt to be caused by *Chlamydia trachomatis*, which can be identified by tissue culture or serologic tests, such as indirect immunofluorescence. Possibly, *Ureaplasma urealyticum* is incriminated. Such forms of urethritis, without penile discharge, are seen in men and likely have a similar origin.

Suppressed Infections. A single dose of antibiotic is usually sufficient to sterilize the urine temporarily. Therefore, physicians must make certain that the urine is collected before the therapy is administered. They should also be alert to the possibility of self-medication or of antibiotics prescribed for other purposes, for example, tetracycline prescribed for acne.

Genitourinary Tuberculosis. When a patient has pyuria, and urine cultures are negative, the physician should look for mycobacteria by urine culture.

Obstruction. That urinary tract obstruction sometimes prevents the appearance of bacteriuria should be kept in mind in patients with severe upper urinary tract infections, especially with fever, toxicity, and exquisite lumbar pain. Intravenous pyelography reveals a silent kidney. Urinary obstruction is

ESCHERICHIA COLI

This bacterium is the most common organism in urinary tract infections. Because it accounts for more than 90% of the commensal aerobic flora of the gastrointestinal tract, it is frequent in the perianal and perineal areas. *E. coli* is a motile, gram-negative bacillus with an average size of 4 × 1.2 µ. It can be cultured easily between 30 and 42° C, with an optimum temperature of 37° C. After 18 hours on nutrient agar, the bacterium produces opalescent, round, and smooth colonies about 3 to 5 mm in diameter. Certain strains produce more mucoid colonies. Each colony, grown from a single bacterium, consists of an aggregate of approximately 10^{10} bacteria. In a nutrient broth, *E. coli* produces a homogeneous turbidity, starting on the third hour of the culture and reaching a maximum density of 10^9 bacteria/ml in about 6 hours.

The identification of *Escherichia coli* is simple and is based on biochemical positive characteristics such as fermenting lactose and, most particularly, indole production, as well as characteristics common to all the Enterobacteriaceae, for example, glucose fermentation with production of gas, absence of oxidase, and facultative anaerobic metabolism. Various selective media are used for identifying and isolating *E. coli* colonies. These media usually contain lactose with an indicator dye for detecting lactose-positive colonies and various substances to inhibit the growth of cocci, gram-positive rods, and fungi. The culture medium most commonly used today is MacConkey's medium.

Escherichia coli has a bacterial wall, a capsule, and flagella, all three of which are antigenic. The O or somatic antigen (Ag) is part of a complex molecule whose lipid portion is the endotoxin. One can use 157 different O Ag for serotyping. In addition, 52 different types of H or flagellar Ag are seen, but they do not occur consistently and may even be lacking in motile bacteria. The K or capsular Ag is composed of the A, B, and L Ag of the capsule; 93 different types are seen. This K Ag is of interest because its presence has been associated with certain disorders. Thus, K Ag has been demonstrated in 84% of all cases of neonatal *E. coli* meningitis and in 39% of *E. coli* pyelonephritis. The antigen cross-reacts with type B meningococcus and, in some cases, with type B *Haemophilus influenzae* (K_{100} Ag) and serotype 3 pneumococcus (K_7 Ag).

In addition to flagella, *Escherichia coli* has filaments called pili or fimbriae that play an important role in the adhesion of the bacterium to certain human cells with specific receptors. In certain experimental models that make it possible to study these properties of adhesion, two types of adhesive surface structures can be distinguished through D-mannose inhibition; the mannose-resistant sites are the most important for the attachment of *E. coli* to human urinary epithelial cells.

Recent studies have shown that coliform bacilli isolated from symptomatic, as opposed to asymptomatic, acute urinary tract infections have two or more of the following virulence factors: K A, lipopolysaccharide (complete O A), mannose-resistant or mannose-sensitive adhesion, resistance to the bactericidal effect of serum, and production of hemolysin.

KLEBSIELLA

Klebsiella inhabits the digestive tract of the normal host and represents under 5% of the aerobic flora. The bacterium secretes a beta-lactamase that hydrolyzes all degradable penicillins, such as penicillin G, ampicillin, and carbenicillin, and is often seen in the superinfecting flora of the oropharynx of patients taking penicillin.

Klebsiella pneumoniae is a gram-negative, nonmotile rod belonging to the Enterobacteriaceae, of which it shares all the characteristics. The bacterium, about 2 to 6 µ long and 1 µ across, has a pronounced bipolar Gram staining. It grows readily on all usual bacteriologic media, and after 18 hours of culture produces colonies approximately 4 to 6 mm in diameter, larger and more opaque than those of *Escherichia coli* and often liquid or mucoid. The organism can be identified easily in 18 hours by fermentation with production of the gas of most carbohydrates; the basic reactions are a positive Voges-Proskauer test, a positive lysine decarboxylase test, the presence of a slow urease, and growth on Simmons's citrate agar.

Eight principal biotypes of klebsiella have been identified, with a few subgroups. A particularly frequent biotype is *Klebsiella pneumoniae*, var. *oxytoca*. Other species closely related to *K. pneumoniae* and less frequently encountered are *K. ozaenae* and *K. rhinoscleromatis*. The capsule of *K. pneumoniae* is much thicker than that of *Escherichia coli*; it is a mucopolysaccharide capsule that seems to play an important role in the virulence of the bacterium, as with other encapsulated bacteria such as pneumococci, meningococci or *Haemophilus influenzae*. The 80 different capsular antigens currently known constitute the basis for an epidemiologic classification of the various serotypes.

---

an emergency and often calls for immediate surgical intervention.

Renal Abscesses. Abscesses or carbuncles of the kidney complicate some cases of pyelonephritis or are secondary to septicemia, particularly of staphylococcal origin. Sometimes, these abscesses are not accompanied by bacteriuria. Clinically, both fever and lumbar pain are present. Confirmation of the diagnosis is often difficult. Intravenous pyelography is not usually helpful, but radioactive isotope studies, gallium scans, in particular, may provide more information.

Urinary Tract Schistosomiasis. This dis-

PROTEUS

The genus proteus includes different species, such as *Proteus mirabilis* and *P. vulgaris*, closely related to the morganella-providencia group of bacteria. Proteus species, which also belong to the Enterobacteriaceae, are thin, gram-negative bacilli, 0.5 μ wide and variable in length. Their biochemical identification is simple because of the presence of a tryptophan desaminase characteristic to this group and a rapid urease production (not present in providencia).

Proteus and related species are saprophytes in the gastrointestinal tract and represent about 5% of the aerobic flora. They are often part of the superinfecting flora in hospitalized patients. *Providencia rettgeri, Stuartii* and *Morganella Morganii*, which are generally resistant to antibiotics, are often found in hospital-acquired superinfections.

Proteus infections are frequently associated with staghorn calculi (Fig. 21–1). The alkalinization of urine during proteus infections, along with their active urease production, promotes the formation of calculi. Other organisms are also associated with renal calculi, however.

Proteus species are motile and swarm over the culture media. This property gives certain species, such as *Proteus mirabilis* and *P. vulgaris*, a characteristic appearance. Over 100 O and H antigens of proteus are known; therefore, serotyping is not common. Proteus cross-reacts, sometimes to an extreme, with certain other microorganisms. Thus, in some rickettsial diseases, the serum of the patient agglutinates a strain of proteus OX 19 or OXK or OX2 (Weil-Felix reaction).

GROUP D STREPTOCOCCUS (ENTEROCOCCI)

Enterococci are streptococci belonging to group D. These small, nonmotile, gram-positive cocci are approximately 0.6 μ in diameter, are ovoid in shape, and occur in short chains. They possess no catalase or oxidase. These bacteria grow preferentially on blood agar, but they can grow on MacConkey's medium. Enterococci are tolerant bacteria that can grow in a 5% saline solution and at temperatures of up to 45° C. These cocci colonize the gastrointestinal tract, urethra, skin, and mucous membranes. They characteristically produce urinary tract infections with low bacterial colony counts. Certain enterococci produce a beta hemolysis on blood agar, owing to a hemolysin coded by a plasmid.

OTHER ORGANISMS THAT CAUSE URINARY TRACT INFECTIONS

ENTEROBACTER

Biochemically and morphologically, these bacteria are similar to klebsiella, but they are motile. Enterobacter species produce a potent beta-lactamase that attacks first- and second- and to some extent third-generation cephalosporins.

SERRATIA

Serratia marcescens is morphologically and biochemically similar to Enterobacter. Serratia is identified by the presence of DNase and a lysine and ornithine decarboxylase and, infrequently in clinical specimens, a red pigment and a characteristic heterogenous resistance to colistin. These bacteria, found in hospital-acquired infections, especially in urologic wards and intensive care units, have a natural or readily acquired resistance to many antibiotics. This resistance accounts for the spread of serratia within hospitals. Of serratia antigens, 14 O A and 12 H A have been identified, and on that basis the bacteria can be studied epidemiologically.

CITROBACTER

Citrobacter is morphologically closely related to *Escherichia coli* and has biochemical and antigenic characteristics that resemble those of salmonella. These similarities frequently cause confusion. Citrobacter species differ from salmonella in that they possess a galactosidase, but no lysine decarboxylase. Two important clinical varieties are known: *C. freundii*, which produces H_2S, and *C. diversus*, which produces indole and occurs in the same clinical situations as *E. coli*. Citrobacter is generally a saprophyte in the gastrointestinal tract, but it is sometimes responsible for urinary tract infections and hospital-acquired superinfections as well.

order, common in Africa, also produces pyuria without bacteria. It is confirmed by identifying *Schistosoma haematobium* ova in freshly voided urine.

Viral Cystitis. In most viral diseases with fever, urine protein levels and the number of white blood cells may increase without any functional sign. In children, however, hemorrhagic cystitis is related to certain adenovirus serotypes.

Disorders in Young Women. Two syndromes may be mistaken for urinary tract in-

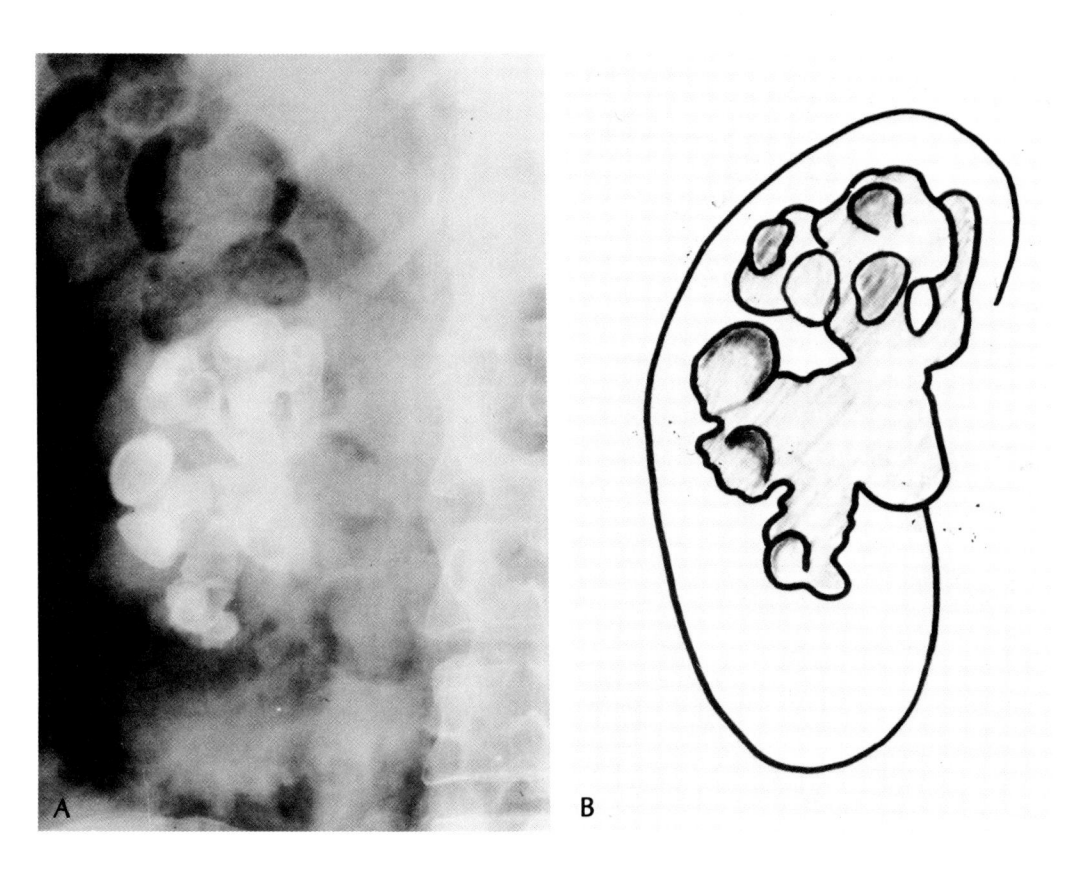

Fig. 21-1. Urinary infection with *Proteus mirabilis* showing calyceal lithiasis. A large kidney stone fills all the pyelocalyceal cavities on this plain roentgenogram. *B*, Schematic view.

fection. One of them, pelvic inflammatory disease, is characterized by severe lower abdominal or pelvic pain, sometimes associated with urinary frequency and pain on urination, and calls for a full pelvic examination and a detailed medical history. The other is the premenstrual syndrome, which is accompanied by less-severe pelvic complaints and is related to the onset of menses. These two syndromes may alternate with genuine urinary tract infections and may confuse both the patient and the physician.

Other Causes of Urinary Tract Infection Without Bacteriuria. Finally, symptoms of urinary tract infection without significant bacteriuria can be observed in patients with renal lithiasis and tumors of the urinary tract. Diabetes mellitus and diuretic treatments are, of course, also accompanied by frequency of urination. The use of "feminine hygiene" sprays can cause burning urination.

> **Objective 21–5. Diagnose a simple cystitis on the basis of laboratory and clinical data.**

An infection exclusively involving the lower urinary tract, a simple cystitis, affects approximately 5% of sexually active women. Cystitis has a tendency to relapse, but it is benign. Because upper urinary tract infections often mimic cystitis, it is important to rule out other possible causes of the symptoms.

The clinical signs and symptoms of cystitis vary in intensity from one patient to another. The patient's temperature and other clinical findings are usually normal. Examination of the urine confirms the infection, which is usually due to *Escherichia coli*. Before accepting the diagnosis of simple cystitis, however, one must ensure that the patient's urinary tract is anatomically sound and the urinary bladder is really the source of the infection. The test for antibody-coated bacteria should be negative, and the patient's bacteriolytic response to therapy should be prompt and sustained. In women, intravenous pyelography is generally not recommended even for a second episode of cystitis, whereas in men, in whom simple cystitis is unusual, the procedure may be considered immediately. Because the incidence of reinfection is high, a follow-up urinalysis should be scheduled just after the end of the treatment, to ensure that the urine is sterile, and again several weeks later.

Relapsing cystitis in young women or in the elderly of both sexes must be distinguished from chronic pyelonephritis. Generally, pyelonephritis reveals itself by bacteriologic relapses with the same strain after the cessation of therapy, whereas urine remains sterile in cystitis for a prolonged period. True relapsing cystitis is often caused by sexual activity ("honeymoon cystitis") and poses difficult therapeutic problems (see Objective 21–11). The long-term prognosis remains good, however, with a few reservations. During pregnancy, women with relapsing cystitis are at high risk of developing pyelonephritis and must be observed carefully and treated promptly.

> **Objective 21–6. Recognize prostatitis.**

Although urinary tract infection in young women is often considered commonplace, the incidence of urinary tract infections in men is not comparable. Infection in males is usually related to an anatomic obstruction: a posterior urethral valve in infants and prostatic hypertrophy in older men. Prostatitis is an important cause of infection. One can distinguish four different entities. Acute bacterial prostatitis, which has obvious symptoms and systemic involvement, is due to the organisms responsible for other urinary tract infections, such as *Escherichia coli* and klebsiella (Table 21–1). Chronic bacterial prostatitis is caused by these same agents and is responsible for recurrent urinary tract infections. Between episodes of urinary tract infection, the patient is usually asymptomatic. The diagnosis of nonbacterial prostatitis is made when the expressed prostatic secretion (EPS) reveals an intense inflam-

Table 21–1. Relative Frequency of Bacteria Responsible for Urinary Tract Infections

Bacteria	First episode or distant reinfection	Recurring infection (closely spaced episodes)	Postoperative or catheterized patients (nosocomial infection)
Escherichia coli	84	75*	20†
Proteus mirabilis	7	—	—
Proteus mirabilis and other related species	—	7	20
Group D streptococcus (enterococcus)	5	5	—
Klebsiella	2	8	35
Staphylococcus epidermidis	1	—	—
Serratia	—	—	8
Enterobacter	—	—	10
Pseudomonas aeruginosa	—	—	4
Other bacteria	1	5	3

*Often resistant to 3 antibiotics
†Resistant to more than 3 antibiotics

matory reaction and the diagnosis of a bacterial prostatitis has been excluded. Prostatodynia is prostatic pain without inflammation.

CLINICAL MANIFESTATIONS OF PROSTATITIS

The diagnosis of prostatitis is easy to suspect, but in older adults, difficult to confirm. The diagnosis should be considered in any young man who has symptoms suggestive of a urinary tract infection. More specifically, the diagnosis is indicated by symptoms of painful urination, pelvic pain characterized by perineal heaviness and often intensified by defecation, and, occasionally, high fever, chills, toxicity, and retroscrotal pain.

On rectal examination, the prostate is typically exquisitely painful, enlarged, and boggy, but prostatitic tenderness may be minimal or absent in patients with chronic cases.

Prostatic infection can also complicate a pre-existing disorder, such as benign hypertrophy or cancer of the prostate, although it usually appears without apparent antecedent.

DIAGNOSTIC TESTS FOR PROSTATITIS

In acute prostatitis, microscopic examination of the urinary sediment and urine culture support the diagnosis by the presence of a frank leukocyturia and, in half the patients, by a bacteriuria of 10^5 bacteria/ml. In difficult cases, unless pain is an obstacle, one should culture prostatic secretions following massage of the prostate, in particular with the Stamey maneuver.

The test for bacteria-coating antibodies by indirect immunofluorescence is positive. Voiding urethrography during intravenous pyelography or after bladder puncture makes it possible to study the morphologic features of the posterior urethra and to observe any lesions present in the bladder. Direct puncture of the prostate, sometimes advocated, is difficult to perform. Retrograde catheterization and radiologic examinations should be proscribed because of the risks of injury and dissemination of infection.

Objective 21–7. Diagnose an acute pyelonephritis.

Acute pyelonephritis (Fig. 21–2) is a bacterial inflammation of both the renal parenchyma and the renal pelvis. It usually follows an ascending infection, though a hematogenous origin is not impossible. This disorder is most serious when it complicates a renal obstructive disease. The onset of acute pyelonephritis is usually sudden, and the patient seeks medical attention early for lumbar pain and fever. The characteristic pain is usually

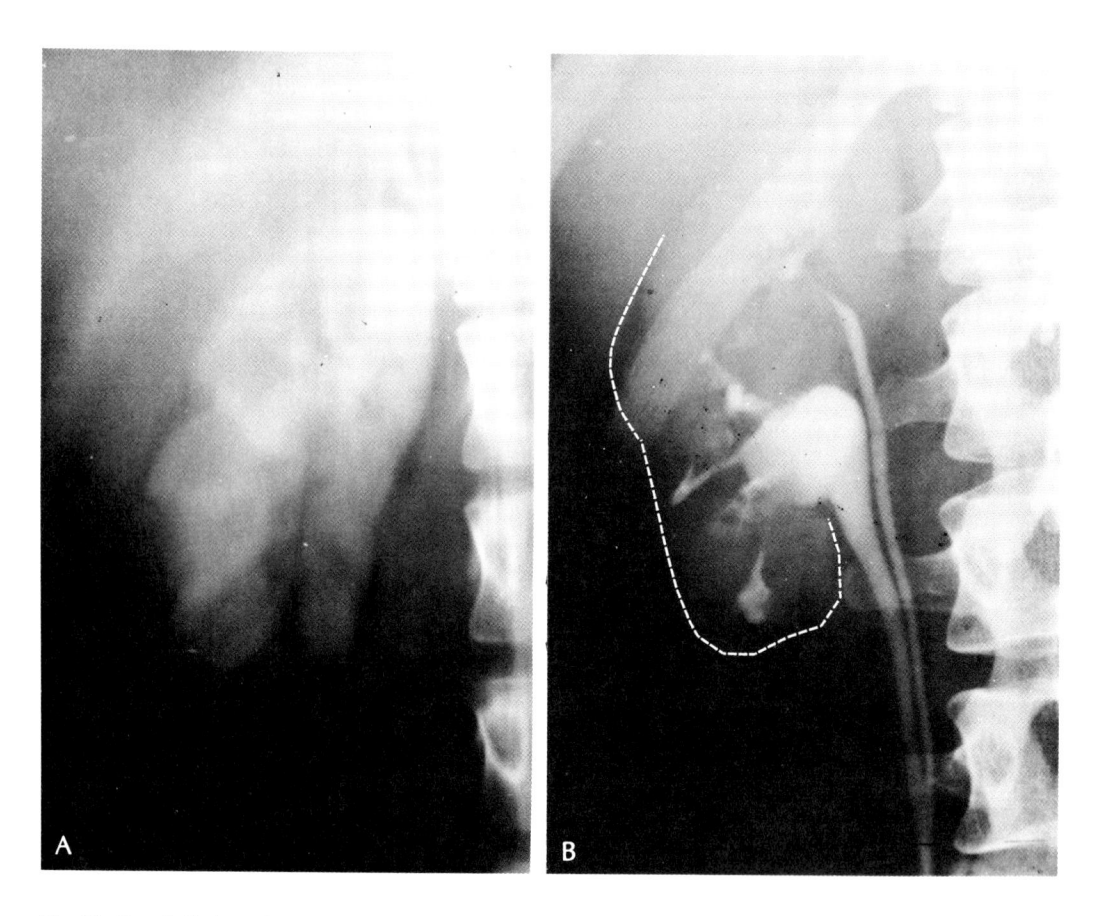

Fig. 21–2. *A,* Early nephrotomography during an intravenous urogram. The kidney is small with irregular contours interrupted by two deep notches. *B,* Same patient 10 minutes after injection of the contrast medium. The inferior calyx is convex and borders the cortical region.

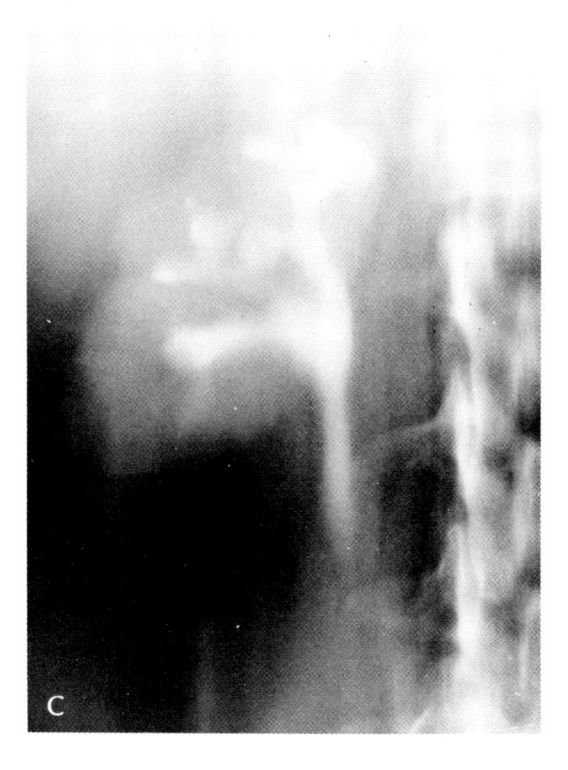

Fig. 21–2. C, Pyelonephritis; note the irregular thinning of the cortical substance and the ball-shaped calyces.

unilateral with a descending radiation, although atypical localizations, bilateral involvement, or even absence of pain are possible. An elevated, fluctuating fever, shaking, chills, malaise, and toxicity suggest an associated septicemia.

The physical examination reveals a painful costovertebrae angle or lumbar fossa. One rarely finds an enlarged kidney on palpation, but local guarding is often noted. The patient may have a past history of renal infection or disease, previous symptoms or signs of lower urinary involvement, or a contributing factor such as pregnancy. Direct microscopic examination of the urine, however, usually provides important objective evidence in the form of large numbers of bacteria, pyuria with clumps of white blood cells, and granular and white blood cell casts. Provided the urine culture is taken before the start of therapy, the culture confirms the bacteriuria the next day and makes it possible to identify the organism and to determine its antibiotic susceptibility. The blood culture is frequently positive in severely ill patients.

Antibody-coated bacteria, present in 88% of patients with acute pyelonephritis, usually indicate an exacerbation of chronic pyelonephritis. Conversely, in an initial episode of acute pyelonephritis, for example in a pregnant woman, the search for antibody-coated bacteria may be negative, probably because of the short duration of the infection. In experimental pyelonephritis in the rabbit, it takes 8 to 21 days to detect the presence of antibody-coated bacteria. Recent studies of the biochemical approach to the diagnosis of acute pyelonephritis have been encouraging. The urinary levels of C-reactive protein, $beta_2$-microglobulin, and S-lactate dehydrogenase appear to be elevated in acute pyelonephritis.

The broad differential diagnosis includes many other diseases such as cholecystitis, appendicitis, salpingitis, perinephric abscess, and perirenal hematoma. Most important, urinary obstruction must be ruled out immediately. The physician must keep in mind that an obstruction and an infection may coexist and may increase the risk to the patient. Whenever the slightest suspicion of obstruction exists, and when no contraindication, such as pregnancy, prevents it, an emergency intravenous pyelogram should be requested.

Antibiotic treatment should begin immediately after cultures are taken (see Objectives 21–10 and 21–11).

> Objective 21–8. Recognize a chronic pyelonephritis in a patient with persistent bacteriuria.

The diagnosis of chronic pyelonephritis is difficult but important. It is difficult because full convincing evidence is usually lacking, and important because of the lengthy treatment, the low rate of success, and the danger of chronic renal insufficiency.

Histologically, chronic pyelonephritis is characterized by interstitial lesions with radial bands of injured tissue running from cortex to medulla and alternating with healthier tissue. An inflammatory infiltrate with mononuclear cells and a destructive sclerosis are seen in the affected areas. These abnormalities are also observed in interstitial nephritis, with various lesions of vascular or congenital origin, in which an infectious factor is not involved. This nonspecificity makes pathologic study difficult.

Frequently, a persistent or relapsing bacteriuria, such as following acute pyelonephritis, draws the physician's attention. Episodes of acute pyelonephritis may complicate the otherwise silent course of chronic pyelonephritis, and they often constitute the first sign of the chronic disorder. The patient's medical history thus becomes valuable evidence.

Specific symptoms are few or are lacking, and the patient's general health is not impaired, unless significant renal failure has already occurred. In some patients, the disease produces polyuria with polydipsia (a sign of renal tubular disorder) or hypertension. This silent disease may, however, become fulminant and may rapidly destroy renal function.

DIAGNOSIS OF CHRONIC PYELONEPHRITIS

The diagnosis is confirmed by many tests. That these tests are so numerous is an indication that their interpretation is difficult. Several diagnostic clues exist, as follows:

1. The Same Bacteria Persist Despite Treatment. Previously (Objective 21–5), we saw that relapsing cystitis is generally due to reinfection; therefore, in each episode, the organism ought to be different each time. In chronic pyelonephritis, however, the same organism, in terms both of biotype and usually of antibiotic sensitivity, persists. This organism can be verified by means of precise biochemical identification and serologic typing. The identity of two bacteria cannot be stated with absolute certainty, however; the only possible certainty is that of a difference. Another difficulty arises because the antibiotic susceptibility pattern of a specific bacterium can change with time.

2. The Bacteria Originate in the Kidney. Pyelonephritis can be suspected from the presence of white blood cell casts and round cells (probably renal), a high urine white cell count (more than 5 per high-power field), and a marked proteinuria, although these findings are not entirely specific.

An upper urinary tract origin may be demonstrated by catheterizing the ureters, but the dangers of infection often make this procedure unpractical, and several expedients have been suggested to obtain similar information with less risk. Lavage of the bladder consists of placing a catheter in the bladder and establishing the basal bacterial count. The bladder is then filled for 30 to 45 minutes with a saline solution containing an aminoglycoside to which the bacteria are susceptible. After rinsing, serial urine cultures are performed every 10 minutes; in lower urinary tract infection, bacteriuria disappears, but it persists when the kidney is infected. Unfortunately, aberrant results are seen, and bladder catheterization carries its usual risks and disadvantages.

The bacterial count during water loading, for example, 200 ml water orally, then 1000 ml/hr intravenously for 3 hours, has been proposed as a diagnostic procedure. Theoretically, the bacterial count could be reduced in cystitis, whereas in pyelonephritis, bacteriuria increases up to a maximum (diuresis apparently mobilizes the intrarenal microorganisms) before decreasing slowly. In this situation also, possible errors limit the significance of the test.

Positive blood cultures during an acute episode of urinary tract infection definitely suggest pyelonephritis because bacteria from urinary infections spread into the blood only under specific circumstances, including urinary instrumentation or other surgical procedures, acute prostatic abscess, obstructive uropathies, and pyelonephritis. Blood cultures are normally negative in lower urinary tract infections such as cystitis.

3. The Bacteria Produce an Immune Response. Broadly speaking, during cystitis, the infection does not cross the mucosa, but remains superficial, outside the parenchyma, and does not trigger the usual immune response. In contrast, the interstitial involvement of pyelonephritis does elicit an immune response, and this reaction can be of some help diagnostically. The physician can look for urinary bacteria coated with antibodies. The sediment should be washed thoroughly and spread on a slide. A human antiglobulin antibody conjugated with fluorescein is placed on the slide. When the bacteria are covered with host antibodies, the antiglobulin attaches itself; when the slide is rinsed, the bound antiglobulin fluoresces on microscopic examination under ultraviolet light. Several studies have shown a correlation between this technique and the results of bladder lavage and ureteral catheterization. The interpretation is not that simple. Other tissue infections such as prostatitis can also give positive test results.

A determination of the urinary IgG is perhaps simpler because pyelonephritis is often accompanied by high levels of urinary IgG. The search in the patient's blood for serum antibodies to the microorganism found in the urine is an attractive idea, but is not currently practiced.

Pyelography can be a key diagnostic technique when one of the patient's kidneys is severely infected. Typically, the pyelogram shows a small kidney whose contour has a dented appearance. The cortex is thin; the calyces are dilated, with a loss of their usual pattern and a ballooning out of their usual flower shape. Actually, such roentgenographic pictures are seldom seen, and other renal disorders, such as obstructive disease or noninfectious interstitial nephropathies, can give a similar picture. A frequent error is to label all such findings, too readily, as chronic pyelonephritis.

Renal functional impairment is a late sign indicative of other complications. The urine-concentrating ability is the first to be reduced. When the blood creatinine and urea levels become elevated, the disease is already advanced. Hyponatremia due to the loss of sodium in the urine and hyperchloremic acidosis may be observed; they are signs of tubular and interstitial involvement, which are unusual in the other forms of renal insufficiency.

4. Underlying Contributing Factors Exist. Chronic pyelonephritis is often secondary to a local or systemic disease. The contributing factors are innumerable, but they usually involve obstruction or severe vesicoureteral reflux. Noninfectious interstitial nephritis, for example caused by phenacetin, is also said to facilitate infection. Diabetes is felt to worsen the progression of the disease, but not to increase its incidence.

From the foregoing, the reader will understand that this diagnosis is difficult to confirm. One should remember that chronic pyelonephritis is infrequent in young adults and evolves slowly. If any doubt exists, it is better to keep the patient under observation for some months with repeated urine examinations than to undertake a long, costly, and irrelevant treatment.

> **Objective 21–9. Confirm the diagnosis of urinary tuberculosis.**

Urinary tuberculosis is now a rare disease, but it should be considered in a number of circumstances. The disease begins in one kidney and, if diagnosed early, is easy to treat and to cure before it spreads to the entire urinary tract and the genital organs.

The initial manifestation of urinary tuberculosis may be as a refractory cystitis without bacteriuria and accompanied by persistent pyuria, hematuria, proteinuria. The disease may also be diagnosed during a routine examination of a patient with no apparent impairment of general health. In men, it may produce epididymitis or prostatic involvement, whereas in a women it may cause sterility, endometritis, metrorrhagia, or even peritoneal spread with ascites.

DIAGNOSTIC TESTS

The diagnosis of urinary tuberculosis can be confirmed by bacteriologic, roentgenographic, and histologic means.

Culture. Bacteriologically, *Mycobacterium tuberculosis* can be cultured from three successive morning urine samples.

Direct examination can be performed on the centrifuged sediment of about 10 ml urine. One should search for the acid-fast bacilli, either after staining by the Ziehl-Neelsen method or, more conveniently, by fluorescence in ultraviolet light after auramine staining. The results may be deceiving because it requires the presence in the urine of large numbers of *Mycobacteria tuberculosis* organisms, and such is rarely the case. Furthermore, contamination by saprophytic mycobacteria often results in a false-positive result. The first suspicious colonies appear around the fourteenth day and become characteristic in 3 weeks. Inoculation to the guinea pig is obsolete as a diagnostic method.

Radiography. Intravenous pyelography is often the technique by which the disease is discovered in asymptomatic patients. The first lesion observed in tuberculosis of the kidney is the constriction of the calyceal neck, whose contours become indistinct. Later, these contours become distended and are transformed into an irregular cavity that may no longer be visible because it is filled with caseous material. When the neck of the renal pelvis narrows (Fig. 21–3), the entire group of calyces dilates and produces a daisy-like appearance. Still later, all the calyces lose their shape, and the picture resembles hydronephrosis. Finally, in old, untreated infections, pus in the different cavities becomes calcified, to give a characteristic picture called putty kidney. When the infection spreads to the ureter, it produces a series of strictures with proximal dilation that have a beaded appearance; the borders are irregular, with a sawtooth edge.

In contrast, involvement of the urinary bladder is most often radiologically undetectable. Occasionally, in advanced cases, such involvement is evidenced by an irregular mucosal outline, with a reduced capacity of the bladder and reflux into the contralateral ureter as yet uninfected. Again, in advanced cases of urinary tuberculosis seldom seen today, fistulization into the intestine or retroperitoneal cavity with abscess formation may be observed.

Needle Biopsy. Biopsy of the tuberculous kidney is rarely performed because of the risk of secondary fistulization. The procedure is indicated only when a strong clinical suspicion of tuberculosis exists and when radiologic and bacteriologic studies fail to produce the expected evidence. Needle biopsy can be performed either transcutaneously or during an exploratory laparotomy. The diagnosis of renal tuberculosis is confirmed by the presence of a granuloma consisting of epithelioid cells and giant cells (see Fig. 8–6), occasionally with central caseous necrosis. Ziehl-Neelsen staining can demonstrate acid-fast bacilli at the center of the granuloma, but because of the limited number of organisms

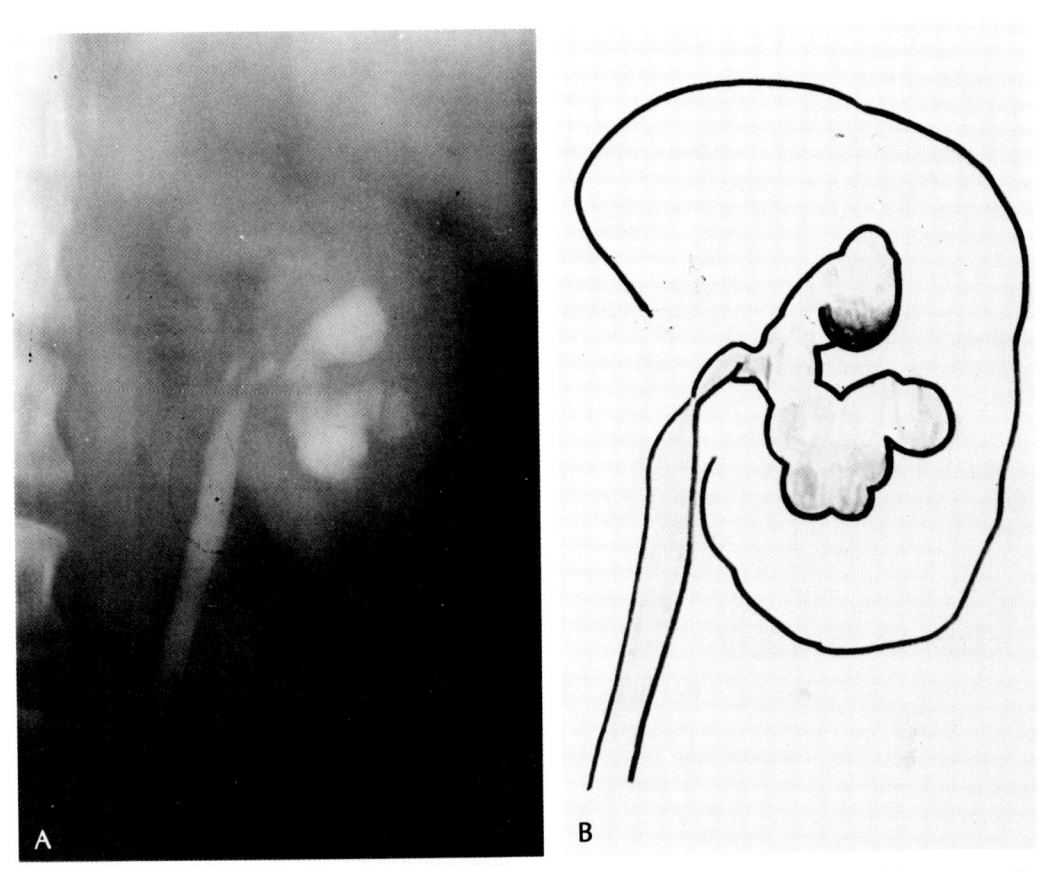

Fig. 21–3. *A*, Renal tuberculosis as seen by intravenous urography. The neck of the renal pelvis is narrowed, the medial and inferior calyces are distended, and the stem of the upper calyces is amputated. *B*, Schematic view.

in the granuloma and the thinness of the tissue slice, these bacilli are seldom seen.

> **Objective 21–10. Outline the general principles for the treatment of urinary tract infections.**

The objectives of therapy of urinary tract infections are first to sterilize the urine and then to prevent future reinfection. Although antibiotics may eradicate bacteria, they cannot repair the underlying anatomic lesions. Even then, such agents are minimally effective when obstruction exists.

The principal antibiotics currently available are listed in Table 21–2.

Antibiotic combinations are seldom recommended in urinary infections, although they may be useful in disorders caused by *Pseudomonas aeruginosa*, in mixed infections when one single product does not cover the whole spectrum of bacteria, or in severe infections in which a synergistic combination of antibiotics may be superior in vitro.

DURATION OF TREATMENT

The duration of treatment depends on several clinical and anamnestic factors related to the disease, such as the site of the infection, associated general symptoms, lesions of the urinary tract, the immune response, underlying diseases, and the frequency of relapses.

A brief treatment lasting 3 days or even a single-dose treatment is intended for uncomplicated infections of the lower urinary tract, or asymptomatic bacteriuria (Table 21–3).

This brief treatment consists of an oral antibiotic given either in a single administration or in 1 or 2 daily doses for 3 consecutive days. In the case of a single daily dose, the antibiotic should probably be given in the evening. The advantages of this type of treatment are minimal side effects, little change in the commensal floras, and reduced cost to the patient. Treating a urinary tract infection briefly with ethically acceptable chances of success presupposes a precise selection of patients. The most appropriate type of patient for this therapy is an otherwise healthy young woman without a history of repeated urinary tract infections and with an uncomplicated infection of the lower urinary tract. In this type of infection, the brief treatment has an 80 to 90% chance of success. Of course, the patient should be monitored, with urine cultures at the end of the treatment and then a week later. This approach is useful diagnostically in that failure of therapy causes the physician to investigate the patient further.

Conventional short-term treatment ranges from 3 to 7 days and is also intended for uncomplicated lower urinary tract infections.

Treatment of 10 days and more is indicated for all patients in whom the urinary tract infection is not limited to the bladder or in those who risk renal involvement. In an uncomplicated upper urinary tract infection, such as acute pyelonephritis, treatment for 10 to 15 days is sufficient. If an anatomic or functional obstacle to the flow of urine is present, or in the case of chronic pyelonephritis or prostatitis, treatment should last much longer, perhaps 2 to 4 months.

Prophylactic treatment is considered in patients with recurrent infections.

GENERAL MEASURES

The patient's intake of fluids should be increased because dilution of the urine and frequent voiding promote sterilization of the urine. Various dietary regimens have not proved their value, but proper hygiene is useful.

> **Objective 21–11. Treat the various types of urinary tract infection.**

CYSTITIS IN YOUNG WOMEN

Simple cystitis in a healthy young woman is the only type of urinary tract infection for which treatment may be initiated without waiting for the results of antibiotic sensitivity tests. The offending organism is *Escherichia coli* in most cases. The treatment is of short duration, from 3 to 5 days, administered or-

Table 21-2. Principal Antimicrobial Agents in the Treatment of a Urinary Tract Infection

Drug	Route of administration	Daily dose*	Comments and Indications
Ampicillin	Oral	1–2 g	Broad indications; risk of selection and superinfection by resistant bacteria, particularly klebsiella
Amoxicillin	Oral	1–2 g	Similar to oral ampicillin (see above)
Penicillin G	IM	2–4 million U	Indicated for streptococcal urinary tract infections
Carbenicillin			Second-line drug in infections caused by Enterobacteriaceae resistant to ampicillin and cephalosporins, i.e., Pseudomonas infections, in combination with aminoglycosides
Asymptomatic and mild infections	IV	9–15 g	
Serious infections with septicemia	IV	20–30 g	
Ticarcillin	IV	10–20 g	Same indications as carbenicillin
Azlocillin, mezlocillin and piperacillin	IM/IV	5–10 g	Same indications as carbenicillin
Cephalexin Cephradine	Oral	1–3 g	Sometimes indicated for lower urinary tract infections caused by Enterobacteriaceae resistant to ampicillin; weak bactericidal action
Cefazolin	IM/IV	1.5 g	Indicated for organisms resistant to ampicillin; monitoring of renal function if the product is used in combination with aminoglycosides
Cefotaxime	IM/IV	1–2 g	Active against many gram-negative bacilli
Moxalactam	IM/IV		
Cefoperazone	IM/IV	2–4 g	Active against pseudomonas and some gram-negative bacilli; indications not established yet
Gentamicin Tobramycin Netilmicin	IM	3–5 mg/kg	First-line antibiotic in *Pseudomonas aeruginosa* infections, pyelonephritis, and infections with multiple resistant strains; ototoxic and nephrotoxic
Amikacin	IM	0.5–1 g	Should be reserved for bacteria resistant to other aminoglycosides; ototoxic and nephrotoxic
Tetracycline	Oral	1–2 g	None of the tetracyclines are first-line drugs for urinary infection
Doxycycline Minocycline	Oral	200 mg	Good prostatic diffusion, justifying their use in prostatitis
Erythromycin	Oral	2–3 g	Use limited to gram-positive cocci infections and some nonfermenting gram-negative bacilli (except *Pseudomonas aeruginosa*); good prostatic diffusion; first choice in prostatitis caused by susceptible organisms
Nitrofurantoin	Oral	300–500 mg	Indicated for lower urinary tract infections and prophylaxis of recurrent urinary tract infections through short-term reinfection in normal urinary tracts; Antagonism with quinolines

Table 21-2. Continued

Drug	Route of administration	Daily dose*	Comments and Indications
Intermediate-action sulfonamides (sulfamethoxazole)	Oral	2-3 g	Indicated for lower urinary tract infections; frequent resistant strains
Trimethoprim-sulfamethoxazole	Oral	160/800 mg	Probably drug of first choice for initial therapy of lower urinary infections; broad indications as curative "changeover" or prophylactic treatment of recurring lower urinary infections through reinfection; good prostatic diffusion of trimethoprim; treatment of choice in prostatitis
Nalidixic acid	Oral	2-4 g	Not first-line broad therapeutic agents and prophylactic indications; may be combined with an aminoglycoside; high risk (about 20%) of selection for resistant strains during therapy

*For an adult whose renal function is normal.

Table 21-3. Factors Precluding Short-Term Treatment of Urinary Tract Infections

Status of the Patient	Underlying Conditions	Nature of Infection and Clinical Characteristics
Male sex	Structural abnormalities	Fever
Infancy and young childhood	Lithiasis and foreign bodies	Frequent recurrences
Old age	Kidney disease	Infecting organisms such as pseudomonas or candida
Pregnancy	Renal transplantation	Antibody-coated bacteria
	Impaired host defenses (diabetes)	Duration of more than 5 days
	Neurogenic bladder	
	Recent surgical manipulation or instrumentation	
	Bladder catheterization	

ally, and should consist of a sulfonamide or a trimethoprim-sulfamethoxazole combination. Even though the disease is benign, the physician should explain to the patient the risk of a recurrence and the measures to be taken when the current episode is over (see Objective 21-12).

ANATOMIC MALFORMATION IN YOUNG CHILDREN

In view of the problems of urine sample collection, the definitive diagnosis should be established on the basis of at least two successive specimens, without catheterization. An underlying anatomic malformation, such as a posterior urethral valve in small infants, should always be suspected, and pyelography should be performed. The type and duration of the treatment depend on the cause and on accessibility to surgical correction.

PROSTATITIS

Recent pharmacokinetic studies have demonstrated the adequate diffusion of only three groups of antibiotics in prostatitis thanks to their liposolubility:

1. Trimethoprim, alone or synergistically with sulfonamides, as in a trimethoprim-sulfamethoxazole combination, gives satisfactory prostatic levels.
2. Erythromycin and macrolides in general are reliable; the alkaline pH (7.2 to 7.8) favors the action of erythromycin.
3. Tetracyclines provide acceptable prostatic levels.

Another essential point in the treatment of prostatitis is its duration: at least 1 and often 3 months. The disease responds slowly, and relapses are frequent.

> **REQUIREMENTS FOR AN OPTIMAL URINARY ANTIBIOTIC***
>
> 1. The agent should be active against the bacterial species usually responsible for urinary tract infections.
> 2. The antibiotic must be eliminated in the urine in an active form.
> 3. Sufficiently high concentrations should be attainable in both the renal parenchyma and the urine.
> 4. The drug should be as independent as possible of the surrounding physicochemical conditions, such as pH, osmolarity, and ionic composition. In certain cases, the pH has to be changed to permit an antibiotic to exert its maximum effect: for example, alkaline pH for aminoglycosides and macrolides, acid pH for penicillins and tetracyclines.
> 5. The antibiotic should not be affected by the density of the bacteria. Certain products, such as polymyxins, and especially the antipseudomonal penicillins such as carbenicillin, lose part of their activity in the presence of a dense inoculum, as found in most urinary tract infections (generally $> 10^7$ bacteria/ml).
> 6. The agent should induce a low rate of bacterial mutations. Because of the many bacteria possibly implicated in urinary tract infections, selection of resistant mutant strains is likely, and treatment may fail. An example is rifampin.
> 7. The drug should induce the smallest possible number of resistant intestinal bacteria because most reinfestations originate from the gut.
> 8. The antibiotic should be suitable for the individuals most often exposed to urinary infections: pregnant women, older people, surgical patients, and those in renal failure. In cases of renal failure, the route of elimination has to be taken into account, and eventually, the dose must be reduced according to the degree of renal failure.

*This discussion does not include urinary antiseptics for which no reliable criterion of activity in vitro exists (quinoline derivatives, methenamine mandelate, or nitrofurantoins).

INFECTION IN ELDERLY PATIENTS

The high frequency of urinary tract infections in the aged is related to an underlying lesion of the lower or upper tract, or perhaps to a decrease in abdominal, perineal, and bladder muscle strength, and to the problem of incomplete micturition, which causes residual urine and facilitates infection. Abstention from medical therapy is usually justified, particularly in patients with asymptomatic bacteriuria. Treatment is indicated only when urinary tract signs and fever appear. Then, the decreased renal function in this age group must be taken into account, and more prolonged treatment than in younger patients should be prescribed also.

RECURRENT INFECTIONS IN WOMEN

As stated earlier, two types of relapsing infections are seen: (1) recurrences, in which the same bacterium is found during different infectious episodes; and (2) reinfections, in which each episode of infection is due to a different bacterium.

When treating reinfection, the aim is to control the present infection and to prevent further episodes. For prophylaxis, the most widely used products are nitrofurantoin or the trimethoprim-sulfamethoxazole combination, given at half the normal dose, to avoid side effects related to long-term therapy, two or three times a week, at night or after sexual intercourse. Reinfections can thus be suppressed for the duration of treatment. The disorder does reappear with unchanged frequency after the cessation of therapy, however.

ACUTE PYELONEPHRITIS

The physician's efforts are directed at controlling the infection as quickly as possible and limiting the risk of chronic pyelonephritis by means of a bactericidal agent usually administered parenterally. The most commonly used medications are ampicillin or related agents, although the risk of bacterial resistance is high. Another choice is an aminoglycoside such as gentamicin, tobramycin, or netilmicin, but care must be taken because of the nephrotoxicity of these agents. The third-generation cephalosporins (cefotaxime, etc.) look promising at this time. Therapy is later modified on the basis of the antibiotic sensitivity test results and the clinical response. The duration of treatment varies from 10 to 15 days, and as stated earlier, subsequent examinations of the urine are of particular importance.

Urinary obstruction must be completely released as rapidly as possible. Total or partial obstruction can rapidly produce severe sepsis with shock, may destroy renal function in the affected kidney, requires immediate surgical treatment, such as nephrostomy.

URETHRITIS

In a presumed chlamydial urethritis, tetracyclines for 10 to 15 days give satisfactory results. Erythromycin is an alternative and is preferred during pregnancy. As with all sexually transmitted diseases, the treatment of all partners must be considered, to avoid reinfection.

> **Objective 21–12. Follow up treatment of a urinary tract infection.**

In over 80% of patients, clinical signs of urinary tract infection regress in 24 to 48 hours, even in chronic pyelonephritis that later relapses. Effective therapy sterilizes the urine in under 8 hours. A verification culture or a urine Gram stain can be performed 24 hours after the start of therapy, to make sure that the antibiotic is producing the desired effect. If the patient's urine is not sterile in 24 hours, several possibilities may be considered: misinterpretation of antibiotic sensitivity test results, growth of a resistant mutant, poor compliance of the patient, renal failure and poor renal antibiotic levels, poor adjustment of urinary pH to the chosen antibiotic (for instance, gentamicin is notably less active at an acid pH), and the presence of a foreign body, such as a calculus or a catheter, in the excretory channel. If the organism differs from the one originally identified, one should consider the possibility of an unsuspected mixed infection, improper collection from a urine collection bag, or even superinfection.

Again, the urine is checked 3 to 5 days from the end of treatment to detect early recurrences, then 2 weeks later, and possibly 30 days later, when a recurrence is likely to be a reinfection. In cases of pyelonephritis, these examinations should extend over a longer period; for example, monthly checks for 6 months.

Pyuria in uncomplicated urinary infections disappears within 4 to 6 days of the beginning of the treatment. The persistence of an abnormal leukocyturia beyond the tenth day is abnormal and may be due to inadequate treatment, uropathy or underlying lithiasis, concomitant urethritis, or undetected urinary tuberculosis.

> **Objective 21–13. Manage a patient with a urinary catheter.**

These are most often urethral catheters, and far more rarely transvesical catheters. Despite all possible precautions, it is estimated that after 6 days, 90% of bladder catheters become infected. The risk is even greater in the case of bladder irrigation.

GUIDELINES FOR CATHETER MAINTENANCE

Strict rules should be observed in connection with the use and maintenance of a urinary bladder catheter, as follows:

1. A bladder catheter should be used only in case of absolute necessity and for the shortest possible time.
2. The catheter should be placed by trained personnel using sterile equipment.
3. The patient's urinary meatus should be cleaned with soap at least once daily.
4. The drainage system of the catheter should be kept closed and sterile; sterile techniques must be used whenever the system is opened, as for a change of bag or irrigation.
5. One must ensure proper drainage by placing the collection bag well below the level of the patient's bladder, and by verifying that the urine can flow freely.
6. Urine specimens are collected with a syringe in the initial portion of the catheter, after local disinfection with alcohol containing iodine, for example.
7. A urinary catheter should not be left in place for more than 14 days, even in the absence of overt infection.

Infection is generally caused by bacteria from the hospital floor that are usually multiply resistant; examples are *Proteus rettgeri*, serratia, *Pseudomonas aeruginosa*, enterobacter, and acinetobacter. Treatment only results in the replacement of one organism with another. As with any infected foreign body in the urinary system, sterilization of urine or cure of a urinary infection while a catheter is in place is wishful thinking and leads to a waste of antibiotics and the appearance of adverse reactions. Therapy consists of refraining from treating the patient who tolerates the catheter and the bacteria well. Only in the event of complications, such as orchiepididymitis, acute pyelonephritis, and septicemia, should treatment be undertaken. In such a case, treatment should be instituted when the catheter is changed or, better yet, removed. Of course, when the catheter has been removed, the patient should be treated with appropriate antibiotics for 14 days.

SUGGESTED READINGS

Kass, E.H.: Pyelonephritis and bacteriuria. A major problem in preventive medicine. Ann. Intern. Med., 56:46, 1962.

Kass, E.H.: Bacteriuria and diagnosis of infections of the urinary tract. Arch. Intern. Med., 100:709, 1957.

Kaye, D.: Urinary Tract Infection and Its Management. St. Louis, C.V. Mosby, 1972.

Kunin, C.M.: Duration of treatment of urinary tract infections. Am. J. Med., 71:849, 1981.

Kunin, C.M.: Detection, Prevention and Management of Urinary Tract Infection. Philadelphia, Lea & Febiger, 1972.

Platt, R., Polk, B.F., Murdock, B., and Rosner, B.: Mortality associated with nosocomial urinary tract infection. N. Engl. J. Med., 307:637, 1982.

Sanford, J.P.: Hospital acquired urinary tract infections. Am. Intern. Med., 60:903, 1964.

Stamey, T.A.: Urinary Infections. Baltimore, Williams & Wilkins, 1972.

Stamm, W.E.: Guidelines for prevention of catheter-associated urinary tract infections. Ann. Intern. Med., 82:386, 1975.

Stamm, W.E., et al.: Causes of the acute urethral syndrome in women. N. Engl. J. Med., 303:409, 1981.

Thomas, V., Shelokov, A., and Forland, M.: Antibody-coated bacteria in the urine and the site of urinary tract infection. N. Engl. J. Med., 290:588, 1974.

CHAPTER 22

Genital Infections

G. Murray, J.M. Hubrecht, P.C. Gosselin,
J. Robert, and J.C. Pechère

> **Objective 22–1.** Explain the attitude and measures for improving the epidemiologic control of venereal infections.

Even though effective diagnostic tools and treatment are available for most sexually transmitted infections, the incidence of these disorders has not decreased in most countries. Classically, many factors are mentioned in explaining this paradox, including urbanization, increased travel and immigration, and changes in sexual habits. We shall discuss other reasons that may involve the medical practitioner more directly.

RELATIONSHIP BETWEEN PATIENT AND PHYSICIAN

The physician, generally unprepared by his training and background, is too often reserved, embarrassed, or even hostile during conversations with the patient about the anxieties and symptoms related to venereal diseases.

In this dominant-dominated type of relationship, the patient is made to feel ill-at-ease because the physician often considers him unreliable and a legitimate target for moralization, even if this view is reflected only in the physician's general attitude. The procedure for single-dose "immediate" therapy, in which the patient is asked to swallow medications in front of a witness, is an eloquent illustration of the mistrust that exists. This type of consultation should be subject to the same rules that govern consultations for other disorders. The patient can be relied upon in as much as the physician has the proper attitude. In his embarrassment, the patient often conceals or glosses over the facts when describing the situation. The different details must be approached clearly, and the characteristics of the sexual practices should be specified (genitogenital, genito-oral, or genitoanal), as should be the predominant orientation (heterosexual, bisexual, or homosexual) and the number and nature of the partners. Certain microbiologic risks of transmission can then be evaluated (Table 22–1). For example, certain infections are favored by ano-oral sexual transmission; belonging to certain social groups, especially prostitutes and the gay community, can predispose a patient to particular venereal infections. This categorization is, of course, rarely possible when no mutual respect and confidence exists between the patient and the physician.

FOLLOW-UP OF INFECTED PATIENTS

The follow-up of patients with venereal disease is another key to epidemiologic control.

303

Table 22-1. Sexually Transmitted Diseases

	Microorganisms	Diseases
Bacteria	Calymmatobacterium granulomatis	Granuloma inguinale
	Chlamydia trachomatis	Urethritis, cervicitis, epididymitis, pelvic inflammatory disease, conjunctivitis, lymphogranuloma venereum, proctitis (?)
	Gardnerella vaginalis	Vaginitis
	Haemophilus ducreyi	Chancroid
	Mycoplasma hominis	Salpingitis (?), urethritis
	Neisseria gonorrhoeae	Urethritis, epididymitis, cervicitis, endometritis, salpingitis, oophoritis, pelvic inflammatory disease, peritonitis, perihepatitis, Bartholinitis, proctitis, gonococcemia, arthritis, pharyngitis, conjunctivitis
	Salmonella	Intestinal infections (fecal-oral transmission)
	Shigella	Intestinal infections (fecal-oral transmission)
	Staphylococcus aureus	Bartholinitis, urethritis (?), vulvitis
	Streptococcus (group B)	Urethritis (?), vaginitis (?)
	Treponema pallidum	Syphilis
	Ureaplasma urealyticum	Urethritis
Viruses	Cytomegalovirus	Cervicitis (?)
	Epstein-Barr virus	Infectious mononucleosis (oral-oral transmission)
	Hepatitis A virus	Hepatitis (fecal-oral transmission)
	Hepatitis B virus	Hepatitis (more frequent in some homosexual groups)
	Herpes simplex virus 1 and 2	Genital herpes
	Molluscum contagiosum virus	Molluscum contagiosum
	Papillomavirus	Condyloma
Parasites	Entamoeba histolytica	Amebiasis (fecal-oral transmission)
	Enterobius vermicularis	Oxyuriasis
	Giardia lamblia	Intestinal infection (fecal-oral transmission)
	Phthirus pubis	Pediculosis pubis ("crabs")
	Sarcoptes scabiei	Scabies
	Trichomonas vaginalis	Vaginitis, cervicitis, urethritis
Fungi	Candida albicans	Vulvovaginitis, urethritis (?)

An individual who has been treated cannot be considered free of infection or cured on the sole basis of the disappearance of the symptoms. It was formerly believed that women, in particular, had asymptomatic infections, but this risk is also shared by men; thus, 39 to 77% of males infected with *Neisseria gonorrhoeae* may be asymptomatic at some time during the course of their infection. Healthy carriers actually constitute a huge reservoir, which the lack of microbiologic follow-up continues to feed iatrogenically. This neglect contributes to the selection of bacterial strains that are less sensitive to therapy. Thus, pharyngeal gonococcal infections, often overlooked, fail to be eradicated by the "classic" therapy, particularly by spectinomycin, cefoxitin, or erythromycin. Occasionally, such as in travelers and migrants, the patient's case cannot be followed locally, and the physician should therefore ask the patient to seek another examination later. Most patients are motivated to have such a follow-up examination when they return home. In general, people are sufficiently concerned with their genital function that they usually follow such advice.

CONTACTS OF INFECTED PATIENTS

A prescription for the treatment of a sexually transmitted disease should not be an isolated measure, but rather should be accompanied by an effort to detect the patient's known sexual contacts retroactively. The possibility of back-and-forth reinfection between sexual partners is a convincing argument for the most reticent individuals. Actually, however, this type of screening is often too little and too late: instead, one should undertake a real, prospective screening in which the treated individual has a special place. He is in the best position to notify his present and potential partners and to understand not only the problems related to the infection, but also the advantages of maintaining good venereal health. The physician and other health personnel then become a support and a resource in this endeavor, which requires an open-minded approach.

Any sexually active person should submit to an adequate history of sexual contacts, particularly when the partners are anonymous and numerous and when the patient already has a previous history of venereal disease. Individuals at high risk are found especially in certain target groups, notably those who have previously been infected, that is, who are already in contact with health professionals and, it is hoped, have found the experience to be positive. Prostitution, travel, migrations, and any sexual contact with a new partner are potential risk factors. Prospective screening is most useful in these situations.

Information on certain risks, and on the use of protective measures such as condoms must be disseminated at least as rapidly as the infection itself, if not more quickly.

REPORTS TO HEALTH AUTHORITIES

Some patients wish to preserve the intimate and confidential aspect of their sexual activities. Encouraged by the physician who is annoyed by bureaucratic interference, they often ask that the case not be reported to the health authorities. Yet, these reports are one of the most useful tools for epidemiologic control. Anonymous reporting, as accepted and practiced in some countries, has not lessened the effectiveness of a prospective contact screening program; indeed, quite the contrary.

> **Objective 22–2.** Recognize and localize a female genital infection.

Female genital infections have many causes and take many forms. Reasons for consulting the physician include leukorrhea, pelvic pain, or sometimes, the search for an infection in an asymptomatic woman when venereal disease is diagnosed in one of her sexual contacts. In any event, the procedure followed by the physician is essentially the same in all three situations. First, one must localize the infection and determine its origin, to treat it properly.

PATIENT'S MEDICAL HISTORY

Women who complain of vaginal discharge, with or without pruritus or pelvic discomfort, do not necessarily have a pelvic infection. The problem may be due, for example, to vaginal atrophy or to an allergy to a "feminine hygiene" product. Some amount of vaginal discharge is even considered physiologic. Thus, symptoms have to be accurately described both qualitatively and quantitatively (Table 22–2).

The following questions are relevant to the diagnosis:

1. Are the leukorrhea and pruritus associated?
2. Is vulvovaginal burning present?
3. What is the color of the discharge?
4. Is the discharge distinctly malodorous?
5. Is the discharge sufficiently profuse to necessitate wearing a pad or changing underclothing?
6. What is the duration of the symptoms and what is their relation to the phase of the menstrual cycle (early, middle, late, during menstruation)?
7. Are urinary symptoms associated, such as frequency or burning, or intestinal symptoms, such as diarrhea and constipation?
8. Is (are) the patient's sexual partner(s) symptomatic?

The experienced physician can often make or rule out the diagnosis of an infection by the patient's medical history alone.

GYNECOLOGIC EXAMINATION

The physician looks for inguinal adenopathy, vulval and anal edema, ulceration, fis-

Table 22–2. Clinical Diagnostic Clues to Female Genital Infections

Patient's Medical History	Sexual habits, pregnancies, surgical procedures, diseases, drugs taken, pruritus, leukorrhea (color, odor, quantity, duration), pain
Gynecologic Examination	Inguinal region and lymph nodes, vulva and vagina (redness, excoriations, ulcerations, warts, condylomas, leukorrhea), cervix (inflammation, nabothian cysts, ulcerations), uterus and adnexa (size, masses, pain), anus (hemorrhoids, fissures)
Specimens	Cytologic study, microscopic examination (trichomonads, yeasts, clue cells), Thayer-Martin medium or equivalent (endocervix, urethra, anus), transport medium to laboratory

sures, and warts or condylomas. The vaginal examination follows that of the external genitalia. The speculum should be inserted without lubricant, so as not to interfere with the direct examination or the culture results. On the other hand, the speculum should be moistened with warm water to facilitate insertion. Is the leukorrhea greenish and frothy, grayish, or white, or is it curd-like and adherent to the walls of the vagina? The absence of leukorrhea could be due to a vaginal douche just prior to the examination. Is the cervix edematous, inflamed, or ulcerated?

The microbiologic and cytologic specimens should be taken at this moment, prior to the bimanual examination. This examination makes it possible to assess the size of the uterus and the presence of any tubo-ovarian mass. Are the cervix and uterus freely movable? Is the palpation painful?

By the end of the examination, an infection can generally be localized anatomically, and sometimes, its origin can be suspected on the basis of the site and the clinical appearance. Nevertheless, microbiologic support is indispensable.

Objective 22–3. Identify the cause(s) of a gynecologic infection.

Like all the other mucosal surfaces, the vagina is inhabited by multiple bacterial species. These organisms vary from one woman to the next and, in the same person, from one period to another, with age, pregnancy, menopause, and phase of the menstrual cycle. This usual endogenous flora includes bacteria without known pathogenic activity, as well as opportunistic bacteria that are not ordinarily pathogenic but may become so when local conditions favor their growth. Some bacteria, such as lactobacilli, colonize more than 75% of women during their child-bearing years. Other bacteria, found only in a small percentage of the population, in no way affect their hosts and thus are considered saprophytes (Table 22–3). *Gardnerella vaginalis* and the fungus *Candida albicans* are considered saprophytes and are classified among the organisms of the usual vaginal flora, although they may cause disease. The parasite *Trichomonas vaginalis* and the bacterium *Neisseria gonorrhoeae* are pathogens, even when they do not cause apparent disease. Thus, the presence of *Candida albicans* is not synonymous with a candidal vaginitis. Indeed, the vaginal flora must be considered an ecosystem that can be modified by many factors, such as antibiotic therapy, surgical intervention, pregnancy and delivery, hormonal therapy, foreign bodies, personal hygiene, and sexual relations.

In light of these observations, interpretation of Gram stains and cultures must take into account both the number and the types of the microorganisms found, and this information must be compared with the clinical findings (Table 22–4).

SPECIMEN COLLECTION METHODS

The accuracy of the diagnosis depends, above all, on the adequacy of the specimen. To begin with, the samples have to be taken

Table 22–3. Causes of Female Genital Infection, by Pathogenicity

1. *Saprophytes without recognized pathogenicity*
   Diphtheroides
   Lactobacillus
   Neisseria (saprophytic)
   Staphylococcus epidermidis
   Alpha-hemolytic streptococci
2. *Saprophytes with potential pathogenicity*
   Actinomyces bovis
   Bacteroides
   Candida albicans and other yeasts
   Clostridium
   Cytomegalovirus
   Escherichia coli and other Enterobacteriaceae
   Gardnerella vaginalis (formerly *Corynebacterium vaginalis*, *Haemophilus vaginalis*)
   Herpesvirus hominis
   Listeria monocytogenes
   Molluscum contagiosum virus
   Mycoplasma
   Papillomavirus
   Peptococcus and Peptostreptococcus
   Staphylococcus aureus
   Streptococcus groups B and D
3. *Exogenous organisms with high pathogenic potential*
   Calymmatobacterium granulomatis
   Chlamydia trachomatis
   Haemophilus ducreyi
   Mycobacterium tuberculosis
   Neisseria gonorrhoeae
   Treponema pallidum
   Trichomonas vaginalis

---

before the administration of any local or systemic antimicrobial therapy. In screening for gonorrhea, the best site for culture is the endocervix, although urethral and anal swabs also are recommended. The urethral culture is taken by pressing the urinary meatus against the symphysis pubis to press secretions from the small urethral glands. The anal swab is collected in the crypts above the anal verge. A pharyngeal culture may be added as well. Cotton-tipped swabs are often employed, but small alginate swabs are preferable for endourethral specimens. If disseminated gonococcemia is suspected, blood cultures are obviously necessary, and when arthritis is associated with the disorder, culture the synovial fluid may be considered. Other important causes of vaginitis, such as *Trichomonas vaginalis*, *Gardnerella vaginalis*, and *Candida albicans*, can be identified microscopically in vaginal secretions collected with a swab.

In abscesses, for example, in a Bartholin's gland abscess, it is preferable to take the specimen by puncture with a syringe, to avoid contamination with the vaginal flora and to culture properly for anaerobic organisms. Aspiration of the endometrial cavity is the best means of collecting microbes responsible for endometritis, whereas collection of menstrual blood or products of uterine curettage must be used to demonstrate *Mycobacterium tuberculosis*. Genital ulcerations, such as seen in syphilis, genital herpes, chancroid, granuloma inguinale, and lymphogranuloma venereum, are caused by agents that grow poorly, if at all, on usual culture media (Table 22–5), but microscopic examinations of the material collected by scraping the lesions is sometimes helpful.

MICROSCOPIC EXAMINATIONS

It is a good idea to examine a fresh slide of vaginal secretions before any trichomonads can lose their motility. A drop of vaginal secretions, collected in the blade of the speculum, is deposited on a slide, is mixed with a drop of physiologic saline solution, is covered with a coverslip, and then is examined under a microscope at a magnification of 10 or 40 times, with the condenser lowered for greater contrast.

Trichomonas vaginalis is a pear-shaped flagellate protozoon the size of a leukocyte. It is identified by its motility and, at the higher magnification, by its undulating membrane and flagella (Fig. 22–1).

In addition, direct examination makes it possible to detect the presence of yeasts and pseudomycelia (Fig. 22–2), as well as clue cells (defined in the following paragraph.)

Gram staining permits a rough, semiquantitative estimation of different bacterial morphologic features. Gram staining of the cervical drainage can be of prime importance in quickly diagnosing *Clostridium perfringens* endometritis. This entity, rare nowadays, represents a true gynecologic emergency, and it is simply not possible to wait for culture

Table 22–4. Associations Between Site of Infection and Microbial Causes of Female Genital Infections

Cause	Vulva and accessory glands	Anus	Urethra	Vagina	Cervix	Endometrium	Fallopian tube
Anaerobic bacteria	+	+ +	0	0	0	+ +	+ +
Calymmatobacterium granulomatis	+	0	0	0	0	0	0
Campylobacter	0	0	0	+?	0	0	0
Candida albicans	+ +	+ +	0	+ +	+	0	0
Chlamydia trachomatis	+	0	+ +	+	+ +	+	+ +
Enterobacteriaceae	+	+ +	+	+	0	+	+ +
Gardnerella vaginalis	0	0	0	+ +	0	0	+
Haemophilus ducreyi	+	+	0	+	+	0	0
Herpes simplex virus 2	+ +	0	0	+ +	+ +	0	0
Molluscum contagiosum	+	+	0	0	0	0	0
Mycobacterium tuberculosis	0	0	0	0	0	+	+
Mycoplasma	0	0	+?	0	0	+?	+?
Neisseria gonorrhoeae	+	+ +	+ +	+	+ +	+	+ +
Enterobius vermicularis	0	+ +	0	+	0	0	0
Papillomavirus	+	+	0	0	0	0	0
Phthirus pubis	+	0	0	0	0	0	0
Staphylococcus aureus	+	+	0	+	+	+	+
Streptococci	+	+	0	+	+	+ +	+ +
Treponema pallidum	+	+	0	+	+	0	0
Trichomonas vaginalis	0	0	+	+ +	+ +	0	0

0, Exceptional cause, if ever; +, possible cause; + +, frequent cause.

results. In contrast, in a case of a fulminating postpartum or postabortum endometritis, the appearance of *C. perfringens* is sufficiently characteristic on the Gram stain for a positive diagnosis to be made. Because *Gardnerella vaginalis* is a fastidious organism and is not always looked for routinely by the laboratory, the Gram stain and direct examination of the vaginal secretions may be the only means available to the physician to support the diagnosis. *G. vaginalis* vaginitis is characterized by the absence of leukocytes and a preponderance of small bacilli adhering in large numbers to epithelial cells, the clue cells (Fig. 22–3).

On the other hand, Gram staining may be misleading in making the diagnosis of gonorrhea in women, unlike in men, because the frequent presence of saprophytic neisseria or other bacteria, such as acinetobacter, which are easily mistaken for *Neisseria gonorrhoeae* (Fig. 22–4), confuse the picture.

Dark-field microscopic examination is the usual procedure for the recognition of *Treponema pallidum*, an organism that cannot be routinely cultivated. In granuloma inguinale, a Giemsa stain of a sample of granulation tissue allows the demonstration of diagnostic Donovan bodies.

CULTURE

Specimens for culture must be dispatched to the laboratory immediately and then inoculated quickly, to ensure the survival of delicate microorganisms such as *Neisseria gonorrhoeae* and *Trichomonas vaginalis*. If a delay between collection and inoculation is unavoidable, one should use a special transport medium and keep the specimen at room temperature. Drying and refrigeration are harmful to gonococci and trichomonads; the latter lose their motility and can be confused with leukocytes.

Neisseria gonorrhoeae requires chocolate agar or similar media, and a carbon dioxide atmosphere for growth. To inhibit the associated vaginal flora, antibiotics not active against gonococci are incorporated into the culture medium, for example, Thayer-Martin medium. For best results, the selective medium should be warmed to 37° C and should be inoculated immediately on taking the culture. If this procedure is not possible, one must use transport media, such as Stuart or

Acknowledgments

This color section is made possible by generous contributions from the following companies:

       Glaxo Canada, Ltd.
       Merck Frosst Canada, Ltd.
       Pfizer Canada, Inc.
       Rhône-Poulenc Pharma, Inc.
       Roussel Canada, Inc.
       Schering Canada, Inc.
       Upjohn Canada, Ltd.
       Bristol Myers Pharmaceutical Group

Plate 1

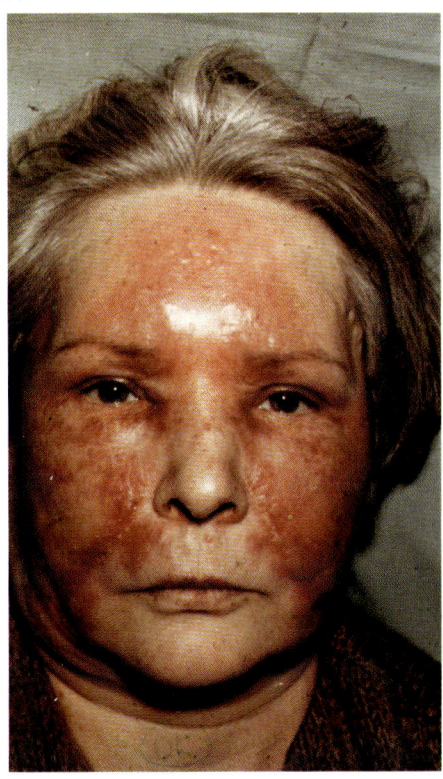

A, Facial erysipelas. The onset of this infection was astonishingly abrupt and produced toxicity, chills, and a high fever in a few hours. The infection started on the internal corner of the right eye and rapidly spread in a centrifugal fashion, out to the forehead and the cheeks in about 2 days, to cause the "butterfly" pattern. The edge of the lesion was sharply defined, especially on the cheeks.

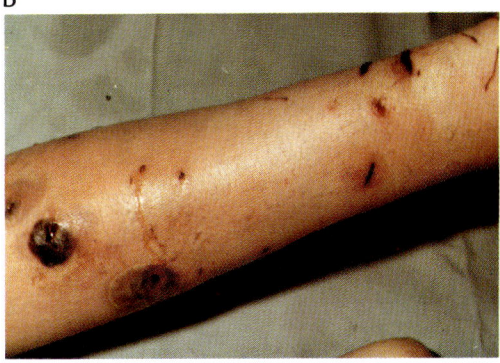

B, Cellulitis due to *Pasteurella multocida*. The diagnosis was suggested by the cat scratches and bites still visible in the photograph. *P. multocida* was isolated from the lesions.

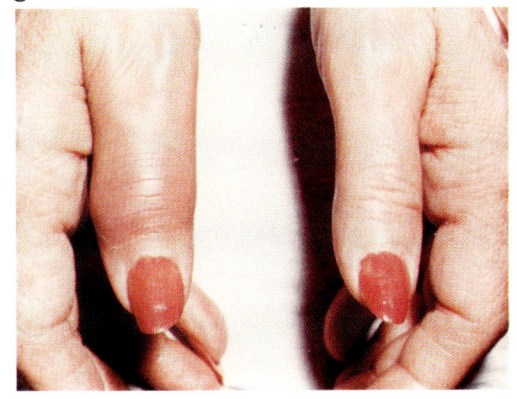

C, Subacute infections due to *Pasteurella multocida*. The diagnosis was not immediately suggested in this case because the initial lesion was inapparent and the circumstances of the infection (bite by the household cat) were omitted by the patient. The bacteriologic diagnosis was made from material obtained by needle puncture, after injection of a small amount of sterile physiologic saline solution.

Plate 2

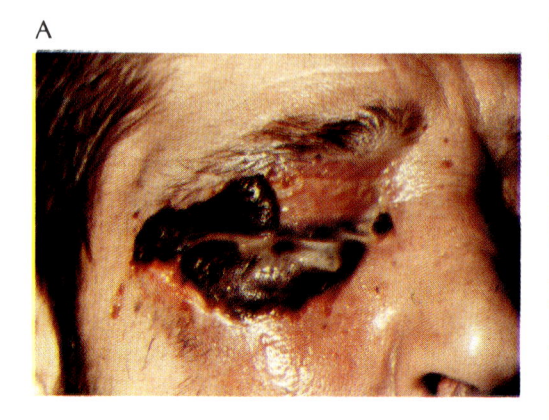

A, Anthrax in a longshoreman who had carried Indian gunnysacks on his right shoulder about a week before. The lesion was accompanied by high fever, an inconstant feature in this illness, and the blood culture yielded *Bacillus anthracis*. The response to penicillin therapy was good.

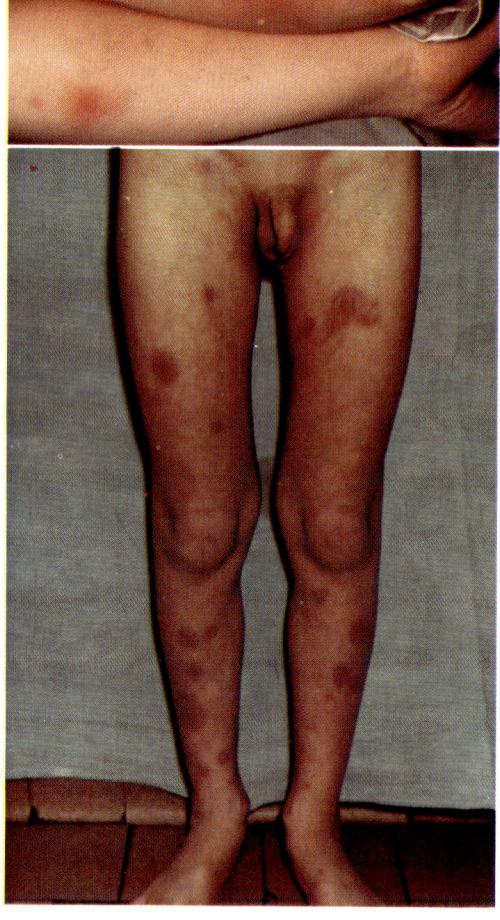

B, Erysipelothrix infection showing characteristic features. This lesion occurred about a week after the patient, a cook, pierced his hand with a fishbone. The infection progressed centrifugally, the border of the lesion was sharply defined, and no fever was present. The bacteriologic diagnosis was confirmed as in Plate 1*C*. The lesion healed rapidly following oral penicillin administration.

C and *D*, Erythema nodosum is generally a clinical diagnosis and is considered an allergic response. Many causes are possible, including streptococcal infections, primary tuberculosis, cat scratch disease, lepromatous leprosy, histoplasmosis, coccidioidomycosis, and diarrheas due to *Yersinia enterocolitica*, not to mention nocardiosis or adverse drug reactions, such as to sulfonamides. The nodules, which occur mainly on the extensor surface of the limbs, may be palpated as indurated and slightly tender areas. Initially pink or red, the nodules later darken as if they were bruises.

Plate 3

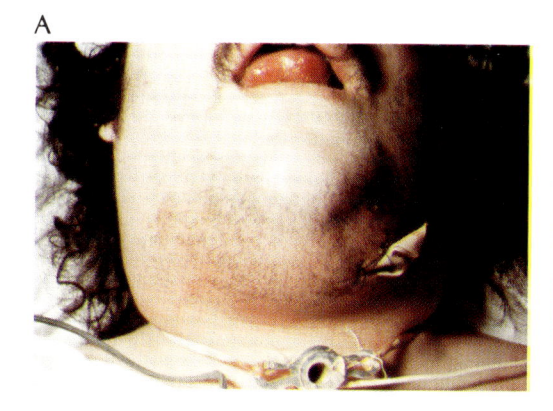

A, Ludwig's angina in a young man with poor oral hygiene. The infection is always impressive in both its sudden onset and its severity. The photograph was taken after the drainage of about a cup of foul-smelling pus. Dyspnea required a tracheostomy. Note the swelling of the floor of the patient's mouth and the position of the tongue that made closing the jaws impossible. The bacteriology of the pus revealed a mixture of aerobes and anaerobes (buccal flora). Treatment with pencillin G was successful.

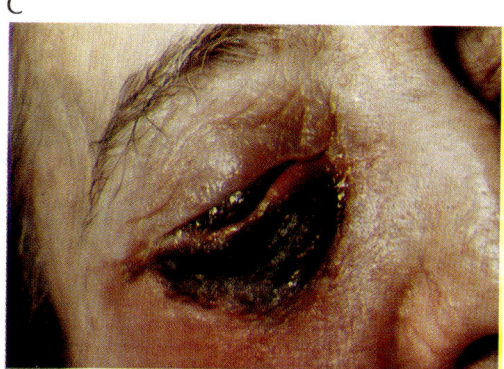

C, Ecthyma gangrenosum due to *Pseudomonas aeruginosa*. This 72-year-old patient had acute agranulocytosis from a reaction to phenacetin. *P. aeruginosa* was found in blood cultures and in the lesion. Cure was achieved with synergistic antibiotic therapy with carbenicillin and gentamicin at high doses, as well as by surgical excision of the lesion. The agranulocytosis spontaneously remitted. Note the clear-cut borders of the ecthyma and the feebleness of the inflammatory reaction. Note also the interesting analogy with the lesion in Plate 2A, and remember that the cutaneous lesions of bacteremia are characteristic of more than one organism.

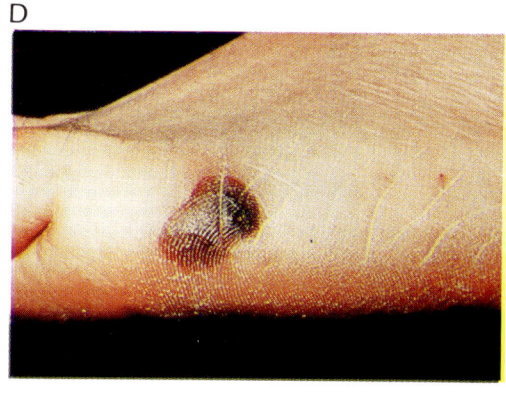

D, Staphylococcal septicemia with purpuric necrotic lesions, predominantly on the extremities (see also Fig. 13–1). These features should suggest an associated underlying endocarditis.

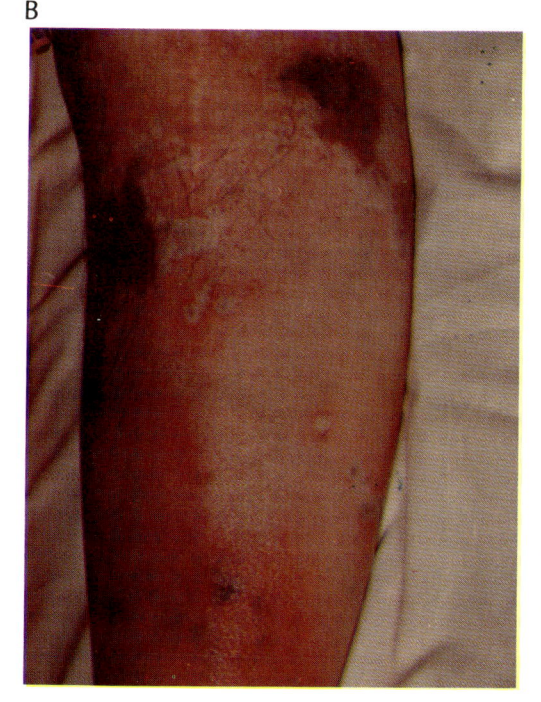

B, Nosocomial bacteremia due to gram-negative bacilli that started as a phlebitis from an intravenous catheter in the arm. Three blood cultures were positive for *Klebsiella pneumoniae*. A rapid demise occurred with a picture of intravascular coagulopathy.

Plate 4

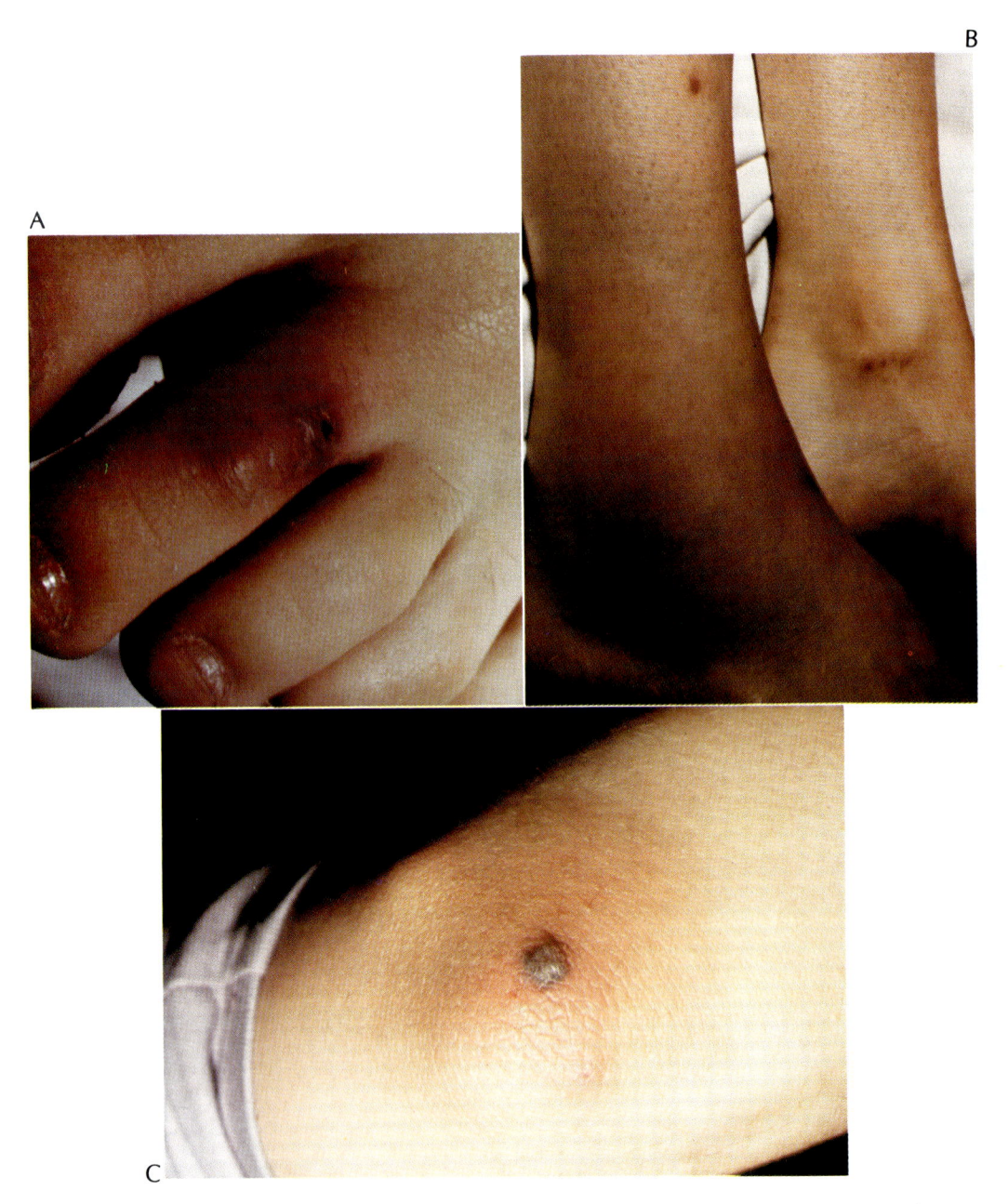

A to *C*, Disseminated gonococcal infections. The most characteristic are pustules, sometimes with a necrotic center resting on an erythematous base. These lesions are scanty and are distributed mainly on the extremities, sometimes over a joint. In *B*, the lesions coexist with an arthritis of the ankle. Microscopic examination or culture of the sample from the lesion may permit the definitive diagnosis.

Plate 5

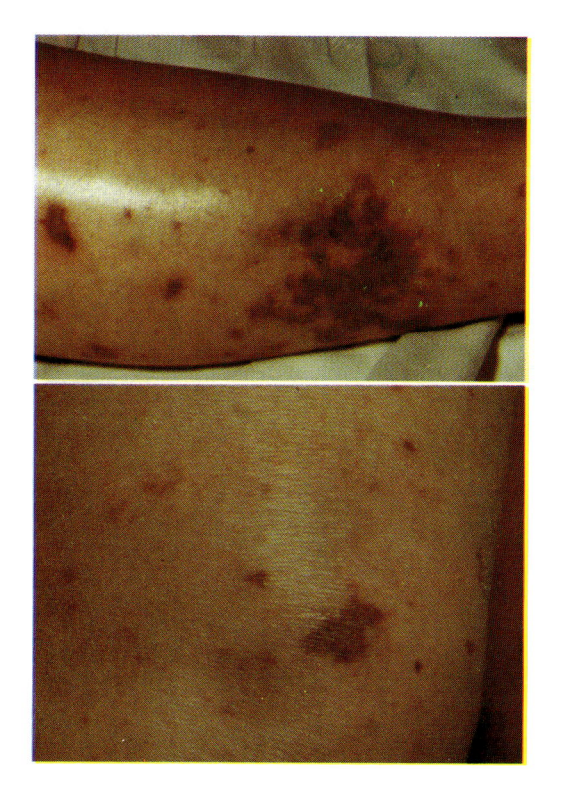

A and *B*, Meningococcemia. *Neisseria meningitidis* can produce an acute vasculitis or local responses of the Shwartzman type that clinically manifest themselves as petechia, purpura, or ecchymoses. Lesions develop on the trunk and legs in zones of pressure, such as caused by stockings or elastic garters; these lesions may be spectacular in appearance and may include gangrene of the extremities.

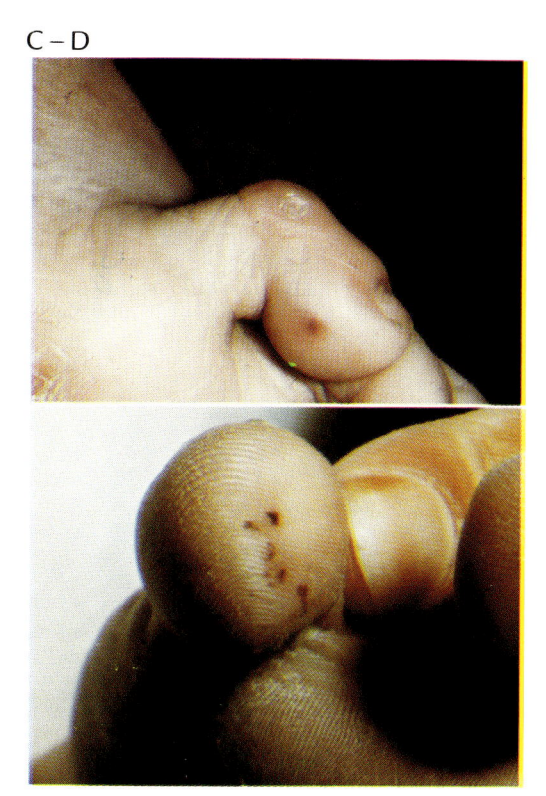

C and *D,* Osler's nodes seen in a patient with endocarditis due to group H streptococci. An Osler's node consists of an inflammatory nodule, warm and slightly tender. Osler's nodes and Janeway lesions were once considered to be of embolic origin, but are now considered to be due to vasculitis.

Plate 6

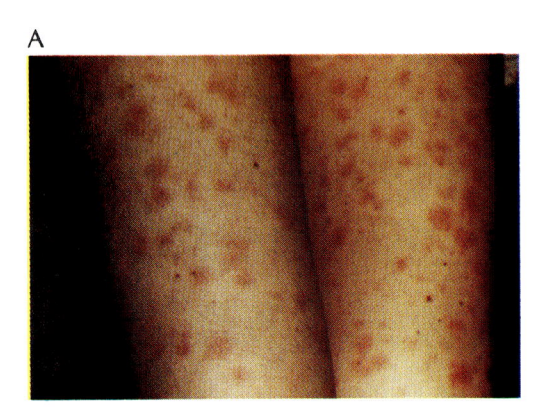

A, Syphilitic roseola. These rosy red macules, which spread over the trunk, shoulders, and thighs, are not pruritic and fade in about 2 weeks.

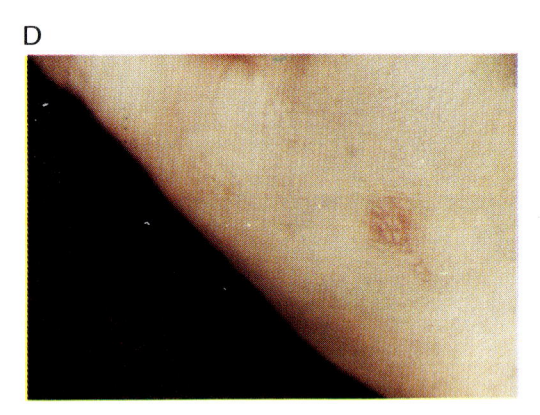

D, Inoculation chancre in cat scratch fever.

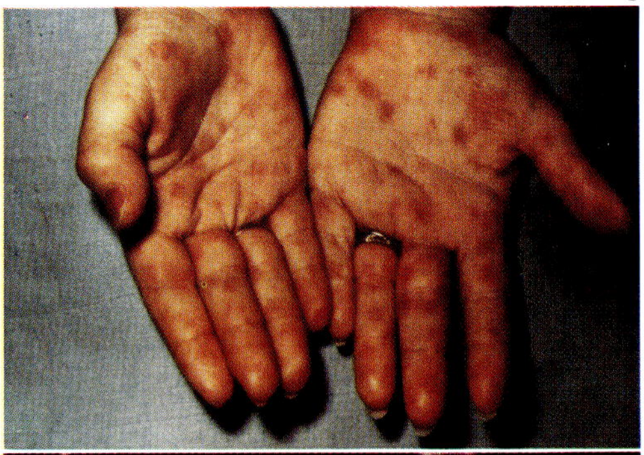

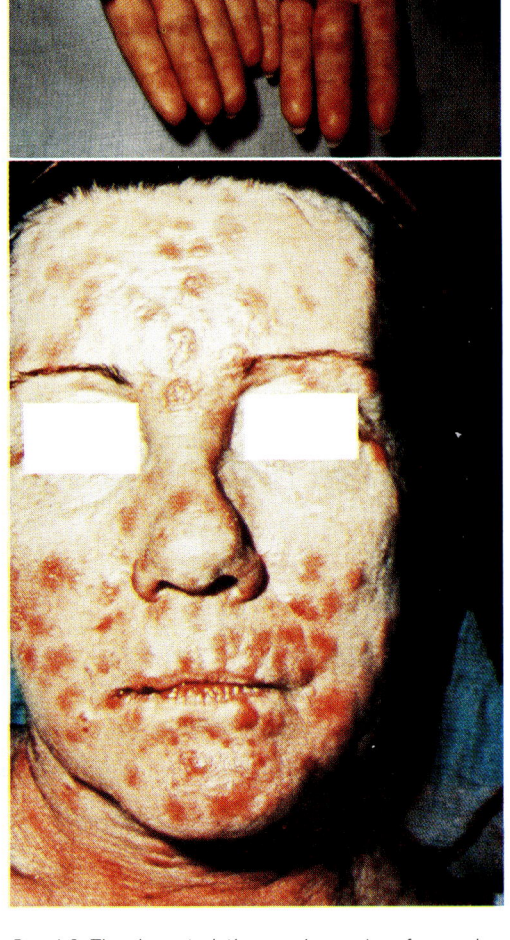

B and *C,* The characteristic maculopapules of secondary syphilis are dry, scaling, noncontagious or only slightly contagious, and nonpruritic. They are most common on the face, chest, back, abdomen, and upper arms; their occurrence on the palms and soles is also an important diagnostic finding. Syphilis should be suspected in all adults with a rash marking the palms and soles, even if other disorders share this characteristic, such as disseminated gonococcal infection, rickettsiosis, hand-foot-and-mouth disease, and drug reactions.

Plate 7

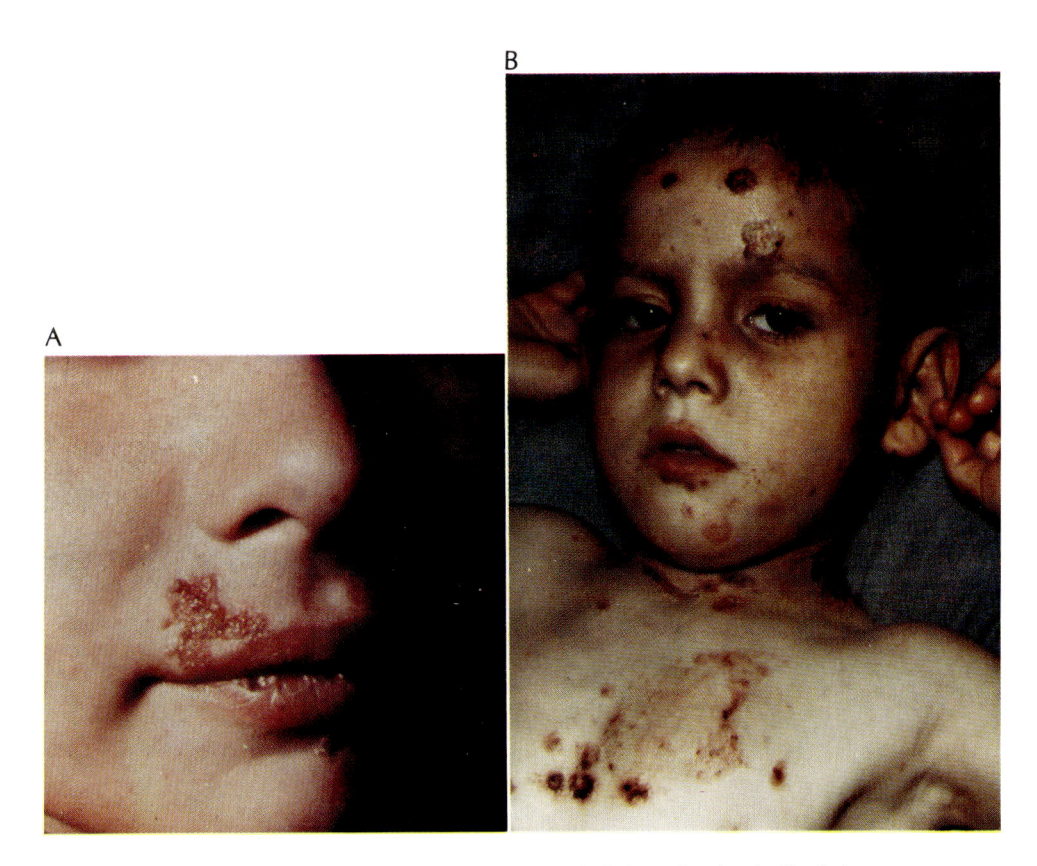

A, Typical aspect of impetigo due to group A streptococci. *B*, Impetigo due to *Staphylococcus aureus*.

Plate 8

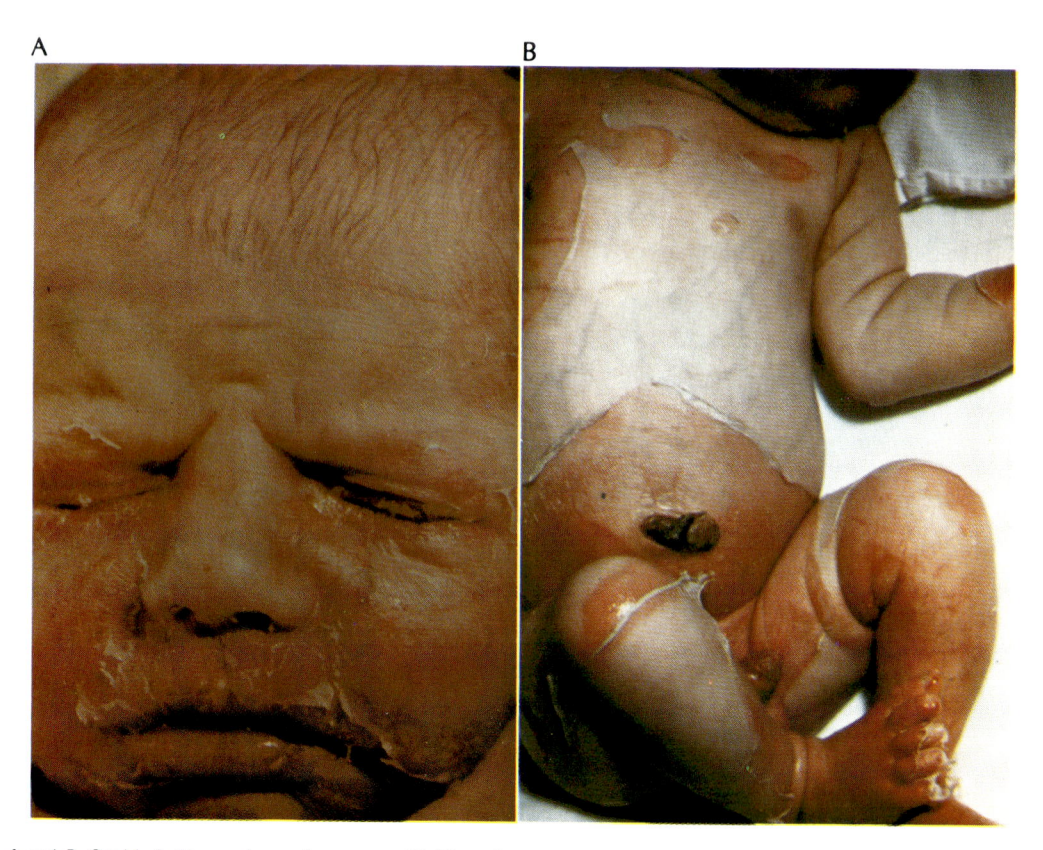

A and *B,* Scalded skin syndrome (compare with Plate 9*A* and *B*). According to one current theory, this disease is due to toxigenic *Staphylococcus aureus.* The skin layers are split superficially, and the mucosa is not affected. The patient's general condition and the prognosis are good.

Plate 9

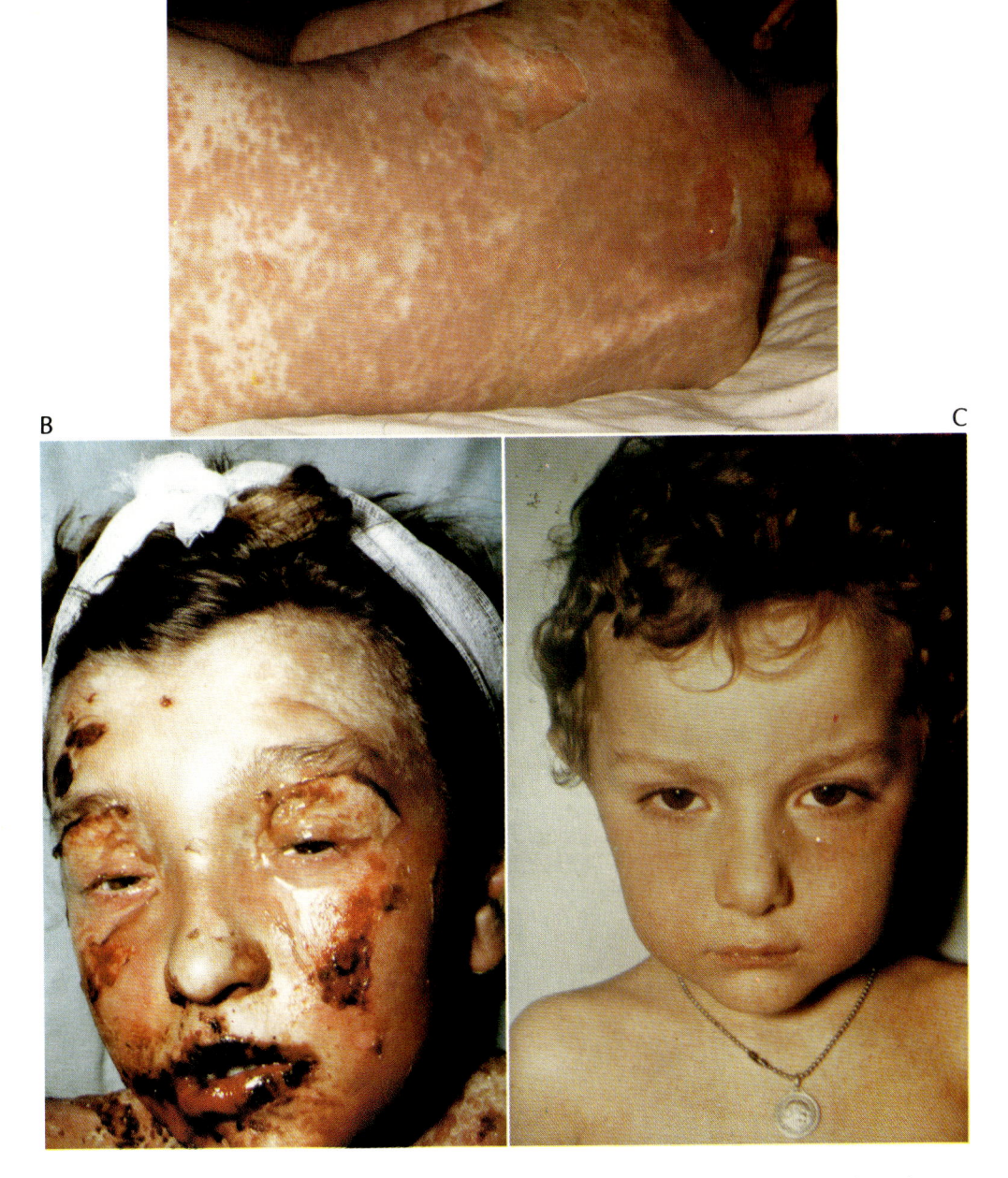

A and *B*, Toxic epidermal necrolysis, an adverse side effect of sulfonamide therapy. In this patient, the oral mucosa was involved, and the Nikolsky sign was positive even on apparently normal skin. This disease is more severe than the scalded skin syndrome.

C, Measles. Initially the rash is sparse and limited to the forehead, hairline, behind the ears and the upper neck; the conjunctivae are infected and photophobia is present.

Plate 10

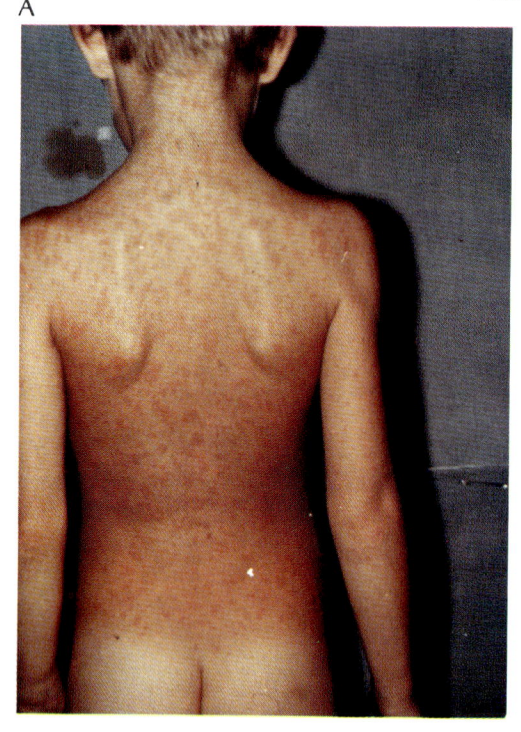

A, In measles, the rash spreads to the remaining portions of the body, progressing downward.

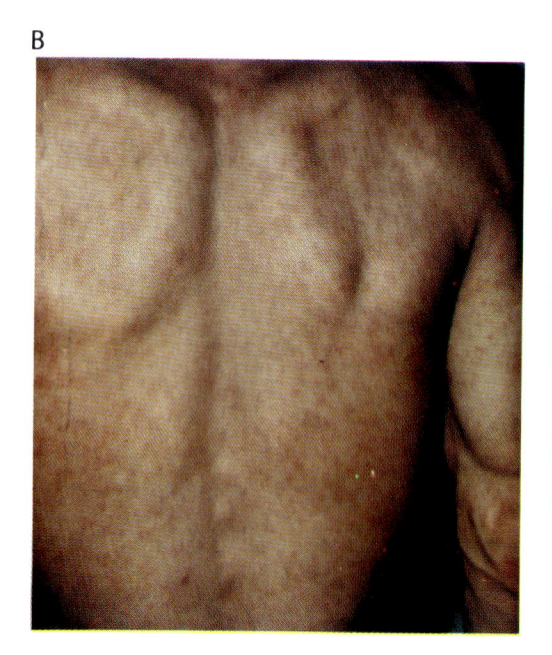

B, Rubella in an adult. In children over 10 years and in adults, the maculopapular rash starts on the face, but is more marked on the trunk, where it has a morbilliform appearance. The diagnosis depends partly on a history of contact with a known case of rubella, but mainly on the results of serologic tests.

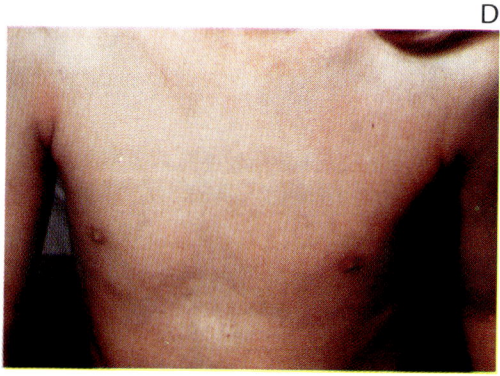

C and *D*, In scarlet fever, the tongue at first is thick and coated. It loses its coating in 2 to 4 days, from the lips to base, then takes on a "peeled strawberry" appearance, papules uncovered. *C* shows a peeled tongue at the third day of the disease. A strawberry tongue is also observed in Kawasaki's syndrome and in the toxic shock syndrome. *D*, The erythema is maculopapular with a granular appearance without an interval of normal skin, at least in the areas affected.

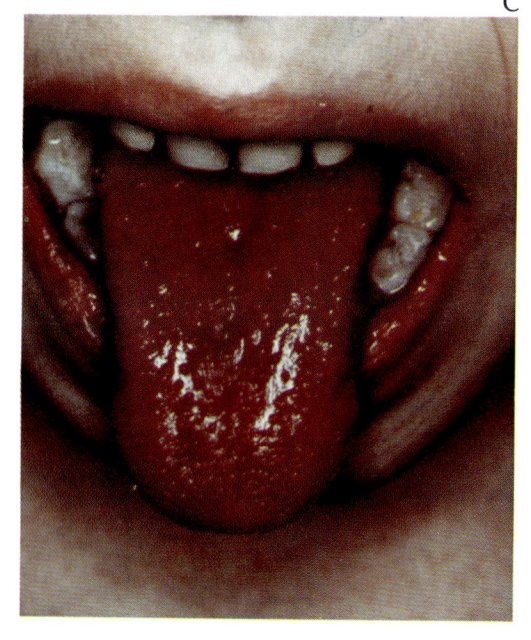

Plate 11

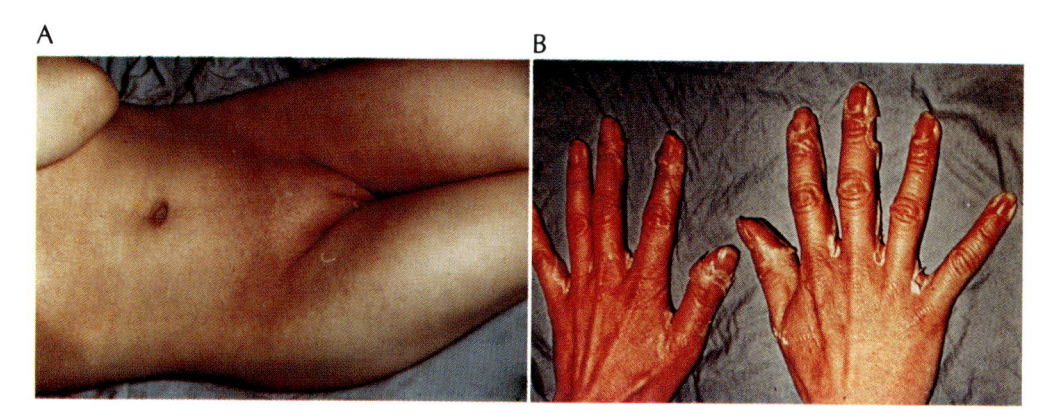

A and *B,* Scarlet fever. The erythema predominates on the trunk (see Plate 10*D*), on the pelvis (*A*), and on the skin folds. At about the tenth day of the illness, a cutaneous desquamation can be observed, sometimes impressive on the extremities (*B*), a feature also seen in Kawasaki's syndrome and the toxic shock syndrome.

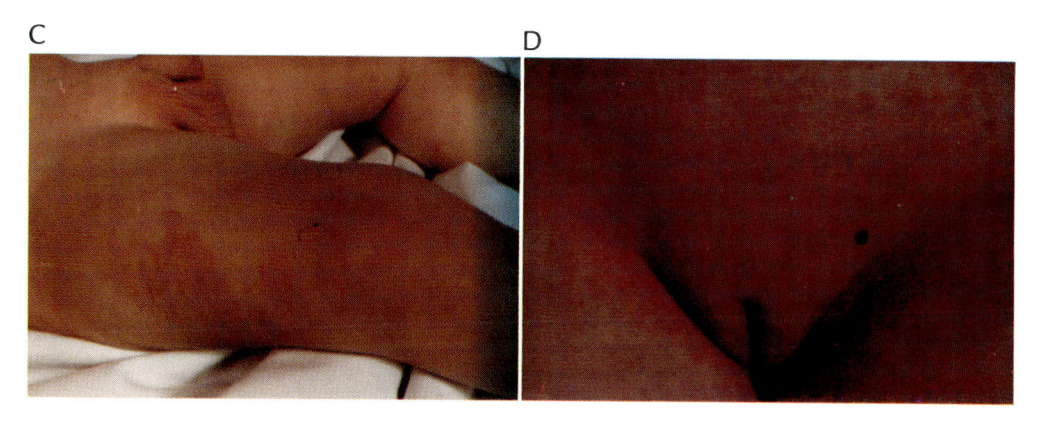

C and *D*, Kawasaki's syndrome, an acute febrile illness of unknown origin, may cause an erythematous rash, a strawberry tongue, and desquamation. Specific laboratory abnormalities are noted, but the diagnosis rests upon clinical features. The child, almost always under age 5, must meet 5 of the 6 following criteria: (1) fever persisting for more than 5 days; (2) conjunctival infection, (3) oropharyngeal mucous membrane changes; (4) distinctive desquamative change in the hands and feet; (5) rash; and (6) lymphadenopathy.

Plate 12

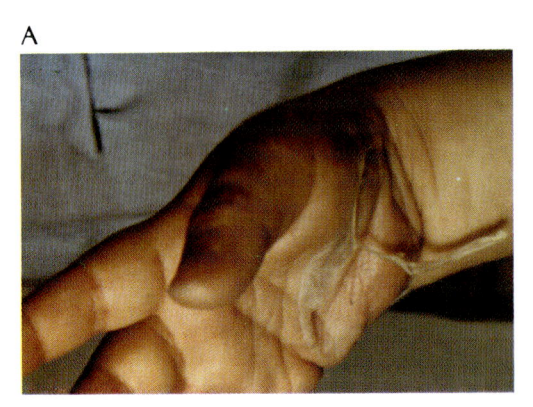

A, Desquamation in Kawasaki's syndrome.

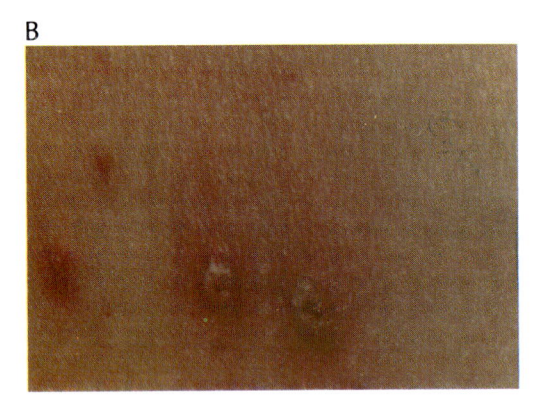

B, Chickenpox. The vesicles are superficial and thin-walled; as they evolve, crusts form in the center of the lesion. Erythema around the base of the vesicle is slight at first, but may worsen. Lesions may be found in varying stages of development at any given moment.

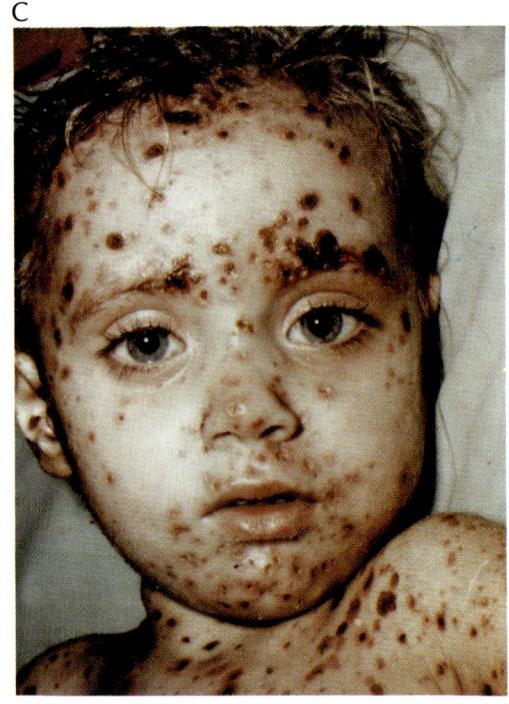

C, Chickenpox may be severe in individuals with immunologic deficiency. This child had acute leukemia, and his chickenpox was simply an aggravation of the normal clinical picture, notably with an impressive rash. Other cases may even progress to the point of shock and intravascular coagulation.

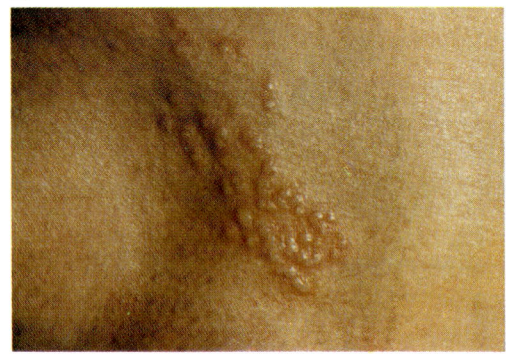

D, Disseminated herpes simplex virus 1 infection during the course of Hodgkin's disease. The definitive diagnosis was established by growth of the virus from the vesicular liquid. The differential diagnosis with disseminated varicella-zoster can be made by a Tzanck smear of a scraping from the base of an unroofed vesicle.

Plate 13

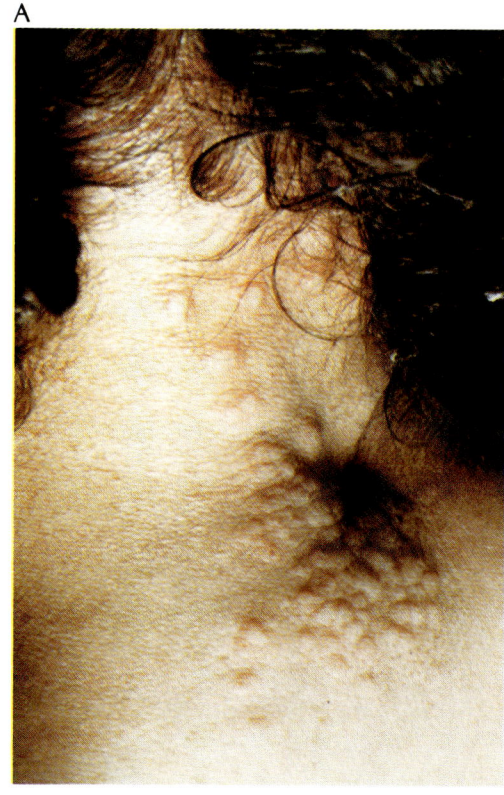

A, Disseminated infection with herpes simplex virus 1. Same patient as in Plate 12*D*.

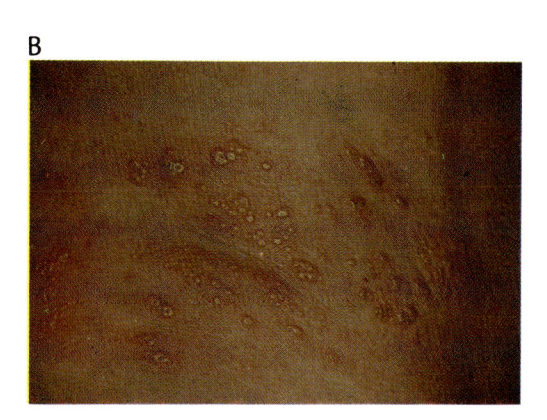

B, Typical intercostal zoster. Vesicles are similar to those of chickenpox (see Plate 12*B*), but their distribution follows the territory of a nerve root.

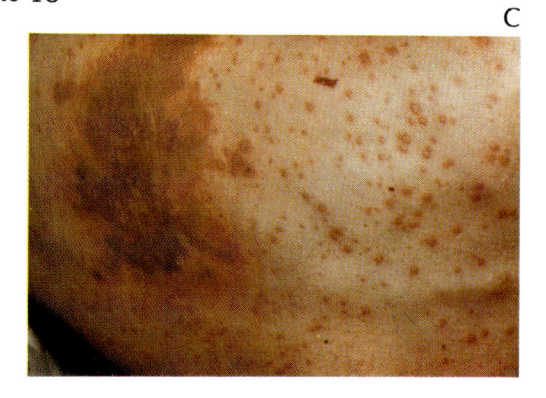

C, Disseminated varicella-zoster. In the immunosuppressed host, in this case with Hodgkin's disease grade 4, the lesions may disseminate in crops to all areas of the skin. Acyclovir, 5 mg/kg every 8 hours for 7 to 10 days in an adult, shows promise in the treatment of this infection.

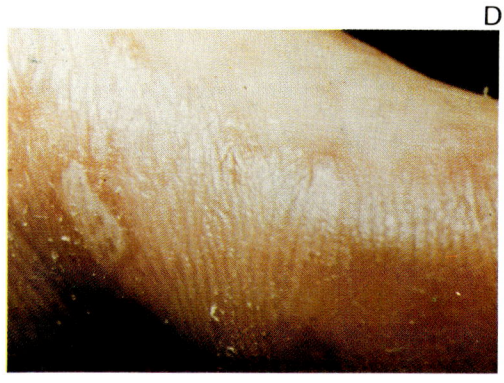

D, Hand-foot-and-mouth disease; details of the lesions.

Plate 14

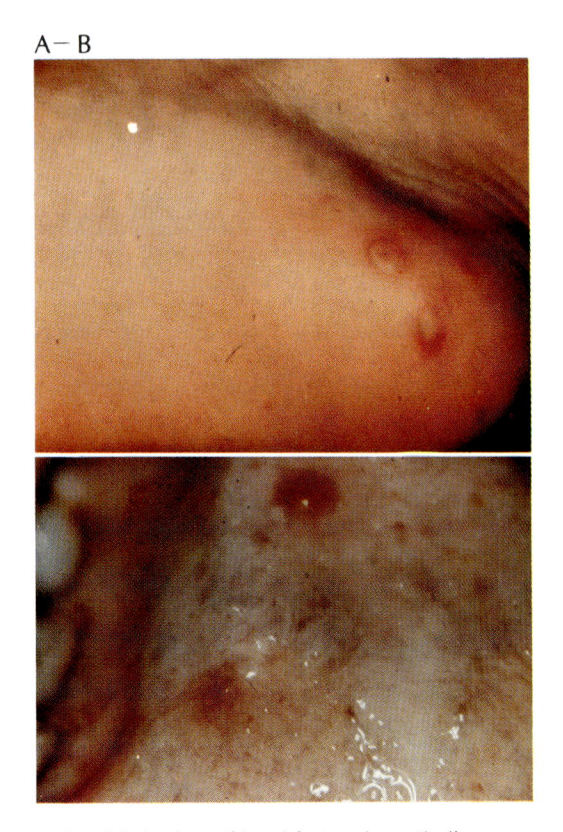

A and *B*, Lesions of hand-foot-and-mouth disease.

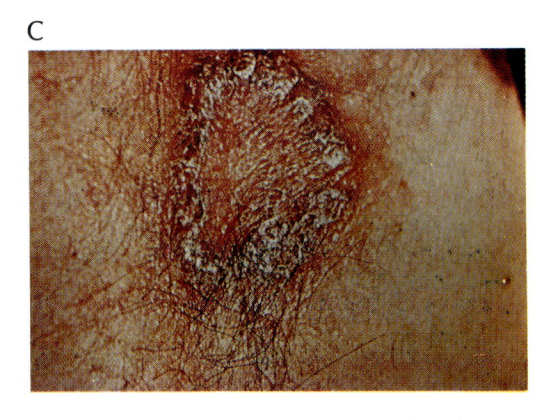

C, Cutaneous leishmaniasis (oriental sore).

Table 22–5. Genital Ulcers

	Syphilis	Genital herpes	Chancroid	Lymphogranuloma venereum	Granuloma inguinale
Agent	*Treponema pallidum*	Herpes simplex virus 2	*Haemophilus ducreyi*	*Chlamydia trachomatis*	*Calymmatobacterium granulomatis*
Incubation period	10–90 days (average 3 weeks)	3–6 days	1–5 days	7–80 days (average 12 days)	8–12 weeks
Clinical features	Painless ulcer; inguinal lymphadenopathy	Pruritus and pain; cervicitis and leukorrhea; vesicles and ulcers	Painful ulcer; inguinal lymphadenopathy	Painless ulcer; inguinal lymphadenopathy	Painful ulcer
Diagnosis	Dark-field examination; repeated VDRL and FTA-ABS tests	Cell culture; cytologic examination (nuclear inclusions)	Culture on special media; Gram staining?	Complement fixation and Frei skin tests	Giemsa staining on granulation tissue (Donovan bodies)
Treatment	(1) Benzathine penicillin G, 2,400,000 U (2) Tetracycline, 500 mg orally 4 times a day for 15 days	Symptomatic; acyclovir cream in primary infection	(1) Erythromycin, 2 g/day for 14 days (2) TMP-SMX 160/800 mg twice a day for 14 days	(1) Tetracyclines, 2 g/day for 14–21 days (2) Sulfamethoxazole, 2 g/day for 21 days	(1) Tetracyclines, 2 g/day for 14 days (2) Gentamicin, 10 mg IM for 14 days
Special considerations	Danger during pregnancy > 5 months	Danger during late pregnancy	Frequent superinfection by anaerobes	Cicatricial changes; rectal stricture	Superinfections

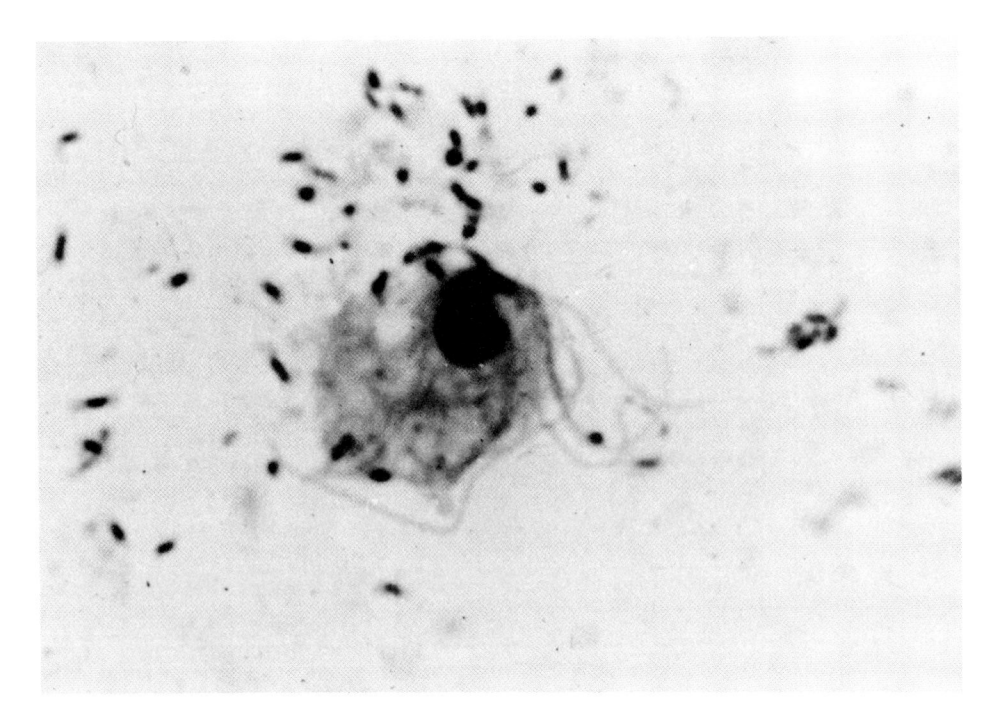

Fig. 22–1. *Trichomonas vaginalis.*

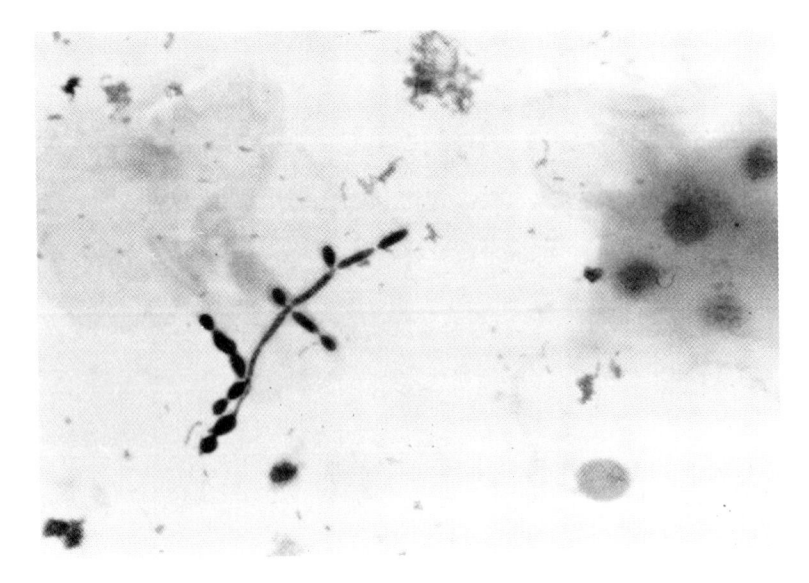

Fig. 22–2. *Candida albicans* from a vaginal smear.

Genital Infections 311

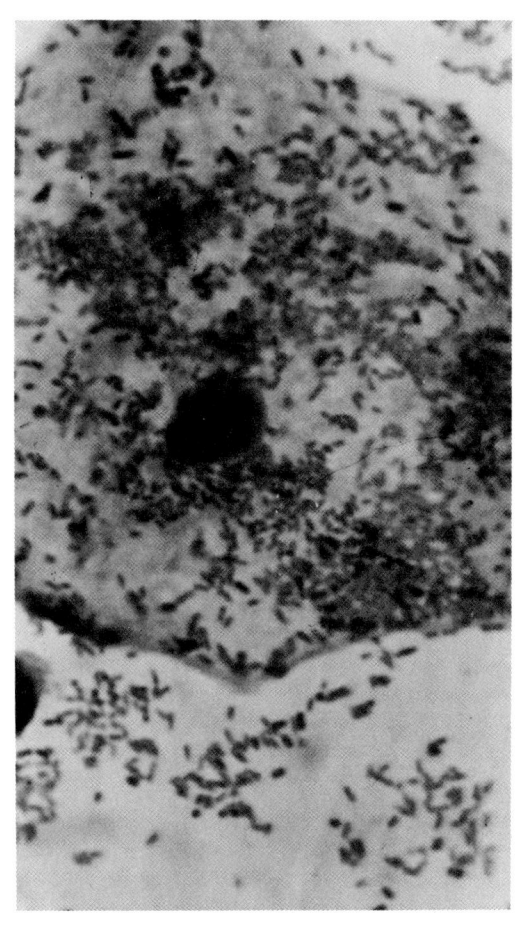

Fig. 22–3. Clue cell.

Amies, in which *N. gonorrhoeae* can survive for 6 to 8 hours. Alternatively, culture bottles containing Thayer-Martin medium and carbon dioxide are commercially available.

For the culture of bacteria other than *Neisseria gonorrhoeae*, the number and kinds of media used vary with the laboratory. These media should be suitable to grow the principal bacteria of the endogenous flora as well as the pathogenic species most likely to be encountered. Identification of anaerobic flora is time-consuming and difficult, so it should be restricted to certain clinical situations such as abdominopelvic sepsis, postpartum uterine infections, and septic abortions. The best specimens in this situation are obtained by direct puncture with a syringe or by endocervical aspiration in the uterine cavity. It is essential to use a closed syringe or an anaerobic transport medium and to dispatch the material immediately to the laboratory, to avoid loss of the anaerobes from the pus, wasted effort, and an erroneous interpretation of the results.

The culture of trichomonads (90% positive) is more sensitive than direct examination (75% positive) when the trichomonads are not abundant. This supplementary procedure does not replace the simple direct examination, however.

> Objective 22–4. Determine the major causes of vaginitis and cervicitis and treat appropriately.

GONORRHEA

Gonorrhea is transmitted almost exclusively by sexual contact, although transmission by contaminated objects has been reported. That the incubation period ranges from 2 to 10 days is academic because in most women, the symptoms remain limited to a "common" leukorrhea or a vague pelvic discomfort. The infection is usually multifocal, but the cervix seems the principal site. Upon examination with the speculum, one may see a thick, purulent discharge flowing out from the endocervix. Anal infection occurs by contiguity, even without direct inoculation, in about half these patients. Most of these patients remain asymptomatic anal carriers, and only a few complain of symptomatic proctitis, characterized by pruritus, tenesmus, and a sensation of rectal fullness.

True gonococcal vulvitis and vaginitis are rare, except in children. Dysuria reflects urethritis or an infection of Skene's glands. Involvement of Bartholin's duct can manifest as a painful mass lateral to the vaginal introitus. More often, the infection spreads upward to the uterus (endometritis), the fallopian tubes (salpingitis), the ovaries (oophoritis), and may lead to peritonitis. In the same context, acute pleuritic right-upper-abdominal pains, with hepatomegaly and a mild elevation of liver

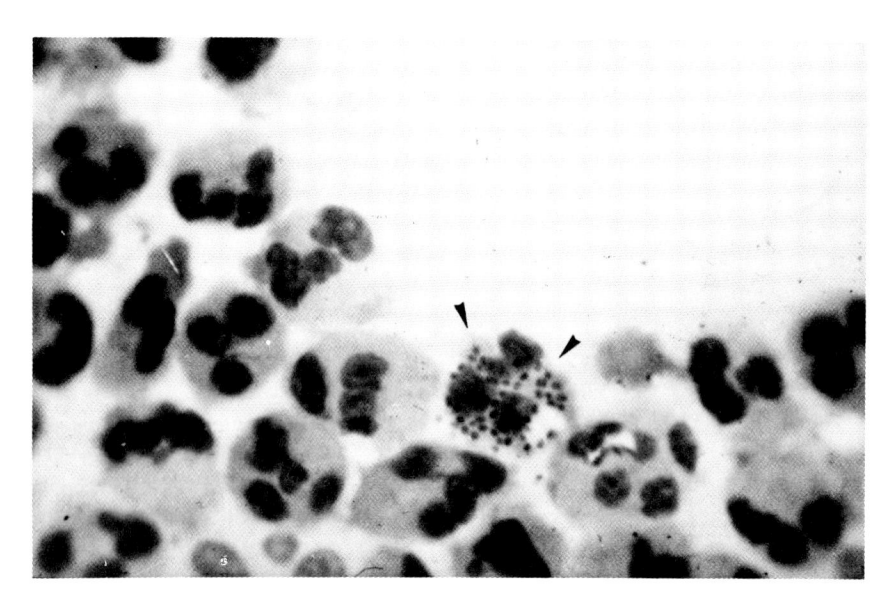

Fig. 22–4. *Neisseria gonorrhoeae* (arrows); Gram stain of an endocervical specimen.

enzyme levels, suggests the well-known but rarely seen diagnosis of perihepatitis (Fitz-Hugh-Curtis syndrome).

Other areas of gonococcal involvement include pharyngitis, generally secondary to orogenital practices, and conjunctivitis. The appearance of scattered cutaneous papules or petechiae, tenosynovitis, or arthritis (see Objective 13–3) with fever should suggest gonococcemia, which occurs in 1 to 3% of these infected women, probably from an endocervical focus and often during menstruation. The culture of *Neisseria gonorrhoeae* in the described sites (see Objective 22–3) confirms the diagnosis. Because one venereal disease can accompany another, it is important to order a serologic test for syphilis; one must, however, take into account the different incubation periods.

Penicillin G or ampicillin is still recommended in many cases of gonorrhea (Table 22–6), despite the larger doses now required and the increasing frequency of penicillinase-producing *Neisseria gonorrhoeae* (PPNG). Tetracycline has the advantage of probable effectiveness against *Chlamydia trachomatis*, often found in patients with gonorrhea. The substitutes for penicillin are spectinomycin for uncomplicated disease or doxycycline. Second-line drugs at this time include cefoxitin and cefotaxime, especially for disseminated infections due to PPNG strains and in patients allergic to penicillin. These secondary agents should be administered as initial therapy in areas where or in populations in which PPNG are frequently encountered. Of course, careful follow-up of the patient and examination and treatment of the patient's sexual partners are mandatory (see Objective 22–1).

CHLAMYDIAL CERVICITIS

Some serotypes of *Chlamydia trachomatis* are sexually transmitted and are responsible for urethritis in males and endocervicitis in females. These organisms can also cause inclusion conjunctivitis and pneumonia in the newborn, who contract the infection at birth during passage through the infected cervix, as well as a follicular conjunctivitis of adults (see Table 32–6) that is acquired by indirect or direct inoculation of the eye. Chlamydiae are also implicated in the production of the urethral syndrome (see Objective 21–4) and, recently, in the so-called pelvic inflammatory disease (PID) (see Objective 22–5). The genital tract is the major reservoir of these serotypes.

Chlamydial cervicitis has an incubation period of 1 to 2 weeks. The infection may produce purulent leukorrhea and cervicitis with erosion, but apparently it is usually asymptomatic and remains latent for years if left untreated. As with other venereal diseases, the incidence varies with sexual activity; the organism is present in 1 to 10% of the general population, but reaches up to 80% in some venereal disease clinics, in mothers of children with conjunctivitis, and in women whose sexual partner has urethritis. The disorder is frequently associated with *Trichomonas vaginalis* and *Neisseria gonorrhoeae*. Although chlamydiae are bacteria susceptible to antibiotics and possess DNA, RNA, and a cell wall, they have no energy of their own and thus have become obligate intracellular parasites. That they grow exclusively in cell culture or in fertile egg culture makes their diagnosis inaccessible to the ordinary bacteriology laboratory. The preservation of these organisms requires a special transport medium and freezing to −60° C.

Giemsa staining of an endocervical or urethral smear is still the simplest tool for bacteriologic diagnosis, but it is disappointing because of frequent false-negative results. Chlamydiae appear in epithelial cells as red paranuclear inclusions on a blue background. Their identification requires experience and is a tedious procedure because of the few inclusions per slide. Immunofluorescence techniques are more sensitive, but they require adequate antisera and equipment. A microimmunofluorescence serologic test, also available, serves primarily as an epidemiologic tool, but it can document a recent infection by seroconversion.

Treatment consists of the administration of tetracycline, 2 g/day for 14 to 21 days. A valid alternative is erythromycin. As with other venereal infections, it is important to treat the patient's sexual partners, to prevent relapses or "ping-pong" reinfections.

VAGINITIS

Candida albicans. *Candida albicans* vaginitis is characterized by a thick, whitish discharge adherent to the walls of the vagina. Patients often complain of burning. In severe cases, the vulva may be erythematous, edematous, and excoriated because of itching.

Because *Candida albicans* belongs to the normal vaginal saprophytic flora, a positive culture must be interpreted in light of the clinical picture. The presence of many yeasts in the vaginal secretions, either upon direct examination or on the Gram stain, constitutes a major clue. *C. albicans* vaginitis is sometimes difficult to treat, and relapses are frequent. To limit these failures of treatment, underlying factors may have to be corrected. Oral antibiotics and contraceptives, pregnancy, and uncontrolled diabetes are believed to stimulate the overgrowth of *C. albicans.*

Standard treatment includes intravaginal application of nystatin once or twice daily for 10 to 14 days; this local treatment is effective in 60% of cases. Imidazole derivatives, such as clotrimazole, miconazole, and econazole (the last not available in the United States), are 80% effective when applied for 3 to 14 days, depending on the product. It may be necessary to continue the use of a vaginal agent for a complete menstrual cycle. Oral administration of nystatin at a dose of 500,000 U 4 times daily for a week has been recommended for reducing an intestinal reservoir of candida. Although this infection is not necessarily sexually transmitted, in that altered host resistance seems to play a larger role, the patient's sexual partner(s) may contribute to recurrences. Therefore, at least when these partners are symptomatic, with balanitis, for instance, they should also apply nystatin cream to the infected regions. In particularly severe or tenacious cases, when the recommended treatments have failed and

Table 22-6. Recommended Treatment for Gonococcal Infections

Diagnosis	Recommended regimens (*not* listed according to an order of preference)	Also likely to be effective against: Chlamydial infection	Incubating syphilis[a]
Uncomplicated genital infections in either sex	1. Aqueous procaine penicillin G, 4.8 × 10⁶ U IM at 2 sites, with probenecid, 1 g orally OR	No	Yes
	2. Amoxicillin, 3 g orally (or ampicillin, 3.5 g orally), with probenecid, 1 g orally[b] OR	No	Yes
	3. Doxycycline, 100 mg orally twice daily for 7 days[c,d] OR	Yes	Yes
	4. Tetracycline HCl, 500 mg orally 4 times daily for 7 days[c,d]	Yes	Yes
	5. Spectinomycin, 2 g IM[f]	No	No
Treatment failure[e] Anorectal infection in men	Regimen 1 or 5	No	Yes, according to regimen 1 or 5
Pharyngeal infection in either sex	Regimen 1, 3, or 4	Yes, according to regimen 3, or 4	Yes, according to regimen 1, 3, or 4
Penicillinase-producing *Neisseria gonorrhoeae* (PPNG)[g]	Regimen 5 OR	No	No
	6. Cefoxitin, 2 g IM, with probenecid, 1 g orally OR	No	Not established
	7. Cefotaxime, 1 g IM Regimen 1, 2, or 5 Regimen 4	No	Not established
Gonorrhea in pregnancy		Yes	Yes
Acute pelvic inflammatory disease (mild)	8. Doxycycline, 100 mg orally twice daily for 10–14 days, with regimen 1, 2, or 6 OR	Yes	Yes
Acute pelvic inflammatory disease (severe)[h]	9. Cefoxitin 2 g IV 4 times daily, with doxycycline, 100 mg twice daily for at least 48 hours after defervescence; then doxycycline, 100 mg orally twice daily to complete 10–14 days	Yes	Yes

Disseminated gonococcal infection	OR 10. Combinations such as aminoglycoside plus clindamycin or doxycycline plus metronidazole	No	Yes
	11. Aqueous crystalline penicillin G, 10 × 10⁶ U IV/day until clinical improvement, followed by amoxicillin or ampicillin, 500 mg orally 4 times daily to complete 7–10 days of treatment	No	Yes
	OR 12. Regimen 2, followed by amoxicillin or ampicillin as in regimen 11	No	Yes
	OR Regimen 4	Yes	Yes
	OR 13. Cefoxitin, 1 g q6h IV for at least 7 days	No	Not established
	OR 14. Cefotaxime, 500 mg q6h IV for at least 7 days	No	Not established
	OR 15. Erythromycin, 500 mg orally 4 times daily for at least 7 days	Yes	Yes
Asymptomatic sexual partner of a patient with gonorrhea	Patient should be examined, culture should be taken, and patient should be treated at once with regimen 1, 2, 3, or 4		

[a] All patients treated for gonorrhea should have serologic test for syphilis, and, if needed, appropriate treatment (Objectives 23–2 and 23–4).
[b] Ineffective against anorectal and pharyngeal infections.
[c] Compliance of the patient is necessary; risk of emergence of tetracycline-resistant strains; contraindicated during pregnancy.
[d] Ineffective against anorectal infections in men.
[e] Possibility of reinfection has to be considered; post-treatment isolates should be tested for resistance pattern, according to the first regimen prescribed (e.g., penicillinase production, resistance to tetracycline).
[f] Ineffective against pharyngeal infection.
[g] For patients with proved PPNG or who are likely to have acquired gonorrhea in areas of high PPNG prevalence.
[h] Treatment of choice not established.

after correction of favoring factors, systemic treatments should be considered. The administration of 5-fluorocytosine, 100 mg/day orally for 1 or 2 weeks, or better, ketoconazole, 200 mg/day orally for 1 or 2 weeks, has had some success, provided the strains of candida are susceptible. Further clinical studies are needed to confirm the actual indications of these new drugs, however.

Trichomonas vaginalis. *Trichomonas vaginalis* produces a frothy, yellowish, malodorous discharge. Pruritus occurs frequently, and petechiae are sometimes found on the uterine cervix. The symptoms frequently begin during or immediately after menstruation. This phenomenon can be explained by the rise in the vaginal pH, then related to the menstrual blood, which favors the growth of trichomonads.

Oral metronidazole, at a dose of 250 mg 3 times daily for 7 days and administrated simultaneously to the patients and their partners, is usually sufficient to eradicate *Trichomonas vaginalis*. According to recent studies, a single dose of 2 g metronidazole orally is equally effective. As in gonorrhea, the single-dose treatment is a minimal form of therapy.

Gardnerella vaginalis. In vaginitis caused by *Gardnerella vaginalis*, the secretions are typically grayish, malodorous, and again adherent to the wall of the vagina. The current treatment for this vaginitis is metronidazole, 500 mg twice daily for 7 days. Simultaneous treatment of the partner(s) is necessary to avoid reinfection. The effectiveness of metronidazole in the treatment of vaginitis may be due not only to the susceptibility of gardnerella, but also to the activity of this drug against associated anaerobic flora. Ampicillin, 2 g daily for 7 days, is a second choice.

General Considerations. In conclusion, the clinical presentations are rarely clear-cut, primarily because of the frequency of mixed infections and the abundance of the accompanying flora. The microbiologic diagnosis is essential for the selection of the proper treatment. When a presumptive pathogen cannot be identified, general measures should be taken to correct causes of local irritation, such as tight clothing, poor hygiene, and overuse of douches and other feminine hygiene products, rather than launching blindly into antibiotic treatment. Organisms such as *Escherichia coli*, enterococcus, or group B streptococcus are rarely implicated in vaginitis. Their overgrowth often disappears spontaneously when the vaginal microbiologic ecology is restored.

> **Objective 22–5. Treat female pelvic infection according to the greatest bacteriologic likelihood.**

Usually, the choice of antimicrobial therapy for endometritis, salpingitis, or pelvic inflammatory disease is based more on clinical judgment than on available bacteriologic results. According to pathogenesis and clinical presentation, three entities are considered in this discussion.

ENDOMETRITIS

Infections occurring after direct trauma to the uterine cavity as a result of curettage, abortion, delivery, or neoplasia consist essentially of endometritis, which may be accompanied by high fever and chills. These infections produce mild to severe pelvic pains and often a putrid vaginal discharge. The patient's uterus appears large and tender. Lymphatic or hematogenous dissemination is the major complication. Bacteremia, demonstrable in over half the patients, often involves two or more different bacteria. These infections are generally polymicrobial, and the causative organisms come from the vaginal flora. Anaerobic and microaerophilic bacteria, including, among others, bacteroides species, clostridium species, and streptococci, today outnumber facultative bacteria such as *Streptococcus pyogenes* (a classic in the epidemics of puerperal sepsis), *Escherichia coli*, and even *Staphylococcus aureus* or *Neisseria gonorrhoeae*. It is difficult to obtain a satisfactory bacteriologic sample because the vaginal secretions also contain bacteria that take no part in the infectious process itself. Antibiotic treatment must reflect the broad bacterial spectrum: clindamycin, metronidazole, or chloramphenicol in combination with an aminoglycoside, or cefoxitin alone, for instance. That evacuation of the uterus, when indicated, is essential to therapy was known in the preantibiotic era.

POSTOPERATIVE INFECTIONS

Postoperative infections can follow a cesarean section, hysterectomy, or other gynecologic surgical procedures. Such infections include wound and pelvic abscesses, which occur most frequently at the level of the vaginal section and in the cul-de-sac of Douglas. The organisms responsible for the infection come from the skin and the vagina: anaerobes, staphylococci, streptococci, and Enterobacteriaceae. Surgical drainage is essential in the treatment of these infections, and antibiotics often play only a secondary role.

PELVIC INFLAMMATORY DISEASE

Pelvic inflammatory disease (PID) complicates a sexually transmitted genital infection. This disorder is, by far, the most frequent pelvic infection, and its incidence, both in Canada and the United States, is estimated at 2% of females between the ages of 15 to 30 with, a peak between ages 20 and 24. Half these patients require hospitalization. A hysterosalpingogram, the presence of an intrauterine contraceptive device, or a previous history of PID are known risk factors. The clinical manifestations vary from patient to patient. The most frequent symptom is lower pelvic pain, usually bilateral. Vaginal discharge, fever, toxicity, and the presence of an adnexal mass are possible signs. The infection may cause abscess formation, tubal obstruction, or sterility and has a tendency to relapse. Hospitalization is recommended in the following cases: if the diagnosis is unclear between a salpingitis and another condition that might necessitate an emergency operation, such as appendicitis or ectopic pregnancy; in the presence of an adnexal mass; when the physician suspects a pelvic abscess; in pregnancy, when the degree of toxicity suggests the risk of septic shock; and when the physician is unable to follow the patient's outpatient treatment, or after failure of same. Any intrauterine device should be removed, and another method of contraception should be prescribed.

In all cases of PID, one should look for *Neisseria gonorrhoeae* in the patient's cervix, urethra, and anus. The organism is found in nearly one-third of patients. The failure of *N. gonorrhoeae* to grow does not rule it out as the causative agent, however, nor does its presence prove that it is the sole agent. In fact, all organisms of the normal flora can be involved in PID. Then the infection must be considered polymicrobial, especially when the patient has repeated episodes. After neisseria, the organisms most often found are *Escherichia coli*, anaerobes including *Bacteroides fragilis*, various streptococci, and *Chlamydia trachomatis*. A blood culture is indicated in a patient showing signs of toxicity. In view of the multiplicity of organisms, the difficulty in obtaining valid bacteriologic specimens, and the absence of distinct clinical signs to enable one to distinguish gonococcal infection from the others, presumptive empirical antibiotic therapy is instituted as soon as the proper specimens have been collected. Tetracycline is a rational choice in mild cases because it is active against both *N. gonorrhoeae* and *C. trachomatis*. Worsening of symptoms or a lack of improvement after 72 hours of antibiotic treatment dictates the use of more aggressive diagnostic procedures, such as laparoscopy, ultrasonography, and scanning, to confirm the diagnosis or to demonstrate the presence of an abscess requiring surgical intervention. Tetracycline is then replaced by the combination of an aminoglycoside with clindamycin, chloramphenicol, or metronidazole, or by cefoxitin alone, to cover a wider range of bacteria.

Recently, medical attention has been drawn to subacute, tenacious infections due to *Actinomyces bovis* in patients with an intrauterine contraceptive device. To treat these infections, the intrauterine device must first be removed, and the best antimicrobial treatment is penicillin G.

> **Objective 22–6. Distinguish among the major male genital infections by means of the patient's medical history and the clinical examination.**

Male patients who have genital infections consult a physician for many different reasons. Urethral discharge, ulceration of the penis, development of condylomas, and scrotal tenderness each immediately suggest a diagnosis. On the other hand, burning on urination, frequent urinations, perineal or lower back pain, and skin eruption are less diagnostic. As odd as it may seem, some patients consult a physician when they have no symptoms because they are afraid that they may have contracted an infection during a sexual contact they feel questionable. After obtaining a description of the symptoms, the physician should seek to reconstruct the patient's medical history, including previous examinations and treatments. Without evasion or false modesty, the epidemiologic history of sexual contacts must be elicited: previous genitourinary disease and recent and present sexual activity in terms of frequency, number of partners, and type of contact. Even though the male genital system frequently becomes infected by venereal transmission, one may also see systemic infections, such as epididymo-orchitis in mumps or tuberculosis, or infections following a surgical procedure, such as epididymo-orchitis following prostatectomy.

The examination of the genital area includes the perineal, anal, and inguinal regions and involves a search for cutaneous and mucosal lesions and adenopathies. The foreskin, if present, should be drawn back to permit a complete examination of the glans penis. The urinary meatus is inspected for sticking of the sides, edema, spontaneous discharge or discharge obtained by "stripping" the urethra, or distal intraurethral lesions, such as condyloma, chancre, or herpes vesicle. The urethra is palpated over its entire length, as are the inguinal regions, spermatic cords, epididymides, and testes. The size and consistency of the prostate and any tenderness felt by the patient during the rectal examination are also noted.

MALE GENITAL INFECTIONS

The clinical information thus obtained generally makes it possible to diagnose and distinguish among male genital infections.

Urethritis. This disorder is characterized by urethral discharge and burning on urination, generally without inguinal lymphadenopathy. It may be associated with prostatitis or with epididymo-orchitis. (See also Objective 22–7.)

Prostatitis. The patient has perineal or lower back pain, difficulty on urination, urethral discharge in some cases, and an enlarged and tender prostate that is sometimes so painful that a rectal examination cannot be performed. Fever, dysspermia, or hemospermia may also be present. (See also Objectives 21–11 and 22–8.)

Genital Ulcerations. In spite of symptomatic differences discussed later, the precise diagnosis is often difficult to make on a purely clinical basis. Ulcerative lesions are often accompanied by inguinal lymphadenopathy. (See also Objective 22–9.)

Venereal Warts. Condyloma acuminatum and molluscum contagiosum are characterized by these lesions. (See also Objective 22–11.)

Epididymo-orchitis. This disorder causes enlargement of the epididymis or testis, which is usually extremely painful and tender. (See also Objective 22–10.)

> **Objective 22–7. Identify the cause of urethritis and define the treatment.**

Because a variety of microbial agents (Table 22–7) can cause urethritis, one must try to identify these agents individually, to ensure appropriate treatment. The diagnosis is not always easy because the infection may have several associated causes and processes and the laboratory diagnosis of some agents is difficult. The clinical presentation is also unclear; urethritis may occur without discharge, or the discharge may be secondary to prostatitis.

The etiologic investigation is based primarily on the microbiologic examination of the urethral discharge. In patients with a profuse discharge, one should collect a drop of secretion to look for gonococci. If no discharge is present, a fine swab can be inserted 3 to 4 cm into the urethral canal to collect a culture specimen for chlamydia.

The sample is best collected in the morning before the first urination, or at least an hour after urination. Microscopic examination for trichomonads should immediately be performed on a fresh specimen, with Gram staining for neisseria. Other procedures are discussed later in this chapter. In the absence of a visible discharge, at least five polymorphonuclear leukocytes per high-power field of unspun urine are required for a diagnosis of urethritis.

Bacterial culture can be done either directly or on transport media. For direct culture, Thayer-Martin medium or the equivalent is generally used. Such a medium is selective for *Neisseria gonorrhoeae*, that is, it prevents the growth of most other organisms.

Chocolate agar allows other bacteria to grow, but these organisms may overwhelm the gonococci. When the culture medium or the incubator is not immediately available, transport media, such as Stuart or Amies media, will enable the gonococci to survive for 6 to 8 hours at room temperature.

If gonococcal infection is suspected, one should obtain swabs from the tonsillar fossae and the folds of the anal verge. In addition, the patient's sexual partner or partners should be examined as well (see Objective 22–1).

GONOCOCCAL URETHRITIS

Clinical Manifestations. Gonococcal urethritis is usually clinically suspected when a frankly purulent discharge is associated with burning on urination. Less frequently, other sites of gonococcal infection are seen: erythematous pharyngitis, proctitis, arthritis, or a skin eruption, such as described in Objective 13–3. Some patients have a much less characteristic clinical picture; for example, urethritis without discharge but with burning on urination. The infection is nearly always the result of sexual contact, whether genital, anogenital (homosexual and heterosexual) or orogenital. Transmission by sponges, towels, and toilet items is exceptional, although it has been "incriminated" in infections in children from economically deprived homes who contract their parents' disease. The incubation period varies from 2 to 10 days.

Microbiologic Features. Microscopic examination typically reveals gram-negative cocci resembling coffee beans, some of which are found intracellularly within the large numbers of polymorphonuclear leukocytes on the slide. To the experienced microscopist, this picture is diagnostically reliable, but a negative examination does not rule out the possibility that the culture may subsequently prove positive. Even when the diagnosis seems sure on the basis of the microscopic examination, culture can be recommended, if only to determine the strain's antibiotic sensitivity.

Treatment. So far as treatment of gonorrhea is concerned, generally accepted recommendations exist in different countries, including the guidelines of the Public Health Service Center for Disease Control in the United States (see Table 22–6). In cases of anogenital gonorrhea, the preference is for

Table 22–7. Causes of Urethritis in Males.

1. *Neisseria gonorrhoeae*
2. Nongonococcal
    Microbial
        Chlamydia trachomatis
        Ureaplasma urealyticum
        Herpesvirus
        Trichomonas vaginalis } usually asymptomatic
        Candida albicans
        Various unknown agents
    Mechanical, allergic?
    Unknown: some respond to antibiotics

penicillin and single-dose therapy. The limitations of this therapy must be emphasized, however. In various parts of the world, the minimum inhibitory concentration of antibiotics against neisseria varies; the schedules apply only to recent and uncomplicated infections in which resistance is not a problem. Therefore, we must consider this type of schedule as the minimum prescription, and the physician should consider each patient individually, rather than rely on a formula. The existence of strains of neisseria resistant to penicillin through the production of a beta-lactamase illustrates this point, and when this type of resistance is present in the community, the physician must rely on certain cephalosporins (cefoxitin or cefotaxime), spectinomycin, or, in Europe, thiamphenicol. In any case, the probability of bacteriologic cure, at best, does not exceed 95%; for this reason, a microbiologic examination a week after completion of the treatment is the only way to prevent the existence of iatrogenic, healthy carriers.

Ancillary therapeutic measures include the use of condoms when sexual abstinence until the time of the follow-up culture is unlikely, to prevent further spread of the disease.

After treatment, a so-called "postgonococcal" urethritis syndrome, characterized by serous discharge and a mild urethral discomfort, may persist or appear. This syndrome may be the result of a residual inflammation or superinfection, or an underlying prostatitis, or a nongonococcal urethritis acquired simultaneously and appearing later because of a longer incubation period. In practice, it is difficult to choose among these possibilities, but the physician should keep in mind that this syndrome often regresses spontaneously in a few weeks, and if not, treatment with tetracycline can cure it.

NONGONOCOCCAL URETHRITIS

As its name indicates, nongonococcal urethritis is a diagnosis of exclusion. After an incubation period of 5 to 30 days, dysuria appears, together with a mild, limited, serous discharge, which may be opaque or even purulent. Occasionally, inguinal lymphadenopathy is seen.

Chlamydia trachomatis. Of the several causes of nongonococcal urethritis, *Chlamydia trachomatis* appears to be responsible for at least half of the cases (Fig. 22–5). In Western countries, the incidence of this infection now seems to be greater than that of gonococcal urethritis. Chlamydiae, whose current classification is shown in Table 22–8, are metabolically deficient bacteria that are obligate intracellular parasites. Unlike viruses, chlamydiae contain both types of nucleic acids, have a wall, and are susceptible to certain antibiotics. The chlamydia is phagocytized by the host cell, in which it produces a colony in the form of an elementary (inclusion) body 0.3 μ in diameter and located close to the nucleus in a vacuole.

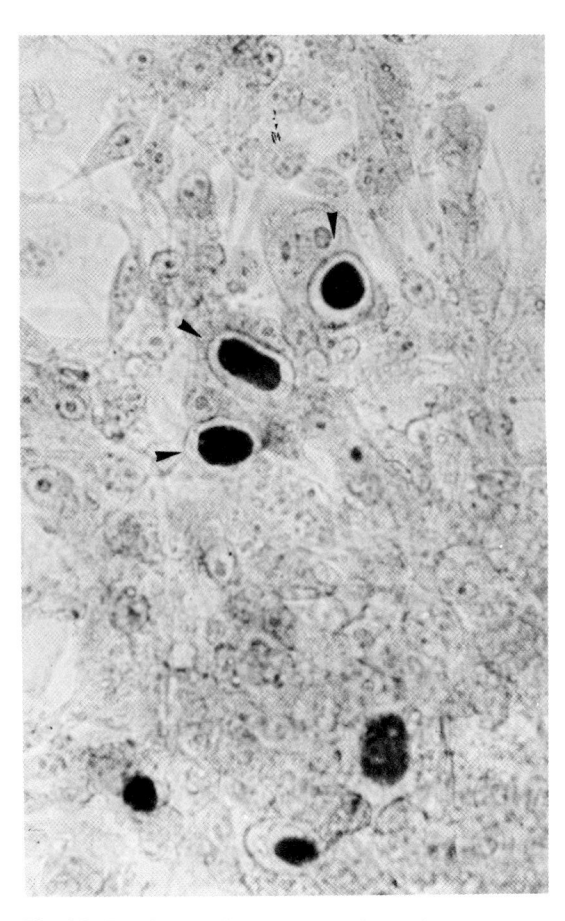

Fig. 22–5. *Chlamydia trachomatis* (arrows).

Table 22–8. Classification of Chlamydiae according to Serotypes and Disorders

Genus Chlamydia	Serotypes	Disorders
Chlamydia trachomatis (subgroup A)	A, B, Ba, C (trachoma serotypes)	Trachoma
		Hyperendemic blindness
	D, E, F, G, H, I, J, K (paratrachoma serotypes)	Inclusion conjunctivitis
		Urethritis and proctitis
		Cervicitis
		Salpingitis
		Peritonitis
		Endocarditis
		Neonatal conjunctivitis
		Pneumonia
	L_1, L_2, L_3	Lymphogranuloma venereum
Chlamydia psittaci (subgroup B)	several biotypes	Psittacosis
		Ornithosis

In chlamydia urethritis, as in cervicitis, direct examination of a stained smear is, in practice, unhelpful and time-consuming. The principal value of the microscopic examination of urethral secretions is to demonstrate the abundance of leukocytes and the relative absence of bacteria, in particular the absence of intracellular neisseria. A positive diagnosis can only be obtained from tissue culture, which is often unavailable. When tissue culture is available, intraurethral epithelial cells are carefully removed as described previously, and the specimen is placed in a special culture medium containing a phosphate buffer enriched with sugar and fetal calf serum (10%), gentamicin, and amphotericin B. When inoculation is done within 24 hours, this medium is kept at $+4°$ C; otherwise, it must be stored at $-70°$ C. Later, the specialized laboratory inoculates live cells weakened by irradiation (McCoy cells (Fig. 22–6), for example) or by a cytostatic agent.

After a few days of incubation, growth of the organism is determined by the presence of intracellular inclusions (Fig. 22–7). Because of the many asymptomatic carriers, culture of the organism in the absence of appropriate clinical indications does not make the diagnosis.

Ureaplasma urealyticum. Formerly called Mycoplasma T (tiny), this organism derives its name from its ability to metabolize urea and is believed to be responsible for 5 to 10% of the cases of nongonococcal urethritis. *U. urealyticum* can be found in the urethra of 40 to 50% of sexually active men in some clinics, particularly men who change sexual partners frequently. Considering this prevalence, the pathogenic role of this organism in urethritis has been doubted, but it has recently been confirmed by inoculation experiments in volunteers and in monkeys. *U. urealyticum* has no real cell wall structure and therefore does not take the usual bacteriologic dyes. Bacteriologic diagnosis by culture is performed only in certain specialized laboratories. For transport, a Stuart-type medium is suitable.

Trichomonas vaginalis. This organism is thought to be implicated in fewer than 2% of the cases of nongonococcal urethritis. *T. vaginalis* may produce a purulent urethral discharge, but more often, it merely colonizes the male urethra without producing symptoms. This organism can be detected by direct examination in a fresh specimen; a phase-contrast microscope is helpful. Papanicolaou staining is also suitable; better yet are acridine orange staining and reading under an ultraviolet microscope. A culture medium is also available, for example, trichomonas broth oxoid.

Candida albicans. Candida is more likely to produce balanitis than urethritis in uncircumcised males.

Miscellaneous Bacterial Causes. *Gardnerella vaginalis*, *Clostridium difficile*, *Streptococcus agalactiae* (group B), *Staphylococcus saprophyticus*, and *Escherichia coli* are sometimes discussed in the literature as

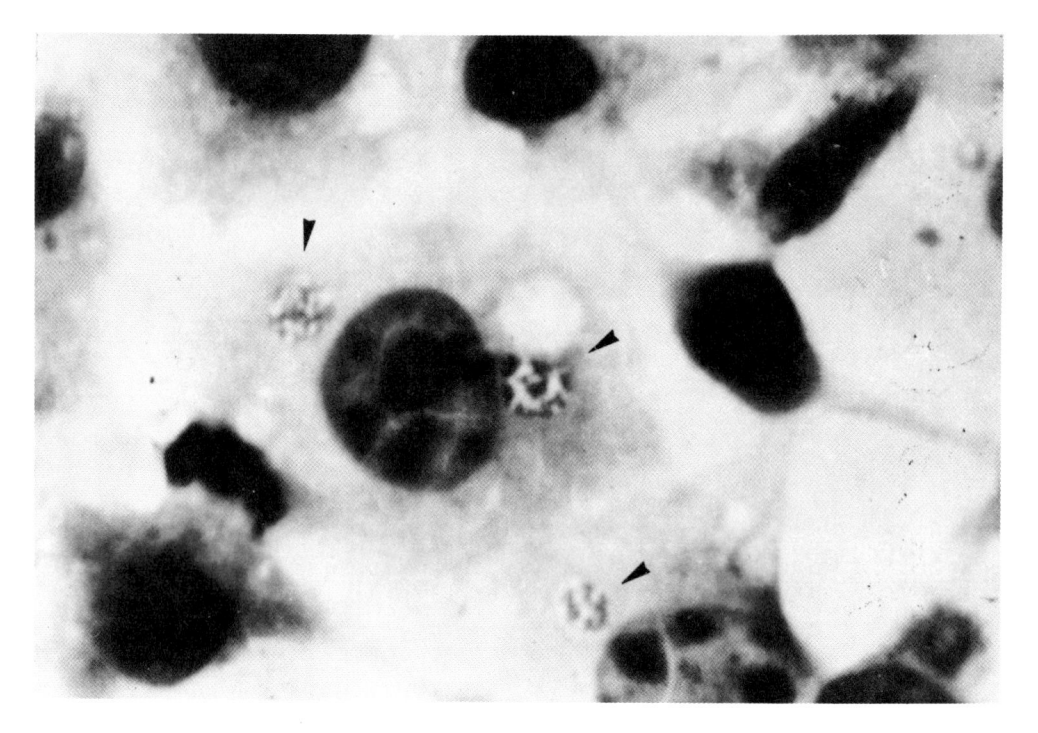

Fig. 22-6. McCoy cells (arrows indicate chlamydia inclusions).

causes of nongonococcal urethritis, and the evidence is suggestive. In practice, these organisms can be taken into consideration when they are abundant, clearly predominant, or found in a pure culture, with no other apparent cause.

Herpesvirus hominis. This virus can produce intraurethral vesicles and causes symptoms of urethritis.

Reiter's Syndrome. This disorder is the association of urethritis with conjunctivitis or uveitis, arthritis, and less frequently, mucocutaneous manifestations such as balanitis and keratoderma blennorrhagicum (see Objective 29–11). Some investigations have shown that *Chlamydia trachomatis* is often isolated from the urethra in these patients; in addition, the serologic test for chlamydiae is sometimes positive. This clinical entity remains a separate syndrome, however, that has been associated with other pathologic findings such as ulcerative colitis and shigellosis, in addition to the HLA-B27 histocompatibility group.

Treatment. Therapy of nongonococcal urethritis carries a degree of uncertainty, both because of the many possible causes, as discussed previously, and because of the general unavailability of confirming bacteriologic tests. Nevertheless, the reputation of this infection for therapeutic failure and relapse is undeserved when we take into account that these complications are probably due to reinoculations from untreated partners or are related to an underlying prostatitis. In practice, the physician's choice is simple because tetracycline, with erythromycin as an alternative, cures more than 80% of all patients, and more than 90% of patients according to some studies.

Various oral treatment schedules can be established, such as tetracycline, 500 mg 4 times daily for 10 days, minocycline, 100 mg once daily for 6 days, doxycycline, 100 mg twice daily for 10 days, or erythromycin ethylsuccinate, 500 mg 3 times daily for 7 to 14 days.

In conclusion, in the majority of cases, only

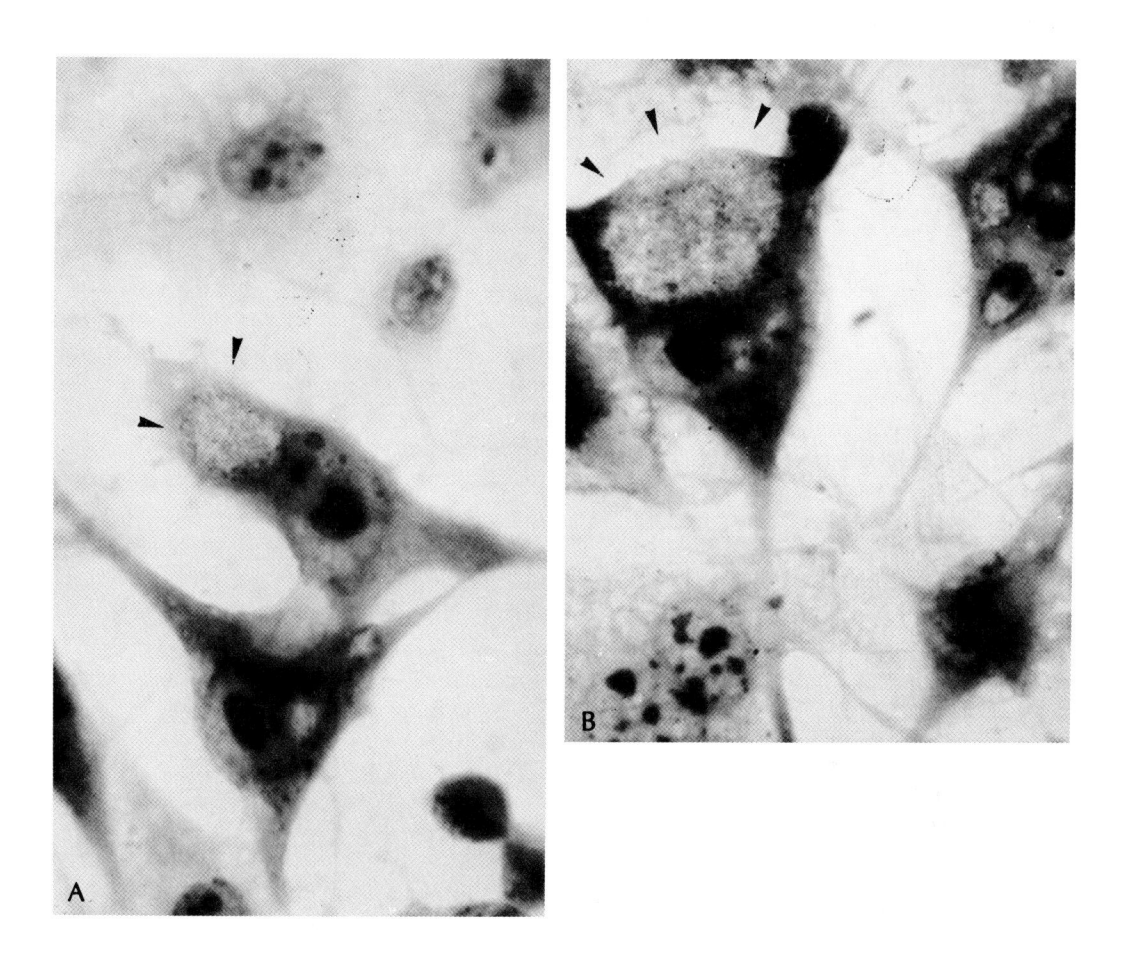

Fig. 22–7. *A* and *B*, *Chlamydia trachomatis* inclusions (arrows).

the gonococcus is directly sought, and Gram staining is the most widely used technique. If the results of the examination are positive, treatment for gonorrhea is instituted. When the result is doubtful or negative, tetracycline is usually prescribed. Special microbiologic studies are usually reserved for resistant or relapsing urethritis that cannot be accounted for by prostatitis or reinoculation.

> Objective 22-8. Identify and treat the various causes of prostatitis.

Some confusion surrounds the term prostatitis. The infectious or inflammatory diseases of the prostate gland fall into four clearly distinguishable syndromes: (1) acute bacterial prostatitis, (2) chronic bacterial prostatitis, (3) nonbacterial prostatitis, and (4) prostatodynia.

ACUTE BACTERIAL PROSTATITIS

General symptoms such as fever and myalgia generally precede the disturbances of micturition, which include dysuria, increased frequency of urination, nocturia, and sometimes even urinary retention. A urethral discharge is usually present, as well as perineal, suprapubic, or low back pain.

On rectal palpation, the patient's prostate is enlarged, tender, and even extremely painful. Massage of the prostate to obtain secretions from such patients presents a real danger of septicemia. The origin of acute prostatitis is nearly always bacterial. Most infections involve gram-negative bacteria, such as *Escherichia coli*, klebsiella, proteus, and pseudomonas, or more rarely, gram-positive organisms, such as *Streptococcus faecalis* or *Staphylococcus aureus*. The possible role of anaerobes is not yet clearly established.

CHRONIC BACTERIAL PROSTATITIS

This disorder is characterized by a clinical picture similar to that of the acute infection, although far less pronounced. Chronic bacterial prostatitis is caused mainly by gram-negative organisms and is usually associated with recurrent bacteriuria (see Objective 21-6). Many of these patients are the sexual partners of women who suffer from relapsing urinary infections.

Although it is now rare, one should consider the possibility of tuberculous prostatitis, especially when the patient has another focus of tuberculosis.

ABACTERIAL PROSTATITIS

Many cases reported in the literature as "chronic prostatitis" actually fall into the category of abacterial prostatitis. These disorders constitute the majority of cases of prostatitis, and the only evidence of an infectious process is the presence of polymorphonuclear leukocytes in the patient's prostatic secretion or semen following massage; the routine bacterial cultures are negative. Both mycoplasma

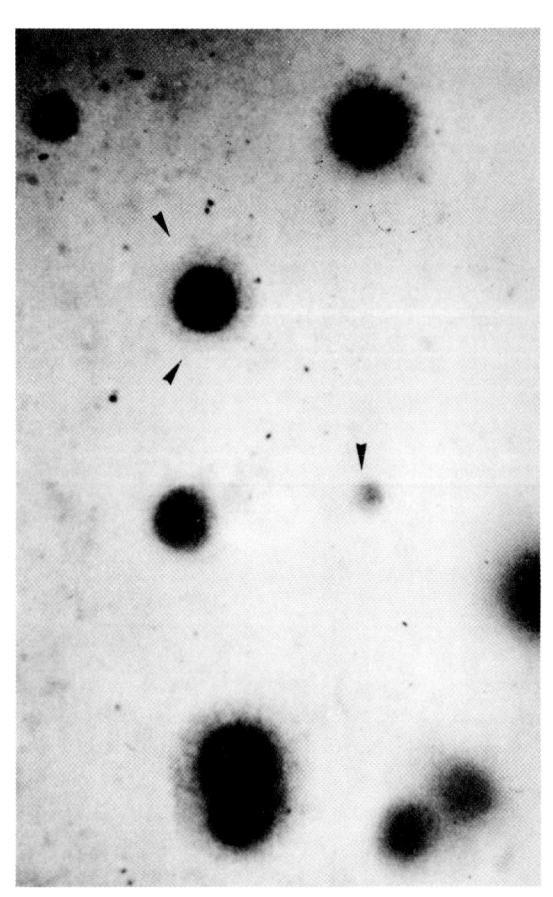

Fig. 22–8. *Mycoplasma hominis* (arrows).

(Fig. 22–8) and chlamydia have been incriminated in such cases, although without convincing proof. The many symptoms of abacterial chronic prostatitis appear to be influenced by the psychologic status of the patient. These complaints are sometimes minor and are limited to perineal discomfort, often experienced while the patient is sitting or driving a car, but occasionally they may include pains in the perineum, lower abdomen, suprapubic region, or lower back, as well as pain during urination or sexual intercourse. Rectal palpation is not always helpful in the diagnosis. Other symptoms include dysuria, increased frequency of urination, and a urethral discharge.

PROSTATODYNIA

When a patient has symptoms of prostatitis without polymorphonuclear leukocytes or bacteria in the prostatic fluid, his condition is described as prostadynia. In this disorder, psychologic factors are often of great importance. The origin of this "autonomic urogenital syndrome" is unknown. The presence of mucous filaments in the urine, sometimes mentioned by the patient, must be verified by microscopic examination because it does not automatically imply exudation and the presence of polymorphonuclear leukocytes.

DIAGNOSIS

The diagnosis of prostatitis is based primarily on the microbiologic examination of the urine and prostatic fluid. To locate the focus of infection, Stamey has proposed the use of fractional cultures. This technique involves the culturing of the following samples:

Fraction I. Initial portion of the urinary stream (5 to 10 ml), considered to be contaminated by the urethral flora (VB*$_1$).

Fraction II. The midstream specimen (VB$_2$). Micturition is then interrupted so that prostatic massage can be performed.

Fraction III. The secretion obtained after massage, or expressed prostatic secretion (EPS).

Fraction IV. The initial portion of the stream (5 to 10 ml) after prostatic massage (VB$_3$).

The four specimens are cultured, and the number of colonies per milliliter is calculated. If VB$_1$ contains more bacteria than VB$_3$, an abundant urethral flora, or even urethritis, is present. If EPS or VB$_3$ contains at least 10 times more bacteria than VB$_1$, the diagnosis of prostatitis should be considered. Some biochemical tests suggest a diagnosis of bacterial prostatitis; examples are a pH above 8, a reduced concentration of zinc, cholesterol, spermine, and citric acid, and an increase in ceruloplasmin level and fraction C3 of complement. Biopsy of the prostate is not often performed or recommended in this condition.

TREATMENT

Acute bacterial prostatitis. In this disorder, all antibiotics appear to penetrate into the prostate to an acceptable degree, and the choice of treatment is based on the antibiotic sensitivity of the organism isolated. When this information is lacking, a cephalosporin or an aminoglycoside is generally administered. When the patient has an abscess, one must also consider surgical drainage.

Chronic bacterial prostatitis. The choice of antibiotic is also guided by sensitivity tests, but other factors must be considered because many antibiotics penetrate poorly into the prostate, except in acute infections, for reasons of pH and liposolubility. In practice, the satisfactory antimicrobial agents are erythromycin, trimethoprim, and, less dependably, tetracyclines, chloramphenicol, its derivative thiamphenicol (not available in North America), and clindamycin. In absolutely refractory bacterial prostatitis, intraprostatic injections of a cephalosporin-aminoglycoside combination by the transperineal approach have been reported to be beneficial. The combination of an antibiotic with an anti-in-

---
*VB, Void bladder.

flammatory agent is believed to increase the effectiveness of the antibiotic therapy as well as improve the subjective condition of the patient. The addition of a mucolytic agent such as acetylcysteine may be beneficial. Surgical treatment is disappointing.

Prostatodynia. The only treatment available is the anti-inflammatory or mucolytic agents (acetylcysteine); some patients improve with prostatic massage.

> **Objective 22–9. Diagnose and treat ulcers of the male genitalia.**

A number of sexually transmitted infectious agents are responsible for genital ulcers. The specific etiologic diagnosis is often difficult to make solely on the basis of the clinical findings. Inguinal lymphadenopathy usually accompanies these ulcerative lesions or may be present alone in some stages of syphilis or lymphogranuloma venereum.

SYPHILITIC CHANCRE

This lesion is produced by the local inoculation of the spirochete, *Treponema pallidum* (see Chap. 23). The incubation period is 2 to 4 weeks after sexual contact. After this time, a hard, painless chancre appears at the site that constitutes the portal of entry of the organism. The lesion, which can be situated on the glans penis, prepuce, shaft, scrotum, or perineum, for example, is sometimes tiny and difficult to detect. Many atypical lesions may be found, notably on mucosal and moist areas. The development of this chancre is slow. In a few days, inguinal lymphadenopathy is a constant finding.

Diagnosis. A small amount of exudate is expressed from the chancre, and a drop is taken for dark-field microscopic examination or for Fontana or Giemsa staining.

Serologic tests include a combination of studies, such as Venereal Disease Research Laboratory (VDRL) or *Treponema pallidum* hemagglutinating antibodies (TPHA) and fluorescent treponemal antibody absorption (FTA-ABS) and Rapid Plasma Reagin (RPR). By means of these tests, one can detect a considerable proportion of cases.

When the chancre is present, the FTA-ABS test has the greatest chance of being positive (90% of cases). Beginning at the secondary stage, which occurs 2 to 4 weeks later and is characterized by mucocutaneous eruptions, the TPHA, RPR, and VDRL tests are positive in 100% of cases.

CHANCROID (SOFT CHANCRE)

This lesion is caused by *Haemophilus ducreyi*, a gram-negative bacillus. After an incubation period of 1 to 5 days, a rapidly ulcerating vesicle or papule appears. Around it, other ulcerations may develop later by autoinoculation. ("The chancroid lives surrounded by its young.") Subsequently, a painful inguinal adenopathy gradually develops; in half these patients, a purulent fistula appears. Half the patients have systemic symptoms such as fever and headaches. The ulceration may gradually enlarge and erode. The thin base of the ulcer bleeds easily; no induration is present—hence the name soft chancre. The disease is transmitted almost exclusively by sexual contact, and exposure does not confer immunity.

Diagnosis. The bacteriologic diagnosis of chancroid is not easy. Direct microscopic examination (Giemsa staining) of pus from the bubo or material obtained by scraping the edges of the ulceration may show bipolar-staining coccobacillary forms resembling a safety pin. Culture is laborious because the organism requires increased levels of carbon dioxide at which to grow.

The therapy of first choice is still the long-acting sulfonamides, 500 mg daily for 10 days, or the combination of trimethoprim and sulfamethoxazole, 80/400 mg twice a day; these agents are not treponemicidal. In case of failure of the sulfonamides, perhaps because of resistance, one should administer tetracycline, which is also active against syphilis, at a dose of 2 g daily for 15 days, or an aminoglycoside such as streptomycin or kanamycin, 1 g daily for 8 days. Many strains of *Haemophilus ducreyi* carry genes for beta-lactamase production, and ampicillin is therefore not an agent of choice.

GENITAL HERPES

Lesions are usually caused by herpes simplex virus 2 (HSV-2) or, more rarely, (10 to 20% of cases) by herpes simplex virus 1 (HSV-1) (Fig. 22–9) (see Table 4–2). Clinically, two sorts of genital herpes infections can be distinguished: primary and recurrent.

Primary Infection. When clinically apparent, primary infection is more severe than recurrences. Not only the external genitalia (glans penis, prepuce, collum glandis penis, penile shaft, and scrotum) and the skin may be infected, but also the urethra, buttocks, thighs, extremities, and the mouth and throat. Pain is a constant feature. Systemic signs, such as fever and malaise, may be present. Bilateral inguinal lymphadenopathy is common. The primary infection may be complicated by meningitis, transverse myelopathy, and sacral radiculopathies; however, herpetic encephalitis is improbable with HVS-2. Recent research has shown that the virus can be found in prostatic and seminal secretions, and viral excretion lasts for about 11 days. Altogether, the duration of this initial episode is about 20 days.

Recurrences. The frequency of recurrences in individuals who have had an initial episode of this infection seems to depend on the patient's sex (more frequent in males), the type of virus (more frequent with HSV-2), and, no doubt, on the immunologic response of the subject at the time of the first infection. A recurrent genital herpes infection generally occurs on the skin of the external genitalia and does not last as long as the primary infection; it is less often accompanied by systemic reactions, and the time of elimination of the virus also appears shorter. The frequency of recurrences decreases with time, but varies from one individual to the next; in some, it exceeds six a year and may have a major psychologic impact on the individual.

Diagnosis. Cytologically, giant multinucleated cells with specific inclusions, Cowdry type A cells, can be seen in scrapings from the base of the ulcer, by Papanicolaou staining or the Tzanck test.

The virus can be cultured from the vesicular lesions. HSV-1 and HSV-2 are antigenically different and can be serotyped in the laboratory; they produce clinically identical lesions. An appropriate medium must be used to transport the specimen to the virology laboratory.

Serologically, the initial infection is manifested by the appearance and rising titers of antibodies to HSV-2 or HSV-1. During recurrences, the level of antibodies generally remains stable.

Treatment. Treatment of genital herpes infections is difficult, but innumerable regimens have been proposed. For recurrent infection, a solution of alcohol and ether (50:50) can be applied and allowed to dry in air; the ether dries and destroys the lipid capsule of the virus, and the alcohol reduces the burning when ether is applied. Acyclovir cream is moderately effective in primary herpes infection, provided the cream is applied early. It is important to caution the patient that this agent has no influence on relapses. During recurrences, patients are contagious for seronegative partners. The presence of antibodies to HVS-2 in persons who have not had symptomatic genital herpes seems to limit the probability of their acquiring a symptomatic infection from an individual who is a carrier of HSV-2. It is also possible that individuals who have a recurrent herpes labialis HSV-1 infection are also less likely to acquire genital herpes.

GRANULOMA INGUINALE

This disorder, which is caused by *Calymmatobacterium granulomatis*, a gram-negative bacillus, is rare in developed countries; it is characterized by a chronic granulomatous infection of the skin and subcutaneous tissues in the genital and perineal region. The incubation period is from 2 to 3 months. The disease begins with papular formations that develop into irregular ulcerations with a beefy-red base. The lesions are painless.

Diagnosis. The diagnosis of granuloma in-

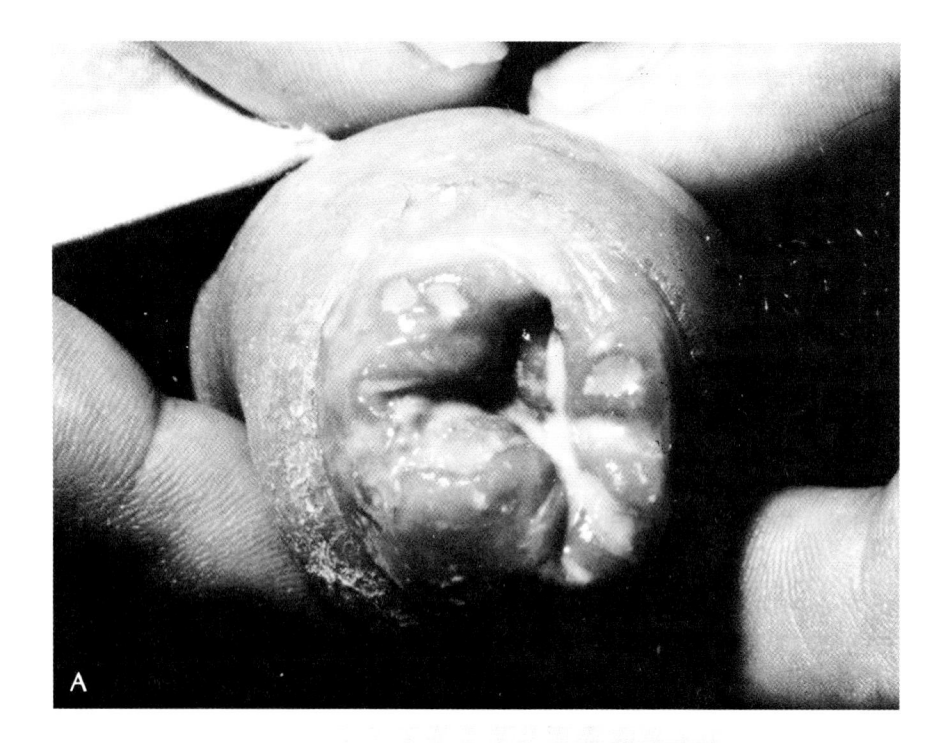

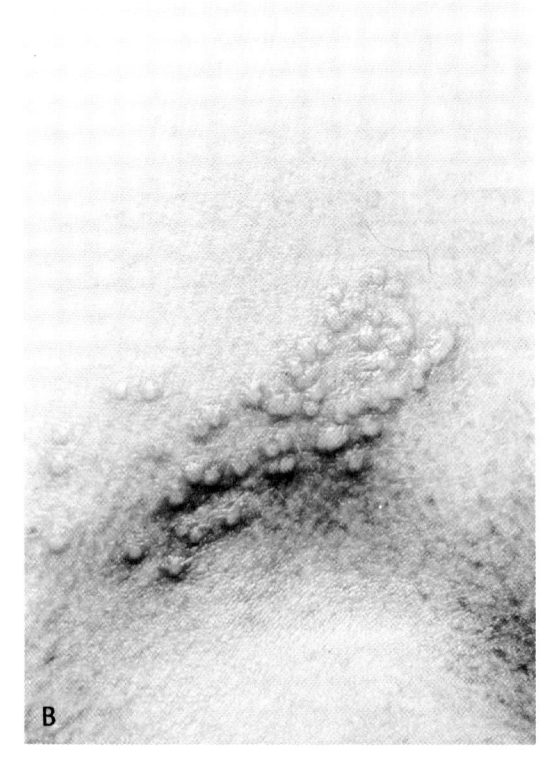

328 *Infections: Recognition, Understanding, Treatment*

Fig. 22–9. *A*, Genital herpes. Strong inflammatory reaction and phymosis, *without* bacterial infection. *B*, Vesicles of herpes simplex virus type I. (Compare with intercostal zona of Plate 12*B*).

guinale is established by direct microscopic examination using Giemsa staining for the Donovan bodies formed by bipolar-staining intracellular and extracellular gram-negative bacilli. Biopsy of the border of the ulceration for histologic study usually makes the diagnosis. Malignant tissue has been reported in chronic lesions.

Treatment. The tetracyclines give excellent results, but the aminoglycosides and chloramphenicol are also effective.

LYMPHOGRANULOMA VENEREUM

Lymphogranuloma venereum (LGV) (Durand-Nicolas-Favre disease, tropical bubo) is caused by *Chlamydia trachomatis* serotypes L_1, L_2, L_3, and sometimes by other serotypes of the paratrachoma group, such as type K (see Chap. 32 and Table 22-8). Both in vitro and in vivo, these particular serotypes are characterized by rapid growth and invasiveness. These serotypes are also lethal for mice on intracerebral inoculation, in contrast to the other serotypes. The chlamydiae that belong to the paratrachoma serotypes (D to K) are usually limited to mucous membranes, whereas the LGV serotypes penetrate more deeply and produce systemic disease (see Table 22-8). In the developed countries of the temperate zone, LGV is less frequent and causes a milder disease than in South America or southern Asia. Good hygiene and an adequate diet may inhibit the spectacular development of the disease.

LGV begins with a vesicular lesion that ruptures and usually becomes ulcerated within 2 weeks of the onset of the infection. This primary lesion is infrequently noticed, especially in women. Then, 2 or 3 weeks later, inguinal adenopathy develops. It is often initially minor and difficult to detect. Fever may also be seen at this point. In Western Europe and in North America, severe complications are rare; the disease is often limited to a painful inguinal adenopathy which may drain for weeks or months under treatment.

Diagnosis. Direct microscopic examination after Giemsa staining of pathologic genital specimens is rarely helpful. Cell culture techniques make it possible to isolate these organisms, but one requires a specialized laboratory. The positive diagnosis is based on culturing material from a primary lesion or from fluid obtained by puncture of the lymph nodes.

The newer serologic tests have reduced the value of the classic Frei skin test. The antigen used was simply purified pus from lymph node lesions. Later, the antigen obtained from a chlamydial culture in the yolk sac of chick embryos was used. The test becomes positive between 8 days and 6 months after infection. In some patients, however, it may never become positive, and the value of the test is thereby limited.

Immunofluorescent serologic testing is the most useful procedure. IgM antibodies are the first to appear and persist for at least 6 weeks. IgG antibodies appear later and persist longer. In nearly all patients, the presence of IgM or of a seroconversion of IgG (elevation of titers at least four-fold) is considered significant. These antibodies differ from those detected by the complement fixation reaction, now used infrequently because it is less sensitive. Patients with inguinal buboes develop antibodies against serotype (L and often also against serotypes D, E, and K). Immunofluorescent serologic testing for LGV may be performed in any case of unexplained inguinal adenopathy, whether or not ulceration is present. If the disease is suspected, biopsy should be avoided because it produces chronic fistulas, and the diagnosis should be made solely be serologic means.

Treatment. For 21 days, the usual treatment includes a tetracycline such as doxycycline, 100 mg twice daily, or tetracycline, 500 mg 4 times daily, or sulfamethoxazole, 1 g twice a day. Surgical treatment is sometimes required to repair fistulas and strictures.

Objective 22-10. Identify the causes of epididymo-orchitis and take appropriate measures.

EPIDIDYMO-ORCHITIS

Enlargement of the epididymis or the testicle accompanied by pain suggests epididymitis, orchitis, or epididymo-orchitis. Acute forms of the disorder are manifested by severe pain, swelling, and fever. In subacute or chronic forms, areas of induration or cyst formations are found on palpation; the patient feels little pain and has no fever.

Diagnosis. The differential diagnosis includes neoplasm, trauma, torsion of the spermatic cord, and strangulated inguinal hernia. The infectious causes of epididymo-orchitis are legion.

In the context of a systemic infection, one might first consider a localization of the disease. Viral causes include mumps, in particular. The diagnosis of mumps should be considered in a postpubertal individual without a history of the disease, with predominant testicular involvement and minimal involvement of the epididymis and with other localizations, such as the parotid glands, or in someone with a known contact with mumps. Coxsackieviral orchitis has also been reported. Epididymo-orchitis may be the metastatic focus of disseminated brucellosis or meningococcal or pneumococcal septicemia.

In sexually active persons, especially those under 35 years of age, an infection caused by *Neisseria gonorrhoeae* or *Chlamydia trachomatis* deserves first consideration. One may confirm the diagnosis by means of the patient's medical history, the finding of urethritis, and special examination of the urethral discharge. Rectal examination and the Stamey test may also be helpful by demonstrating an associated prostatitis. When *Chlamydia trachomatis* is the causative agent, however, confirmation of the diagnosis may be particularly difficult.

After the age of 35, gonococcal and chlamydial epididymo-orchitis become less frequent, whereas infection with gram-negative bacteria, such as *Escherichia coli*, klebsiella, and pseudomonas, originating from a urinary disorder or sometimes from prostatitis becomes more common. An obvious precipitating cause, such as a urinary catheter or recent urologic intervention, is sometimes found. The urine culture is usually positive.

In patients of any age, the differential diagnosis should include tuberculosis, although now rare, especially when the cause of the epididymo-orchitis remains obscure, when the course of the illness is protracted, and when other factors are suggestive, for example, a history of pulmonary tuberculosis. In such a case, one often sees an overlying tubercular focus, either prostatic or renal. The means available for confirming this diagnosis are discussed in Objective 21–9.

Treatment. The treatment of epididymo-orchitis includes measures for relieving the pain and inflammation, such as the use of an athletic supporter and the limitation of activity. Surgical drainage of an abscess is rarely required. Therapy depends on the cause of the disorder. Penicillin or its substitutes are indicated for urethritis in gonococcal infections (see Table 22–6), tetracycline is indicated for chlamydial infections, and ampicillin, aminoglycosides, or third-generation cephalosporins are indicated for infections caused by gram-negative organisms.

Objective 22–11. Diagnose condyloma acuminatum, molluscum contagiosum, and pediculosis pubis, and counsel patients in whom these conditions are found.

BENIGN TUMORS CAUSED BY VIRUSES

Condyloma acuminatum, also known as verruca acuminata or venereal wart, is caused by a papillomavirus (papovavirus group) that has not yet been cultured. The disorder is often associated with other sexually transmitted diseases. The incubation period is at least 3 months. Condylomas (Figs. 22–10 and 22–11), usually situated in the urethral meatus or the collum glandis penis, may regress spontaneously.

Molluscum contagiosum is a rare viral infection characterized by umbilicated, hemispheric, wart-like lesions. The lesions may multiply rapidly by autoinoculation.

Diagnosis. Generally, the diagnosis of condylomas and molluscum lesions is based on clinical appearance. When in doubt, patho-

NEISSERIA GONORRHOEAE

Neisseria gonorrhoeae, the gonococcus, is a small, gram-negative coccus occurring in pairs, resembling coffee beans, and infecting man. Biochemical tests distinguish it from the other species of the family Neisseriaceae, which includes other pathogens important to man such as *Neisseria meningitidis* (meningitis, septicemia), *Branhamella catarrhalis* (chronic bronchitis), moraxella (conjunctivitis, and acinetobacter (hospital-acquired infections). On smears of exudate, some *N. gonorrhoeae* are observed characteristically within polymorphonuclear leukocytes, whereas others are extracellular.

The gonococcus is a fragile and fastidious aerobic organism. Because it is delicate, it must be inoculated rapidly after collection, or a transport medium must be used; because it is fastidious, it requires rich nutrient media and a suitable moist atmosphere enriched in carbon dioxide. Selective media are employed because the presence of other bacteria may inhibit its growth. Thayer-Martin medium, used in culture of *N. gonorrhoeae,* is a chocolate agar containing colistin, vancomycin, and nystatin to inhibit the normal flora of the urethra, oral cavity, and vagina.

For some time, bacteriologists have identified 4 or even 5 sorts of colonies (T_1 to T_5); this finding is of medical interest because only T_1 and T_2 seem to be pathogenic. Pathogenicity has been related to the presence of filaments called pili at the surface of the organisms; the cocci constituting colonies T_3, T_4, and T_5 have no such filaments. The pili, whose length may exceed 4 μ, appear to be necessary for the attachment of the gonococci to the host cells and particularly to the urethral and pharyngeal epithelium. *Neisseria gonorrhoeae* also has a capsule and surface lipopolysaccharides (endotoxin). In addition, it is capable of secreting an enzyme that splits IgA and is believed to be important in the organism's virulence.

The susceptibility of gonococci to antibiotics has varied in time. Initially, sulfonamides were active; however, no doubt after their widespread use in treating gonorrhea and other ailments, these agents became less effective. When penicillin was introduced, the minimum inhibitory concentration (MIC) ranged between 0.003 and 0.03 U/ml; 150,000 U were sufficient to cure most cases. By the end of the 1950s, these MICs gradually rose and it became necessary to increase the doses to current levels. This slow phenomenon of reduced susceptibility is not due to the production of a beta-lactamase, but is probably caused by the progressive selection of more resistant bacterial strains.

In 1975, the first case of much greater resistance to antibiotics was reported. These resistant strains have since multiplied and are found worldwide. In this instance, resistance is the result of the production of a TEM type of beta-lactamase, similar to that of *Haemophilus influenzae* and coded by a plasmid. This beta-lactamase inactivates not only penicillin G, but also ampicillin and the first-generation cephalosporins, and hence makes it necessary to prescribe other products such as spectinomycin, cefoxitin, cefotaxime, or tetracycline. With tetracycline also, however, a shift toward resistance has been observed. To conclude on a practical note, penicillin still remains the drug of first choice in most areas of the world, and the susceptibility of the gonococcus to an antibiotic cannot be taken for granted. Antibiotic sensitivity tests are of value, and follow-up cultures taken after treatment are even more so, even though the patient is asymptomatic.

---

logic examination of a biopsy specimen confirms the nature of the formations. Examination by electron microscope may demonstrate the presence of the condyloma virus in the nuclei of infected cells. Antigenic differences are believed to exist with the verruca viruses. Sixty percent of the sexual partners of affected patients may develop condylomas.

Treatment. To treat condyloma acuminatum, one should carefully apply 20% podophyllum resin, which has antimitotic activity, leave it in place for 4 hours, then wash, and apply an antibiotic cream. One must be careful of burns. The treatment should be repeated regularly. For large clusters of lesions or in case of treatment failure, surgical cauterization is recommended.

To treat molluscum contagiosum, excision by curettage is preferred. Otherwise, electrofulguration may be performed under local anesthesia.

PEDICULOSIS PUBIS

Phthirus pubis, the pubic louse, differs from the head and body lice, *Pediculus humanus capitis* and *Pediculus humanus corporis,* in that it is more squarish, has a wider thorax, and measures approximately 1 mm in length. The second and third pairs of legs are much longer than the first; at the extremity of the limbs are pincers that give these creatures the name "crabs."

These lice are found in pubic hair, but in hairy individuals they may also occur in the armpits, eyelashes, mustache, and beard. The lice are seen more clearly when they are gorged with blood and take on a rust color.

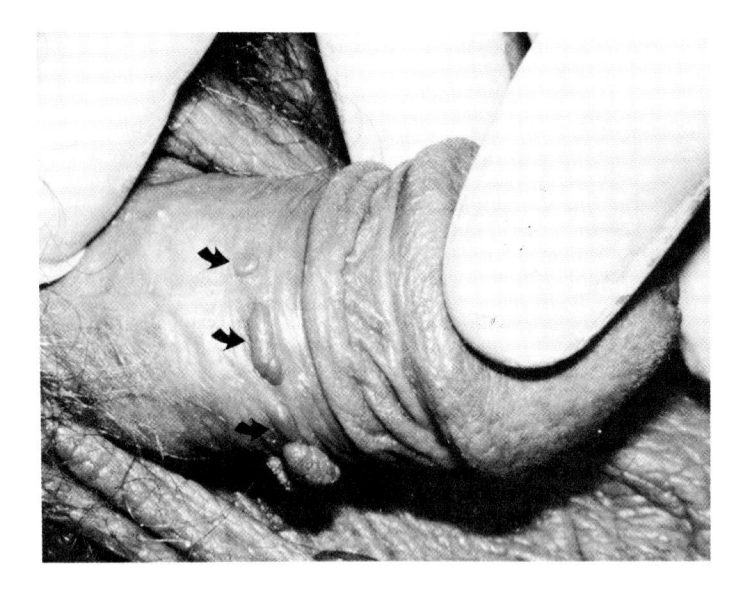

Fig. 22–10. Acuminate condylomas.

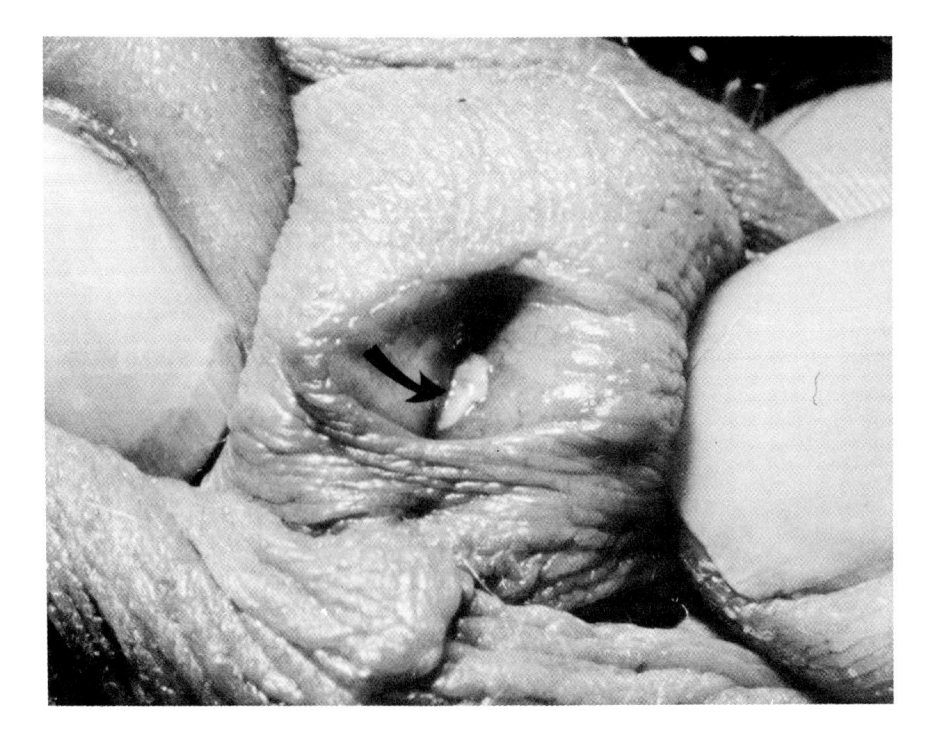

Fig. 22–11. Intraurethral acuminate condyloma mimicking chronic urethritis.

Their life span is estimated at one month, and they multiply rapidly. Essentially, patients complain of pruritus. The excoriations readily become superinfected, and related lymphadenopathy is common.

Pediculosis pubis is contracted principally during sexual intercourse, but is can also be contracted from sanitary facilities, undergarments, and borrowed sports equipment. The parasite can survive for about 24 hours outside the host.

Diagnosis. The diagnosis is based on the search for nits (eggs) attached to the roots of the patient's hair or to moving adult lice. The duration of infestation can be evaluated approximately by the distance that separates the nit from the patient's skin. Microscopic examination is performed by observing an adult louse pressed on a slide.

Treatment. Shaving the patient's pubic hair is not necessary. Lindane (gamma benzene hexachloride) 1% is used in the form of a lotion or shampoo or in powder form. One thorough application is usually sufficient.

SUGGESTED READINGS

Female Genital Infections

Burkman, R.: Association between intrauterine device and pelvic inflammatory disease. Obstet. Gynecol., 57:369, 1981.

Charles, D.: Infections in Obstetrics and Gynecology. Philadelphia, W.B. Saunders, 1980.

Dans, E.P.: Gonococcal anogenital infection. Clin. Obstet. Gynecol., 19:103, 1975.

Eschenbach, D.A.: Epidemiology and diagnosis of acute pelvic inflammatory disease. Obstet. Gynecol., 55(Suppl.):142S, 1980.

Eschenbach, D.A.: Acute pelvic inflammatory disease: etiology, risk factors and pathogenesis. Clin. Obstet. Gynecol., 19:147, 1976.

Goldacre, M.J., et al.: Vaginal microbial flora in normal young women. Br. Med. J., 1:1450, 1979.

Hansfield, H.: Disseminated gonococcal infection. Clin. Obstet. Gynecol., 18:131, 1975.

Hill, G.B.: How bacterial flora of the genital tract relates to infection. Contemp. Ob/Gyn, 15:113, 1980.

Holmes, K.K., Eschenbach, D.A., and Knapp, J.S.: Salpingitis: overview of etiology and epidemiology. Am. J. Obstet. Gynecol., 138:893, 1980.

Larsen, B., and Galask, R.P.: Vaginal microbial flora: practical and theoretic relevance. Obstet. Gynecol., 55(Suppl.):100, 1980.

Ledger, W.J.: Laparoscopy in the diagnosis and management of patients with suspected salpingo-oophoritis. Am. J. Obstet. Gynecol., 38:1012, 1980.

Leger, W.J.: Infection in the Female. Philadelphia, Lea & Febiger, 1977.

Monif, G.R.G.: Significance of polymicrobial bacterial superinfection in the therapy of gonococcal endometritis-salpingitis-peritonitis. Obstet. Gynecol., 55(Suppl.):154, 1980.

Monif, G.R.G.: Infectious Diseases in Obstetrics and Gynecology. Hagerstown, MD, Harper & Row, 1974.

Per-Anders, M.: An overview of infectious agents of salpingitis, their biology, and recent advances in method of detection. Am. J. Obstet. Gynecol., 138:933, 1980.

Pheifer, T.A., et al.: Nonspecific vaginitis. Role of Haemophilus vaginalis and treatment with metronidazole. N. Engl. J. Med., 298:1429, 1978.

Rein, M.F., and Chapel, T.A.: Trichomoniasis, candidiasis and the minor venereal diseases. Clin. Obstet. Gynecol., 18:73, 1975.

Spiegel, C.A., et al.: Anaerobic bacteria in nonspecific vaginitis. N. Engl. J. Med., 303:601, 1980.

Sweet, R.L.: The case for a polymicrobial etiology of acute salpingitis. Contemp. Ob/Gyn, 15:93, 1980.

Sweet, R.L., and Ledger, W.J.: Cefoxitin: single agent treatment of mixed aerobic-anaerobic pelvic infections. Obstet. Gynecol., 54:193, 1979.

Sweet, R.L., Draper, D.L., Schachter, J.: Microbiology and pathogenesis of acute salpingitis as determined by laparoscopy: what is the appropriate site to sample? Am. J. Obstet. Gynecol., 138:985, 1980.

Washington, A.E.: Update on treatment recommendations for gonococcal infections. Rev. Infect. Dis., 4(Suppl.):758, 1982.

Weström, L.: Incidence, prevalence, and trends of acute pelvic inflammatory disease and its consequences in industrialized countries. Am. J. Obstet. Gynecol., 138:880, 1980.

Male Genital Infections

Alani, M.D., et al.: Isolation of Chlamydia trachomatis from the male urethra. Br. J. Vener. Dis., 53:88, 1977.

Bowie, W.R.: Etiology and treatment of nongonococcal urethritis. Sex. Transm. Dis., 5:27, 1978.

Bowie, W.R., Alexander, E.R., and Holmes, K.K.: Etiologies of postgonococcal urethritis in homosexual and heterosexual men roles of Chlamydia trachomatis and Ureaplasma urealyticum. Sex. Transm. Dis., 5:151, 1978.

Drach, G.W.: Prostatitis and prostatodynia. Urol. Clin. North Am., 7:79, 1980.

Grayston, J.T., and Wang, S.P.: New knowledge of Chlamydiae and the diseases they cause. J. Infect. Dis., 132:87, 1975.

Hafiz, S., McEntegart, M.G., Morton, R.S., and Maitkins, S.A.: Clostridium difficile in the urogenital tract of males and females. Lancet, 1:420, 1975.

Hallen, A., Ryden, A.C., Schwan, A., and Wallin, J.: The possible role of anaerobic bacteria in the aetiology of non-gonococcal urethritis in men. Br. J. Vener. Dis., 53:368, 1977.

Holmes, K.K., et al.: Etiology of non-gonococcal urethritis. N. Engl. J. Med., 292:1199, 1975.

Hubrechts, J.M., Baltus, J., Weiser, M., and Butzler,

J.P.: Chlamydia associated urethritis. Acta Clin. Belg., 32:211, 1977.

Hubrechts, J.M., et al.: Isolation of Chlamydia trachomatis in lymphogranuloma venereum. Acta Clin. Belg., 35:2, 1980.

Nilsen, A.E., et al.: Efficacy of oral acyclovir in the treatment of initial and recurrent genital herpes. Lancet, 2:571, 1982.

Oriel, J.D., et al.: Chlamydial infection. Isolation of Chlamydia from patients with non-specific genital infection. Br. J. Vener. Dis., 48:429, 1972.

Perroud, H.M., and Miedzybrodzka, K.: Chlamydial infection of the urethra in men. Br. J. Vener. Dis., 54:45, 1978.

Pfau, A., Perlberg, S., and Shapira, A.: The pH of the prostatic fluid in health and disease. Implications of treatment in chronic bacterial prostatitis. J. Urol., 119:384, 1978.

Ripa, K.T., Mardh, PPA., and Thelin, I.: Chlamydia trachomatis urethritis in men attending a venereal disease clinic: a culture and therapeutic study. Acta Derm. Venereol., 58:175, 1978.

Schachter, J., and Dawson, C.R.: Human Chlamydial Infections. Littleton, MA, S.G. Publishing, 1978.

Swartz, S.L., et al.: Diagnosis and etiology of non-gonococcal urethritis. J. Infect. Dis., 138:445, 1978.

Taylor-Robinson, D., Csonka, G.W., and Prentice, M.J.: Chlamydia and ureaplasma-associated urethritis. Lancet, 1:903, 1977.

Taylor-Robinson, D., et al.: Ureaplasma urealyticum and Mycoplasma hominis in chlamydial and non-chlamydial urethritis. Br. J. Vener. Dis., 55:30, 1979.

Treharne, J.D., Darougar, S., and Jones, B.R.: Modification of the microimmunofluorescence test to provide a routine serodiagnostic test for chlamydial infection. J. Clin. Pathol., 30:510, 1977.

Wallin, K., and Forsgren, A.: Group B streptococci in venereal disease clinic patients. Br. J. Vener. Dis., 51:401, 1975.

CHAPTER 23

Syphilis

M.F. Rein

> **Objective 23–1.** Describe the clinical situations in which syphilis should be suspected.

Syphilis is a specific infection caused by the spirochete *Treponema pallidum*. The disease has a chronic course with subacute periods separated by asymptomatic intervals, during which the diagnosis can be made only serologically. *T. pallidum* remains sensitive to penicillin, and treatment is effective. The major problem facing the clinician, therefore, is recognizing syphilis and maintaining a high index of suspicion in a setting where the disease has become uncommon.

SEXUAL PARTNERS OF PATIENTS WITH SYPHILIS

The moist lesions of early syphilis contain large numbers of treponemes that can be transmitted during intimate contact. Thus, primary and secondary syphilis are considered infectious stages of the disease. In venereal disease clinics, syphilis has been found in about one half of the sexual partners of patients with early syphilis. Sexual partners who have had repeated exposure to the infected patient are at particularly high risk of infection, as high as 90% in some series. Although not every sexual exposure transmits the infection, the risk of infection in sexual partners is so high that such patients should be treated on first presentation. Clinical and serologic evidence of syphilis usually does not develop until about 3 weeks after acquiring the infection, but the incubation period may be as long as 90 days and may be prolonged by subcurative doses of antibiotics. Thus, patients who have been sexually exposed to persons with primary or secondary syphilis within the past 90 days should be treated even if the initial physical examination and serologic testing fail to give evidence of the disease. Treating a patient before lesions develop prevents further transmission of infection. Patients whose infections are cured before their serologic tests become reactive are likely to remain seronegative.

Patients who have been infected for more than 90 days are unlikely to remain seronegative. If, therefore, a patient is seen more than 90 days after sexual exposure to early syphilis, the physician need only order a serologic test (see the discussion later in this chapter). If this test is nonreactive, one can assume that the patient did not acquire syphilis from that exposure and need not be treated.

PRIMARY SYPHILIS

Genital Lesions. At the end of the incubation period, usually about 3 weeks after

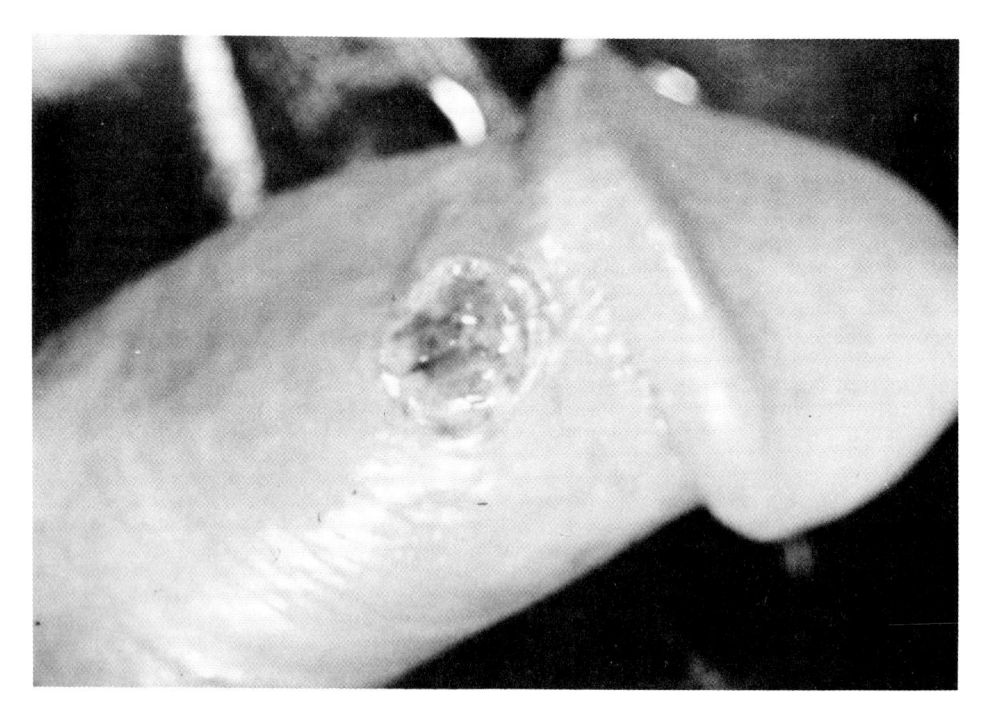

Fig. 23–1. Syphilitic chancre.

exposure to syphilis (the range is 10 to 90 days), the patient develops a lesion called a chancre at the point of initial inoculation and multiplication of the spirochete (Fig. 23–1). The chancre begins as a papule, which erodes to form a gradually enlarging ulcer with a clean base and an indurated edge. Although it is generally painless, some patients do experience discomfort. Syphilis should be suspected in a patient with a clean, ulcerated lesion of the genitalia. Although the classic chancre of primary syphilis is a single lesion, in recent series, almost half the patients with proved primary syphilis had more than one penile ulcer.

The morphologic features of chancres are variable, and the differential diagnosis of ulcerative lesions of the genitalia may be difficult. For example, herpes genitalis usually occurs initially as grouped, umbilicated vesicles on an erythematous base. These vesicles subsequently ulcerate to form clusters of painful lesions. Patients often describe a prodrome of itching or burning of the affected skin, beginning about 12 hours before the vesicles appear. The incubation period for primary herpes infection is usually about 7 days, shorter than the incubation period for syphilis. Chancroid may produce multiple ulcerations of the genitals. The ulcerations are usually ragged, have a necrotic base, and have elevated edges that form a crater. Induration is generally less marked than with syphilis. The incubation period for chancroid may be as short as 72 hours.

Extragenital Lesions. Extragenital chancres are most frequently observed around or in the mouth and may involve the gingiva or tonsil. Perianal and rectal chancres occur in women as well as in homosexual men who practice receptive anal intercourse. Chancres about the nipple are also recognized. In the past, dentists occasionally developed chancres of the finger following examination of patients with oral lesions, and neonates developed chancres of the eyelid resulting from passage through an infected birth canal. In general, the clinician should consider syphilis as part of the differential diagnosis of ulcerative lesions anywhere on the body.

> **PATHOGENESIS AND STAGES OF SYPHILIS**
>
> *Treponema pallidum* can penetrate intact mucous membranes or may infect by tiny cuts or abrasions in cornified epithelium. Even before the first lesion appears or the blood test becomes reactive, the spirochetes have entered the blood and lymphatic systems and have become widely disseminated.
>
> The initial lesion of syphilis, the chancre, appears when spirochetes have multiplied to about 10^7/gm of tissue. The slow rate of the organism's division explains the usual 3-week incubation period. Patients with a lesion only at the site of inoculation and with regional adenopathy are said to have primary syphilis. These manifestations resolve spontaneously. The early dissemination of the organisms sets the stage for secondary syphilis, generally manifested by involvement of the skin, viscera, and more rarely, the central nervous system. These manifestations also resolve without treatment. The patient then progresses through a prolonged asymptomatic period, although about 25% have relapses resembling secondary syphilis during the first year or so following infection. The asymptomatic period is called latent syphilis. About one-third of patients spontaneously cure their infections, about one-third remain infected but asymptomatic, and about one-third develop the features of late syphilis. About 15% of untreated syphilitics develop late benign syphilis, which consists of granulomatous (gummatous) involvement of the skin and bones. These granulomas are destructive to surrounding tissue, but the process is promptly arrested by adequate therapy.
>
> About 10% of patients develop late cardiovascular manifestations. *Treponema pallidum* may directly affect the aortic endothelium and may produce a characteristic irregularity reminiscent of tree bark. Rolling and thickening of the aortic valve cusps may lead to aortic insufficiency, which may be made worse by the weakening and dilatation of the aortic valvular ring. Aortic insufficiency decreases coronary perfusion, and the coronary arteries may themselves be directly involved; this endarteritis may lead to coronary occlusion. Involvement of the vasa vasorum weakens the aortic tunica media, and the aorta may then develop an aneurysm.
>
> About 8% of untreated patients have late syphilitic involvement of the central nervous system. This complication may result from direct granulomatous involvement of brain tissue or from vascular insufficiency produced by syphilitic endarteritis.
>
> Syphilis is characterized by an obliterative endarteritis manifested as endothelial proliferation and perivascular infiltration primarily with mononuclear cells, a process that may impair blood flow. Syphilitic infection may also elicit a granulomatous reaction called a gumma. Gummas may appear in any organ and are probably a manifestation of delayed hypersensitivity in the immune host. Antigen-antibody complexes have been detected in the blood of patients with secondary syphilis and may be responsible for some manifestations, such as glomerulonephritis and the Jarisch-Herxheimer reaction.

Regional Adenopathy. Painless, usually bilateral inguinal adenopathy (satellite bubo) appears in 50 to 70% of patients with primary syphilis of the genitalia. Painless regional adenopathy may follow development of a chancre at an extragenital site. For example, cervical adenopathy may accompany a syphilitic lesion of the oral cavity. The affected lymph nodes usually occur in a chain and are discrete, firm, and movable.

The differential diagnosis of regional adenopathy is extensive. Tender adenopathy accompanies many acute infections and is characteristic of brucellosis, tularemia, cat-scratch disease, and infection with pyogenic cocci; such adenopathy also accompanies the genital lesions of chancroid and herpes genitalis. Tender adenopathy is characteristic of lymphogranuloma venereum.

Course of Primary Syphilis. Even without treatment, the syphilitic chancre heals completely within about 4 to 6 weeks, and the regional adenopathy resolves. Spontaneous resolution of the manifestations of infection may erroneously suggest a cure and may delay the patient's seeking appropriate medical attention. Spirochetemia actually precedes development of the chancre. From 2 to 8 weeks, but occasionally as long as 6 months, after the appearance of the chancre, the patient may develop the manifestations of secondary syphilis.

SECONDARY SYPHILIS

The signs of secondary syphilis are variable and have contributed to the status of syphilis as the "great imitator." Secondary syphilis often begins with illness characterized by sore throat, malaise, headache, arthralgias, and fever. This complex of symptoms is nonspecific and usually suggests an acute viral illness. The suspicion of secondary syphilis, therefore, generally depends on the subsequent development of more specific features.

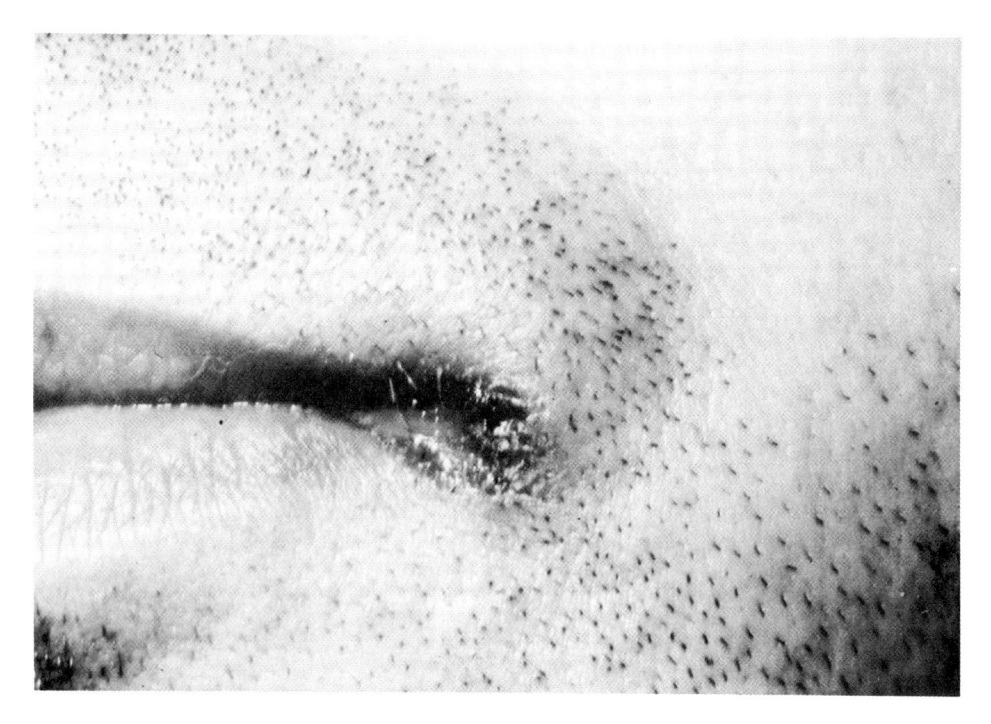

Fig. 23–2. Syphilitic papule on the lips.

Generalized Rash. Skin lesions (Plate 6A to C) are found in 80% of affected patients but they vary in type and appearance, and diligent examination is often required. Macular lesions, the most common, are found in about one-third of patients. These lesions frequently involve the patient's thighs, abdomen, and trunk. They are usually bilaterally symmetric, follow lines of skin cleavage, and have a coppery or "boiled ham" color. Mild-to-moderate pruritus is compatible with the diagnosis. The rash almost invariably involves the genitalia and is frequently prominent on the palms of the hands and soles of the feet, a distribution that suggests syphilis. Indeed, a generalized rash that completely spares the genitalia and oral mucous membranes is unlikely to be syphilitic. Maculopapular lesions are seen in about 12% of patients with syphilis (Fig. 23–2), and about 5% manifest follicular lesions, particularly on the back and extensor surfaces of the extremities.

Less-common skin lesions include annular lesions, which appear principally around the face, and pustular lesions, which are seen in only about 2% of patients. Vesicles or bullae are rare in secondary syphilis in adults, although they may be seen in congenital syphilis.

The dry skin lesions of syphilis are generally negative to dark-field microscopic examination and are minimally contagious.

Mucous Membrane Lesions. The mucous membranes are involved in about 60% of cases of secondary syphilis. The lesions may be subtle and limited to one area, for example, to the undersurface of the tongue. About one-third of patients develop mucous patches (Fig. 23–3). These patches are painless, oval ulcerations usually covered by a grayish or yellowish membrane. Inflammation around the lesions is minimal, and they are easily differentiated from aphthous stomatitis. Mucous patches contain large numbers of spirochetes and should be considered contagious. Careful dark-field microscopic examination is often diagnostic, but it may be difficult to differentiate *Treponema pallidum* from the normal spirochetal flora of the oral cavity. A generalized rash completely sparing

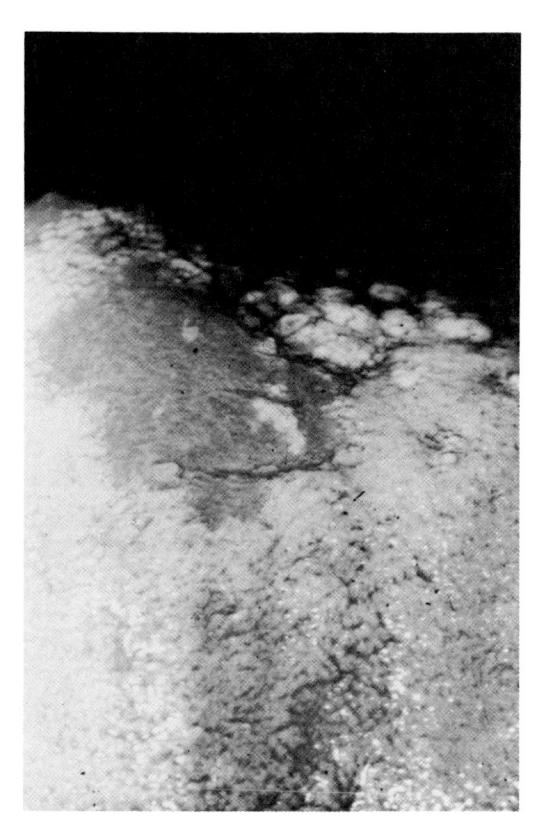

Fig. 23–3. Syphilitic mucous plaques on the tongue.

the patient's mouth and genitalia is unlikely to be syphilitic.

Condyloma Latum. This flat, hypertrophic lesion resembles a wart and develops in moist areas. These condylomas are frequently found around the anus or vagina, but they have also been described in the axilla and other moist areas. The lesions do not represent points of inoculation, but result from hematogenous dissemination of spirochetes. Like other moist lesions of syphilis, condylomas may be shown by dark-field microscopic examination to contain large numbers of spirochetes.

Alopecia. Patchy, nonpruritic alopecia of the scalp, beard, or eyebrows may be syphilitic, but common fungal infections must first be excluded as a diagnosis.

Generalized Lymphadenopathy. This complication is observed in about 75% of patients with secondary syphilis. The groups of lymph nodes most frequently involved are the inguinal, suboccipital, posterior auricular, and cervical (posterior more frequently than anterior). Epitrochlear adenopathy should be sought because it is suggestive of syphilitic infection, although this type of adenopathy is also seen in other conditions, including sarcoidosis, infectious mononucleosis, and lymphoma. The generalized adenopathy, like the regional lymph node involvement in primary syphilis, is not usually painful, and the affected nodes remain discrete.

Course of Secondary Syphilis. Hepatitis and immune complex glomerulonephritis occasionally accompany secondary syphilis. Uveitis and osteitis are rarely observed. The manifestations of secondary syphilis usually resolve within 2 to 6 weeks even in the absence of therapy. Some of the skin lesions may heal with scarring.

Acute Lymphocytic Meningitis. The central nervous system is asymptomatically involved in about one-third of patients with secondary syphilis, but central nervous system symptoms accompany only about 2% of cases. The cerebrospinal fluid may contain 500 white blood cells/ml, primarily mononuclear, and the protein level is frequently elevated. The symptoms are those of a basilar meningitis, often including meningeal and cranial nerve signs. Meningovascular syphilis usually occurs within the first 10 years after the acquisition of syphilis and may also become manifest as an acute basilar meningitis. The differential diagnosis of lymphocytic meningitis is extensive and includes viral, mycobacterial, and fungal diseases. Almost all affected patients have a positive Venereal Disease Research Laboratory (VDRL) test (see the discussion later in this chapter) on cerebrospinal fluid. This finding should be regarded as diagnostic of syphilitic meningitis because false-positive reactions in the cerebrospinal fluid are rare.

Cerebrovascular Accident in a Young Person. Meningovascular syphilis most frequently results from syphilitic endarteritis and usually manifests as seizures or a stroke. In the absence of hypertension, a stroke in a young person should prompt a search for meningovascular syphilis.

TERTIARY SYPHILIS

Dementia (General Paralysis). The causes of dementia are varied, and a detailed diagnostic workup is usually fruitless. Serologic tests for syphilis do, however, sometimes reveal an arrestable pathogenesis and general paresis. This condition develops because of direct spirochetal involvement of brain substance and usually becomes manifest 15 to 20 years from the time the patient acquired syphilis. A variety of disorders of higher cerebral function, personality changes, and delusional states may be demonstrated. One sometimes sees the Argyll-Robertson pupil, which is small and further constricts with accommodation, but does not react to light. This finding is suggestive of neurosyphilis. The patient's cerebrospinal fluid is generally abnormal, as characterized by small numbers of lymphocytes and a slightly elevated protein level, and the VDRL test on cerebrospinal fluid may be reactive. Unfortunately, nontreponemal tests in blood are sometimes nonreactive in patients with paresis. The fluorescent treponemal antibody absorption (FTA-ABS) test (see the discussion later in this chapter) should be performed on serum, but this test may also be nonreactive in patients with paresis.

Posterior Column Disease and Peripheral Neuropathy. Tabes dorsalis results from syphilitic involvement of the posterior columns and dorsal roots of the spinal cord. The condition is so characteristic that the diagnosis can be made clinically. Affected individuals often manifest losses of vibration sense and proprioception that result in a broad-based gait. Patients frequently complain of paresthesias, described as severe, sharp pains that may affect any part of the body. Impotence and bladder dysfunction are common. Optic atrophy is seen in one-quarter of affected individuals, and the Argyll-Robertson pupil is more prevalent than in paresis. Many patients with tabes dorsalis have normal cerebrospinal fluid, and some have nonreactive nontreponemal tests for syphilis on serum and cerebrospinal fluid. Thus, the FTA-ABS test is useful in confirming a diagnosis of tabes dorsalis and should be performed even if the nontreponemal tests on blood are nonreactive. The differential diagnosis includes combined systems disease and diabetic or alcoholic peripheral neuropathy.

Destructive Skin and Bone Lesions. About 15% of untreated syphilitics eventually manifest granulomatous lesions of skin and bone. These lesions, called gummas, are gradually progressive and destructive. Distributed asymmetrically about the body, gummas are often indurated and painless. They may heal at one edge and advance at another. Active lesions usually have sharp margins, and ulcers may have a punched-out appearance, with peripheral hyperpigmentation. These gummas often heal as atrophic, superficial scars. Lesions in the shape of segments of circles suggest syphilis. Skin lesions may be confused with malignant disease or with infection by atypical mycobacteria or fungi.

Bones are frequently involved and may show periostitis with localized increases in bone density or destructive lesions surrounded by sclerosis. The tibia is involved in about half the patients, and the clavicle, skull, or fibula is involved in about 25% each.

Biopsies of skin or bone are nonspecific and reveal granulomas. Organisms are only rarely seen. Serologic tests for syphilis are almost invariably reactive, and the lesions heal rapidly after appropriate treatment. Scarring may be significant.

Proximal Aortic and Aortic Valvular Disease. About 10% of untreated syphilitics eventually develop cardiovascular disease, usually involving the aortic valve and the proximal aorta. The second sound of the aorta is altered; it is sometimes described as having a tambour-like quality. Symptoms of aortic insufficiency develop later. An aortic diastolic murmur in a person without hypertension or a history of rheumatic heart disease should prompt a consideration of syphilis. Aortic insufficiency murmurs, with a peak intensity at the third or fourth intercostal space at the right sternal border, correctly suggest syphilis about 50% of the time. Later, patients often develop congestive heart failure or angina pectoris. Syphilis should be considered in the differential diagnosis in young people who develop angina pectoris without other predisposing factors. Weakening of the aorta may result in aneurysm. About half of syphilitic aneurysms occur in the aortic arch; another 40% involve other parts of the thoracic aorta. The abdominal aorta is involved in only 10% of syphilitic aneurysms.

CONGENITAL SYPHILIS

Babies with congenital syphilis may be completely asymptomatic at birth, but they sometimes have stigmas suggestive of the disease. Affected children may develop disseminated lesions of the skin and mucous membranes resembling those of secondary syphilis. The nasal mucous membranes are particularly susceptible, and syphilitic involvement results in snuffles, a persistent, mucopurulent nasal discharge containing large numbers of spirochetes. This involvement may progress to hemorrhagic rhinitis, which suggests the diagnosis of congenital syphilis. Condyloma latum is also seen in some patients. The skin lesions of congenital syphilis sometimes localize to a diaper rash distribution. Vesicles and bullae, rare in adults, are common in children with congenital syphilis.

Nearly all affected children have radiologic evidence of bone involvement. Long bones show a characteristic area of provisional calcification of the epiphysis, beneath which is seen an area of rarefaction. Tongues of moth-eaten calcification involve the metaphysis. Periostitis causes concentric layers to form in subperiosteal bone; the shafts of the long bones thus have a layered appearance. Skeletal involvement may be painful and may result in voluntary splinting of an extremity.

Congenital syphilis should also be considered in neonates manifesting hepatosplenomegaly, lymphadenopathy, jaundice, or hemolytic anemia. These findings are much less specific, however, and may accompany a variety of diseases.

From 75 to 90% of cases of congenital syphilis are diagnosed in patients over the age of 10 years.

Certain dental, ocular, and auditory findings comprise Hutchinson's triad, which is pathognomonic of congenital syphilis. Hutchinson's teeth are secondary incisors, which are usually barrel-shaped, shorter, and narrower than normal, and have a notch in the center of their edge. Distortion of the 6-year molar may yield a mulberry-like appearance. Interstitial keratitis usually appears between 5 and 20 years of age and is characterized by photophobia, eye pain, blurred vision, and tearing. Examination reveals mild injection of the iris and limbus and grayish infiltrates of the cornea. Nerve deafness may occur.

Fissuring around the mouth and anus, called rhagades, is a rare finding. Hypertrophic skeletal lesions include anterior bowing of the tibia, known as saber shins, or enlargement of the medial end of the clavicle. Erosive lesions occasionally result in perforation of the palate; syphilis was once the most common cause of this defect. Collapse of the nasal bones may produce a saddle-nose deformity.

> Objective 23–2. Confirm a diagnosis of syphilis by laboratory methods.

DARK-FIELD MICROSCOPIC EXAMINATION

The syphilitic nature of a genital or extragenital ulcer is best documented by demonstrating *Treponema pallidum* in fluid from the lesion by dark-field examination. The physician should wear gloves for this procedure. The surface of the lesion is cleaned by abrasion with a gauze pad until the sore begins to bleed. The lesion is then blotted until blood flow ceases. Pressure on the sides of the lesion usually brings forth a small amount of blood-free fluid, which can be picked up on the surface of a glass microscope slide,

---
TREPONEMA PALLIDUM

Treponema pallidum is a fine, spiral organism approximately 0.15 μ wide and 6 to 15 μ long. The organism is poorly visualized with routine microbiologic and histologic stains, but it may be seen in tissue with a variety of silver stains and is identified by dark-field microscopy in fluid recovered from lesions or lymph nodes. When observed in the living state, the organism displays 6 to 14 regular spirals, which are maintained during its movements. *T. pallidum* has a trilaminar outer membrane similar to that seen in gram-negative bacteria. Unlike these bacteria, however, *T. pallidum* probably does not possess a biologically active endotoxin.

The spirochete is microaerophilic and survives poorly in atmospheric oxygen. This property and its sensitivity to drying and to extremes of temperature explain in part its almost exclusively venereal mode of transmission. At present, *Treponema pallidum* cannot be cultured on artificial media, although its viability and virulence can be maintained by serial passage in susceptible animals, principally rabbits. Fortunately, *T. pallidum* has remained sensitive to the antibiotics used for the treatment of syphilis.
---

covered with a coverslip, and examined by dark-field illumination. The dark-field condenser angles the light so that no light passing directly through the preparation enters the microscope's lens. Objects are thus visualized by reflected, rather than by transmitted, light and appear bright against the dark background. An adequate dark-field preparation should reveal tiny, bright particles subjected to Brownian movement and should be almost free of erythrocytes. The preparation is carefully examined for *T. pallidum*, which can be recognized by its characteristic shape and movements. The organism maintains 6 to 14 regular spirals during its movements, it rotates in corkscrew fashion along its long axis, it moves forward and backward along this axis, and it bends at the midpoint. Experience is necessary for accurate interpretation of dark-field microscopic preparations. Patients who have taken even small quantities of antibiotics may fail to have a positive dark-field examination.

Dark-field microscopic examination of oral lesions is difficult because saprophytic oral spirochetes may closely resemble *Treponema pallidum*. Careful cleansing and isolation of the lesion are necessary. The dry skin lesions of secondary syphilis are rarely dark-field positive, but an examination of material from condyloma latum usually reveals organisms. Snuffles of congenital syphilis are dark-field positive, as is material aspirated from syphilitic lymphadenopathy.

SEROLOGIC TESTS

Patients with syphilis develop antibodies directed against a poorly defined lipid, which may be a component of the spirochete. Cross-reacting lipids are found in a variety of normal tissues and serve as the basis for the nontreponemal tests for syphilis, which generally employ a lipid extracted from beef heart as an antigen. The antigen is mixed with the patient's serum, and the clumping of the antigen particles is observed by techniques that vary with each specific test. Nontreponemal tests are technically easy to perform and are inexpensive. Those currently in common use are the VDRL test, the rapid plasma reagin (RPR) test, and the automated reagin test (ART). These nontreponemal tests may be positive in a variety of diseases other than syphilis, such as the following: acute viral illnesses including varicella, hepatitis, and infectious mononucleosis; bacterial infections such as leprosy, tuberculosis, and leptospirosis; and conditions such as parenteral drug abuse and collagen vascular diseases, which are associated with the formation of abnormal immunoglobulins.

Nontreponemal tests may be quantitated, and the results are expressed as the highest dilution of serum yielding a reaction. The RPR and ART tests may yield antibody titers two to eight times higher than the VDRL on the same serum. Because changes in antibody titer have considerable clinical significance, patients should be followed over time with the same nontreponemal tests.

Patients with syphilis also develop antitreponemal antibodies, which can be detected by a variety of procedures employing *Treponema pallidum* as the antigen. The principal treponemal test in current use is the FTA-ABS test in which antitreponemal antibody is detected by indirect fluorescence of spirochetes attached to a slide. The FTA-ABS test, the current standard for the diagnosis of syphilis, is the most sensitive serologic test in all defined stages of syphilis. The microhemagglutination test for *Treponema pallidum* (MHATP) uses treponemal antigens attached to the surface of erythrocytes, which agglutinate when mixed with serum from patients with syphilis. The use of this test is becoming more widespread, but it is less sensitive in primary syphilis than is the FTA-ABS test.

The *Treponema pallidum* immobilization (TPI) test, an expensive and technically difficult procedure, is no longer routinely available. Because it is less sensitive than the FTA-ABS test, a negative TPI test result does not rule out syphilis in a patient with a positive FTA-ABS test result.

Treponemal tests are generally used to confirm the diagnosis of syphilis in patients with reactive nontreponemal tests. They are not routinely quantified and so are reported only as reactive or nonreactive.

Incubating Syphilis. Reactivity with the nontreponemal tests for syphilis generally begins about 3 weeks after acquisition of the infection, but it may take as long as 90 days. The interval may be prolonged by subcurative antibiotic treatment. Thus, syphilis cannot be reliably ruled out until at least 90 days after the suspected exposure. It is therefore routine practice to treat those who have had sexual contact with infectious syphilis within the past 90 days, no matter what their current serologic status.

Primary Syphilis. Fifty percent of patients have not synthesized adequate levels of antibody to react to the nontreponemal tests by the time the chancre first appears. When the chancre has been present for days to weeks, the majority of patients have a reactive nontreponemal serologic test. In primary syphilis, the overall sensitivity of the nontreponemal tests is about 75%; that of the treponemal tests is about 90%. Thus, negative serologic tests for syphilis do not exclude a diagnosis of primary syphilis, particularly in patients who have had a chancre for a short time. The diagnosis can usually be confirmed, however, by retesting the patient a week after the initial examination.

When the clinical setting is suggestive of primary syphilis, it is probably unnecessary to confirm a reactive nontreponemal test with a treponemal test.

Secondary Syphilis. Almost all patients with secondary syphilis are reactive to all serologic tests for syphilis. Thus, a diagnosis of secondary syphilis can be essentially ruled out by a nonreactive quantitative nontreponemal test result. Rarely, patients with secondary syphilis have such high levels of nontreponemal antibody that the qualitative nontreponemal tests may be falsely nonreactive (prozone phenomenon). This problem is obviated by ordering quantitative nontreponemal tests on such patients, so the serum is tested in higher dilutions.

Latent Syphilis. By definition, the diagnosis of latent syphilis depends entirely on serologic evidence. Because of the low prevalence of syphilis in the general population and the high frequency of false-positive reactions to the nontreponemal tests, a reactive nontreponemal test result is not sufficient evidence of latent syphilis. All patients with a positive nontreponemal test should have the diagnosis confirmed by a treponemal test, preferably the FTA-ABS test. Unfortunately, as discussed previously, even a reactive treponemal test result does not absolutely confirm the diagnosis of syphilis.

Late Syphilis. The sensitivity of the nontreponemal tests drops as low as 50% in some stages of late syphilis, particularly with tabes dorsalis. In investigating suspected cases of late syphilis, an FTA-ABS test should be ordered even if nontreponemal test results are nonreactive.

A reactive VDRL test result on cerebrospinal fluid suggests the diagnosis of neurosyphilis, but false-positive reactions are encountered, although rarely. The FTA-ABS test is so sensitive that results are positive on cerebrospinal fluid in the absence of a true central nervous system infection because any blood contamination of cerebrospinal fluid produces a false-positive result. The test cannot be used to differentiate neurosyphilis from syphilis without central nervous system involvement.

Syphilis in Pregnancy. The seriousness of congenital syphilis makes serologic screening of pregnant women advisable. The risk of congenital syphilis is greatest in patients who acquire syphilis during pregnancy. Thus, women with multiple sexual partners should be re-examined serologically at intervals during pregnancy to detect newly acquired cases of syphilis.

Congenital Syphilis. Both the nontreponemal and treponemal tests detect IgG antibodies, which freely cross the placenta. Thus, seroreactivity in umbilical cord blood does not necessarily confirm a diagnosis of congenital syphilis, but may merely indicate transplacentally acquired maternal antibody. These possibilities can be differentiated by following the antibody titer of nontreponemal tests in the baby. If the baby is not infected, then the titer of the nontreponemal tests should fall at a rate consistent with the elimination of maternal immunoglobulin. Serologic tests for syphilis should be nonreactive by 4 months of age. On the other hand, if the titer of nontreponemal antibody remains stable or rises after birth, the baby is synthesizing antibody in response to in utero infection. Unfortunately, the stigmas of congenital syphilis may develop during the interval, or the baby may be lost to follow-up.

The FTA-ABS test can be made specific for IgM. Because IgM does not cross the placenta, IgM antitreponemal antibodies detected in the baby's serum indicate fetal antibody synthesis in response to true infection. Unfortunately, the test has not lived up to its initial promise. It is nonreactive in many asymptomatic newborns with congenital syphilis and has been falsely positive in the presence of other in utero infections.

Because of the uncertainties of serologic diagnosis of congenital syphilis in the asymptomatic baby, it is probably prudent to treat such children at birth.

> **Objective 23–3.** Interpret positive serologic tests in a patient with no clinical evidence of syphilis.

The diagnosis of syphilis may be suspected clinically when the disease manifests as primary syphilis, secondary syphilis, or late syphilis. During longer periods, however, the patient has neither signs nor symptoms of the disease. Such patients are said to have latent syphilis, which can be diagnosed only through the reactivity of serologic tests.

DIAGNOSIS OF LATENT SYPHILIS

The manifestations of early syphilis often go unnoticed because they resolve without treatment, may be masked by intercurrent antibiotic therapy, or may be comparatively mild. Therefore, many patients with latent syphilis do not give the physician a medical history suggestive of early syphilis. The clinician is frequently faced with the problem of an asymptomatic patient who is found on routine screening to have a reactive serologic test for syphilis. A reactive nontreponemal test result should be confirmed with the FTA-ABS or MHA-TP test. If the treponemal test result is nonreactive, the result of the reactive nontreponemal test can be considered a false-positive, and the diagnosis of syphilis can be largely excluded. Because the FTA-ABS test is the most sensitive test for all stages of syphilis, no other serologic test can be used to rule out the diagnosis once the result of the FTA-ABS test is positive.

All serologic tests for syphilis are subject to false-positive reactions, and the clinician is faced with less than complete certainty that the patient truly has syphilis. The physician's approach should include careful and sympathetic questioning of the patient concerning any possible history of early syphilis or of prior positive serologic tests for syphilis, such as in the military, during prior hospital admissions, in premarital blood tests, and in previous pregnancies, and sexual history. A history of homosexual contact increases the likelihood that the patient has syphilis and also that the clinical manifestations of primary syphilis may have gone unnoticed. A history of collagen vascular disease or parenteral drug abuse increases the likelihood of false-positive serologic reactions. The patient should then be examined carefully for subtle manifestations of syphilis, including scars from healed genital lesions, regional or generalized lymphadenopathy, subtle oral lesions, hair loss, or the late manifestations of congenital syphilis. Any of these findings supports a diagnosis of syphilis.

The probability that a patient with a reactive serologic test for syphilis actually has the disease is called the predictive value of a positive test (PVpos). Unfortunately, even with accurate tests like the FTA-ABS, the predictive value of the test drops rapidly in a population with a low prevalence of syphilis. Consider, for example, a test having 95% sensitivity (reactive in 95% of all patients with syphilis) and 99% specificity (correctly nonreactive in 99% of patients who do not have syphilis) applied to a population where only 1 in 1000 people tested actually has the disease. In this setting, PVpos equals .087. Only 9 of every 100 patients with a reactive serologic test actually have syphilis. Thus, the clinician must be cautioned that when applying even excellent tests to a population of patients with a low prevalence of disease, the overwhelming majority of reactive tests are false-positive.

Clinicians therefore face a difficult dilemma. On the one hand, they cannot rule out syphilis in the patient, but on the other hand, the diagnosis is far from certain. In this setting, it seems prudent to explain the uncertainties carefully to the patient, but to recommend treatment because the risks of treatment are low and the course of untreated syphilis is potentially disastrous.

The nonvenereal treponematoses such as yaws, pinta, and bejel cause a serologic reactivity in nontreponemal and treponemal tests that is indistinguishable from that caused by venereal syphilis. These diagnoses should be considered in patients who have resided in areas where such diseases are endemic and who have reactive serologic tests for syphilis.

ASYMPTOMATIC NEUROSYPHILIS

The asymptomatic patient with a positive serologic test result for syphilis may have asymptomatic neurosyphilis. By definition, such patients display none of the clinical features of syphilitic involvement of the brain or spinal cord; they may nonetheless be infected. Because the diagnosis is based on examination of the cerebrospinal fluid, this fluid should be examined in all patients with untreated syphilitic infection of unknown duration or in untreated or inadequately treated patients known to have been infected for more than a year. The cerebrospinal fluid in patients with asymptomatic neurosyphilis generally has a normal glucose concentration. The protein concentration is usually only minimally elevated; 35 to 60% of patients have normal values, and only 5 to 20% of patients have a protein level higher than 100 mg/dl. Pleocytosis of the cerebrospinal fluid is often minimal as well; 70% of patients have between 5 and 10 cells/mm^3, and only about 10% of patients have more than 10 cells/mm^3; about 60% of affected patients have a lymphocytic predominance. A reactive VDRL test result in cerebrospinal fluid is a strong indicator of neurosyphilis, but it may be nonreactive in the spinal fluid of some affected patients. The FTA-ABS test is of no value in examining the cerebrospinal fluid.

Objective 23–4. Treat syphilis.

Penicillin G remains the treatment of choice for all stages of syphilis in patients who are not hypersensitive to the drug. The duration of therapy is important. Treatment for early syphilis usually consists of benzathine penicillin G, which produces low serum levels persisting for 3 weeks following a single

> **NONVENEREAL TREPONEMATOSES**
>
> Infections with other organisms of the genus *Treponema* are acquired nonvenereally. These infections are most common in areas of poverty, poor hygiene, and overcrowding, and are usually acquired before puberty. Each infection results in reactive nontreponemal and treponemal tests for syphilis. All such infections are successfully treated with long-acting penicillins.
>
> Yaws occurs principally in tropical areas. From 3 to 4 weeks after infection with *Treponema pertenue,* the patient develops a papule that enlarges to form a raised, crusted lesion, the "mother yaw." Nontender, regional adenopathy is common. Then, 3 to 4 weeks later, the patient develops a diffuse papular eruption with lesions that become crusted. The patient's bones are often painfully affected with osteitis and periostitis, and many years later, destructive lesions of the skin and bones may develop.
>
> Pinta, infection with *Treponema carateum,* is found only in Central and South America. An initial, papular lesion appears 1 to 3 weeks after exposure and extends to become a scaly, mildly pruritic patch accompanied by regional lymphadenopathy. From 3 to 9 months later, the patient develops a generalized, scaly rash. The lesions characteristically progress through a variety of color changes, including blue, violet, brown, and, finally, white. Bones and viscera are not greatly involved. In 1 to 3 years, the depigmented lesions appear principally on the wrists and ankles.
>
> Bejel occurs in drier, cooler areas, including the Balkans, the Eastern Mediterranean, and Northern Africa. Three weeks after infection, one occasionally sees a transient, painless oral lesion. Patients then develop mucous patches, condyloma latum, and generalized adenopathy. These late lesions involve skin and bone.
>
> When a patient has a reactive serologic test for syphilis, the physician should look for a history of residence in an area endemic for nonvenereal treponemal disease.

intramuscular injection. Primary or secondary syphilis, or syphilis known to be of less than a year's duration, can be adequately treated with a single administration of 2.4 million U benzathine penicillin G. Alternatively, one can administer aqueous procaine penicillin G, 600,000 U intramuscularly daily for 8 days. This alternate regimen, although effective, is less convenient than the single-dose treatment, both for the physician and the patient. Patients allergic to penicillin may be treated with tetracycline hydrochloride or erythromycin (stearate, ethylsuccinate, or base), 500 mg orally 4 times a day for 15 days. Erythromycin is particularly appropriate for penicillin-allergic pregnant women, in whom tetracycline should be avoided.

For syphilis of more than a year's duration, or for infections of unknown duration, with the possible exception of neurosyphilis, one may prescribe benzathine penicillin G, 2.4 million U intramuscularly weekly for 3 successive weeks or aqueous procaine penicillin G, 600,000 U intramuscularly daily for 15 days. Patients allergic to penicillin may be treated with tetracycline or erythromycin as previously mentioned, but the drug must be administered for 30 days.

NEUROSYPHILIS

Neurosyphilis presents special problems because of the low levels of penicillin found in cerebrospinal fluid following the administration of benzathine penicillin G. The best treatment of symptomatic or asymptomatic neurosyphilis is probably the administration of at least 10 million U aqueous crystalline penicillin G intravenously daily for at least 10 days. Infants with congenital syphilis but without evidence of central nervous system involvement (normal cerebrospinal fluid examination) can be treated with a single administration of benzathine penicillin G, 50,000 U/kg intramuscularly. Patients with abnormalities of the cerebrospinal fluid should, however, be treated with higher doses, such as aqueous crystalline penicillin G, 50,000 U/kg intramuscularly or intravenously daily in 2 divided doses for a minimum of 10 days. Anaphylactic reactions to penicillin are not described in neonates.

JARISCH-HERXHEIMER REACTION

Beginning about 1 to 6 hours after treatment with penicillin, a patient with syphilis may have an abrupt onset of fever, chills, myalgias, headache, flushing, and, occasionally, hypotension. In addition, one may ob-

> **EPIDEMIOLOGY OF SYPHILIS**
>
> The venereal nature of syphilis has been recognized since the earliest descriptions of the disease. Disease is known to develop in 30 to 50% of the sexual contacts of patients with primary or secondary syphilis, but the risk of a single exposure has not been determined. Syphilis is most prevalent in sexually active populations and age groups; the highest age-adjusted rates for early syphilis reported in the United States are found in men and women between the ages of 20 and 24. The prevalence of infection is also increased in homosexual men, who account for over half the cases reported in larger cities.
>
> The World Health Organization estimates that 50 million new cases of syphilis are acquired annually throughout the world. Reported cases of syphilis diminished rapidly after the introduction of penicillin in the late 1940s and reached a nadir in 1955. Although the prevalence of late syphilis has continued to decrease in developed countries, the incidence of early syphilis began to rise again in the early 1960s.
>
> Nonvenereal acquisition of syphilis is reported, but is uncommon. The infection can be acquired by kissing someone who has an active oral lesion. Acquisition by blood transfusion is no longer a significant problem because serologic tests are routinely performed on donated blood, and *Treponema pallidum* does not survive current methods of prolonged blood storage. Children have been reported to acquire syphilis by sharing a bed with an infected parent. The presence of acquired syphilis in a child should, however, raise the question of child abuse in the mind of the examiner. The most important nonvenereal mode of acquisition occurs in utero.

serve transient exacerbation of rashes and increased tenderness of the patient's adenopathy. This reaction is felt to be caused by rapid lysis of spirochetes by penicillin with the formation of antigen-antibody complexes in the blood, although others believe it results from endotoxin blue. The reaction, which develops in about 50% of patients treated for primary syphilis and in up to 90% of patients treated for secondary syphilis, is usually mild, resolves within 24 hours, and is adequately treated with aspirin. More serious complications can develop in pregnancy or with neurosyphilis or cardiovascular syphilis, but fortunately, these complications are rare. In these patients, prior treatment with corticosteroids can eliminate the reaction.

SEROLOGIC RESPONSE TO THERAPY

In the months following adequate therapy for syphilis, one should observe at least a fourfold drop in antibody titer of the early nontreponemal tests; for example, from 1:64 to 1:16. By 24 months after therapy, the VDRL test is nonreactive in about 95% of patients treated for primary syphilis and in about 75% of patients treated for secondary syphilis. Fewer than half the patients who have had syphilis for more than 2 years become seronegative within 5 years. Thus, initially, one should follow the quantitative nontreponemal tests monthly until a fourfold drop in antibody titer is documented. Thereafter, the patient should be followed serologically every 3 months until the titer has stabilized. Determining this lowest antibody titer in addition to documenting the initial fourfold drop is important because subsequent rises in titer may indicate a need for retreatment, either on the basis of relapse or reinfection. Because the RPR and ART tests yield titers 2 to 8 times higher than the VDRL test on the same serum, sequential studies should be performed on patients with the same nontreponemal serologic tests. Switching from test to test may produce spurious drops or elevations in antibody titer.

Seroactivity with the treponemal tests persists in most patients despite adequate therapy. Thus, a reactive treponemal test in a patient previously treated for syphilis is not itself an indication for retreatment or for examination of the cerebrospinal fluid.

SUGGESTED READINGS

Anonymous: Sexually transmitted diseases. Treatment guidelines. Morbid. Mortal. Weekly Rep., 31(Suppl.):50, 1982.

Brown, S.T.: Update on recommendations for the treatment of syphilis. Rev. Infect. Dis., 4(Suppl.):837, 1982.

Chapel, T.A.: The signs and symptoms of secondary syphilis. Sex Transm. Dis., 7:161, 1980.

Chapel, T.A.: The variability of syphilitic chancres. Sex Transm. Dis., 5:68, 1978.

Fiumara, N.J., Fleming, W.L., Downing, J.G., and Good, F.C.: The incidence of prenatal syphilis at the Boston City Hospital. N. Engl. J. Med., 247:48, 1952.

Jaffe, H.W.: The laboratory diagnosis of syphilis: new concepts. Ann. Intern. Med., 83:846, 1975.

Jaffe, H.W., and Kabins, S.A.: Examination of cerebrospinal fluid in patients with syphilis. Rev. Infect. Dis., 4(Suppl.):842, 1982.

Kampmeier, R.H.: The late manifestations of syphilis: skeletal, visceral and cardiovascular. Med. Clin. North Am., 48:667, 1964.

Lee, T.L., and Sparling, P.F.: Syphilis: an algorithm. JAMA, 242:1187, 1979.

Morrisson, R.E.: Syphilis. In Current Therapy. Edited by H.F. Conn. Philadelphia, W.B. Saunders, 1982.

Sparling, P.F.: Diagnosis and treatment of syphilis. N. Engl. J. Med., 284:642, 1971.

Stokes, J.H., Beerman, H., and Ingrahm, N.R.: Modern Clinical Syphilology. Philadelphia, W.B. Saunders, 1944.

Waring, G.W.: False-positive tests for syphilis revisited: the intersection of Bayes' theorem and Wassermann's test. JAMA, 243:2321, 1980.

CHAPTER 24

Infection and Pregnancy

B. Grenier

> Objective 24–1. Explain why systematic screening for asymptomatic bacteriuria is required in pregnant women.

Several controlled studies have established a relationship between symptomatic bacteriuria and gestational complications, both in the mother and the infant. The prevalence of bacteriuria, which varies according to the study, the population, and the urine culture technique, appears to be at least 4 to 7% in a majority of surveys. This disorder is much more common in lower socioeconomic groups. These bacteriurias are asymptomatic most of the time and produce no significant consequences if treated and monitored properly. On the other hand, when untreated, these infections cause cystitis or acute pyelonephritis during pregnancy in more than 20% of patients. These observations justify the systematic culturing of urine in pregnant women, but other data also reinforce this position. When significant bacteriuria persists throughout pregnancy, pathologic sequelae can often be found after delivery: 30 to 80% of the cultures remain positive, the urine concentrating capacity is reduced in 14 to 40% of the patients, and an intravenous urogram is abnormal in 10 to 30% of the patients. Moreover, although not all prospective studies agree, it seems that toxemia, premature delivery, and low birth weight in infants are more frequent in untreated bacteriuric women than in nonbacteriuric or successfully treated women.

We are far from understanding the mechanisms by which urinary infections lead to reproductive disorders. Although numerous questions remain unanswered, the systematic detection and treatment of bacteriuria during pregnancy is imperative. Thus, a culture should be taken during the first or second trimester in all pregnancies. If bacteriuria is detected using the proper technique and is eventually confirmed by a second culture, a short course of therapy, usually 5 to 10 days, sterilizes the patient's urine in more than 80% of cases. Shorter treatments of only 1 to 3 days, successful in lower urinary tract infections, have not been evaluated in this particular condition.

The antimicrobial agent is chosen on the basis of the antibiotic sensitivity of the organism, usually a sensitive *Escherichia coli*, and the potential toxicity of the drug. A sulfonamide, such as sulfisoxazole, 1 g 2 to 4 times daily for 5 to 8 days, is preferred by most physicians if the pregnancy is more than 2 weeks from term. Amoxicillin, 250 mg 3 to 4 times daily for 5 to 8 days, and nitrofurantoin, 100 mg 2 to 4 times daily for 5 to 8 days, represent possible alternatives. These women should be followed up regularly with urine cultures during pregnancy and, when indicated by persistent bacteriuria, with renal function tests and intravenous urography after delivery.

> Objective 24–2. Identify infections that may affect the fetus across the placenta, to take preventive action.

Certain infections, when acquired during pregnancy, cross the placenta and affect the fetus. The abbreviation TORCH groups bring together the diseases that, because of their frequency and the seriousness of their consequences, have a considerable socioeconomic impact: *toxoplasmosis, rubella, cytomegalovirus,* and *herpes; other* infections include, in particular, syphilis and listeriosis (Table 24–1). When, in the pregnant woman, a bacterium, virus, or parasite disseminates hematogenously, it may cross the placenta and develop within the fetus. The consequences of the intrauterine infection may be any of the following (Tables 24–2 and 24–3): resorption of the ovum, abortion, stillbirth, malformation because of an arrest of organogenesis at a crucial stage, delay in intrauterine growth, prematurity, infection persisting beyond birth or congenital disease, or latency of or total recovery from the infection, with the birth of a healthy infant.

CONGENITAL TOXOPLASMOSIS

Toxoplasmosis, one of the most widespread infections in the world, is essentially a zoonosis for which the specific host is the domestic cat and probably the other members of the cat family. When a nonimmune gravid woman is infected, the toxoplasma can invade the fetus across the placenta with greater and greater ease during the course of pregnancy (Table 24–4). In the first trimester of pregnancy, congenital infections appear to be less common (17%) but more severe than during the last trimester, when they are more frequent but asymptomatic or mild.

Diagnosis. The physician cannot rely on clinical signs in diagnosing a primary infection in a pregnant woman. Polyadenopathy, fever, and mononucleosis (see Objective 25–4) occur in combination in fewer than 10% of patients; in practice, the diagnosis is serologic. Several tests are available. The Sabin-Feldman dye test, which used to be the reference, has now been replaced by the indirect fluorescent antibody (IFA) test or the indirect hemagglutination (IHA) test. An enzyme-linked immunosorbent assay (ELISA) and a radioimmunoassay allow for automation. In an attempt to standardize data, the World Health Organization has recommended expressing the results of these tests in International units (IU) rather than in dilution titers. The detection of IgM antibodies

Table 24–1. Prevalence of Maternal, Fetal, and Neonatal Infections

Organism	Mother (per 1000 pregnancies)	Fetus (per 1000 live births)	Newborn* (per 1000 live births)
Cytomegalovirus (CMV)			
during pregnancy	16–130	5–15	—
at delivery	110–280	—	50–100
Rubella virus			
epidemic	20–40	4–30	0
interepidemic	0.1–1.0	0.2–0.5	0
Toxoplasma gondii	1.5–6.4	1.3–7	0
Herpes simplex virus	1–10	rare	0.1–0.5
Herpes varicella-zoster virus	0.2	?	variable†
Treponema pallidum (Syphilis)	0.2	0.1	0
Streptococcus, group B	50–250	0	1–2
Escherichia coli	common	0	1–2

*Infection acquired at delivery or shortly afterwards.
†According to the epidemic situation.

Table 24–2. **Major Consequences of Intrauterine Infections**

Infecting Organism	Prematurity	Retardation of Intrauterine Growth	Malformation	Congenital Disease	Persistent Postnatal Infection
Virus					
Rubella	−	+	+	+	+
Cytomegalovirus	+	+	+	+	+
Herpes simplex	+	−	−	+	+
Herpes varicella-zoster	−	(+)	(+)	+	+
Mumps	−	−	−	(+)	+
Measles	+	−	−	+	−
Coxsackie B	−	−	(+)	+	−
Poliovirus	−	−	−	+	−
Hepatitis B	+	−	−	(+)	+
Bacteria					
Treponema pallidum	+	−	−	+	+
Listeria	+	−	−	+	−
Campylobacter	+	−	−	+	−
Mycobacterium tuberculosis	+	−	−	+	+
Protozoans					
Toxoplasma	+	(+)	+	+	+
Plasmodium (malaria)	(+)	+	−	+	+

−, Infections not producing anomalies.
+, Sequelae have been demonstrated.
(+), A causal relation is uncertain.

(IgM-IFA) is of special value here, because it permits early detection of the disease. The IgM antibodies become detectable as soon as 5 days after infection and disappear within a few months. By contrast, the rise in IgG antibodies is slow; it often takes 2 months to reach maximum titers with the IFA and the dye test and 4 to 6 months with the IHA test. Moreover, the persistence of IgG antibody titers for years adds a further potential for ambiguity.

The serologic diagnosis rests either on a seroconversion, indicating the importance of systematic screening at the beginning of pregnancy, or on a serial 2-tube rise in titer when sera drawn at 3-week intervals are run in parallel. The presence of IgM at a significant titer or a strongly positive IgG test, for instance, 300 IU in the IFA test, are only presumptive evidence.

Therapy. When primary toxoplasmosis is recognized in a pregnant woman, antibiotic therapy can be recommended. Sulfonamides such as sulfadiazine can be given safely at the beginning of the pregnancy and are effective in animal models. Pyrimethamine should be avoided because of its potential teratogenicity.

Spiramycin, a macrolide antibiotic not available in the United States, is given 2 to 4 g/day in 4 divided doses every day until delivery. This treatment is said to reduce the number of children born with infections, but not the number of newborns clinically affected by the disease. The only other alternative available to a woman infected during early pregnancy, when the risk of malformation is greatest, is therapeutic abortion. The decision must ultimately be made by the well-informed patient herself.

Prevalence and Prevention. Should we order a serologic test for toxoplasmosis at the beginning of all pregnancies? The answer may depend on the risk of congenital infections, which varies from one population to another. The prevalence of nonimmune pregnant women is 68% in New York, 71% in London, 14% in Paris for the French population, and 30% in Paris for Spanish and North African immigrants. These impressive variations are said to be related to the different methods of meat preparation, although other as yet unknown reasons may exist. The incidence of primary infections occurring during gestation is around 1.3% in the United States and Great

Table 24–3. Clinical Manifestations of the Major Prenatal and Neonatal Infections

Clinical signs	Rubella virus	Cytomegalovirus	Toxoplasma gondii	Herpes simplex	Treponema pallidum	Coxsackie virus B	Streptococcus group B
Hepatosplenomegaly	+	+	+	+	+	+	+
Jaundice	+	+	+	+	+	+	+
Adenopathy	+	–	+	–	+	+	–
Pneumonia	+	+	+	+	+	+	+
Skin							
Petechiae	+	+	+	+	+	+	+
Vesicles	–	–	–	++	+	–	–
Exanthem	–	–	+	+	++	+	–
Central Nervous System							
meningoencephalitis	+	+	+	+	+	+	+
microcephaly	–	++	+	+	–	–	–
hydrocephaly	+	–	++	+	–	–	–
intracranial calcification	–	++	++	–	–	–	–
deafness	+	+	–	–	+	–	–
Heart							
myocarditis	+	–	+	+	–	++	–
malformation	++	–	–	–	–	–	–
Bone lesions	++	–	+	–	++	–	–
Eye							
glaucoma	++	–	–	–	–	–	–
cataract	++	–	+	+	+	–	–
chorioretinitis or retinopathy	–	+	++	+	–	–	–
optic atrophy	–	+	+	–	–	–	–
microphthalmia	+	–	+	–	–	–	–
uveitis	–	–	+	–	+	–	–
keratoconjunctivitis	–	–	–	++	–	+	–

–, Not seen or rarely seen.
+, Routine in this infection.
++, Has some value as a pathognomonic sign of this infection.

FETAL DEFENSES AGAINST INFECTION

The first defense against blood-borne infection of the fetus is the so-called placental barrier. Once infectious agents gain access to the intervillosal spaces of the placenta, the agents may be destroyed or may produce only a localized placental infection without affecting the fetus. Such "barrier" effects have been observed during the course of infections such as tuberculosis, syphilis, malaria, rubella, and cytomegalovirus (CMV). In some circumstances, however, the microorganisms infect the fetus.

A second line of protection may be provided by immunologic defenses progressively acquired by the fetus during its development. The maturation of the specific and nonspecific immunologic response begins between the eighth and twelfth weeks of intrauterine life. The two populations of lymphocytes differentiate between themselves at this point. The T lymphocytes, thymus-dependent, provide cellular immunity and protection, particularly against fungal and viral invaders. By gestational week 20, the B lymphocytes produce immunoglobulins of the IgM type, especially if stimulated by an infection such as rubella, CMV, or toxoplasmosis. On the other hand, a rubella infection in the first trimester of pregnancy can compromise the development of the immune system and may create a serious congenital immunologic deficit.

The acquisition of phagocytic and polymorphonuclear neutrophil activity is gradual. The faculties of chemotaxis and phagocytosis in the neonate's cells are said to be equivalent to those in adult cells, but bactericidal properties connected to the formation of peroxide are still imperfectly developed. Both newborns and, to an even greater extent, fetuses are more susceptible than infants to bacterial infections, especially infections with staphylococci and enteric bacteria.

Finally, the fetus benefits from the transfer of maternal immunoglobulins, especially IgG. This active transport process across the placental barrier uses a specific receptor on the Fc fragment of the IgG molecule. Immunoglobulin transfer begins early in development and reaches maximum intensity in the second half of gestation. At birth, IgG plasma concentrations are equal in the mother and child, with a half-life in the latter of 20 to 30 days.

When a fetal infection occurs, several responses are possible, depending on the gestational age of the fetus. An infection occurring in the first trimester of pregnancy, when fetal immune defenses are just beginning to develop, is likely to have serious consequences, such as death of the fetus, arrest of embryogenesis, or major malformations. Sometimes an antigen, the rubella virus for example, persists for prolonged periods in an infected infant, both intra- and extracellularly, because of a stage of immunotolerance that renders the host incapable of responding to this antigen. The immunologic and inflammatory responses of the fetus in the second half of pregnancy often generate serious inflammatory lesions, which may be treatable. Thus, when a fetus is infected with syphilis before the fifth or sixth month of gestation in the absence of an inflammatory response, no tissue lesions are produced. If the infection occurs after this time, the fetal lymphocytes and plasmocytes respond and produce severe tissue damage, such as pneumonia alba, the white fetal pneumonia of syphilis. An analogous picture is seen in a rubella infection occurring in the last part of gestation.

The suppression or alteration of the expression of the disease is also possible, especially when the infection occurs in the latter part of pregnancy or during the perinatal period and thus involves an already immunocompetent host. These defenses still remain incomplete, however; for instance, the newborn is without maternal IgM, specifically important in immunity against gram-negative bacteria. This lack contributes to the susceptibility of the newborn to devastating infections with bacteria such as *Escherichia coli*.

Table 24–4. Incidence of Congenital Infection Toxoplasmosis by Trimester of Maternal Infection in 145 Pregnancies

Congenital Toxoplasmosis	First		Second		Third		Total	
Severe illness	3		6		0		9	
Mild illness	1	(17%)	5	(25%)	2	(65%)	8	(34%)
Asymptomatic infection	1		9		22		32	
No infection	24	(83%)	59	(75%)	13	(35%)	96	(66%)
Total	29	(100%)	79	(100%)	37	(100%)	145	(100%)

(Modified from Desmonts, G., and Couvreur, J.: Toxoplasmosis in pregnancy and its transmission to the fetus. Bull. N.Y. Acad. Med., 50:146, 1974.)

Britain and about 7.5% in France. The actual incidence of congenital toxoplasmosis remains uncertain, however. Approximations have been proposed as follows (per 1000 live births): Vienna, 6 to 7; Paris, 3; New York City, 1.3.

When a toxoplasmosis test is performed at the beginning of pregnancy, a positive result implies protection for the mother; a woman who has had toxoplasmosis at any time before gestation will not deliver an infected child. On the other hand, the absence of antibodies at the beginning of the pregnancy indicates a risk of primary infection, and certain recommendations should be made: eat only well-cooked meat; avoid direct contact with cats; do not handle earth potentially soiled by cat feces without gloves, for example, while gardening; and repeat the tests at the end of the first two trimesters of pregnancy.

CONGENITAL RUBELLA

In general, rubella infections are simple. Complications such as arthritis, thrombocytopenic purpura, and encephalitis remain uncommon. Unfortunately, when rubella occurs in a nonimmune, pregnant woman, the viremia that occurs 10 days after contact and continues for 5 to 8 days may infect the fetus with serious consequences. The timing of the fetal infection determines the type of teratogenic effect. As pregnancy progresses, the risk and the severity of congenital rubella diminish. Among infants who have contracted the disease during intrauterine life, the frequency of malformations and disabilities identified in the first 4 years of life is as follows: 0 to 8 weeks of gestation, 85%; 9 to 12 weeks of gestation, 52%; 13 to 20 weeks of gestation, 16%; after 20 weeks, no malformations.

TOXOPLASMA GONDII

Toxoplasma gondii is an obligate intracellular protozoan, classified among the Sporozoa. This parasite exists in three forms: trophozoite, cyst, and oocyst. The trophozoite, which can invade nearly any mammalian cell, is the form involved in acute disseminated infection. Trophozoites are shaped like a crescent or a bow and measure 4 to 8 μm in length and 2 to 3 μm in width.

The cysts' dimensions (10 to 100 μm) vary according to the number of organisms each contains, from several to 3000 merozoites. Cysts are found in the tissues of infected animals and man, most often in the brain, skeletal muscles, and myocardium. When these cysts are ingested, peptic or tryptic digestive fluids disrupt the cyst wall, and viable *Toxoplasma gondii* are released. These parasites may infect the new host. Cysts do not usually cause symptoms, but they survive for a long time in the host; persistent latent infections in tissues are in the form of cysts.

The oocysts are excreted exclusively in the stool of cats or members of the cat family, 3 to 5 days after eating infected meat. The sexual reproductive phase of the life cycle of *Toxoplasma gondii* begins within the epithelial cells at the tips of the ileal villi. The fusion of a micro- and macrogametocyte forms the ovum, or oocyst, which is then excreted in the host's feces. The excretion rate may reach 10 million/day and can continue for 1 to 3 weeks. To become infective, the oocysts must undergo maturation or sporulation; the egg or zygote divides into 2 sporoblasts, which are surrounded by a membrane and constitute the sporocyst. Inside each membrane, the sporocyst divides twice. The cyst, now sporulated and infectious, has a diameter of about 10 μm and contains 8 sporozoites that, on ingestion, release infectious trophozoites. The duration of maturation varies from 2 to 21 days, depending on the ambient temperature and oxygenation. The sexual cycle of toxoplasmosis, with the formation of gametes and the excretion of oocysts, occurs completely only in the cat. In all other animals and in man, the life cycle comes to a dead end; after a phase of hematogenous dissemination of the trophozoites, the organisms establish themselves in the tissue in the form of cysts.

Man can be infected by the following principal routes (Fig. 24–1):
1. Ingestion of oocysts from food soiled with dust contaminated by vectors such as flies and roaches or containing particles of earth contaminated with cat feces. This exclusive source of transmission for herbivores may be the most common route of infection in human populations.
2. Ingestion of cysts contained in infected animal tissue. The cysts, which remain infectious for 2 months at 4° C, are destroyed by freezing and thawing the meat and by cooking at temperatures greater than 70° C. This means of transmission is the rule for carnivores; it may also be frequent in human populations that ordinarily consume raw or superficially cooked meat.
3. Maternal-fetal transmission in the course of pregnancy.
4. Transmission by fresh blood or by granulocytes or organ homografts.

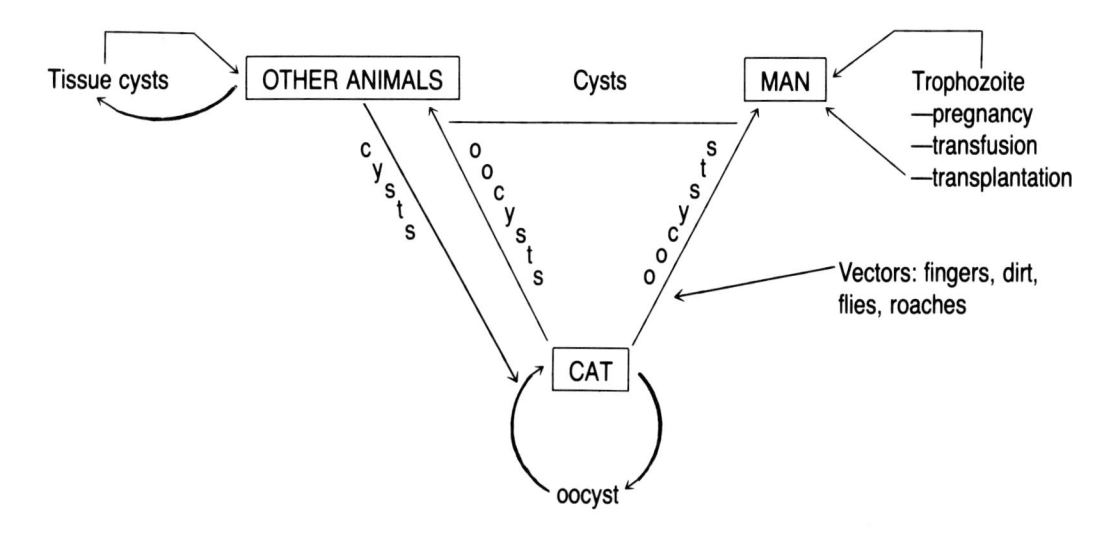

Fig. 24–1. Transmission of *Toxoplasma gondii*.

Risk of Infection. The risk of congenital rubella in a given population is a function of the proportion of seronegative women of childbearing age. In Europe and North America, rubella infection occurs primarily before puberty, and therefore only 10 to 20% of women between 20 and 35 years of age remain unprotected. In other areas of the world, such as Central America and Japan, up to 70% are unprotected. Widespread vaccination of the susceptible population should decrease these figures. The risk of infection is especially great for young seronegative women in daily contact with young children, such as nurses and employees of nurseries, schools, hospitals, or maternity clinics.

Diagnosis. In general, clinical evidence of rubella in the pregnant woman is unreliable (see Objective 27–6), and the diagnosis, as in toxoplasmosis, depends mainly on serologic testing. After a primary infection, the first immune response is in the form of IgM antibodies, which reach a peak approximately 14 days after contact and disappear about 2 months later. IgG antibodies begin to appear about 18 days after contact; hemagglutination-inhibition antibodies reach their highest titer in a week, followed by immunofluorescent and neutralizing antibodies. Complement-fixing antibodies rise more slowly, with a peak about 2 months after the start of the infection.

At the time of a reinfection, limited viral proliferation can occur in the pharynx, but apparently without viremia and therefore without risk to the fetus. When the level of antibody is low, a rapid anamnestic response, exclusively of IgG, can be observed. Thus, the presence of IgM represents a reliable criterion for the diagnosis of a primary infection.

One cannot overemphasize the importance of determining the rubella-immune status of all young women before they become pregnant and, in the absence of antibody, of immunizing them. Effective contraception is necessary for 1 or 2 months following the vaccination.

If a nonimmune woman has already become pregnant, immunization is contraindicated. The physician's responsibility then becomes the ongoing clinical and, more important, serologic surveillance of the grávid patient. To establish the diagnosis of a primary rubella infection with certainty, a seroconversion alone does not suffice; a significant elevation of antibody titers (at least fourfold) and the presence of IgM-specific antibodies are required.

During a pregnancy that has proceeded less than 20 weeks, the discovery of IgM antibodies, direct evidence of a primary infection, has serious implications and may lead the physician to recommend an abortion. It is unwise to let the diagnosis depend on a single determination. The denaturation of IgM by 2-mercaptoethanol, although simple and inexpensive, is not an entirely reliable reaction. The reference technique, which involves separation of IgM by ultracentrifugation in a sucrose gradient, is, however, long, difficult, and costly.

Prevention. Even a large dose of standard

RUBELLA VIRUS

The virus of rubella belongs to the family Togoviridae. Spherical, with an icosahedral symmetry, and measuring 60 nm in diameter, the virus contains RNA and is surrounded by a lipoprotein envelope essential for its infectivity; it is destroyed by heat, formaldehyde, ether, and other lipid solvents. In a medium containing little protein, such as serum or albumin diluted 1:100, the virus preserves its infectivity for at least a week at 4° C and indefinitely at −70° C. Freezer temperatures from −10° C to −20° C or a high or low pH rapidly degrade the infectious capacity of rubella virus. Thus, all specimens and tissue samples submitted for isolation of this virus should be preserved and transported at 4° C in ice, rather than frozen or covered with dry ice.

The virus contains an antigenic hemagglutinin directly linked to its infectivity that is active at 4° C and at 25° C, but not at 37° C. The serologic test most often used for the diagnosis depends on this antigen, namely, the hemagglutination-inhibition assay (HIA). Man also responds to rubella infection with the production of neutralizing and complement-fixing antibodies.

The virus itself can be cultivated in a number of cell lines.

gammaglobulin given to a pregnant woman who has just been exposed to rubella does not reliably prevent fetal infection. Such an injection of at least 20 ml, considering it is mainly wishful thinking, is only justified in a woman who refuses to consider interruption of the pregnancy. In fact, a so-called therapeutic abortion is the only effective measure. Prevention of rubella essentially depends, therefore, on active immunization with a single injection of attenuated live virus vaccine. This method of prevention naturally raises some as yet unanswered questions concerning efficacy and toxicity.

How long does the immunity conferred by the vaccine last? Antibodies produced in response to vaccination are detectable for several years, but the duration of protection is briefer than that provided by antibodies produced in response to the natural disease. Rubella reinfections are at least ten times more frequent in vaccinated subjects than in those with natural immunity (1 to 3% of the naturally infected population), but these lead to a booster response with a rapid rise in IgG antibody and therefore neither a viremia nor a fetal infection occurs.

Immunization, with multiplication of the vaccine virus, produces some minor symptoms in 15% of susceptible individuals: mild fever about the fifth to sixth day, adenopathy, a brief exanthem, and, more important, arthralgias that may be prolonged for several weeks, particularly in young women. Viral multiplication in the pharynx is insufficient to contaminate other susceptible individuals in contact with the vaccinate; therefore, vaccination of children in contact with pregnant women is apparently not dangerous. On the other hand, the vaccine produces a viremia with a potential risk of transplacental contamination of the fetus. No experimental or clinical evidence has yet to link the vaccine-induced viremia with any malformation, possibly because the infecting dose is too small, or attenuation of the virus limits its pathogenicity, or the virus favors the production of interferon. Nevertheless, rubella immunization is considered contraindicated during pregnancy. Active immunization is therefore recommended before puberty or concurrent with effective contraceptive protection.

Mass vaccination of the entire population of children could theoretically eliminate all risk of infection for pregnant women by interruption of the natural transmission of the virus. At present, however, direct prevention is limited to systematic vaccination of girls, if possible before puberty, and by serologic surveillance of pregnant women at risk.

INFECTION WITH CYTOMEGALOVIRUS (CMV)

Incidence. The incidence of infection with CMV is, on average, 1 per 100 live births (0.5 to 2.2 per 100). The most severe forms of congenital infection are manifested by hepatosplenomegaly, icterus, thrombocytopenic purpura, similar to that seen in the congenital rubella syndrome, and central nervous system involvement such as intracranial calcifications, microcephaly, chorioretinitis, deafness, and mental retardation. At least 10 times more frequent, however, are infections that are clinically latent at birth and become apparent in later years in the form of hearing difficulties, behavioral problems, and minimal cerebral dysfunction. No specific treatment or prevention exists.

DIAGNOSIS OF CONGENITAL RUBELLA

Clinical features of congenital rubella are varied. The malformation syndromes may include cardiac lesions such as ductus arteriosus, coarctation of the aorta, pulmonary and aortic stenosis, and atrial and ventricular septal defects, ocular lesions such as cataracts, glaucoma, and chorioretinitis, deafness, micrencephaly, and mental retardation. Acute infections can be characterized by thrombocytopenic purpura, hepatitis, interstitial pneumonitis, encephalitis, myocarditis, and radiolucencies of the long bones; the differential diagnosis includes toxoplasmosis, cytomegalovirus infection, and syphilis. Most congenital rubella infections, however, remain subclinical and require laboratory diagnosis, which is easy. The nasopharynx of a newborn with the disease contains a considerable amount of rubella virus that can be isolated on tissue culture. Increasing IgM titers in serum during the first weeks of life are also found.

The number of pregnant women excreting CMV is much higher than the number of fetal infections with CMV. In the United States, in the course of a normal pregnancy, CMV is present in the cervical os of 2% of women in the first trimester and 28% of women in the last trimester of pregnancy. At delivery, the virus is present in the urine of 4 to 5% of parturient women and in the milk of 25% of women who are seropositive. In comparison to this large number of women who excrete the virus, the incidence of congenital infections is low (see Table 24–1).

Transplacental maternal-fetal transmission of CMV occurs only when a primary infection takes place during pregnancy. In fact, the first child of a young woman is often affected. Several reports have noted CMV infection in two successive children of the same mother, however. In each of these cases, the first child was clinically affected, but the second had an asymptomatic infection. The maternal infection is generally latent and is rarely accompanied by prolonged fever, relapsing pharyngitis, adenopathy, asthenia, or the mononucleosis syndrome seen in some primary infections. Chronic infection in the mother generally does not result in fetal infection.

Viral Transmission. It seems that viral transmission in healthy individuals requires close contact. In all populations, the prevalence of CMV infection increases abruptly after puberty and during adolescence and is statistically linked to sexual activity. Direct infection by saliva or sexual intercourse probably plays a determining role. The frequency of cervical contamination has been mentioned, and the presence of the virus in sperm has also been demonstrated for 11 weeks in a patient recovering from a CMV-induced mononucleosis syndrome. Fresh blood less than 72 hours old is another recognized source.

Thus, the possibility of fetal infection depends on the prevalence of maternal immunity and on the risk of acquiring an infection during pregnancy. The prevalence of immunity in children between 6 months and 14 years increases most rapidly in the lowest socioeconomic groups and in institutionalized children. In Europe and the United States, 85 to 90% of young women are immune to CMV.

During a primary infection, viral particles carried by the lymphocytes first infect the placenta and then gain access to the fetal circulation. As with toxoplasmosis and rubella, the timing of the fetal infection is probably an important determinant of the gravity of fetal involvement; the earlier the infection, the more serious it is. The frequent infection of infants by contact with the cervix during delivery is not harmful.

Diagnosis. As with toxoplasmosis and rubella, the clinical diagnosis of CMV is a difficult task because the clinical signs are nonspecific and unreliable. The most frequently used techniques in serologic diagnosis are direct immunofluorescence and complement fixation. The IFA test permits IgM antibody identification and can therefore give evidence of a primary infection. Electron microscopy or culture of the urine sediment or blood cells identifies only the presence of the virus and not the timing of the infection. Cytologic study of the urine sediment, to look for inclusions in the epithelial cells, yields the same information and is easier to perform, but is less sensitive. Isolation of the virus in tissue culture from blood, urine, throat washings, or tissues of an infected neonate is usually possible.

Prevention. To conclude, the only available preventive measure is nonspecific. Pregnant seronegative women should avoid working with children, for example, in a pediatric intensive care unit, and they should not be transfused with fresh blood less than 72 hours old.

OTHER INFECTIONS CAPABLE OF TRANSPLACENTAL TRANSMISSION

The following are much less frequent causes of transplacental infection.

Herpes Simplex Virus 2. This virus is responsible for severe neonatal infections, but the newborn appears to acquire the disease

CYTOMEGALOVIRUS (CMV)

Cytomegalovirus, a member of the Herpesviridae, is surrounded by an envelope, contains an icosahedral nucleocapsid of DNA, and has a total diameter of 180 to 250 nm. The virus is unstable: outside a cell, at 37° C, its infectivity falls to half within 45 minutes; at 60° C, its infectious power is unstable. Stability of the virus may be increased by the addition of 70% sorbitol before freezing. In urine preserved or transported at 4° C, the infectivity of CMV is maintained for at least a week. Visualization of the viral particle in cells or urine is possible by electron microscopy, although the particle cannot be distinguished from that of the other herpes viruses such as Herpesvirus hominis, varicella-zoster, or Epstein-Barr. CMV is the most commonly isolated, however.

Although many epithelial tissues can support viral proliferation in vivo, human fibroblast cell lines are used for a culture of the virus in vitro. The cytopathogenic effect extends slowly from cell to cell in the form of clusters that progressively enlarge to take over the entire cell layer in 2 to 4 weeks. From 1 to 3 days after inoculation, the early antigens of CMV can be identified in the cluster of foci of infected cells using specific immunofluorescent techniques.

The antigenic activity of the virus gives rise, in vivo, to the appearance of antibodies that may be demonstrated using various techniques, such as neutralization, complement fixation, indirect immunofluorescence, agglutinization, and hemagglutination. The existence of two and perhaps three serotypes is not universally accepted.

In vivo, the CMV infected cells are characterized by their large size (25 to 40 μm) and by the presence of a large, eosinophilic intranuclear inclusion that pushes aside the chromatin and is occasionally associated with a basophilic cystoplasmic inclusion (Fig. 24–2).

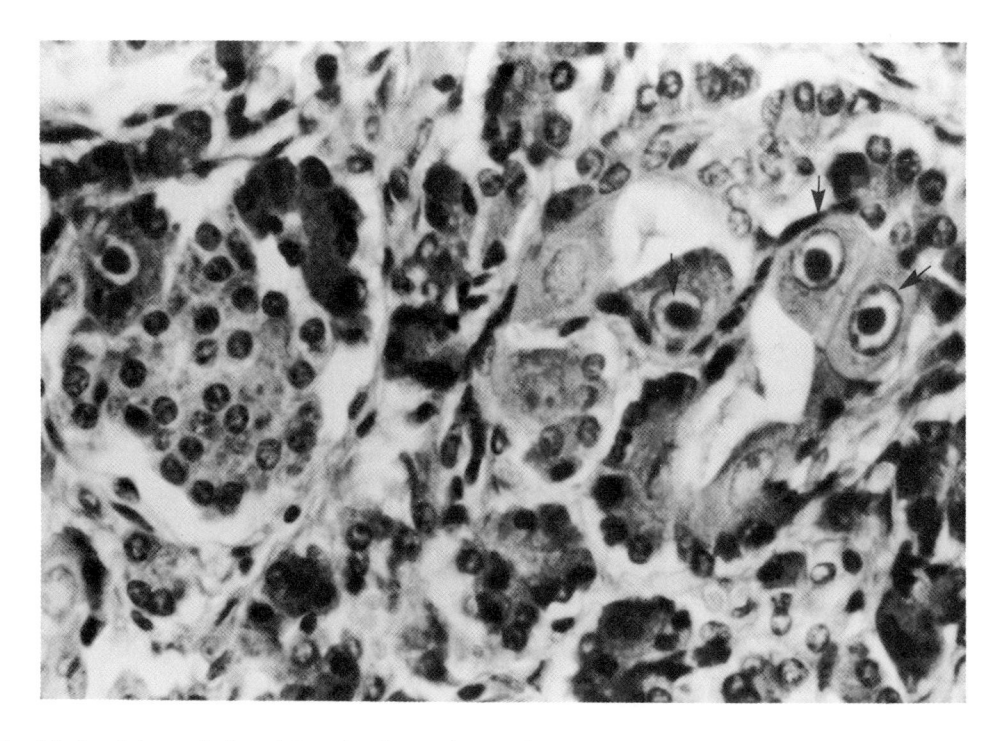

Fig. 24–2. Cytomegalovirus. Infected cells are characterized by their large size and by the presence of a large, eosinophilic intranuclear inclusion.

at delivery during passage through the birth canal of a mother having a genital herpes infection (see Objective 24–4). In some cases, however, transplacental infection may result from a maternal viremia. If infection occurs during the first trimester of pregnancy, the illness may cause fetal death, abortion, or multiple congenital anomalies.

Varicella-Zoster Infections. Several epidemiologic studies have noted 1 case of maternal varicella for every 4000 to 5000 pregnancies. Zoster must be even less common. Contrary to older data, varicella may not have a graver prognosis for pregnant women than for the general population. On the other hand, a specific group of congenital anomalies is observed when maternal varicella occurs in the first trimester of gestation, especially between the eighth and fifteenth weeks. These anomalies include retardation of intrauterine development with low birth weight for gestational age, atrophic and pigmented cutaneous scars, limb hypoplasia, amyotrophy and hypotrophy of the musculature, tendon areflexia, retardation of osseous development, clubfoot, and central nervous system and ocular abnormalities.

When the mother develops varicella in the 17-day period preceding delivery, the newborn is at risk of congenital varicella. The mortality rate is greater than 25% when the rash of varicella appears in the mother less than 5 days before or within 2 days after delivery or when such a rash is seen in the infant between 5 and 10 days of age, that is, when the delivery occurs before the transplacental passage of sufficient maternal IgG antibodies. Curiously enough, congenital varicella appearing during the first 5 days of life is generally benign.

To prevent this risk in the nonimmunized woman near delivery who has been exposed to varicella or zoster, an injection of 5 ml specific zoster immune globulin (ZIG) is recommended within the first 3 days following the contact. If the mother develops varicella during the 5 days before delivery or following the birth, the newborn should immediately receive 2 ml ZIG intramuscularly.

Listeria Bacteremia. This disorder may cause abortion before the fourth month of pregnancy. Acquired later, listeriosis may be the cause of premature delivery and, as seen in Objective 24–4, the organism is likely to infect the neonate at the time of delivery.

It is important to recognize a listeria infection in a pregnant woman, to prevent infection of the infant by means of appropriate antibiotic therapy. Generally, the clinical picture includes an influenza-like fever with chills, headaches, back pain, occasionally pharyngitis and diarrhea, lower abdominal pains, a burning sensation on urination, and sometimes pyelonephritis. The diagnosis is made by positive blood cultures. The isolation of listeria from a vaginal culture must be interpreted with caution because this finding may reflect only an asymptomatic carrier state. Serologic agglutination and immunofluorescence tests are neither practical nor useful. The treatment of choice is ampicillin, 4 to 6 g/day for up to 3 weeks. Because of the wide gap between inhibitory and bactericidal concentrations of ampicillin, some consultants suggest the addition of an aminoglycoside to the therapeutic regimen.

Syphilis. A pregnant woman with syphilis can transmit the infection to the fetus by hematogenous dissemination, specifically, during the primary and secondary stages of the disease. Congenital syphilis is not generally contracted by the fetus until after the sixteenth week of pregnancy. When the infection is untreated, 25% of the fetuses die before birth; another 25% die soon after birth, and the infants who survive have a 40% chance of developing progressive symptomatic syphilis, which includes various malformations of the teeth and bones, interstitial keratitis, neurosensory deafness, arthritis, and neurosyphilis.

The systematic screening of all pregnant women, obligatory in many countries, is thus an important and useful precaution, especially because treatment of the woman before the sixteenth week of pregnancy prevents a congenital infection of the fetus. After the sixteenth week of gestation, treatment of the mother also has an effect on the fetus, but does not repair any previous damage.

Objective 24–3. Direct diagnostic efforts in a patient with fever, rash, or genital infection during pregnancy.

Any infection occurring in the course of pregnancy raises a dual problem: first, determining its origin, and second, assessing the risk to the fetus from the infectious process or its treatment.

FEVER

The potential causes of an episode of fever in pregnancy are innumerable; however, clin-

---
LISTERIA MONOCYTOGENES

Listeria monocytogenes is a small, gram-positive, nonsporulating bacillus that grows easily on a number of different media. It contains both O and H antigens, which permit identification of several different serotypes.

In the United States and Canada, serotype IVb predominates and comprises 60 to 85% of the isolates. In northern and eastern Europe, serotypes Ia and Ib are most common, whereas in France and Western Europe serotypes Ia, Ib, and IVb are isolated with equal frequency. Maternal and neonatal listeriosis appear to be far more common in Europe than in North America.

The modes of transmission remain largely unknown. A risk of infections seems to exist for anyone dealing with animals and animal products. Contaminated food, dust, or soil may also transmit the disease. *Listeria monocytogenes* is commonly found in the intestinal and vaginal flora of normal women as well. Sulfonamides, ampicillin, aminoglycosides including streptomycin, tetracycline, chloramphenicol, and erythromycin are all active against this organism in laboratory testing.

As with group B streptococci infections, neonatal listeriosis can give rise to either (1) early infections, occurring within the first 5 days of life and presenting as a classic granulomatous sepsis of the newborn with a high mortality rate, or (2) late diseases, appearing in the second week of life and manifesting as an acute meningitis with a mortality rate of 1 to 15%. Early infections are due to the same serotype that colonizes or infects the mother, whereas late infections are caused by the serotype IVb in 80% of cases. Treatment is with ampicillin or a combination of ampicillin and an aminoglycoside.

---

ical attention is usually directed to the following:

Urinary Tract Infection. When a pregnant patient has a urinary tract infection, even without major local symptoms, the urine must be cultured. Careful culture technique is essential if reliable results are to be obtained. Once an infection is confirmed, treatment becomes necessary.

Viral Infection. A primary infection with rubella virus, CMV, or *Toxoplasma gondii* must be considered in any pregnant woman shown to be susceptible by previous serologic screening tests. The clinical picture may include adenopathy, a fleeting exanthem, or a mononucleosis syndrome. In practice, the diagnosis depends upon evidence of serologic conversion. If a transfusion is necessary for any reason during pregnancy, it is wise to avoid using fresh blood to reduce the possibility of transmitting CMV.

Other Disorders. Close to term, when a patient has an isolated fever or an influenza syndrome, the possibility of a listeriosis must be considered. The diagnosis is made by blood culture. Also possible are phlebitis or any concurrent infection in which the major problem during pregnancy is the risk induced by the therapy itself.

RASH

In a pregnant patient with an exanthematous rash, one must first consider the possibility of rubella. The diagnosis of rubella is based on either a seroconversion or a demonstration of a significant titer of antibody, which must include the presence of IgM-specific antibody. Occasionally, the rash is caused by secondary syphilis or acquired toxoplasmosis. Other exanthemous diseases and allergic rashes do not in themselves give rise to any special risks during pregnancy.

GENITAL INFECTION

A gynecologic infection in the patient or urethritis in her partner may be caused by the following:

Gonorrhea. This disease may be treated with penicillin G or ampicillin, or for beta-lactamase-producing gonococci, cefoxitin or cefotaxime. Treatment may be accompanied by a syphilis serology.

Chlamydial Infection. An infection with chlamydia, either confirmed by isolation or clinically suspected, should be treated with erythromycin and not with tetracycline.

Trichomonas vaginalis Infection. This infection poses no particular danger to the fetus or the newborn, except in association with other sexually transmissible diseases. One must also keep in mind that the use of metronidazole is contraindicated during pregnancy.

Objective 24-4. Estimate the risks of acquiring a perinatal infection.

RISK FACTORS

The incidence of neonatal infections runs from 5 to 10% of births. Three main routes of contamination can be posited: (1) in utero following an amniotic infection; (2) in the course of delivery through the birth canal (Table 24–5); and (3) after delivery, by means of maternal care and nursing. Conditions that increase the risk are prolonged rupture of the membranes, premature labor, long and difficult delivery, the use of internal instruments to monitor the fetus, prematurity, and low birth weight. Male infants are, for unknown reasons, more susceptible to neonatal infection than females.

The risk of neonatal bacteremia increases markedly when the bacteria carry specific surface antigens, which apparently are virulence factors: 75% of the neonatal meningitis produced by *Escherichia coli*, group B streptococci, and *Listeria monocytogenes* is associated with the presence of the specific surface antigens K, BIII, and IVb, respectively. Polysaccharide B, the same polysaccharide capsular antigen of group B meningococci, prevents phagocytosis by polymorphonuclear cells, slows the clearance of organisms from the blood, and may also allow the concentration of bacteria to reach 1 per mm^3, which is apparently the threshold for the risk of meningeal invasion.

Many organisms can cause perinatal infections. *Neisseria gonorrhoeae*, *Chlamydia trachomatis*, group B streptococci, herpes simplex virus 2, *Escherichia coli*, various other enteric bacteria, and hepatitis B virus are most likely to produce serious consequences. The severity of a perinatal infection varies. For instance, although CMV infections are

Table 24–5. Association between Neonatal Disease and the Vaginal Flora

Microorganisms	Association with Disease
Bacteroides	rare
Campylobacter	rare
Candida albicans	significant
Chlamydia trachomatis	significant
Clostridium	rare
Cytomegalovirus	significant
Escherichia coli	significant
Gardnerella vaginalis	rare
Haemophilus influenzae	rare
Haemophilus parainfluenza	rare
Hepatitis B virus	rare
Herpes simplex virus 2	significant
Klebsiella	rare
Lactobacillus	nonexistent
Listeria monocytogenes	rare
Mycoplasma hominis	rare
Neisseria gonorrhoeae	significant
Neisseria meningitidis	rare
Other anaerobes	nonexistent
Proteus	rare
Pseudomonas	rare
Salmonella	rare
Shigella	rare
Staphylococcus aureus	rare
Staphylococcus epidermidis	nonexistent
Streptococcus (viridans)	nonexistent
group A	significant
group B	significant
group D	rare
Trichomonas vaginalis	rare

common (see Table 24–1), they usually remain asymptomatic. In contrast, nearly all infants infected with herpes simplex virus have clinical disease, and two thirds of them either die or are seriously disabled by it.

Examples of neonatal infections follow in the next few sections.

CONJUNCTIVITIS OR OPHTHALMITIS

Several agents can produce neonatal conjunctivitis or ophthalmitis (Table 24–6). Prophylactic measures were proposed as early as a century ago, and currently, in most countries, it is obligatory to instill a drop of a 1% aqueous solution of silver nitrate, or a penicillin G solution in some places, in each eye at birth.

To avoid the risk of chemical conjunctivitis, the instillation of either penicillin or an aminoglycoside has been advocated, but for several reasons, including the risks of sensitization and increasing resistance, none of these are recommended for routine prophylaxis in most countries.

Chlamydial Conjunctivitis. None of these methods, including the instillation of silver nitrate (called Credé's method after its originator), prevent conjunctivitis caused by *Chlamydia trachomatis*, now the most frequent cause of neonatal eye disease.

Chlamydial conjunctivitis is a mild, self-limiting disease with a long incubation period. It is seen predominantly on the tarsal conjunctiva of the eyelids. The disease usually heals spontaneously within 2 to 4 weeks, but occasionally, several months are required. From 5 to 12% of pregnant women are estimated to be carriers of this sexually transmitted chlamydia, and the risk of neonatal infection is therefore 25 to 50%.

Neonatal transmission of *Chlamydia trachomatis* is also the cause of a serious respiratory infection, with or without conjunctivitis, manifested by cough, dyspnea, and signs of diffuse pulmonary infiltration. The therapy for this pneumonitis is erythromycin parenterally administered. The conjunctivitis responds to local tetracycline instillation or to sulfacetamide eyedrops.

STREPTOCOCCAL INFECTION

Group B hemolytic streptococci (or *Streptococcus agalactiae*) are an increasing cause of serious neonatal infection. The structure of this coccus includes a polysaccharide B antigen common to all its members and type-specific antigens Ia, II, and III, in addition to a serotype Ic containing antigens Ia and Ib. The bacteria usually produce a small zone of beta hemolysis, although the hemolysin is sometimes incomplete and the hemolysis is not apparent unless aided by adjacent staphylococci (CAMP test, Fig. 24–3).

In contrast to group A streptococci, at least 85% of these group B streptococci are resistant to bacitracin and, like listeria, produce two types of infections in the newborn: an early infection almost from birth, and one with a delayed onset, a week or more post partum.

Early Neonatal Infection. The early neonatal streptococcal infection is more easily established in infants of low birth weight or in high-risk, premature infants with amniotic infection or anoxia. The onset of the infection is early, from the first few hours to the third or fourth day of life, and is brutally sudden with respiratory distress, apnea, septic shock, and a high mortality rate. Septicemia is the rule, and the mortality rate is between 40 and 80%. The source of infection is the mother; the serotype of the organism in the infant is

Table 24–6. Neonatal Eye Infections

Cause of Infection	Time of Onset after Birth
Chemical conjunctivitis (silver nitrate)	6–24 hours
Neisseria gonorrhoeae	2–5 days
Chlamydia trachomatis	5–14 days
Staphylococcus aureus, haemophilus, moraxella	4 days–3 weeks
Herpes simplex virus 2	2 days–3 weeks

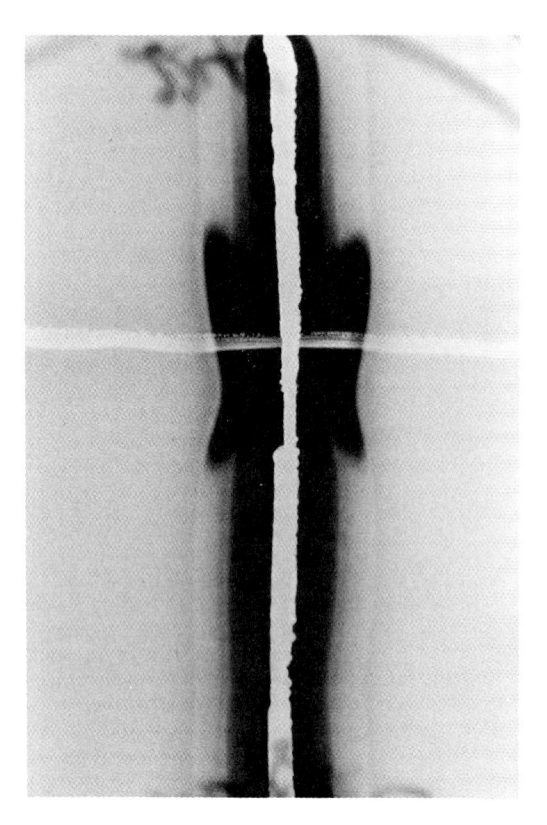

Fig. 24–3. The CAMP test is used to identify group B streptococci on blood agar. The vertical streak is seeded with *Staphylococcus aureus* and the horizontal streak with a group B streptococcus. Hemolysis creates a distinct pattern at the crossing of the two streaks. (Courtesy of Dr. J.C. Pechère.)

identical to that of the mother. Although the prevalence of the vaginal carrier state in pregnant women may run from 20 to 40%, the risk of early neonatal infection is in the neighborhood of 0.3 per 100 infected women. The risk of infection may reach 2 per 100 if the child's birth weight is less than 2000 g and increases for lower weights. In the hope of interrupting the maternal carrier state, various procedures have been advocated:

1. Antibiotic therapy at the end of pregnancy with either penicillin, ampicillin, or erythromycin. This procedure has been shown to decrease the carrier rate temporarily, but it is expensive, carries the risk of provoking allergic reactions, and selects for antibiotic-resistant flora.

2. Immunization of the mother with the B III streptococcal capsular polysaccharide. The rate of neonatal infection is lower in infants of mothers possessing anti-group B streptococcal antibody. The maternal-fetal transfer of protective antibody is not detectable until after the thirty-second week of gestation. Immunization trials of the mother with streptococcal B III capsular polysaccharide or with immunoglobulin for the newborn have not yet been completed. A multitype, capsular vaccine is currently under investigation.

3. Administration of penicillin G to the newborn by a single intramuscular dose of 50,000 U within an hour of delivery. This procedure decreases the incidence of gonococcal ophthalmia as well as infant colonization and early infection with group B streptococci, as compared to control subjects. The usefulness of this treatment has yet to be determined in light of a resulting increase in penicillin-resistant pathogens.

Late Neonatal Infection. Infection of older infants with group B streptococci is different from early infection. It is not clearly related to maternal contamination or to obstetric difficulties. Late neonatal infection is often a focal infection beginning in the second or third week of life that takes the form of a meningitis and occasionally an otitis or septic arthritis. These infections are caused by streptococcus B III in nearly all cases. The mortality rate for late neonatal infection is lower than that for the early infection; however, the risk of neurologic sequelae, such as hydrocephalis after meningitis, is considerable.

NECROTIZING ENTEROCOLITIS

The determinants of necrotizing enterocolitis are multiple. At least four host factors are well recognized:

1. Low birth weight, less than 2500 g in 75% of cases.
2. Anoxia on delivery.
3. Hyperosmolar formula given early in life.
4. An epidemiologic factor, as yet not clearly identified. The transmissible nature of

this disorder is suggested by the occurrence of epidemics in hospital nurseries and the suppression of these epidemics by strict hygienic measures and attention to proper technique.

Although many organisms can cause neonatal diarrhea, such as enteropathic *Escherichia coli* and coronavirus, no specific organism has been identified in this disease. Enterotoxin-producing *Clostridium difficile* is now generally considered responsible for antibiotic-associated pseudomembranous colitis in infants as in adults, but not in neonatal diarrhea.

After a symptom-free interval of several days, the illness begins abruptly with the patient's refusal to eat, vomiting, and abdominal distension, and it continues with diarrhea that is often bloody. Occasionally, gas is seen in the walls of the intestine on abdominal roentgenograms. The mortality rate is high: 50 to 75% within several days.

HEPATITIS B

Current evidence indicates the importance of protecting the infants of mothers who are carriers of hepatitis B (HB) virus from infection with this agent at or shortly after birth, especially if the mother is a carrier of e antigen (HB_e), which probably signifies high infectivity and therefore a high risk of transmission. Prophylactic recommendations for the infant have not yet been completely formulated. Anti-HB specific immunoglobulin, in a dose of 0.5 ml/kg, has been advocated in the first day or so of life; the immunoglobulin should be administered each month at a dose of 0.16 ml/kg for 4 to 6 months (or a multiple of the dose at wider intervals), and concurrent anti-HB virus immunization should be administered. The vaccine is commercially available.

> Objective 24–5. Outline the restrictions on the use of antibiotics during pregnancy and in nursing women.

GENERAL RESTRICTIONS

No special requirements for antibiotic therapy exist during pregnancy, although when needed, such therapy is more urgent because two individuals are at risk. Pregnancy, however, is an important factor in restricting antibiotic use because of the singular sensitivity of pregnant women to the hepatotoxic effects of intravenous tetracycline and because of the potential for injury to the fetus or infant of certain antimicrobials that cross the placenta or are present in breast milk.

SPECIFIC RESTRICTIONS

Beta-Lactam Antibiotics. These agents, not restricted in pregnancy, include penicillin G and the penicillinase-resistant penicillins such as oxacillin, ampicillin, and amoxicillin. Information on the tolerance of carbenicillin and ticarcillin is not available; however, these drugs are probably well tolerated by pregnant patients. The cephalosporins, at least the older compounds, are well tolerated. Preliminary data for the second- or third-generation cephalosporins seem to indicate the same.

Aminoglycosides. These drugs are generally contraindicated in pregnancy. The fetal risk of ototoxicity from streptomycin has been shown; deafness and vestibular damage may occur. Although damage to fetal cranial nerve VIII has not been observed with kanamycin, gentamicin, tobramycin, or amikacin, their use during pregnancy is not recommended because fetal blood levels are about one-half of maternal ones, just as with streptomycin, and a similar level of toxicity could occur.

Antituberculous Agents. If antituberculous therapy must be given to a pregnant woman, neither streptomycin nor ethionamide is advised, whereas isoniazids, ethambutol, and rifampin can be prescribed.

Tetracycline. The administration in a pregnant woman of high doses of tetracycline, such as 2 g/day or more, intravenously, even if the patient's renal function is normal, can provoke a syndrome of hepatomegaly, jaundice, hepatic and renal failure, pancreatic involvement, hematemesis and coma; the mortality rate reaches 80%. Similar toxicity has been noted with lower doses of tetracycline in women with reduced renal function. Moreover, the tetracyclines are even less appro-

Table 24–7. Excretion of Antibiotics in Human Breast Milk

Antibiotics	Maternal Dose and Route	Maternal Serum Concentration	Concentration in Milk	Ratio of Milk to Serum
Penicillin G	100,000 IU, IM	0.29–1.1	0.01–0.04	0.02–0.2
Oxacillin	1 g orally	0.3–5.6	0.2	0.03–0.70
Streptomycin	1 g IM	14–18	0.3–1.3	0.02–0.10
Novobiocin	250 mg orally	12–52	3–5	0.10–0.25
Erythromycin	400 mg orally	0.4–3.2	0.4–1.6	0.50
Chloramphenicol	250 mg orally	26–49	16–25	0.50
Tetracycline	500 mg orally	0.9–3.2	0.5–2.6	0.60–0.80
Nalidixic acid	1 g orally	—	4	—
Isoniazid	5–10 mg/kg	6–12	6–12	1.00
Sulfonamide	500 mg orally	8–9	9	1.00

IM, Intramuscularly.
(From McCracken, G.H., Jr.: In Infectious Diseases of the Fetus and Newborn Infant. Edited by J.S. Remington and J.O. Klein. Philadelphia, W.B. Saunders, 1976.)

priate during pregnancy because they produce 2 undesirable consequences in the fetus: (1) slowing of bone development of up to 40%, especially in the third trimester of pregnancy; and (2) after the fourth month, hypoplasia and staining of the tooth enamel.

Chloramphenicol. This agent has no clearly documented risk in the pregnant woman other than its propensity for producing a rare case of aplastic anemia. The mode of action of this agent in blocking the translation of messenger RNA at the ribosomal level is troublesome, however, and most physicians try to avoid its use in a pregnant woman. The use of chloramphenicol therapy in a neonate, especially a premature infant with inadequate hepatic glucuronide conjugation, can be catastrophic. The accumulation of unconjugated chloramphenicol can lead to an often fatal vascular collapse called the "gray syndrome." Thus, chloramphenicol is inadvisable at the end of pregnancy, close to term, in the newborn, and in nursing mothers.

Sulfonamides. The sulfonamides are well tolerated by pregnant women and by infants. During the perinatal period, however, these agents may, by competetive binding, prevent bilirubin from fixing to serum albumin and hence may increase both the level of unbound, unconjugated bilirubin and the risk of kernicterus even at serum levels that are only moderately elevated. Therefore, prescription of the sulfonamides, especially the long-acting compounds, is not advised near term, in the neonate, and at the beginning of nursing.

In infants with glucose-6-phosphate dehydrogenase deficiency, the sulfonamides, nalidixic acid, and nitrofurantoin can provoke a brusque hemolysis (Table 24–7).

Other Contraindicated Agents. Several anti-infectious agents have shown carcinogenic, teratogenic, or antifolate activity in laboratory animals. These drugs are not indicated in pregnant women, most especially during the first trimester: metronidazole and its derivatives, which are prescribed for giardiasis, trichomoniasis, and anaerobic infections; pyrimethamine, which is prescribed for toxoplasmosis and malaria; and trimethoprim, a constituent of the trimethoprim-sulfamethoxazole combination, and its derivatives.

RECOMMENDED ANTIBIOTICS

In all, three families of agents can be prescribed freely during gestation, nursing, and in the newborn, with the usual precautions and in appropriate doses: the beta-lactams, the macrolides and related agents, and the now infrequently prescribed polymyxins. Among the macrolides, it is inadvisable to prescribe erythromycin estolate because of the greater frequency of its side effects, even though these effects have not been described in the newborn. Although the stools of more than a third of young infants may be colonized by *Clostridium difficile,* the use of clindamycin does not present serious problems in this age group.

SUGGESTED READINGS

Blattner, R.J., Williamson, A.P., and Heys, F.: Role of viruses in the etiology of congenital malformations. Progr. Med. Virol., 15:1, 1973.
Catalano, L.W., Jr., and Sever, J.L.: The role of viruses as causes of congenital defects. Annu. Rev. Microbiol., 25:255, 1971.
Fucillo, D.A., and Sever, J.L.: Viral teratology. Bacteriol. Rev., 37:19, 1973.
Miller, M.J., Sunshine, P.J., and Remington, J.S.: Quantitation of Cord serum IgM and IgA as a screening procedure to detect congenital infection: results in 5006 infants. J. Pediatr., 75:1287, 1969.
Nahmias, A.J., Visintine, A.M., and Starr, S.E.: Viral infections of the foetus and the newborn. In Viral Infections: A Clinical Approach. Edited by L. Drew. Philadelphia, F.A. Davis, 1976.
Remington, J., and Klein, J.O.: Infections of the Fetus and Newborn Infant. Philadelphia, W.B. Saunders, 1977.
Siegel, J.D., and McCracken, G.H., Jr.: Sepsis neonatorum. N. Engl. J. Med., 304:642, 1981.
Wientzen, R.L., Jr., and McCracken, G.H., Jr.: Pathogenesis and management of neonatal sepsis and meningitis. Curr. Probl. Pediatr., 7:1, 1977.

Toxoplasmosis

Alford, C.A., Jr.: Immunoglobulin determinations in the diagnosis of fetal infections. Pediatr. Clin. North Am., 18:99, 1971.
Barbosa, J.C., and Ferreira, I.: Sulfadoxine-pyrimethamine (Fansidar) in pregnant women with toxoplasma antibody titers. In Current Chemotherapy. Proceedings of the Tenth International Congress of Chemotherapy. Washington, D.C., American Society for Microbiology, 1978.
Desmonts, G., and Couvreur, J.: Congenital toxoplasmosis. A prospective study of 378 pregnancies. N. Engl. J. Med., 290:1110, 1974.
Grussman, P.L., Krahenbull, J.L., and Remington, J.S.: In vivo and in vitro effects of trimethoprim and sulfamethoxazole on toxoplasma infection. In Current Chemotherapy. Proceedings of the Tenth International Congress of Chemotherapy. Washington, D.C., American Society for Microbiology, 1978.

Rubeola (Measles) and Rubella

Hanshaw, J.B., and Dudgeon, J.A.: Viral diseases of the fetus and newborn. Philadelphia, W.B. Saunders, 1978.
Krugman, S.: Present status of measles and rubella immunization in the United States: a medical progress report. J. Pediatr., 90:1, 1977.
Philips, C.A., Maeck, J.V.S., Roger, W.A., and Savel, H.: Intrauterine rubella infection following immunization with rubella vaccine. JAMA, 213:624, 1970.
Miller, E., Cradock-Watson, J.E., and Pollock, T.M.: Consequences of confirmed maternal rubella at successive stages of pregnancy. Lancet, 2:781, 1982.
Modlin, J.F., et al.: Risk of congenital abnormality after inadvertent rubella vaccination of pregnant women. N. Engl. J. Med., 294:972, 1976.
Townsend, J.J., et al.: Progressive rubella panencephalitis: late onset after congenital rubella. N. Engl. J. Med., 292:990, 1975.

Herpes simplex

Ch'ien, L.T., et al.: Antiviral chemotherapy and neonatal herpes simplex virus infection: a pilot study experience with adenine-arabinoside (Ara-A). Pediatrics, 55:678, 1975.
Kibrick, S.: Herpes simplex. In Obstetric and Perinatal Infections. Edited by D. Charles and M. Finland. Philadelphia, Lea & Febiger, 1973.
Nahmias, A.J., and Walls, K.: The torch complex: perinatal infections associated with toxoplasma and rubella, cytomegalo- and herpes simplex viruses. Pediatr. Res., 5:405, 1971.
Nahmias, A.J., Josey, W.E., Naib, Z.H., and Freeman, M.G.: Perinatal risk associated with maternal genital herpes simplex virus infection. Am. J. Obstet. Gynecol., 110:825, 1971.

Varicella

Meyers, J.D.: Congenital varicella in term infants: risk reconsidered. J. Infect. Dis., 129:215, 1974.
Savage, M.O., Moosa, A., and Gordon, R.R.: Maternal varicella as a cause of fetal malformations. Lancet, 1:352, 1973.

Listeriosis

Becroft, D.M.O., et al.: Epidemic listeriosis in the newborn. Br. Med. J., 3:747, 1971.
Insley, J., and Hussain, Z.: Listerial meningitis in infancy. Arch. Dis. Child., 39:278, 1964.
Seeliger, H.P.R.: Listeriosis. New York, S. Karger, 1961.

Antibiotic Therapy during Pregnancy

McCracken, G.H., Jr., and Nelson, J.D.: Antimicrobial therapy for newborns. Monographs in Neonatology. New York, Grune and Stratton, 1977.
Sutherland, J.M., and Light, I.J.: The effect of drugs upon the developing fetus. Pediatr. Clin. North Am., 12:781, 1965.

Streptococcus Group B

Headings, D.L., Herrera, A., Mazzi, E., and Bergman, M.A.: Fulminant neonatal septicemia caused by Streptococcus bovis. J. Pediatr., 92:282, 1978.
Hodes, D.L.: Penicillin prophylaxis and neonatal streptococcal disease. Hosp. Pract., 15:115, 1980.
Howard, J.B., and McCracken, G.H.: The spectrum of group B streptococcal infections in infancy. Am. J. Dis. Child., 128:815, 1974.
Ingram, D.L., et al.: Group B streptococcal disease. Its diagnosis with the use of antigen detection, Gram's strain and the presence of apnea, hypotension. Am. J. Dis. Child., 134:754, 1980.
Siegel, J.D., et al.: Single-dose penicillin prophylaxis against neonatal group B streptococcal infections. A controlled trial in 18,738 newborn infants. N. Engl. J. Med., 303:769, 1980.

Chlamydia trachomatis

Alexander, F.R.: Chlamydia: the organism and neonatal infection. Hosp. Pract., *14*:63, 1979.

Hammerschlag, M.R., et al.: Prospective study of maternal and infantile infection with Chlamydia trachomatis. Pediatrics, *64*:142, 1979.

Harrison, H.R., English, M.G., Lee, C.K., and Alexander, E.R.: Chlamydia trachomatis infant pneumonitis. Comparison with matched controls and other infant pneumonitis. N. Engl. J. Med., *298*:702, 1978.

Urinary Infections

Whalley, P.: Bacteriuria of pregnancy. Am. J. Obstet. Gynecol., *97*:723, 1967.

CHAPTER 25

Infectious Adenopathy

J.L. Vildé

Objective 25–1. Identify an isolated swelling as a lymph node.

The identification of an isolated superficial swelling as a lymph node is based mainly on clinical grounds. The site of the swelling is a reliable index: the mass is situated in a likely area for cervical, axillary, inguinal, or epitrochlear lymph nodes. The consistency of the mass, the presence of several lymph nodes in the same region, and the discovery of an inflamed portal of entry in the territory drained by the lymphatic structures constitute further presumptive evidence. Other sources of swelling may be confused with lymph node enlargement, however (Table 25–1). It may be difficult to exclude parotid swelling due to mumps or to a tumor when the swelling is located in the inferior maxillary angle and the retromaxillary region; extension of the swelling to the masseter muscle and an elevated serum amylase level indicate parotid involvement. In the axilla, hidradenitis, a subacute staphylococcal infection of the sweat glands, may be confused with adenopathy. In the neck, certain congenital cysts can be easily mistaken for a suppurative cold adenitis, but the clear fluid removed by puncture is noninflammatory and contains no polymorphonuclear leukocytes.

When in doubt, it is useful to perform a lymph node puncture with aspiration. The only contraindication to this procedure is an aneurysm, which should be suspected when the swelling is pulsatile, expansile, and characterized by a murmur. Lymph node puncture, which becomes mandatory when the adenopathy becomes fluctuant, facilitates the etiologic diagnosis.

Objective 25–2. Determine the infectious cause of cervical or axillary adenopathy.

The lymph nodes are one of the most dependable means of defense against numerous local bacterial infections. They contain all the immunologically competent cells involved in resistance to infection: T cells and macrophages, on which cellular immunity depends, and B cells, which are responsible for the synthesis of antibodies (Fig. 25–1). So-called pyogenic bacteria, obligate extracellular parasites such as the streptococcus or staphylococcus, cannot cross this barrier. Facultative intracellular bacteria such as *Mycobacterium tuberculosis*, brucella, *Pasteurella multocida*, and *Francisella tularensis* are rapidly ingested by the macrophages that play an essential role in their elimination. These microorganisms sometimes remain in a quiescent state within the phagocytes themselves for prolonged periods (Table 25–2).

369

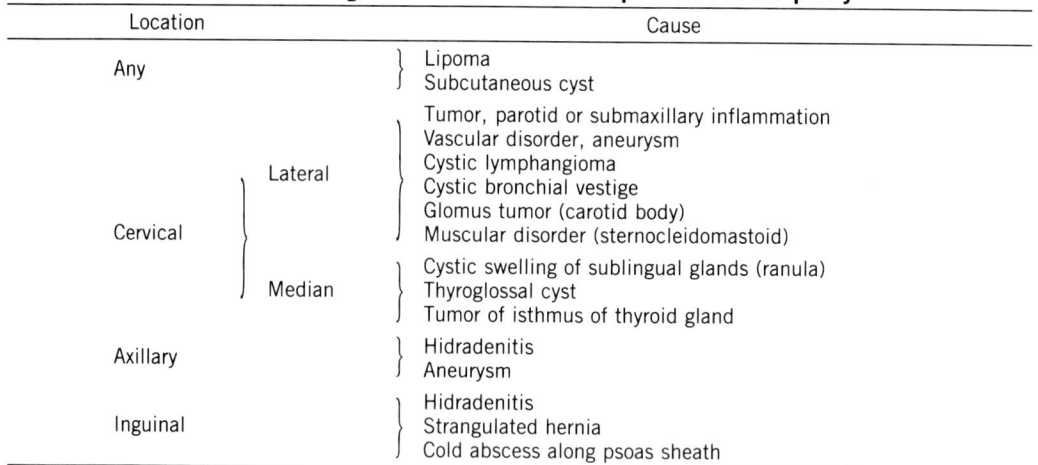

Table 25–1. Differential Diagnosis of an Isolated Superficial Adenopathy

Location		Cause
Any		Lipoma Subcutaneous cyst
Cervical	Lateral	Tumor, parotid or submaxillary inflammation Vascular disorder, aneurysm Cystic lymphangioma Cystic bronchial vestige Glomus tumor (carotid body) Muscular disorder (sternocleidomastoid)
	Median	Cystic swelling of sublingual glands (ranula) Thyroglossal cyst Tumor of isthmus of thyroid gland
Axillary		Hidradenitis Aneurysm
Inguinal		Hidradenitis Strangulated hernia Cold abscess along psoas sheath

---

PUNCTURE OF A LYMPH NODE

The puncture is performed with a fine needle of 0.6 to 0.8 mm (22 to 24 gauge) if the lymph node is soft, or with a finer, intradermal type of needle if the lymph node is hard. Effective aspiration is provided by a tight plastic syringe. Local anesthesia is generally unnecessary, except in anxious patients. After immobilizing the lymph node between two fingers, the physician punctures the node at the upper rather than at the lower part to avoid fistulization and maintains strong aspiration for a few seconds.

The material collected is spread onto slides and is dried rapidly without smearing. The slides are stained with the Giemsa stain to determine the nature and appearance of the cells collected (large numbers of lymphocytes confirm that the material comes from a lymph node in the absence of suppuration), with the Ziehl-Neelsen stain to identify mycobacteria, with toluidine blue or methylene blue to detect pyogenic bacteria, and in some cases with the Gram stain. When the material is purulent or serosanguineous, part of it is sent to a microbiology laboratory for inoculation on chocolate agar, on acid-fast media, or when indicated, on enriched or special anaerobic medium.

Local infection by one of these bacteria results in enlargement of the satellite lymph nodes, often the only symptom of infection.

An isolated infectious adenopathy is often secondary to a mucosal or cutaneous injury or infection. The demonstration of this portal of entry and the circumstances of its occurrence are the keys to identifying the cause. The diagnosis is then confirmed by the presence of pus on lymph node puncture and by a bacteriologic examination.

The investigation is pursued with a blood count, a tuberculin test, and a chest radiogram. In an appropriate context, serologic tests for cytomegalovirus, toxoplasmosis, Epstein-Barr virus, rubella, syphilis, and tularemia are also ordered. If the cause of the adenopathy remains unknown after this first series of investigations, a biopsy may be indicated when the lymph node is large, growing, or painful. This procedure is not always easy, however, notably when the lymph node is small or when it is located in the axillary region. Once the biopsy has been performed, the lymph node is divided into two fragments; sterile technique is essential. One fragment is for bacteriologic analysis, and the other is both for cytologic examination by slide impression and for histologic study after fixation in a 10% neutral formalin solution. Histologic study often provides the evidence of an infectious origin; one may see epithelioid granulomas with necrosis, which could suggest tuberculosis, cat-scratch disease, or tularemia, or an acute inflammatory response from a pyogenic infection.

ADENITIS CAUSED BY PYOGENIC ORGANISMS

This disorder is caused mainly by staphylococci or streptococci and is accompanied by

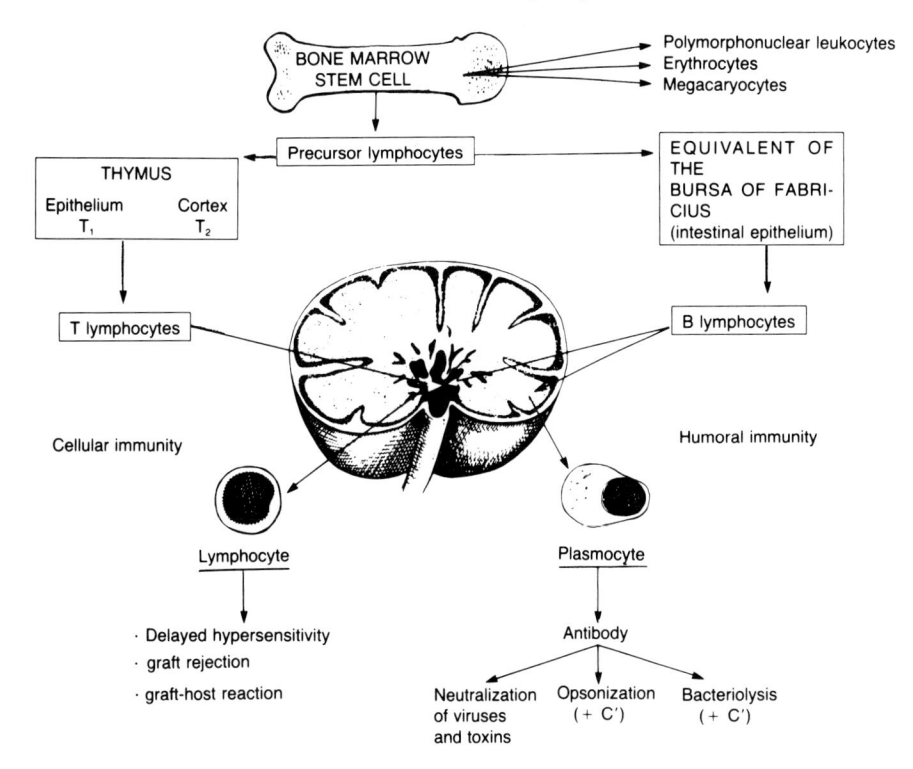

Fig. 25–1. Schematic representation of immunity.

Table 25–2. Facultative Intracellular Parasites: Biologic Properties and Their Meaning

Organisms	
Actinomyces israelii	Histoplasma capsulatum
Blastomyces dermatitidis	Listeria monocytogenes
Brucella	Mycobacteria (*M. tuberculosis* and atypical)
Candida albicans	Nocardia
Coccidioides immitis	Pasteurella multocida
Cryptococcus neoformans	Toxoplasma gondii
Francisella tularensis	

Properties	Meaning
Ability to multiply or persist in macrophages	Tropism for nodes and other lymphatic structures Possible recurrences Necessity for antibiotics characterized by intracellular penetration
Production of cellular type immunity	Vaccination requiring live vaccines
Development of delayed hypersensitivity	Availability of specific intradermal tests Histologic features: epithelioid cells and giant cells with caseous or caseiform necrosis

fever, lymphangitis, and a polymorphonuclear leukocytosis. This type of adenitis is usually secondary to dermatitis, an insect bite, an infected wound of the face or scalp, purulent pharyngitis, a peritonsillar abscess, or an acute dental infection. A phlegmonous adenitis of the neck is occasionally observed and can be caused by a variety of organisms, some of them anaerobic bacteria. Identification of the pathogenic organism after puncture or biopsy guides the antibiotic therapy. If no organism is isolated and if adenitis remains the presumptive diagnosis, therapy with an antistaphylococcal penicillin or a cephalosporin can be attempted.

SUPERFICIAL ADENOPATHY CAUSED BY MYCOBACTERIA

Infection with *Mycobacterium tuberculosis* is still the most common cause of chronic, draining cervical adenopathies; in some countries, 50% of all isolated, chronic, suppurative cervical adenopathies are tuberculous in origin. The cervical site is the most common, although a tuberculous superficial adenopathy may be situated in the axillary fossa. Tuberculous adenitis can be observed at any age, especially in immigrants from underdeveloped countries and certain ethnic groups from South America, North Africa, and Asia.

The course of the disorder is most often subacute or chronic, without systemic infectious signs, when no other site of tuberculous infection is present. The involved lymph node, only moderately painful, becomes fluctuant. Drainage may occur in a few weeks or months by fistula formation through the skin.

The diagnosis of tuberculous adenopathy is suggested by the patient's background. At risk are recent immigrants, individuals living in poor socioeconomic conditions, and patients with a personal or family history of untreated tuberculosis, known or discovered by lung roentgenogram. Tuberculin skin tests are always positive, often large or even bullous. The discovery of another active focus of tuberculosis is additional supportive evidence. The diagnosis of tuberculosis is confirmed by bacteriologic examination of the lymph node material. The search for *Mycobacterium tuberculosis* is made by direct examination with Ziehl-Neelsen staining and culture on special media. *M. tuberculosis* grows in 3 to 6 weeks, after which sensitivity to antituberculous drugs must be determined. Sometimes, microbiologic confirmation is not possible, however, and treatment must be instituted on the basis of the aggregate of clinical and histologic evidence. A biopsy performed when clinical and microbiologic investigations fails to establish the diagnosis shows an epithelioid granuloma with giant cells and caseous necrosis; this appearance is suggestive, but not pathognomonic, of tuberculosis.

The conventional therapy combines two antituberculous agents: isoniazid and ethambutol or rifampin. More recently, a single-drug regimen has been used with success in patients with isolated tuberculous adenitis. According to the present recommendation, the treatment should be maintained for 12 months, but this duration is unnecessarily long in uncomplicated cases. Surgical excision is rarely indicated nowadays.

Bovine Tuberculous Adenopathy. This rare disorder follows oral ingestion of infected materials, such as unsterilized fresh milk from infected cows. Pasteurization, which does not eliminate the bacteria totally, and the tuberculin surveillance of dairy cows have reduced the risk of bovine tuberculosis. The disease is still seen, however, where the law does not require that herds be tuberculin-negative. Although the typical localization is mesenteric, this type of adenopathy may be found in the cervical region with an oral portal of entry, occasionally visible in the form of an ulceration of the inner cheek.

The diagnosis is made by isolating *Mycobacterium bovis*, which can be distinguished from the human variety by its cultural and microbiologic characteristics. The treatment is the same as for adenitis caused by *M. tuberculosis*, and the prognosis is equally favorable.

Superficial Adenopathy Caused by Atypical Mycobacteria. This rare form of adenopathy usually affects children under 3 years of age and is nearly always located in the cervical region. The portal of entry is probably cutaneous rather than buccopharyngeal.

At first, the inflamed lymph node is firm, movable, and barely tender. Then, in 1 to 2 months, it grows fluctuant and may become fistulous in the absence of treatment. Fever is generally absent. On the whole, the course of the illness is shorter and milder than that of *M. tuberculosis* adenitis. In contrast with adenitis caused by *M. tuberculosis*, the tuberculin tests are only weakly positive or even negative in atypical mycobacterial infection. Intradermal tests with specific antigens produce more intense reactions. The identification of atypical mycobacteria in the lymph node specimen is necessary for a definitive diagnosis.

The principal mycobacteria isolated are *Mycobacterium scrofulaceum* of the scotochromogen group, mycobacteria of the Battey group, and, more rarely, *M. kansasii* (see Table 8–1). These mycobacteria are resistant to several antituberculous drugs, but are susceptible to rifampin and ethambutol. Some feel, however, that isolated lymph nodal involvement without dissemination is probably best handled by surgical excision, provided the procedure is performed by a surgeon experienced in the anatomic features of the area. Nevertheless, medical treatment is required when the patient has impaired immunity, when the infection is disseminated, or when it is impossible or risky to remove the involved tissues completely.

Bacille Calmette Guérin (BCG) Adenitis. The only common complication of BCG vaccination, this form of adenitis is more likely to occur in young children, with the use of multiple puncture or wide scarification techniques, and with concentrated vaccine.

The site of adenitis is in lymph node drainage corresponding to the point of penetration of the vaccine and therefore is usually axillary (vaccination on the arm) or, rarely, cervical. Adenitis is observed during the second month following vaccination, frequently even later, when the lesion has healed. The patient may have an inflammatory adenopathy that later resolves; although sometimes it becomes suppurative and fistulous. The course of the illness is then similar to that of tuberculous adenitis, but it is much shorter and without risk of spreading. The fistula is benign and heals spontaneously. A short course of isoniazid therapy to hasten recovery has been proposed, although it is not mandatory.

BCG vaccination is not widely practiced in the United States.

ZOONOTIC ADENOPATHIES

The zoonoses, a varied group of infections transmitted from animals to man, can produce isolated adenopathies. The causative microorganisms are usually facultative, such as *Francisella tularensis* and *Pasteurella multocida*, or obligate intracellular parasites, such as *Toxoplasma gondii* and the agent of cat-scratch disease, and as such involve the reticuloendothelial and lymphatic systems (see Table 25–2).

Toxoplasmosis. Infection with *Toxoplasma gondii*, discussed in Objective 25–4, is occasionally characterized by an isolated adenopathy without fever. The course of the infection is chronic, without suppuration or inflammatory signs, and the principal differential diagnostic consideration may be Hodgkin's disease.

Tularemia. In tularemia, caused by *Francisella tularensis*, the portal of entry is usually the hand, in the form of a cutaneous ulcer; therefore, the epitrochlear or the axillary lymph nodes become involved. If the portal of entry is the conjunctiva, then the preauricular lymph nodes (Parinaud's syndrome) and sometimes the cervical nodes are involved. The incubation period lasts 3 to 4 days, and the infection is often accompanied by systemic signs such as fever and chills. The adenopathy may become inflammatory and fluctuant, and then may drain.

A history of contact with animals during the preceding days suggests the diagnosis. *Francisella tularensis* is harbored by rabbits, hares, and rats. In most cases, the infection is transmitted directly to hunters, cooks, or other persons who have cut up or handled carcasses. Indirect transmission through insect vectors such as ticks, fleas, and mosquitoes has also been reported, as has infection by inhalation (pulmonary tularemia). Human-to-human transmission seems unlikely (Table 25–3). The existence of an animal epidemic and the history of a stay in an infected rural area are, of course, important diagnostic considerations. The usual laboratory tests supply

Table 25–3. Adenopathies in Diseases Transmitted by Animals

Source	Type of Infection	Mode of Transmission	Disorder
Animal	Direct	Bite or scratch	Cat-scratch disease, Pasteurellosis, Rat-bite fever
		Handling	Tularemia, Brucellosis
		Ingestion	Toxoplasmosis, Brucellosis
	Indirect	Insect	Plague, sometimes tularemia
		Contaminated meat	Toxoplasmosis

little information. The blood count and sedimentation rate generally remain normal.

The organism can be isolated from the initial lesion, the lymph node, or the blood culture, but it is difficult to culture and requires selective media (blood agar and cysteine). It is a small, nonmotile, gram-negative rod containing an endotoxin. Histologic examination of the lymph node shows pseudotuberculous formations with epithelioid cells and even caseous necrosis. Serologic diagnosis usually provides the key. Serologic tests may show agglutinins that appear in the first week and rise until the eighth week. To confirm the diagnosis, the highest titer should exceed 1:80; it is often much higher. An intradermal test using organisms killed with phenol produces an intense delayed hypersensitivity in an individual infected by *Francisella tularensis*. This test is positive 2 or 3 weeks from the onset of the infection.

Cat-Scratch Disease. Also known as benign lymphoreticulosis, this subacute adenitis involves several lymph nodes in the same area. The axillary nodes are affected in most cases, but the site of adenitis may be in the inguinal fold, in the crease between the pectoralis major and deltoideus muscles (deltoid-pectoral nodes), or in the greater supraclavicular fossa or the epitrochlear region. The onset of the disorder is progressive and its course extends over several weeks, without fever. The lymph nodes are only slightly tender, with little inflammation. These nodes soften as necrosis develops, and they may become fluctuant and drain. The skin becomes reddish purple in color, and the enlarged nodes become tender.

A known cat scratch from a young cat should give a clue to the diagnosis, but the initial lesion (Plate 6D) has often healed or has become inapparent by the time the adenopathy appears. In many cases, the patient does not remember being scratched, but the presence of a pet cat in the home aids the diagnosis. The disease has also been thought to be transmitted by scratches from plants, such as rosebush thorns, succulent plant thorns, or splinters, after contact with animal debris, such as a bone fragment, or following an injury with a metal object. The results of the usual laboratory procedures, blood count, and sedimentation rate are normal. Sometimes, a slight leukocytosis with granulocytosis occurs. The patient's chest roentgenogram is normal. The presence of deep, mediastinal, or even abdominal adenopathies has been reported, but rarely.

Puncture of a soft lymph node produces a creamy, aseptic pus. This pus should be preserved carefully because the specific antigen used for the intradermal test is prepared from this material. The intradermal skin test with this antigen is an essential means of diagnosis. Intradermal injection of a small quantity of antigen (less than 0.1 ml) produces a delayed hypersensitivity reaction in 48 hours. This injection may also produce a regional reaction with an exacerbation of inflammatory signs in the lymph nodes, or especially at the site of the scratch. The allergic reaction is often intense and can be considered specific when the antigen is prepared by a competent laboratory. This antigen is not commercially available.

Serologic tests for psittacosis (ornithosis) may be positive because of the antigenic cross-reaction with the agent of cat-scratch disease.

Cat-scratch disease is frequently self-limiting. The efficacy of medical treatments such as tetracycline is not established. In rare cases, as in the presence of chronic fistulization, surgical excision is necessary.

Pasteurellosis. *Pasteurella multocida* is responsible for both infectious adenopathies and septicemia following an animal bite. The adenopathies are usually located in the axillary or epitrochlear regions and follow a subacute or a chronic course, without softening or fistula formation. Fever is not usually present, except in the first few days. Articular signs consisting of joint pain or even arthritis are observed in the affected area, as well as inflammation of the wound. The principal complication consists of dissemination of the infection resulting in meningitis, septic arthritis, epiglottal chondritis, and pleuropulmonary infections. A generalized flu-like syndrome constitutes another complication. The diagnosis is considered on the grounds of a history of animal bite shortly before the appearance of the adenopathies. Indeed, cats and dogs harbor *P. multocida* as a buccopharyngeal saprophyte.

The intense pain felt in the wound in the hours that follow the bite is out of proportion to the size of the wound itself. This symptom has diagnostic value. *Pasteurella multocida* can be isolated in the primary lesion, in the lymph node, or in the blood, but puncture is rarely performed because the lymph node remains firm. An intradermal test (not commonly performed in the United States) uses the specific antigen and produces a local, delayed hypersensitivity reaction in 48 hours. With a proper control test, this reaction must be distinguished from early erythemas caused by the medium used as a support for the antigen.

Treatment is as suggested in Table 25–4. If the diagnosis is made when complications such as metastatic foci have already evolved, the dose of penicillin G must, of course, be higher.

Plague. This disease, which by local spread produces buboes in the inguinal region, is discussed in Objective 25–3.

ADENOPATHIES CAUSED BY VIRAL INFECTIONS

Numerous viral infections can be accompanied by cervical adenopathy, and the clinical context may lead one to look for infectious mononucleosis, rubella, or adenovirus infections, among others.

MISCELLANEOUS CAUSES OF ADENOPATHIES

Primary syphilis with a chancre on the tonsils must not be overlooked as a cause of isolated cervical lymphadenopathy; secondary syphilis can cause a generalized adenopathy.

Mycotic diseases bring about isolated lymph node enlargement. Cervicofacial actinomycosis is caused by *Actinomyces israelii*, an anaerobic bacterium. In some patients, the infection is localized in the cervical lymph nodes (Fig. 25–2), but most often affects the adjacent area after spreading by contiguity. Clinically, the disorder causes a mass-like swelling and runs a subacute course. Cervical actinomycosis is usually seen secondary to dental or facial diseases; corticosteroid therapy or other immunosuppressive treatment may also be a contributing factor. The swollen lymph node shows little inflammation, is not tender, does not become immediately fistulous, and is not accompanied by fever. The diagnosis is sometimes made clinically, but more often histologically. An inflammatory reaction with polymorphonuclear leukocytes and histiocytes is accompanied by extensive sclerosis, in which one sees characteristic "sulfur granules" of organisms clumped together (Fig. 25–2). *A. israelii* can be cultured from a biopsy specimen or a puncture. The organism grows slowly, and strict anaerobic conditions are necessary. Tetracycline and penicillin G or related agents are the most effective antibiotics. Tetracycline, at a dose

Table 25-4. Principal Infectious Causes of Isolated Superficial Adenopathies of Animal Origin and their Treatment

	Causative agent	Usual locations	Systemic signs	Laboratory diagnosis: Culture	Laboratory diagnosis: Serologic tests	Laboratory diagnosis: Intradermal tests	Treatment: First choice	Treatment: Alternative
Tularemia	*Francisella tularensis*	Cervical, preauricular, axillary	High fever and chills at beginning	Special media	Yes	Yes	Tetracycline, 0.5 g q6h orally for 21 days	Streptomycin, 0.5 g q12h IM for 10 days
Cat-scratch disease	Unknown	Axillary, epitrochlear, cervical	Generally absent	No	Nonspecific	Yes	Surgical excision in some situations	
Pasteurellosis	*Pasteurella multocida*	Axillary, epitrochlear	Moderate or absent	Usual media	Yes	Yes	Penicillin G, 10 × 10⁻⁶ U/day by IV infusion for 15 days	Tetracycline or ampicillin, 0.5 g q6h orally for 15 days
Plague	*Yersinia pestis*	Inguinal	Very severe	Usual media	Yes	No	Streptomycin, 0.5 g q6–12h IM for 10 days AND Tetracycline, 0.5 g q6h orally for 10 days	Chloramphenicol, 15–20 g/kg q6h (2 g/day) IV for 10 days
Rat-bite fever	*Spirillum minor*	Axillary	Severe	Direct examination, inoculation to guinea pig	No	No	Penicillin G, 10 × 10⁻⁶ U/day by IV infusion for 10 days	Tetracycline, 0.5 g q6h orally for 10 days
Toxoplasmosis	*Toxoplasma gondii*	Cervical, axillary	Moderate or absent	Inoculation to mouse	Yes	Yes, but of little diagnostic value	Pyrimethamine*, 50 mg/day orally for 15 days, AND Sulfadiazine, 1–1.5 g q6h orally	Spiramycin 1 g q8h orally for 1 month

*Contraindicated in pregnant women.
IM, Intramuscularly; IV, intravenously.

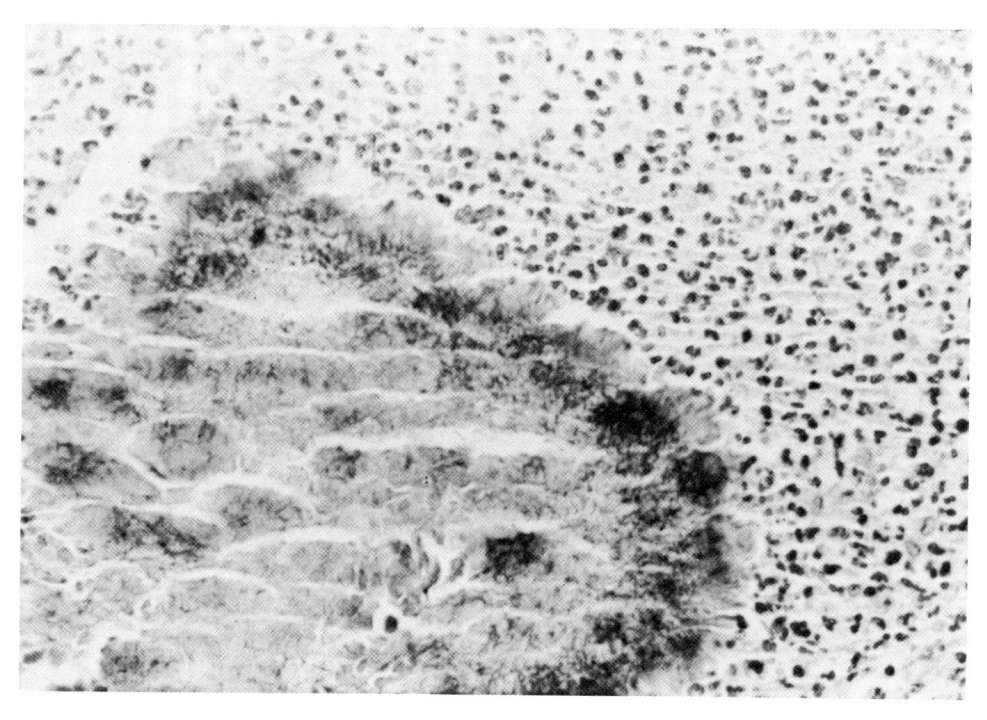

Fig. 25–2. Actinomycosis in a lymph node. The appearance is that of a foreign body in the lymphoid tissue with the typical peripheral filaments. (Courtesy of the Pathology Service, Hôtel-Dieu de Québec, Canada.)

of 500 mg every 6 hours, is often preferred. Alternatives are amoxicillin, 1 to 2 g/day in severe cases, and at the beginning of treatment, parenteral penicillin G at a minimum dose of 4 millions U/day. It is often necessary to continue the prescription for several weeks or months to prevent relapses. Proper oral hygiene is the best prevention for actinomycosis.

Superficial adenitis may occur in patients with phagocytic deficiencies such as chronic granulomatous disease. The principal causative organisms are Enterobacteriaceae and staphylococci, but the clinical appearance of the disorder is much closer to that of tuberculous adenitis. In a child, the diagnosis may be suggested by a history of frequent infectious episodes. This diagnosis is confirmed by demonstrating the leukocytic defect by means of the nitroblue tetrazolium reduction test and the study of the bactericidal activity of the patient's leukocytes.

Objective 25–3. Find the infectious cause of an isolated inguinal adenopathy.

An inguinal adenopathy can be shown to have an infectious cause by the presence of a portal of entry in the area drained by the inguinal lymph nodes. The inguinal lymph nodes drain the lymphatic vessels of the lower limbs, the external genital organs, and the anal canal. One must distinguish between two etiologic groups, according to whether the portal of entry is venereal or nonvenereal (Table 25–5).

DIAGNOSTIC PROCEDURE

The individual's medical history is first obtained, including age, sexual activity, life style and occupation, and place of residence (rural or urban). One should examine the patient's lower limbs, to search for a wound, a breach in the skin, and punctures, and the patient's external genital organs and anus, to

Table 25-5. Infectious Inguinal Adenopathies

	Causative microorganism	Clinical signs	Laboratory diagnosis	Treatment
Nonvenereal				
Acute adenitis	Staphylococcus aureus Streptococcus pyogenes	Wound, lymphangitis, Erysipelas	Hemogram, Blood culture, local specimen	Beta-lactam antibiotic
Drug addiction	Staphylococcus aureus Streptococcus pyogenes and gram-negative bacilli	Venous puncture marks	Hemogram, blood culture, local specimen	Beta-lactam antibiotic
Plague	Yersinia pestis	Severe infectious state	Lymph node puncture Direct examination	Streptomycin
Tularemia	Francisella tularensis	Skin ulceration, variable fever	Serologic tests	Tetracycline
Brucellosis	Brucella		Blood culture, serologic tests	Tetracycline, occasionally rifampin
Cat-scratch disease	Unknown	Scratch marks	Specific Ag intradermal skin test	No antibiotic available
Venereal				
Syphilis	Treponema pallidum	Genital chancre	Direct dark-field examination, serologic tests	Penicillin G
Chancroid	Haemophilus ducreyi	Genital chancre	Direct examination of node material	Sulfas or Tetracyclines
Lymphogranuloma venereum	Chlamydia trachomatis	Genital lesions uncommon	Serologic tests, Frei test (?)	Tetracyclines or sulfas
Herpes	Herpes simplex virus 2	Genital lesion	Tzanck test	
Granuloma inguinale	Calymmatobacterium granulomatis	Chronic genital ulcerations	Biopsy of genital lesion	Tetracyclines

search for a chancre or a simple scar. In women, this examination requires careful inspection with a speculum; cervical or upper vaginal lesions are drained by the deep inguinal and external iliac lymph nodes, which are inaccessible to direct palpation. In men, the medical history may include a healed chancre or even a recent urethral discharge. In most cases, no portal of entry is found, even though the adenopathy is due to venereal disease.

The laboratory tests required depend on the clinical conditions. Although its value is limited, the blood count is helpful in determining (1) leukocytosis with granulocytosis in adenitis caused by a pyogenic organism or in satellite adenitis of a soft chancre and (2) the mononucleosis syndrome sometimes seen in primary syphilis, in lymphogranuloma venereum, or naturally in Epstein-Barr virus infection. Isolated inguinal adenopathy is exceptional, however. If genital lesions are associated with inguinal adenopathy, an investigation for syphilis should always be made, including a dark-field microscopic examination of the serous fluid collected from the chancre or lymph node to identify *Treponema pallidum* and a smear and Gram stain to detect *Haemophilus ducreyi*, which is often difficult to culture. In case of urethral discharge, a smear and a culture are performed to look for *Neisseria gonorrhoeae* and, in some situations, *Chlamydia trachomatis*.

Biopsy of an inguinal lymph node should be avoided. The procedure is associated with long-term complications, and interpretation of the specimen is often difficult because normal individuals with trifling cutaneous wounds and lesions often show a nonspecific inflammatory reaction. In some instances, however, such as to rule out a lymphoma, and as a last resort, one should consider performing a biopsy.

NONVENEREAL CAUSES OF INGUINAL ADENOPATHY

Common Bacterial Infections. The most frequent causes are acute or subacute adenitis due to *Staphylococcus aureus* or *Streptococcus pyogenes*. The source of the infection is often evident, such as an infected wound, a burn, lymphangitis, erysipelas of the lower limb, or chronic dermatitis. Satellite inguinal adenopathy is seen with venous puncture sites in the lower extremities of heroin addicts.

The lower limbs are sometimes a portal of entry for zoonoses, especially in plague.

Plague. Now a rare infection in most countries, plague still must be considered in some instances because of the persistence of a few endemic centers and the development of intercontinental transportation. In the bubonic form of the disease, the onset is usually abrupt and is marked by a rise in temperature, a significant deterioration in the patient's condition including toxicity, and rapid appearance of the bubo. The swollen, inflamed, tender, matted lymph nodes are usually found in the inguinal region and sometimes in the axillary region. The bubo appears within hours, but it may be delayed or absent, thereby making the diagnosis difficult. In the absence of treatment, a grave, toxic infectious syndrome develops, with a 60 to 90% mortality rate. The mortality rate is close to 100% in the primary septicemic form of plague or in the pulmonary form when treatment is delayed.

Aside from a known epidemic or a history of a stay in an area where the disease persists, such as Southeast Asia, India, the Middle East, or California, Arizona, and New Mexico, the diagnosis of plague is based principally on isolation of the organism in the blood, bubo, or lymph node. Direct examination of the lymph node sample permits a rapid diagnosis by demonstrating many small gram-negative rods. *Yersinia pestis*, which grows on the usual aerobic media, is identified and distinguished from *Y. pseudotuberculosis* by its cultural and antigenic characteristics. A search for agglutinins can also be undertaken, but it is of less value and too lengthy.

The domestic or wild rat is historically the principal reservoir of the disease, and epidemic human infection occurs by way of the rat flea, which maintains the infectious cycle in rodents. On the other hand, wild rodents, ground squirrels, prairie dogs, and gophers are responsible for the sporadic cases occurring in the United States.

Emergency antibiotic treatment (see Table 25–4) is instituted, and the case is immediately reported to the health authorities.

Tick-Borne Infections. These infections are accompanied by inguinal adenopathy when the bite occurs in the lower limbs, as is frequent. Ulceration and eschar appear at the site of the bite. Nodules that simulate sporotrichosis may also be observed.

VENEREAL CAUSES OF INGUINAL ADENOPATHY

Inguinal adenopathy is often observed in patients with venereal disease. An adenopathy usually accompanies genital herpes infections and may be seen with urethritis, mainly gonococcal. Some rarer infections should also be considered, however, such as primary syphilis, with a genital or anal chancre. In this case, the enlarged lymph nodes are often bilateral, firm, and nontender, with little inflammation; one side is usually more enlarged than the other. Adenopathy persists more than 3 to 6 weeks after the chancre. *Treponema pallidum* can be identified by dark-field microscopic examination in lymph node fluid collected by puncture. On the other hand, serologic tests are usually positive at this point in the course of the illness (see Objective 23–2).

Chancroid. This disorder, caused by *Haemophilus ducreyi*, is observed mainly in populations with a low standard of living and deficient hygienic conditions, or among certain groups, for example in the armed forces. Most cases occur in men. In women, the lesions may be undetected, and a carrier state may exist. After a period of incubation of 2 to 5 days, the patient develops genital ulcers with irregular edges and covered by a purulent exudate. Unilateral, inflammatory, and tender inguinal adenopathy is accompanied by abscess formation and, sometimes, by the formation of a fistula through the skin. The diagnosis is based primarily on clinical findings because bacteriologic culture is difficult. Smears from the ulcer or, better yet, from lymph node material, are examined for *H. ducreyi*, a small gram-negative rod. Isolation of the organism from a culture of the lymph node specimen is possible, but it is rarely successful. Chancroid can be associated with other sexually transmitted diseases, and serologic tests for syphilis should be performed in the weeks that follow.

Chancroid can be treated with sulfonamides or streptomycin (agents ineffective against syphilis) as well as with tetracycline (active against *Treponema pallidum* or with a tetracycline-sulfonamide combination. Treatment is administered for 2 weeks.

Lymphogranuloma venereum. In this disorder, the adenopathy appears from 5 to 15 days after the infection. In fewer than one-third of patients, the portal of entry is a papular, vesicular or ulcerated lesion on the external genital organs. The enlarged lymph nodes are either unilateral or bilateral; they become tender and fluctuant, with periadenitis. Fistulas may subsequently form through the skin. This adenopathy usually follows a prolonged course. Systemic signs such as fever or leukocytosis or secondary manifestations such as erythema nodosa or hepatitis may be present.

Chlamydial Infection. The isolation of *Chlamydia trachomatis* from a lymph node specimen is difficult, and indeed, the diagnosis is usually based either on the clinical appearance or on the presence of complement-fixing serum antibodies with a titer of more than 1/64. The Frei skin test is neither sensitive nor specific. The possibility of associated syphilis should be kept in mind. Sulfonamides, tetracycline, and erythromycin are active against chlamydia in vitro. Tetracycline is administered in a dose of 2 g/day (0.5 g 4 times daily) for 3 weeks; the response is seldom immediate. Therapeutic puncture should be performed if the lymph node is fluctuant and if spontaneous rupture is imminent.

Granuloma inguinale. This chronic genital infection is caused by *Calymmatobacterium granulomatis* and is manifested by frequently extensive and sometimes hemorrhagic ulcerations that may resemble carcinoma. The infection occurs more frequently in women and in tropical or subtropical regions. Inguinal adenopathy almost always accompanies these lesions; deep adenopathy may also be present when the lesions are located in the cervix uteri. The superficial nodes are inflamed, but not tender. The diagnosis is made primarily on the basis of a careful examination of the biopsy specimens of the ulcerated lesions; an intense histiocytic reaction is observed, and macrophages are found to contain Donovan bodies consisting of *C. granulomatis*. Tetracycline, in a dose of 2 g/day for 4 to 6 weeks, is the most active antibiotic against this organism. Streptomycin is an alternative.

Objective 25–4. Identify the infectious cause of polyadenopathy.

Polyadenopathy accompanies numerous diseases (Table 25–6). The search for a cause must encompass not only infections, but also drug reactions and hematologic disorders such as Hodgkin's disease. When making the diagnosis, the physician should pay special attention to the patient's epidemiologic history, such as a stay in a zone endemic for trypanosomiasis or leishmaniasis, known contact with children, or contact with animals, as well as to such clinical features as fever, rash, pharyngitis, and splenomegaly. The blood smear may rule out hematologic disease, or it may reveal mononucleosis. The lung roentgenogram may show mediastinal adenopathy, suggesting sarcoidosis or lymphoma. A biopsy of the lymph node is also performed when a definitive diagnosis is not otherwise possible.

INFECTIOUS POLYADENOPATHY

Associated with Skin Eruptions. Polyadenopathies accompany skin eruptions in common viral infections such as rubella, measles, chickenpox, infectious mononucleosis, and

Table 25–6. Superficial Polyadenopathies: Infectious Causes and Principal Clinical Signs

Infection	Fever	Rash	Pharyngitis	Splenomegaly
Rubella	Mild	Maculopapular	Mild or absent	Moderate or absent
Secondary syphilis	Mild or absent	Present	Absent	Moderate or absent
Toxoplasmosis	In some cases	Infrequent	Absent	Rare
Brucellosis	Typically undulant	Absent	Absent	Present
Visceral leishmaniasis	Usual and high	Absent	Absent	Extreme
Infectious mononucleosis	Usual	Maculopapular (ampicillin-induced)	Present	Frequent
Cytomegalovirus infection	Usual	Infrequent; maculopapular (ampicillin-induced)	Rare	Moderate or absent

cytomegalovirus infections. Macular rash, splenomegaly, headaches, eventually fever, and a compatible sexual history should lead the physician to suspect secondary syphilis (see Chap. 23).

Associated with Mononucleosis. When mononucleosis is discovered in the course of a polyadenopathy, one should immediately consider certain infections such as infectious mononucleosis, cytomegalovirus infection, toxoplasmosis, rubella, secondary syphilis, chickenpox, brucellosis, and typhoid fever. Mononucleosis is one of the classic causes of febrile polyadenopathy. The patient's lymph nodes are enlarged in all the superficial areas, but especially in the cervical region. Other signs and symptoms are described in Objective 3–8. Primary cytomegalovirus infection in an individual with normal immune response is usually clinically silent. The infection may cause a prolonged febrile syndrome, without significant impairment of the patient's general condition, that is occasionally associated with splenomegaly and superficial adenopathy. The lymph nodes are not tender, inflamed, or particularly enlarged.

Associated with Toxoplasmosis. Superficial adenopathies involve more than two areas in more than half the cases of symptomatic acquired toxoplasmosis. This disorder follows a silent course for several weeks or months, generally without suppuration or marked inflammation. During the initial stage, symptoms such as fever, mild sore throat, and rash may occur. Complications or other localizations, such as hepatic, cardiac, or neuromeningeal, have been observed, especially in immunodepressed patients. The presence of a new pet cat in the home is of diagnostic value, but the infection may also be acquired by eating undercooked meat, especially lamb. The parasite *Toxoplasma gondii* may be identified in the affected lymph nodes after puncture or on a biopsy section. Intraperitoneal or intracerebral inoculation in the mouse causes the parasite to multiply and produces a fatal infection, but the procedure is not recommended for routine laboratories. Serologic tests are the usual methods for confirming the diagnosis. (See Objective 24–2 for additional information on the cycle and the serologic features of *T. gondii* as well as its consequences in pregnancy.)

Most patients with normal immunologic functions do not require specific therapy. Indications for treatment are the presence of severe and persistent symptoms, notably fever, evidence of damage to vital organs such as active chorioretinitis (more often a complication of congenital toxoplasmosis), or impairment of the immunologic defenses.

Treatment consists of the administration of one or more drugs active against the parasite: spiramycin, pyrimethamine, or sulfonamides. The combination of spiramycin, 2 g/day, and pyrimethamine, 50 mg/day, is effective, but pyrimethamine may cause hematologic complications, such as megaloblastic anemia, leukopenia, or neutropenia, which necessitate the simultaneous prescription of folinic acid. Pyrimethamine is therefore contraindicated in pregnant women. The combination of pyrimethamine and sulfonamides is also effective and generally recommended in the U.S.; similarly, the trimethoprim-sulfamethoxazole combination has been proposed, but its action is less reliable. Treatment must be continued for at least a month.

Associated with other Infections. A superficial polyadenopathy is part of the clinical picture of many other bacterial and parasitic infections. Generally, the superficial lymph nodes are not greatly enlarged and do not constitute either an isolated or a predominant sign. Thus, in septicemic acute brucellosis, diffuse lymph node enlargement is associated with splenomegaly. The epidemiologic context, leukopenia or neutropenia, isolation of the organism by blood culture, and an agglutination test confirm the diagnosis of brucellosis.

In the visceral form of leishmaniasis, kala azar, caused by the parasite *Leishmania donovani,* fever and marked splenomegaly are the predominant symptoms. Diffuse lymph node enlargement also occurs frequently. The parasite can be identified in lymph node material.

In African trypanosomiasis (sleeping sickness), caused by the parasite *Trypanosoma gambiense* or *T. rhodesiense,* superficial adenopathy is always present and constitutes one of the major signs of the disease. Other signs include fever, hepatosplenomegaly, and in 10 to 15% of patients, papuloerythematous skin patches called trypanids. Early neuromeningeal signs, headaches, episodes of excitement or lethargy, mental disorders, and various nervous system involvements should bring the diagnosis to mind. This diagnosis is confirmed by a history of a stay in an endemic zone in equatorial Africa, by laboratory signs of an intense inflammatory syndrome with an elevation of IgM levels, by a meningeal reaction with moderate pleocytosis and, later, with an increased protein level in the cerebrospinal fluid, and finally, by the discovery of the trypanosome in the cerebrospinal fluid or lymph nodes. Treatment is with trivalent arsenic derivatives.

NONINFECTIOUS AND NON-NEOPLASTIC INFLAMMATORY POLYADENOPATHY

This type of polyadenopathy is often associated with fever and with various cutaneous or systemic signs that simulate infections. The diagnostic considerations and the investigations prior to lymph node biopsy are similar to those in other adenopathies. A febrile polyadenopathy, with or without associated skin eruptions, may be produced by drug reactions and serum sickness. The patient's medical history is essential to the diagnosis. Passive immunization with heterologous serum is rarely a cause nowadays. Among the drugs responsible for this syndrome are the hydantoins, especially, but also phenobarbital and allopurinol. This syndrome has been also observed after injections of povidone and lipidol, as well as in beryllium poisoning.

Superficial adenopathy of this type is observed in sarcoidosis and in collagen diseases, lupus erythematosus, juvenile rheumatoid arthritis, and Whipple's disease. In this context, we can also mention the Kawasaki syndrome or mucocutaneous lymph node syndrome, first described in children in Japan, and the Destombes syndrome or benign sinus lymphohistiocytosis observed in black children. In these syndromes, the adenopathy is mainly cervical, and only a histologic study confirms the diagnosis by demonstrating macrophages containing large numbers of lymphocytes.

Persistent generalized lymphadenopathy may be part of the acquired immune deficiency syndrome (AIDS), which has been described in certain groups of homosexual men, in Haitians, in patients with hemophilia, in drug addicts, and in sexual partners of these persons (see Chap. 33).

SUGGESTED READINGS

Barton, L.L., and Feigin, R.D.: Childhood cervical lymphadenitis: a reappraisal. J. Pediatr., 84:846, 1974.

Bridges, R.A., Berendes, H., and Good, R.A.: A fatal granulomatous disease of childhood: the clinical, pathological and laboratory features of a new syndrome. Am. J. Dis. Child., 97:387, 1959.

Dajani, A.S., Garcia, R.E., and Wolinski, E.: Etiology of cervical lymphadenitis in children. N. Engl. J. Med., 268:1329, 1963.

Francis, D.P., Holmes, M.A., and Brandon, G.: Pasteurella multocida infections after domestic animal bites and scratches. JAMA, 233:42, 1975.

Greenfield, S., and Jordan, M.C.: The clinical investigation of lymphadenopathy in primary care practice. JAMA, 240:1388, 1978.

Kawasaki, T., et al.: A new infantile acute febrile mucocutaneous lymph node syndrome prevailing in Japan. Pediatrics, 54:271, 1974.

Lincoln, E.M., and Gilbert, L.A.: Disease in children due to mycobacteria other than Mycobacterium tuberculosis. Am. Rev. Respir. Dis., 105:683, 1972.

Quie, P.G., White, J.G., Holmes, B., and Good, R.A.: In vitro bactericidal capacity of human polymorphonuclear leukocytes: diminished activity in chronic granulomatous disease of childhood. J. Clin. Invest., 46:668, 1967.

Spaulding, W.B., and Hennessy, J.N.: Cat scratch disease: A study of eighty-three cases. Am. J. Med., 28:504, 1960.

Von Reyn, C.F., et al.: Epidemiologic and clinical features of an outbreak of bubonic plague in New Mexico. J. Infect. Dis., 136:489, 1977.

Weese, W.C., and Smith, I.M.: A study of 57 cases of actinomycosis over a 36-year period. Arch. Intern. Med., 135:1562, 1975.

Young, L.S., et al.: Tularemia epidemic: Vermont 1968. Forty-seven cases linked to contact with muskrats. N. Engl. J. Med., 280:1253, 1969.

CHAPTER 26

Primary Skin Infections

R. Lessard

> Objective 26–1. Diagnose crusted or bullous lesions as impetigo by means of clinical and microbiologic evidence.

Impetigo is a skin infection that can occur at any age, but it is seen much more frequently in children than in adults. A characteristic case is that of a 5- or 6-year-old child who has been playing in melting snow, sand, or soil, usually in the springtime. Often, the child's parent notices 2 or 3 lesions on the face, wrists, elbows, knees, or thighs (Fig. 26–1) and takes the child to the physician. The lesions may be "clean," that is, pink, shiny, sharply demarcated, and usually round, or they may be oozing and "dirty-looking," with a few crusts of a characteristic, honey-yellow color. At the periphery of the lesion is a ring-like detachment and, occasionally, an intact bullous elevation.

The child's parent usually reports that the lesion began with a small, pruritic, erythmatous spot that the child then scratched. The spot grew larger, began to ooze, and became crusty; a few days later, other lesions appeared. The bullous stage, which is considered characteristic of impetigo, is not usually noticed by the parent.

The site of impetigo is often the face, especially the region around the nose and mouth, the ears, or the scalp. In a scalp infection, the physician should investigate the possibility of its association with pediculosis.

A specimen for the identification of the causative organism can easily be obtained by scraping a lesion with a sterile swab and inoculating agar with the scrapings. The microbial agents responsible for this intraepidermal cleavage are gram-positive cocci, usually *Staphylococcus aureus*, or the group A streptococci (approximately 25% of the cases) (Plate 7A and B), or a combination of the two. Group A streptococci, particularly types 49 and 2, can cause acute glomerulonephritis, a complication not seen in staphylococcal impetigo.

> Objective 26–2. Indicate appropriate prophylactic and therapeutic measures once impetigo has been diagnosed.

Cleanliness is the best way to prevent impetigo. The disease is easily transmitted by family pets, dirty nails, insect bites, playing on the ground outdoors, and of course, by direct contact. Usually, adults contract the disease in barber shops, swimming pools, and sauna baths. Impetigo can also complicate pre-existing lesions, such as scabies, herpes, or dermatitis.

Most lesions respond to antiseptic or topical antibiotic treatment within 2 or 3 days.

385

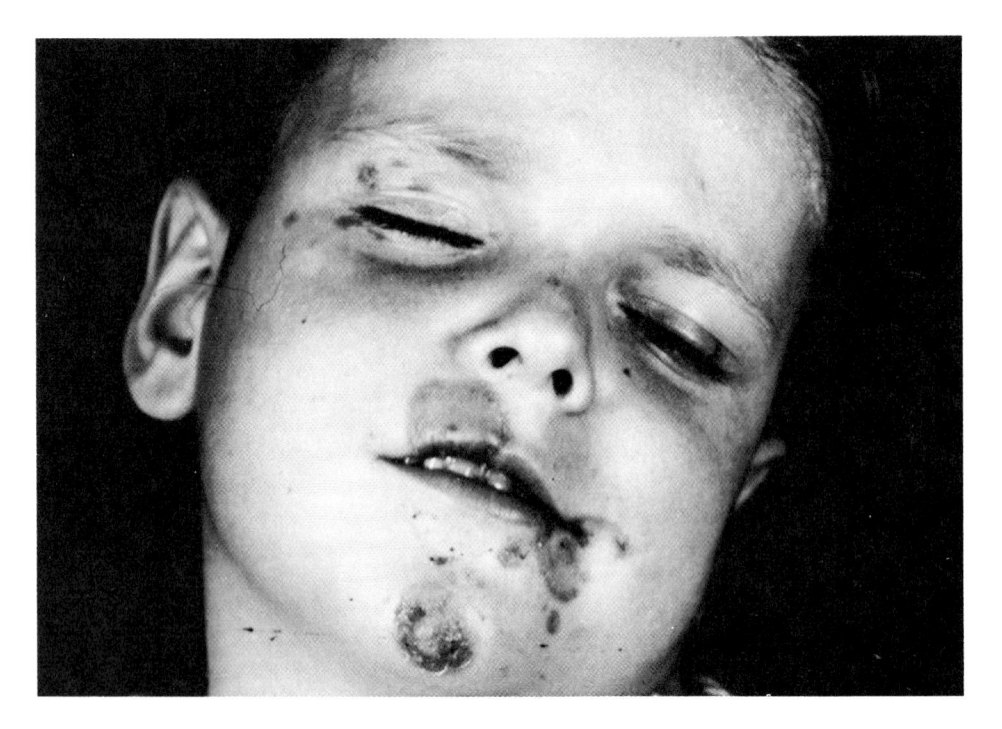

Fig. 26–1. Impetigo. (Courtesy of the Dermatology Service, Hôtel-Dieu de Québec, Canada.)

OPEN AND CLOSED INFECTIOUS LESIONS

Two basic types of skin infections occur, open and closed. Open lesions are infections of the skin surface that are almost always moist and oozing. The serous discharge is yellowish or greenish and forms a hard and thick crust when it clots. Identification of a microbial agent is made from the readily obtained specimen of serous fluid or crusts, but interpretation is difficult because of the inevitable bacterial contamination. Clinical judgment is usually more important than laboratory results in establishing a diagnosis.

Infections with an intact surface are closed lesions. Pustules, folliculitis, furuncles, panniculitis, and cellulitis are examples of closed lesions. In these cases, the lesion must be opened to take a specimen for culture. If proper microbiologic technique is used, the results can be meaningful.

Systemic antibiotic therapy is not called for in the usual, localized, well-tolerated staphylococcal impetigo. Such treatment does become necessary, however, when the lesions are extensive or oozing, when the patient has a fever, or when the infecting organism is a streptococcus.

The usual prescription includes a penicillin, such as penicillin V, 15 to 20 mg/kg/day orally in 4 divided doses for 3 to 5 days, or for 10 days in a streptococcal infection. When a penicillinase-producing staphylococcus is the cause, a semisynthetic penicillin is indicated, such as dicloxacillin, 20 to 30 mg/kg/day orally in 3 divided doses for 3 to 5 days.

Isolation of the patient is not usually necessary, provided the common rules of hygiene are observed and oozing lesions are covered.

Objective 26–3. Explain the benefits and limitations of antibiotic therapy in acne, folliculitis, furunculosis, hidradenitis, felon (whitlow), and paronychia.

These cutaneous lesions differ in their physiopathologic features and clinical appearance (Table 26–1). They all have two troublesome features in common, however; they are widespread, and they persist or recur. Because all

Primary Skin Infections

Table 26–1. Differences Among Acne, Folliculitis, Furunculosis, and Hidradenitis

	Precipitating Cause	Pathogenic Organisms	Site of Predilection	Appearance of Elementary Lesion
Acne	Obstruction of hair follicle	Infection a minor factor; *Pityrosporon ovale, Propionibacterium acnes*	Face, chest	Papulopustule
Folliculitis	Limited infection of hair follicle	*Staphylococcus aureus, S. epidermidis*	Face, buttocks, thighs	Pustule centering around a hair
Furunculosis	Infection and subsequent necrosis of hair follicle and its appendages	*Staphylococcus aureus*	Face, back of neck, hands, buttocks, thighs	Lesion similar to that of folliculitis, but larger
Hidradenitis	Infection and subsequent necrosis of hair follicle and its apocrine gland	*Staphylococcus aureus, S. epidermidis, Proteus mirabilis*	Axilla and groin exclusively	Chronic infection with fistulization, scarring, and cyst formation

these lesions have an inflammatory or suppurative appearance, one is tempted to prescribe an antibiotic, but before doing this, the physician must determine the possible efficacy of the drug by establishing the proper indications.

ACNE

Acne affects the pilosebaceous follicles in areas of skin where sebaceous glands are numerous, such as the face and upper chest. The disorder occurs when these glands are hormonally stimulated at puberty, and they begin to secrete their contents through the hair follicle (Fig. 26–2). The wall of the hair follicle is lined with squamous epithelium, and, for various reasons, including hormonal secretion, these squamous cells may become more adherent and may accumulate in thicker layers. The result is obstruction of the hair

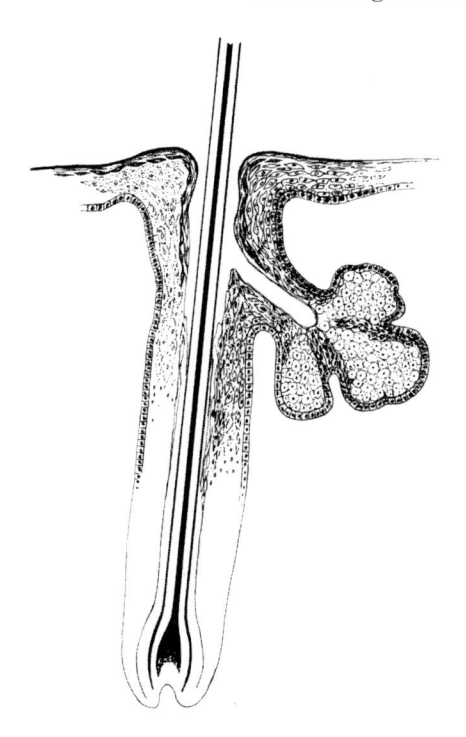

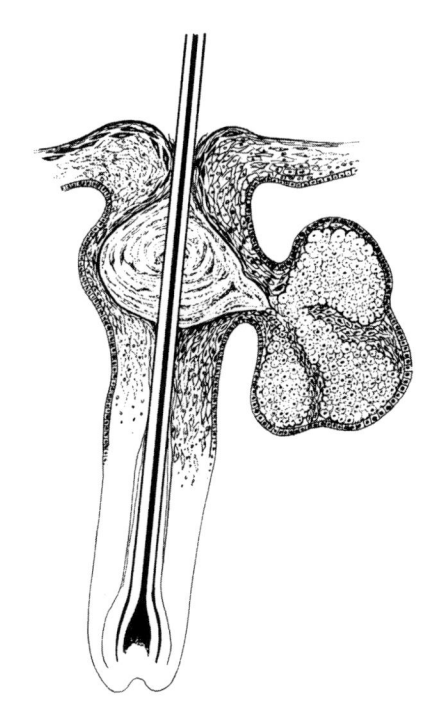

Fig. 26–2. Left, normal follicle. Right, follicle obstructed by squamous debris.

follicle duct. The flow of sebum is, therefore, restricted or slowed, and mechanical obstruction increases. An actual plug, the comedo, then forms in the hair follicle. As sebaceous gland secretion continues proximal to the obstruction, the gland becomes dilated under pressure.

Sebum is composed mainly of triglycerides, but also of squalene and wax esters. The hair follicle contains the saprophytes *Pityrosporum ovale* and *Propionibacterium acnes* and secretes a lipase that can split triglycerides into free fatty acids. The dilatation of the sebaceous gland ultimately creates fissures in the wall of the gland through which free fatty acids, which are irritating to the surrounding tissues, can escape. The tissues subsequently become inflamed from the irritation of the acid. Clinically, these phenomena are manifested in the form of a papule or a papulopustule (Fig. 26–3). It is therefore clear that acne is not initially an infection; the intervention of bacteria is facultative and secondary.

For many years, oral tetracyclines have been used to treat acne. In addition to being active against *Propionibacterium acnes*, these agents are believed to act as lipase inhibitors. The daily doses are small, 250 to 1000 mg, but the treatment must be continued for months. The therapeutic indications should be limited to forms of acne that produce a significant cosmetic problem. Topical antibiotics, such as erythromycin, tetracycline, and clindamycin, also seem to be effective because the use of propylene glycol in these preparations permits sufficient penetration.

FOLLICULITIS

Folliculitis, which affects many hair follicles (Fig. 26–4), is an actual infection in which the most common pathogen is *Staphylococcus epidermidis* or *S. aureus* (see Objective 1–1). This benign disease generally does not require systemic antibiotic treatment, even if the infection is persistent or relapsing.

FURUNCULOSIS

Furunculosis is a staphylococcal infection of the hair follicle and the surrounding tissues. The lesion is larger than in folliculitis and is potentially much more serious. Most of the time, the lesion heals spontaneously after "ripening" (well-limited collection), opening, and discharging a "core," which is the remnant of the destroyed follicle; however, particularly in an individual with deficient host defenses, such as a diabetic, the infection may spread locally. Several adjoining follicles affected simultaneously may form a large suppuration, called a carbuncle. When a furuncle is handled or traumatized, septicemia may result. Systemic antibiotic therapy is therefore indicated under the following conditions:

1. If a patient has depressed immunologic functions.
2. When the infection extends locally.
3. If a carbuncle is present.
4. When fever is present.

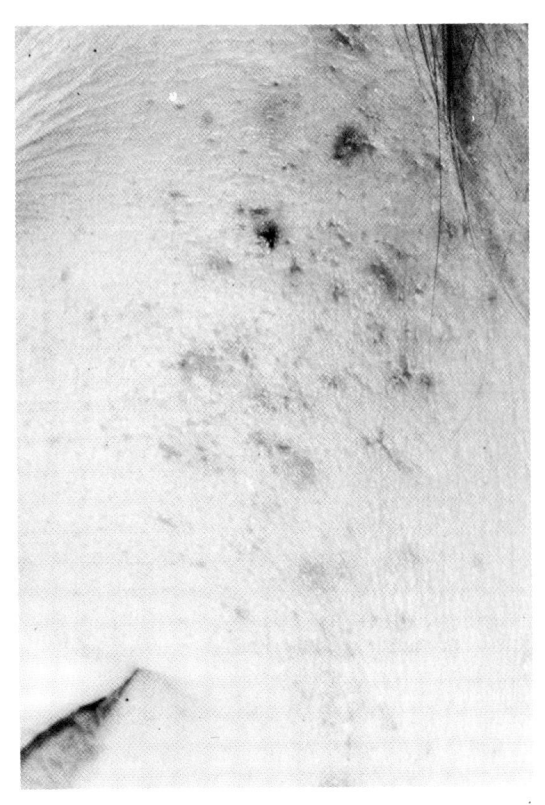

Fig. 26–3. Acne. (Courtesy of the Dermatology Service, Hôtel-Dieu de Québec, Canada.)

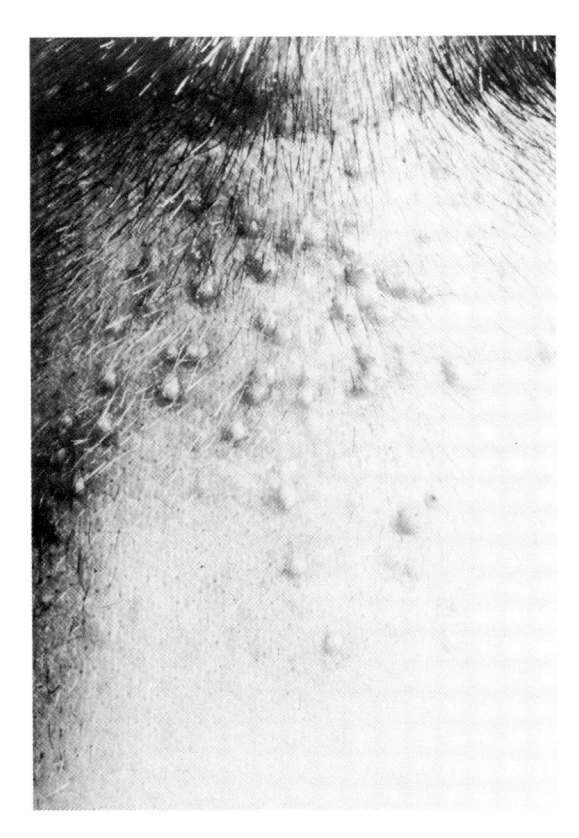

Fig. 26–4. Folliculitis in the back of the neck. (Courtesy of the Dermatology Service, Hôtel-Dieu de Québec, Canada.)

The antibiotic of choice is a semisynthetic penicillin, such as dicloxacillin, 50 mg/kg/day orally, or oxacillin, 100 mg/kg/day intravenously, depending on the severity of the infection. When the staphylococcus does not produce penicillinase, treatment with penicillin G is preferred. Antibiotic treatment of furunculosis does not prevent recurrences.

HIDRADENITIS

The course of hidradenitis, a distressingly protracted infection, is barely altered by antibiotic therapy. Surgical excision may be necessary to cure the disease. When the infection recurs, the physician should investigate the possibility of an immune deficiency.

PARONYCHIA AND FELON (WHITLOW)

Paronychia and felon (whitlow) occur with the introduction of a pathogen, usually *Staphylococcus aureus*, beneath the nail and the nail wall that produces an inflammatory reaction with a red or sometimes violaceous swelling. The reason for the intense pain of a felon is that the structures at the end of the finger, that is, the ungual phalanx and the nail, leave little room for swelling, and consequently, an infection creates intense pressure. A pathogenic organism may easily gain entrance during work or during a manicure. Therefore, it is important to avoid microtraumas of the tissues around the nail as much as possible and to be particularly careful when periungual portals of entry exist. The practical treatment for microbial felon is an antibiotic effective against staphylococcus and the application of moist compresses.

A felon may also be caused by the introduction of a fungus in the periungual tissues. *Candida albicans*, for example, can easily grow in this site if a portal of entry exists. The mode of introduction is the same as for bacteria. A felon caused by a fungal infection is particularly common in diabetics, as well as in kitchen or confectionery workers, and it presents a special problem in individuals with depressed host resistance. Treatment is difficult and consists of the application of nystatin ointment. Systemic antifungal agents such as 5-fluorocytosine and amphotericin B are effective, but are rarely necessary. A careful search should be made for conditions that encourage the development of this infection.

TREATMENT OTHER THAN PHARMACOLOGIC

The specific treatment of folliculitis, furunculosis, and hidradenitis is, as previously explained, limited to antibiotic therapy and, in particular cases, surgical excision. Because of their stubborn nature and their tendency to recur, however, these three diseases present real problems for the clinician, who must understand the patient's desire to obtain a definitive, curative treatment. The physician must recommend certain measures that inevitably appear too simple to the patient.

The first recommendation should be to maintain strict cleanliness of the affected areas. It is usually unnecessary to use antiseptic soaps or liquids; washing under a shower with ordinary soap is the best way to eliminate the offending agents. Because these lesions often appear in moist or closed areas, such as the groin, axilla, and buttock, a second recommendation is to wear loose clothing that provides adequate ventilation. Obviously, a girdle or tight jeans are inadvisable for a person with hidradenitis or folliculitis of the pubis, the inguinal region, or the buttock. Similarly, a truck driver who sits on a leather or plastic seat all day will find that gluteal folliculitis does not heal rapidly. One should not apply ointments to these regions, but rather drying lotions, tinctures, and talcum powder. Antibacterial lotions and creams, which interrupt the carrier state, are temporarily beneficial. In dealing with the family of a patient who has a recurrent staphylococcal infection, the physician should recommend improved hygiene. Pinching of the lesions to drain them is ill advised and even dangerous for the patient because it may spread the infection.

> **Objective 26–4.** Differentiate between a dermatophytosis and a mycosis caused by a yeast in a localized skin lesion.

Fungi often infect the skin. Mycoses are termed deep when the responsible organism is found in the corium, including the reticular layer, or in the internal tissues. These infections are called superficial when the fungus infects the stratum corneum or the keratin of the adnexa, that is, the hair and nails (Table 26–2). Only the superficial mycoses are discussed here.

These mycoses are divided into two groups on the basis of their origin: dermatophytoses, caused by microsporum, trichophyton, and epidermophyton, and yeast infections, caused by candida and pityrosporon. This microbiologic distinction is important in therapy because different drugs are required for the treatment of these two groups of organisms. Clinical considerations are based on the site of the lesion: inguinal folds, glabrous skin, interdigital webs, nails, or scalp.

INGUINAL INTERTRIGO

Inguinal intertrigo clearly illustrates the importance of a precise etiologic diagnosis because incorrect treatment causes the lesions to persist almost indefinitely. The infection usually occurs in an athletic young man with pruritic lesions of the inguinal folds and the internal aspect of the thighs. Examination reveals red, scaly patches that may be either dry or slightly moist.

Causes. Possible causes of this condition are: a traumatic irritation that has become superinfected, generally by gram-positive cocci; psoriasis; erythrasma, an infection caused by *Corynebacterium minutissimum*; dermatophytosis; or candidiasis or monilial infection. The local appearance is sometimes suggestive of the diagnosis. Dry, sharply demarcated patches with a well-defined border suggest a dermatophytosis (Fig. 26–5), whereas an oozing, poorly demarcated lesion is more characteristic of candidiasis.

Diagnosis. A salmon-red fluorescence under Wood's light points to erythrasma. The other skin folds and the rest of the integument should also be examined because one may discover, for example, typical lesions of psoriasis or of athlete's foot. In women, an intense erythema of the vulva and vagina with leukorrhea should remind the physician of the possible spread of a genital candidiasis to the groin.

The distinction between candidiasis and dermatophytosis can be made microbiologically by examining scales taken from the lesion. Using either a surgical knife with a small, curved blade or a stylet, the physician should moisten the periphery of the patch, scrape off the scales, and deposit them on a slide. Then, 1 or 2 drops of 20% potassium hydroxide should be added before the slide is protected with a coverslip. The preparation should be heated gently over an alcohol lamp and should then be examined under a microscope. Generally, a dermatophytosis can be identified by the presence of a number of

Table 26-2. Fungal Infections of Skin and of Various Tissues

Type of Infection	Type of Fungus	Specific Agent	Disorder or Site of Infection
DEEP	Dimorphic fungi	*Blastomyces dermatitidis* *Blastomyces brasiliensis* *Coccidioides immitis* *Histoplasma capsulatum var. duboisii* *Sporothrix schenckii* *Cryptococcus neoformans* *Phialophora* and *cladosporium*	North American blastomycosis South American blastomycosis Coccidioidomycosis Histoplasmosis Sporotrichosis Cryptococcosis Chromomycosis
		Candida, particularly *C. albicans*	Mucous membrane infection: mouth, vagina, digestive tract Skin fold infection: groin, axilla, interdigital webs, commissures of lips, vulva, perianal region Nails: onychomycosis
SUPERFICIAL	Yeasts	*Pityrosporum orbiculare*	Tinea versicolor
	Dermatophytes	*Microsporum* *Trichophyton* *Epidermophyton*	Scalp: ringworm, favus Beard: sycosis Glabrous skin: face, trunk, limbs Skin folds: intertrigo Groin: tinea cruris Axillary infection Interdigital spaces: athlete's foot Nails: onychomycosis

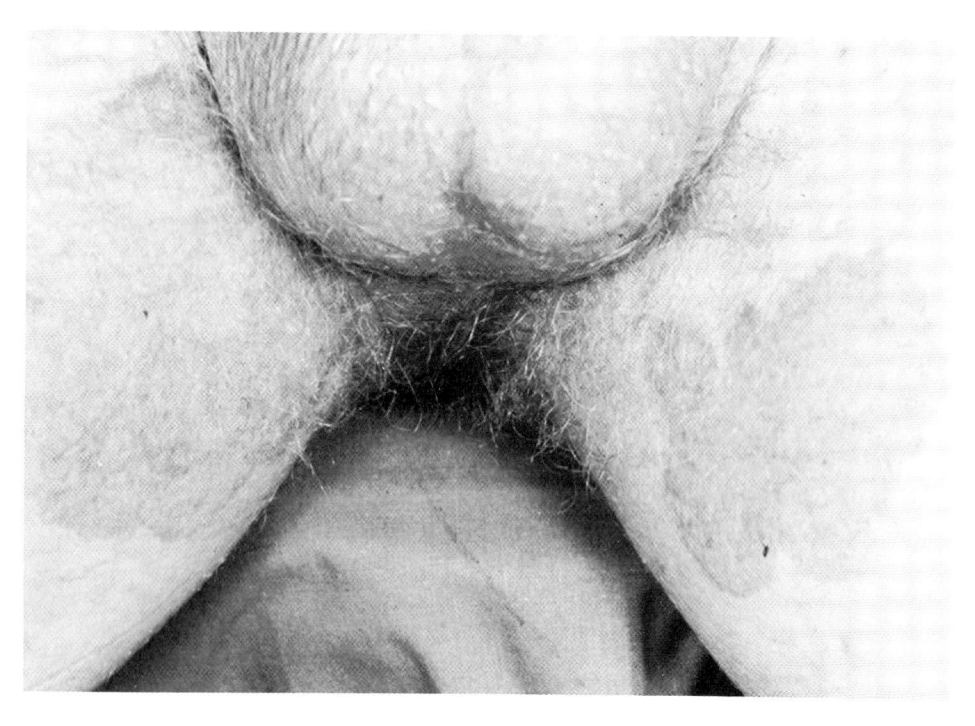

Fig. 26–5. Inguinal dermatophytic intertrigo. (Courtesy of the Dermatology Service, Hôtel-Dieu de Québec, Canada.)

branching, septate hyphae, whereas the presence of nonseptate, irregular pseudohyphae and numerous yeasts indicate a probable candidiasis. A positive diagnosis is obtained on the basis of the cultural characteristics by inoculating scales in Sabouraud's agar. The culture takes a long time for dermatophytosis, but with a yeast such as *Candida albicans*, for example, inoculation in human serum makes identification possible within a few hours because it permits the characteristic chlamydospores to form rapidly.

Treatment. The treatment of inguinal dermatophytosis consists of the topical application of an antifungal agent active against dermatophytes, such as iodinated alcohol, tolnaftate, clotrimazole, or micronazole nitrate, twice a day for 15 or 20 days. Griseofulvin should be reserved for patients in whom the inguinal dermatophytosis has reached the gluteal crease or the perianal region and has spread through annular lesions with a geographic contour on the buttocks, thighs, and other remote areas.

Candida albicans intertrigo is easily treated by local applications of nystatin or other agents, such as miconazole, active against yeasts. Although all areas affected by candidiasis must be treated, there is no point in giving oral nystatin alone to treat cutaneous candidiasis because this antibiotic is not absorbed and remains in the intestine. In rare cases, it may be necessary to prescribe 5-fluorocytosine.

Erythrasma disappears within a few days after treatment with erythromycin at an adult dose of 500 mg every 6 hours. The "automatic" prescription of a cortisone ointment reduces the itching temporarily, but does not inhibit the growth of the fungus. The infection continues for months, and the prolonged application of this ointment, which provides relief but does not cure, eventually produces cutaneous atrophy with striae.

GLABROUS SKIN

Essentially, two mycoses must be considered in this diagnosis: dermatophytosis and tinea versicolor. The distinction is generally easy to make on clinical grounds.

Dermatophytosis (Tinea Circinata). Dermatophytic involvement of the skin of the face, limbs, and trunk is characterized by a red, scaly patch that is active peripherally. The border of the patch is slightly raised and is vesicular; the patch itself extends in centrifugal fashion. This infection is called tinea circinata (Fig. 26–6).

The patches multiply and grow by spreading at the periphery to form extensive areas with a polycyclic contour. If left untreated, tinea circinata can invade almost the entire surface of the skin, but it is usually self-limiting. Microscopic examination of a potassium hydroxide preparation of scale scrapings shows branching, septate, mycelial hyphae. The dermatophyte is positively identified by culture. Treatment consists of applications of topical antifungal agents active against dermatophytes. If the fungal involvement is extensive, it may be necessary to prescribe oral griseofulvin.

Tinea Vesicolor. *Pityrosporum orbiculare* is a pathogenic yeast-like fungus that causes a superficial mycosis of the glabrous skin called tinea versicolor. Tinea versicolor occurs in the form of yellowish or whitish patches of various sizes ranging from less than a millimeter to a few centimeters in diameter (Fig. 26–7A). These macules and patches are distributed mainly over the patient's chest, neck, shoulders, and arms. When left untreated, the lesions may spread over the entire surface of the skin. Examination by Wood's light demonstrates a characteristic fluorescence.

Scraping the lesions with a blunt curette produces a lamellar detachment of the scales. For a positive diagnosis, the scrapings should be placed in potassium hydroxide between a

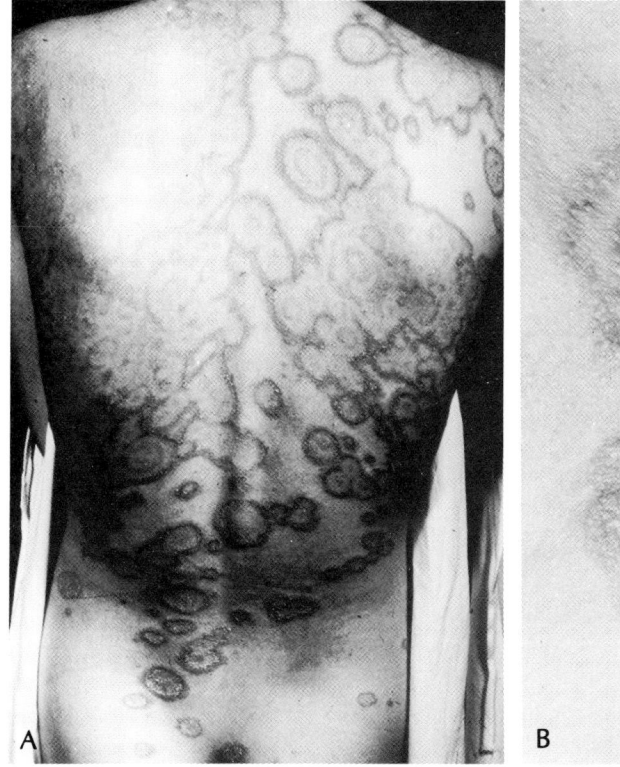

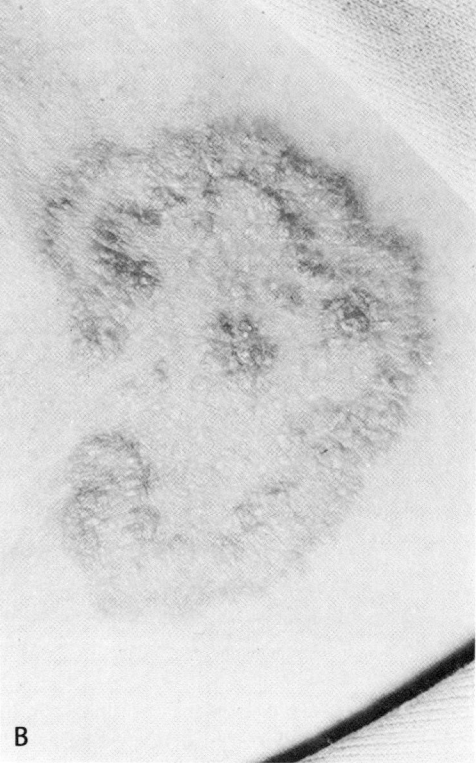

Fig. 26–6. *A* and *B,* Dermatophytosis of glabrous skin. (Courtesy of the Dermatology Service, Hôtel-Dieu de Québec, Canada.)

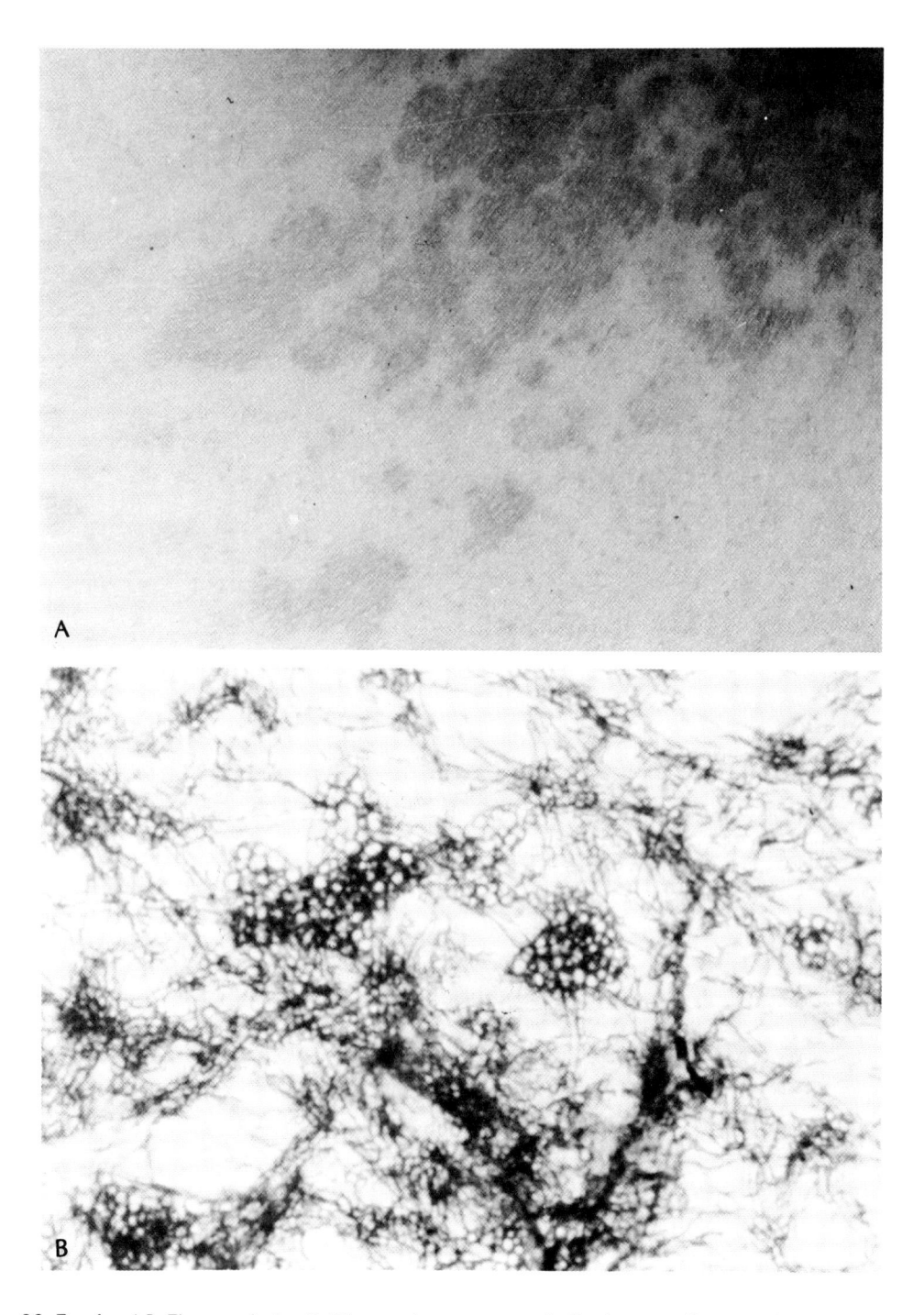

Fig. 26–7. *A* and *B*, Tinea versicolor. *B*, Microscopic appearance of adhesive tape. (Courtesy of the Dermatology Service, Hôtel-Dieu de Québec, Canada.)

slide and coverslip and examined under a microscope. An even simpler procedure is to apply cellophane adhesive tape to a patch of lesions, then transfer the material to a slide. Microscopic examination of this preparation reveals a few mycelial hyphae and numerous clusters of spores (Fig. 26–7B).

A distinctive feature of this disease is that its appearance depends on whether or not the patient's skin is suntanned; hence the name, versicolor. On white skin, the patches appear yellowish on a paler background. The scaly thickening of the lesions serves as a screen to the ultraviolet rays, so the patches do not tan when exposed to sunlight. During the summer when the rest of the patient's skin tans normally, the disease appears in the form of pale patches.

In most cases, the differential diagnosis has to be made between vitiligo and pityriasis alba. The lesions of vitiligo are not scaly. In pityriasis alba, the scaling is fine and powdery, and the patches are poorly demarcated.

Treatment consists of the application of sodium hyposulfite, iodine, and salicylic acid in alcohol or a product containing sulfur, such as selenium sulfide, to cause the patches to scale. Miconazole and clotrimazole are also effective. Because the fungus is localized exclusively in the thick, accumulated scales, the pathogen is eliminated, and the disease is cured by complete desquamation of the lesions. This disease is not contagious or is only mildly contagious, but it is relapsing, and some persons are more likely to contract it than others. Especially predisposed are patients with an immune deficiency or those treated with immunosuppressant drugs.

INTERTRIGO OF INTERDIGITAL SPACES

Lesions of the interdigital spaces of the feet and hands may be caused either by dermatophytes or by yeasts. Involvement of the feet is usually due to dermatophytes, which produce athlete's foot (Fig. 26–8). The lesion usually begins in the fourth interdigital space, where it may remain localized for a long time. The interdigital web is whitish, macerated, and has moist scales. The lesion is well-demarcated and is slightly elevated at the periphery. A moist fissure is often found between the toes. Itching and burning are significant. The lesion may gradually spread to the other indigital spaces, as well as to the sole and the dorsal surface of the toes and foot. In the hands, the lesion is frequently caused by yeasts, and the third interdigital space is principally involved (Fig. 26–9).

The diagnosis is established by obtaining scrapings of the lesions and examining them directly under the microscope. If this search shows no hyphae or yeasts, it must be repeated. Only after several negative examinations may the intertrigo be diagnosed as nonmycotic. If the disorder is not caused by a fungus, it may be a bacterial intertrigo or even psoriasis. A positive microscopic examination is necessary before treatment against dermatophytes or yeasts can be instituted.

INFECTIONS OF THE NAILS (ONYCHOMYCOSIS)

Infections of the toenails and fingernails caused by dermatophytes or yeasts are common. When the infection is caused by a dermatophyte, the nail becomes grayish, yellowish, or whitish, and is thickened, hyperkeratotic, and friable (Fig. 26–10). In a yeast infection, cleavage and disintegration occur at the base and the lateral fold of the nail. Nailbed inflammation due to candida is usually preceded or accompanied by paronychia. A drop of pus may be expressed at this site.

Of course, other diseases of the nails exist besides onychomycosis. Psoriasis or trophic disorders may cause changes that fit the same description. Therefore, a precise etiologic diagnosis should be made by microscopic examination of scrapings, and antimycotic treatment should not be prescribed until positive test results are obtained. If dermatophytes are implicated, the treatment consists of oral griseofulvin for several months. The nail must have time to grow, and all the infected keratin must be eliminated. Griseofulvin does not kill the fungus, but inhibits its growth. Because the administration of this antibiotic for long

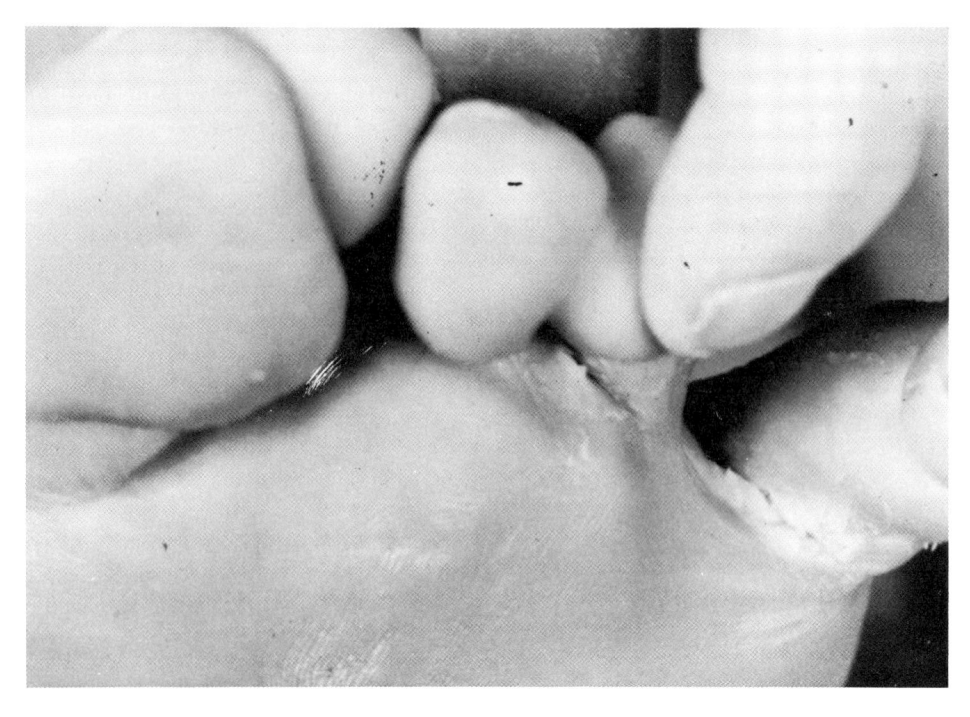

Fig. 26–8. Athlete's foot. (Courtesy of the Dermatology Service, Hôtel-Dieu de Québec, Canada.)

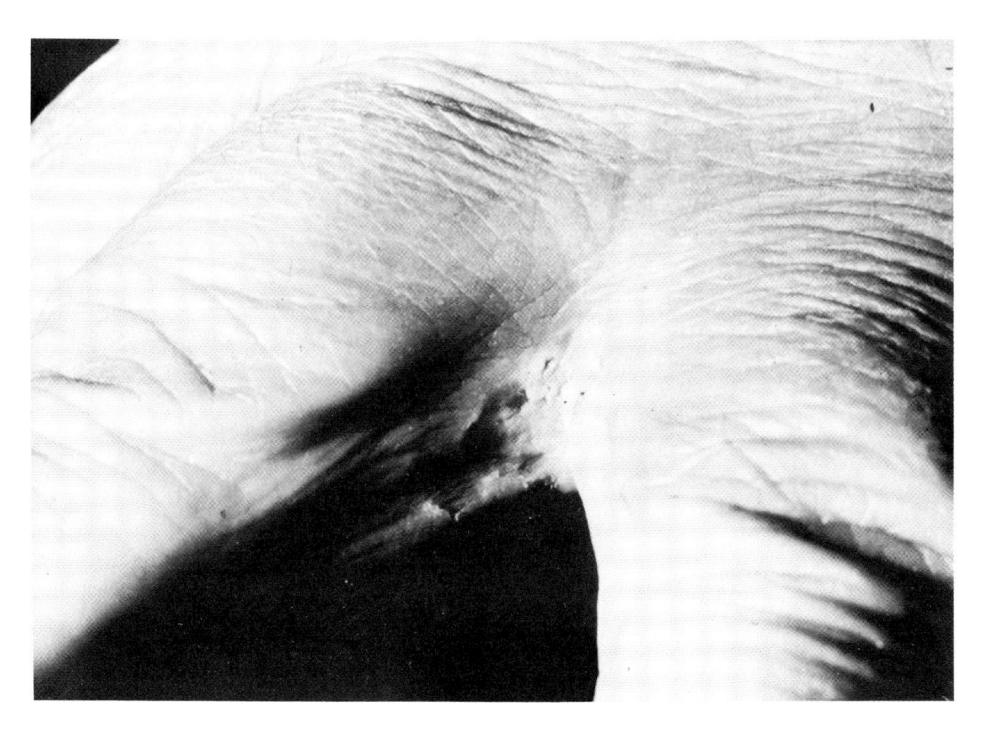

Fig. 26–9. Intertrigo due to *Candida albicans* in the third interdigital space of the hand. (Courtesy of the Dermatology Service, Hôtel-Dieu de Québec, Canada.)

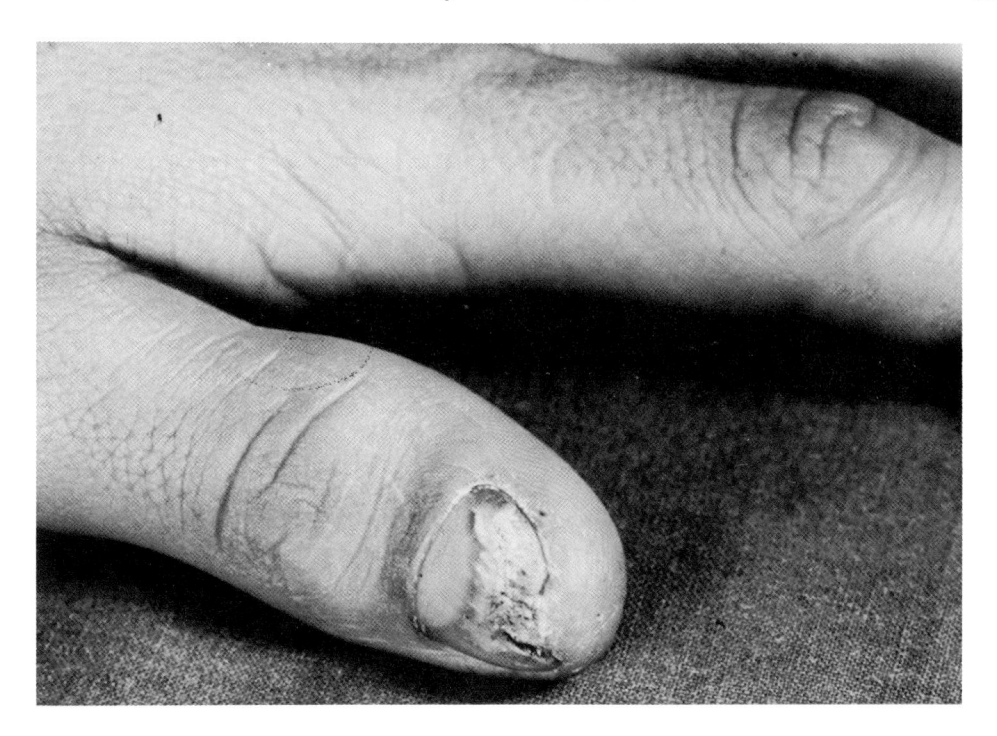

Fig. 26–10. Dermatophytic onychomycosis. (Courtesy of the Dermatology Service, Hôtel-Dieu de Québec, Canada.)

periods entails certain risks of intolerance, particularly hepatic, one must weigh these risks against the benign character of the onychomycosis.

Candida Onychomycosis. This disorder, which is troublesome to the patient because it is inflammatory and painful, can usually be treated by appropriate topical antifungal agents, local antiseptics, and dyes, although sometimes oral 5-fluorocytosine is needed. Of course, predisposing factors, such as poorly controlled diabetes, working with damp materials, sensitivity to foods and detergents, or local traumas, must be eliminated.

SCALP INFECTIONS (TINEA CAPITIS AND FAVUS)

Fungal infections of the scalp are frequent among children, even though large school epidemics disappeared with the advent of griseofulvin. The lesion appears in the form of a bald patch a few centimeters in diameter (Fig. 26–11). Such patches are round or oval, single or multiple, and their surface is grayish or whitish and scaly. The hairs at this site are broken and short, and one may also see red, scaly patches elsewhere on the surface of the skin. Fungal lesions must be distinguished from alopecia areata, also characterized by circumscribed bald patches, although the lesions are not scaly. In alopecia areata, the skin is shiny, tense, and smooth, and remaining hairs are rare, darker, measure only 1 or 2 mm, and have a characteristic terminal thickening or an "exclamation point" formation.

Diagnosis. In tinea capitis, examination in Wood's light produces an obvious and characteristic green fluorescence. The specimen is prepared for examination in potassium hydroxide between a slide and coverslip, as for inguinal dermatophytosis. One sees hair infected with the fungus; the hair shaft is usually surrounded by a mantle of spores, and hyphae are also found within the hair itself.

The source of the infection is often a cat or a dog that also has bald patches on the muzzle, head, or ears. On a farm, the infection

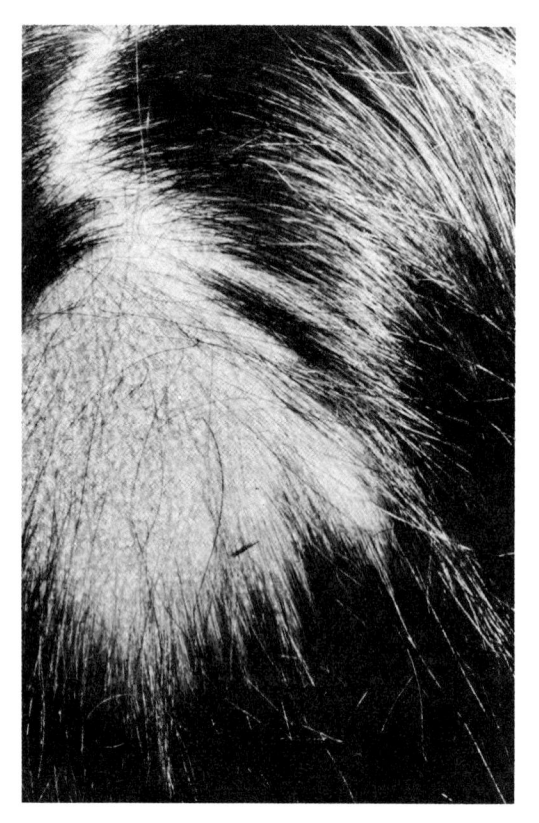

Fig. 26–11. Ringworm of the scalp. (Courtesy of the Dermatology Service, Hôtel-Dieu de Québec, Canada.)

may come from cattle. Adults rarely have scalp involvement, and untreated tinea capitis infections in children heal spontaneously at puberty. Favus, an exception, produces different clinical lesions. In favus, diffuse involvement of the entire scalp is followed by suppuration and scarring.

Treatment. In most cases, the treatment of tinea capitis infections in children requires the oral administration of griseofulvin, 10 mg/kg/day, for a period of at least a month. This regimen must be accompanied by daily local treatment with a topical antifungal agent active against dermatophytes, as well as a medicated shampoo. The patient's hair should be shaved, and the patch should be epilated with forceps.

> **Objective 26–5.** Distinguish among the principal infectious causes of chronic cutaneous ulcers.

Some ulcerating or vegetating skin lesions fail to heal despite antiseptic, or even antibiotic, treatment, and their course is chronic and slowly progressive. These lesions may be grouped under the title of chronic cutaneous ulcerations. They pose an often difficult clinical problem in which the establishment of an etiologic diagnosis becomes an essential condition for specific treatment (Table 26–3).

CLINICAL FEATURES

Usually, these lesions are deep, ulcerating sores measuring from one to several centimeters in diameter. The base of the ulcer is vegetating or granular and contains serofibrinous material, pus, and coagulated blood. The contour of the lesion is often irregular, and its borders have certain distinctive characteristics. They are thick and elevated, with steep edges that are sometimes detached or undermined, as if the ulcer were progressing beneath the edge. The ulcer's contour and periphery are inflamed and are erythematous, violaceous, yellowish, or brownish in color. A yellowish brown color suggests the presence of a granuloma. By pressing down at that site with a clear glass, the physician may judge the quality of the color and may identify the so-called apple-jelly nodules, which suggest the diagnosis of tuberculosis, nontuberculous mycobacterial infection, tertiary syphili, or other granulomas.

DIAGNOSIS

The most useful diagnostic procedure is to take a sample of tissue by biopsy and, after grinding it, to perform a complete microbiologic examination. Direct microscopic examination after routine or special staining may immediately reveal the presence of acid-fast bacilli, clumped cocci, or fungi. Inoculation for culture an ordinary and special media, such as Sabouraud's agar or Löwenstein's medium, at appropriate temperatures

Table 26–3. Chronic Cutaneous Ulcers

Cause	Clinical Characteristics of Lesion	Characteristics of Pathogen	Culture Medium	Serologic or Skin Tests	Treatment
Tuberculosis	Ulcer with irregular contour, detached borders, granulation at base, lupoid infiltrate	Acid-fast bacillus	Löwenstein-Jensen or similar	PPD* test positive	Streptomycin, rifampin, isoniazid
North American blastomycosis	Vegetating and verrucous patch, ulcerous or nonulcerous	Budding yeast (*Blastomyces dermatitidis*)	Sabouraud's agar, 25° C (mycelial form), 37° C (yeast form)	Complement fixation and blastomycin intradermal reaction	Amphotericin B
Tertiary syphilis	Infiltrated patch, ulcer with granulomatous contour, lupoid infiltrate	*Treponema pallidum* cannot be found	Cannot be cultured	VDRL† and FTA‡ tests positive	Aqueous procaine penicillin G
Atypical mycobacterial infection	Vegetating lesion, sometimes ulcerous at inoculation site	*Mycobacterium marinum*, *M. ulcerans*	Löwenstein-Jensen or similar	PPD* test often positive	Tetracycline, rifampin, ethambutol
Botryomycosis	Vegetating patch, rarely ulcerous	Clumped cocci (staphylococcus)	Culture generally negative		Surgical excision; antibiotics according to sensitivity tests
Pyoderma gangrenosum	Ulcer with regular contour and steep, detached edges	Histologic examination shows vasculitis process	All cultures negative		
Varicose ulceration	Ulcer localized on legs, often in malleolar regions	Noninfectious cause			Local antiseptics or antibiotics; debridement in case of superinfection

*PPD, Purified protein derivative (of tuberculin)
†VDRL, Venereal Disease Research Laboratory
‡FTA, Fluorescent treponemal antibody

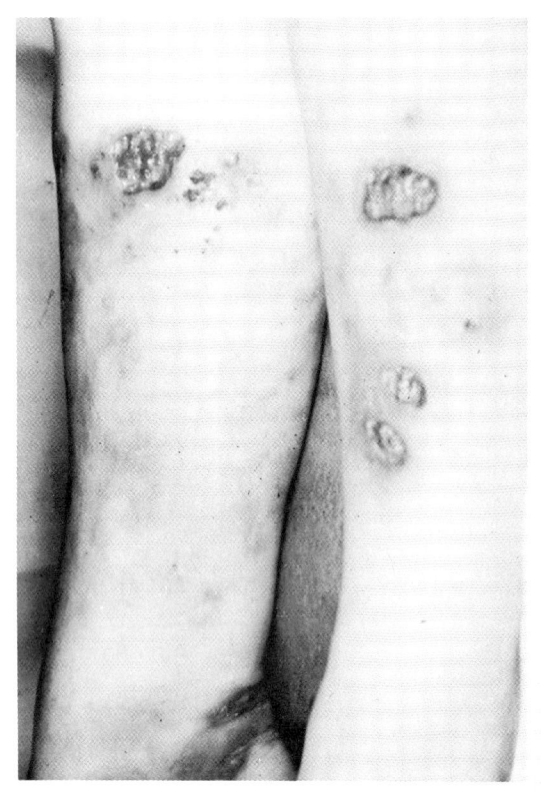

Fig. 26-12. Ulcers of tertiary syphilis. (Courtesy of the Dermatology Service, Hôtel-Dieu de Québec, Canada.)

is probably of vascular origin. It may accompany certain gastrointestinal diseases, particularly ulcerative colitis.

Self-Inflicted Injuries. Malingering patients (dermatitis factitia) have self-inflicted and self-maintained cutaneous ulcers that often look suspicious because of their bizarre contour and unusual location. In addition, a psychologic factor may exist.

Treatment. Once the etiologic diagnosis has been made, a curative treatment can be given: antituberculous drugs, such as streptomycin, rifampin, or isoniazid, for tuberculous ulcers; amphotericin B, by intravenous infusion over a period of several weeks, for North American blastomycosis (Fig. 26-13); aqueous procaine penicillin G in a total dose of 9 million U for ulcers of tertiary syphilis; tetracycline by mouth in a dose of 1 to 2 g/ makes it possible to identify the causative agent precisely. This same material can also be injected into certain sensitive animals, such as a mouse for sporotrichosis, as a further step in a difficult etiologic diagnosis, but such a procedure is seldom necessary.

Syphilis. Failure to perform serologic tests for syphilis is a major error (Fig. 26-12). It is impossible to find *Treponema pallidum* in ulcerous or granulomatous lesions of tertiary syphilis, but the serologic tests (Venereal Disease Research Laboratory, fluorescent treponemal antibody) are positive, usually in high titer. If, in spite of all these efforts, the causative agent is not identified, and if the serologic tests for syphilis are negative, the possibility of pyoderma gangrenosum or of malingering should be considered.

Pyoderma Gangrenosum. This extensive and progressive ulcerative cutaneous disease

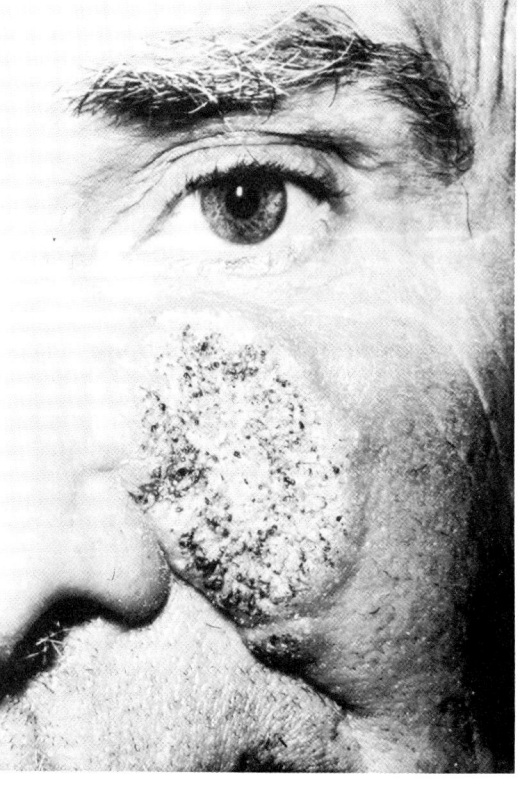

Fig. 26-13. North American blastomycosis. Chronic nonulcerative vegetating patch (diagnosis was confirmed histologically). (Courtesy of the Dermatology Service, Hôtel-Dieu de Québec, Canada.)

day for 2 to 4 months for a *Mycobacterium marinum* infection.

VASCULAR ULCERS

Varicose ulcers and ulcers of the leg due to arterial disease are usually superinfected, but this secondary infection is not the cause of the ulcer. Such an infection however, may cause the ulcer to persist or may even complicate its course. Bacteriologic findings are difficult to interpret because of the usual colonization by species that do not take an actual part in the infectious process.

Treatment. Topical antiseptic or antibiotic treatment, with or without debridement, generally controls the secondary infectious complication; systemic antibiotic therapy can thereby be avoided. Treatment of the vascular ulcers themselves requires more involved therapy, however. An ulcer on a leg affected by varicose veins, edema, or the sequelae of repeated phlebitis heals with difficulty. The ulcer is often covered by an adherent fibrinous and necrotic material that inhibits granulation. The best way to reduce congestion and edema in this instance is by bedrest, with the patient's foot elevated about 10 cm. The patient is permitted to get up only for the toilet and for a short walk each day. The fibrinous material can be removed with forceps, but often only after being "digested" by an ointment or jelly that contains proteolytic enzymes, such as streptokinase or streptodornase, or by products such as dextranomer beads. Subsequently, granulation may be stimulated by means of a dressing containing silver nitrate in a 1% aqueous solution or by the daily application of a gauze pad steeped in 20% benzoyl peroxide.

Some ulcers have a violaceous periphery with hemorrhagic dots and small, porcelainlike, cicatricial areas with a pearly white color. This capillaritis is caused by a hyalinizing vasculitis of the venules of the middle layers of the dermis. In these patients, the peripheral area of the lesion must be carefully protected by a padded dressing because the least trauma can cause an ulcer.

A much more sensitive area for the formation of trophic ulcers of the leg is the internal retromalleolar and submalleolar region. Because the venous system is deficient in this area, it is a propitious site for the formation of a leg ulcer.

A sphacelous ulcer secondary to arterial insufficiency is treated in the same way with the addition of local heat, but granulation and healing are difficult. Peripheral vascular surgical procedures are frequently indicated, for example, sympathectomy, endarterectomy, and arterial transplantation.

MALIGNANT ULCERS

The possibility exists that a chronic, cutaneous ulcer may be malignant. Certain lymphomas or sarcomas have this clinical appearance, and sometimes only repeated biopsies can determine the definitive diagnosis.

SUGGESTED READINGS

Brown, J., Kelm, M., and Bryan, L.E.: Infection of the skin by Mycobacterium marinum: report of five cases. Can. Med. Assoc. J., *117*:912, 1977.

Degos, R.: Dermatologie. Paris, Flammarion, 1981.

King, A., and Nicol, C.: Venereal Diseases. 4th Ed. London, Baillière Tindall, 1980.

Sneddon, I.B., and Church, R.E.: Practical Dermatology. London, Edward Arnold, 1976.

Solomon, L.M., Esterly, N.B., and Loeffel, E.D.: Adolescent Dermatology. Philadelphia, W.B. Webster, 1978.

Stewart, W.D., Danto, J.L., and Maddin, S.: Dermatology: Diagnosis and Treatment of Cutaneous Disorders. 4th Ed. Chicago, C.V. Mosby, 1978.

Touraine, R., and Revuz, J.: Dermatologie Clinique et Vénéréologie. Paris, Masson, 1982.

CHAPTER 27

Infections with Rashes

A. Dachy, A. Kahn, D. Blum, P. Demol and J.C. Pechère

Objective 27–1. Rapidly identify rashes that signal immediate danger.

Rashes often present physicians with diagnostic enigmas. Nevertheless, some cutaneous signs stem from serious diseases and must be recognized upon initial contact with the patient. Four general categories are posited: hemorrhagic rash, macular or maculopapular rash, exfoliative dermatitis, and ecthyma gangrenosum. Table 27–1 provides an overview of the diagnoses discussed.

CUTANEOUS HEMORRHAGIC ERUPTION

The combination of purpura or petechia with a fever is not unequivocal evidence of an infection, but the possibility must immediately be considered. The mechanisms of a cutaneous hemorrhagic eruption are, among others, direct injury to the capillary bed by an infectious agent or by an immunologic process and disseminated intravascular coagulation. A coagulation screen can be performed rapidly to identify and eventually to correct the anomalies found. The principal aim of the investigation, however, is to uncover the cause of the eruption; a number of hypotheses exist (Table 27–1).

Meningococcemia. In the course of a febrile disease of abrupt onset, the discovery of petechiae should suggest meningococcemia even when the meningeal signs are missing. Because a petechial rash is usually limited initially to the palpebral conjunctivae or to parts of the body compressed by clothing or elastic bands, each patient must be undressed and examined thoroughly. At a more advanced stage of meningococcemia, the cutaneous signs are scattered over the entire body and are virtually impossible to miss. These signs are confluent lesions with an ecchymotic appearance or numerous necrotic, purpuric lesions with or without a round pustule in the center. Epidemiologic and clinical evidence of the diagnosis are presented elsewhere (see Objective 30–3). The physician must act rapidly in taking the bacteriologic samples, from blood, cerebrospinal fluid, a throat swab, and occasionally a pustule, in starting the coagulation workup, and in administering penicillin therapy, at 200,000 U/kg/day (1 million U intravenously q2h in adults). The physician must also support the patient's vital functions when necessary; present or imminent shock is a major clinical concern.

Pneumococcal and Gram-Negative Septicemias. Meningococcemia is not the only septicemia that can be accompanied by hemorrhagic skin manifestations. These rashes are also observed in pneumococcal septicemia

Table 27–1. Cutaneous Manifestations of Serious Infectious Disease

Type of Rash or Cutaneous Disorder	Disease
Hemorrhagic	Meningococcemia
	Pneumococcal septicemia in asplenic patients
	Gram-negative septicemias (Enterobacteriaceae, pseudomonas, aeromonas)
	Endocarditis (streptococcal, staphylococcal)
	Borreliosis
	Typhus and Rocky Mountain spotted fever
	Viral hemorrhagic fevers
Macular or maculopapular	Endocarditis and septicemias
	Typhoid and paratyphoid fevers (rose spots)
	Rickettsioses
	Rocky Mountain spotted fever
	Epidemic typhus
	Scrub typhus
Exfoliative dermatitis of presumed staphylococcal origin	Ritter's disease
	Lyell's syndrome
	Toxic shock syndrome
Ecthyma gangrenosum	Gram-negative bacillary septicemias

and in the context of a disseminated intravascular coagulopathy in infants, in alcoholics, and above all, in asplenic patients. Even if this rare disorder is confused with meningococcemia, penicillin is a proper therapeutic choice in either case. In other circumstances, a diagnostic error has far graver consequences; for example, septicemias due to gram-negative bacilli, such as enteric bacteria, pseudomonas, or aeromonas, sometimes give rise to purpura fulminans similar to that seen in meningococcemia, but requiring a different therapeutic approach.

The clinical and pathologic contexts of the two disorders are different. Meningococcemia can be of abrupt onset in infants and young individuals in apparent good health. Occasionally, an epidemic outbreak in the area reinforces clinical suspicion of the disease. In contrast, gram-negative septicemias generally strike more elderly individuals in whom a portal of entry can often be found or in patients of any age in whom an underlying disease favors disseminated infection. Examples of such predisposing disorders are pyelonephritis, especially with obstruction; investigation or manipulation of the urinary tract; gastrointestinal surgical procedures; ascending cholangitis; bronchopneumonia; venous catheters left in place over long periods; extensive third-degree burns; leukemia; lymphoma; and neutropenia or other advanced states of immunosuppression. Microscopic examination of a gram-stained smear of an appropriate material such as the cerebrospinal or pustular fluid, or even buffy coat, sometimes provides immediate and decisive evidence of the cause of the sepsis. Appropriate therapy for a gram-negative sepsis that is either confirmed or strongly suspected is discussed in Objective 13–3.

Endocarditis. Petechiae in moderate numbers can also be seen in some streptococcal and staphylococcal septicemias. Such a finding suggests an endocardial focus of infection. This question is treated in greater detail in Chapter 14, but the importance of a cardiac murmur in support of this diagnostic hypothesis is worth repeating. Besides petechiae, several other cutaneous signs, although infrequent, are compatible with the diagnosis of endocarditis, particularly the classic Osler's nodes and Janeway lesions.

Borreliosis. Much more rarely, a petechial rash is due to borreliosis, that is, the tick- or louse-borne relapsing fever caused by a spirochetal organism in western North America, Central America, and Africa. The high mortality rate can be reduced by appropriate antimicrobial therapy with tetracycline, chloramphenicol, or erythromycin; some strains of tick-borne disease are resistant to penicillin, but penicillin is generally useful in louse-borne fevers.

Viral Infections. Hemorrhagic or petechial skin lesions are not exclusive to bacterial diseases, and various viral infections should also be mentioned. Such routine diseases as measles, rubella, infectious mononucleosis, and varicella are occasionally associated with purpuric rash, although such a rash is not necessarily a serious prognostic sign. The so-called viral hemorrhagic fevers are worth considering when the patient has returned from a trip to an endemic geographic area. The term "viral hemorrhagic fevers" groups together some disparate entities (Table 27–2), which nonetheless all have a viral origin, a specific geographic localization, a similar clinical appearance, and a common grave prognosis. Lassa fever is a descriptive example.

Besides the clinical appearance, the most important diagnostic evidence of viral hemorrhagic fever is a stay in an endemic zone and perhaps the season or the incubation period; this information is found in Table 27–2. Among the most important precautions to be taken with these diseases are isolation of the patient and extreme care in handling laboratory specimens. The risk of interpersonal transmission is considerable.

MACULOPAPULAR RASH

Typhoid or Paratyphoid Fever. Most physicians should be able to recognize rose spots, which are 10 to 20 small macules, 2 to 4 mm in diameter. More pink than red, these spots blanch under pressure and are found characteristically on the upper half of the patient's abdomen. In the clinical context described in Objective 16–1, rose spots suggest either typhoid or paratyphoid fever. Some viral infections, enterovirus in particular, produce an enteritis and a similar eruption, but in these disorders the spots are more numerous and are not similarly localized. Once the cultures are taken, treatment can be begun as described in Objective 16–3 because the lesions in the appropriate clinical context are pathognomonic for the disease.

Rickettsioses. Some rickettsioses must also be considered in life-threatening infectious exanthems, in particular Rocky Mountain spotted fever, epidemic typhus, and scrub typhus. A typhus-like disease due to *Rickettsia canada*, recently discovered but as yet unnamed, can be added to the list. These diseases, usually curable today, are characterized by a high mortality rate if appropriate antibiotic therapy is not administered in time.

In North America, as well as in some South American countries, Rocky Mountain spotted fever should be considered in a patient with a macular or maculopapular rash that first appears around the wrists and ankles. This rash initially blanches under pressure and rapidly spreads. It is then more marked on the extremities than on the trunk. Without being entirely pathognomonic, involvement of the palms and soles supports the diagnosis. At an advanced stage of the disease, the rash looks petechial or ecchymotic, and in its most extreme form, like a purpura. The disease usually appears in the spring and early summer.

The patient, who complains of severe headaches, myalgia, and photophobia, is agitated, irritable, and sometimes confused. The conjunctivae are injected, the neck is stiff, the face and extremities are puffy, and occasionally, mild heptosplenomegaly is present. A small, blackish eschar and an accompanying local adenopathy are excellent diagnostic clues, unfortunately not always present, that correspond to the portal of entry, which is the site of the tick bite. This portal of entry escapes one's attention if it is not looked for, notably on the scalp. The tick is the sole vector of the infection. In the western United States, the brush tick, *Dermacentor andersoni*, is most frequently implicated; in the eastern United States, it is the dog tick, *Dermacentor variabilis*.

Other important diagnostic evidence is exposure in an endemic area 2 to 14 days before the onset of the clinical signs; the average incubation period is around a week. Infection can occur practically anywhere in the United

Table 27-2. Viral Hemorrhagic Fevers

Type of Hemorrhagic Fever	Epidemic Area	Principal Endemic Foci	Origin: Virus and Reservoir	No. of Days	Incubation Most Active Months	Mortality Rate (%)	Contagiousness of the Patient
Associated with rodents							
Lassa	West Africa	Rural nosocomial	Arenavirus (rodent: mastomys)	1–23	Jan–Dec	8–52	Strong (strict isolation)
Argentine	Argentina	Grain fields (corn)	Arenavirus (rodent: calamys)	10–14	Mar–July	5–30	?
Bolivian	Bolivia	Rural familial	Arenavirus	10–14	Feb–Sept	5–30	Weak
Korean-Siberian hemorrhagic nephrosonephritis	1. Korea, Japan, and Siberia 2. Eastern Europe and Scandinavia	Rural areas, forests, hay	Virus, recently identified (voles and mice)	9–35	Mar–July Nov–Sept (Asia); Sept–Jan (Europe)	1–10	Weak or nil
Transmitted by mosquitoes							
Dengue	Indochina, Indonesia, Malaysia, Philippines, South Pacific, and India	Mainly children	Flavivirus (dengue types 1–4) (man)	2–8	Mar–Nov Jan–Dec	5–10	Nil in the absence of a vector
Yellow fever	Africa and tropical America	Jungles and in cities	Flavivirus (man, monkeys)	3–6	Jan–Dec	5–10	Nil in the absence of a vector
Transmitted by ticks							
Crimean	Soviet Union, Bulgaria, central Asia, and central Africa	Rural cattle	Togavirus, not grouped (bovines, small mammals)	3–9	June–Aug	10–50	Nil in the absence of a vector
Kyasanur Forest fever	Province of Mysore (India)	Forest cattle	Flavivirus (cattle, monkeys, rodents, birds)	3–8	Feb–June	3–10	Blood and tissues occasionally contagious
Omsk	Western Siberia	Cattle (summer); muskrats (trappers)	Flavivirus (domestic animals, rodents)	3–8	Jan–Dec	5–10	Blood and tissues occasionally contagious
Other							
Marburg	Central Africa	Uncertain, perhaps monkeys	Marburg virus (vector unknown)	3–8	?	High	Strong (strict isolation)
Ebola	Sudan and Zaire	Uncertain, sometimes nosocomial	Ebola virus (vector unknown)	4–16	?	High	Strong (strict isolation)

LASSA FEVER

Lassa is the location of a Nigerian Protestant mission where this disease was noted for the first time in 1969. The primary, endemic focus of infection appears to be in West Africa, but interhuman transmission of the virus may extend the epidemic possibilities.

The reservoir of the virus is a rodent widespread in Africa, *Mastomys natalensis*. Besides the rat-to-man transmission, which probably occurs through the intermediary of foodstuffs contaminated by rat urine, interhuman spread has already tragically struck the medical personnel in that area of Nigeria. Urine, stool, saliva, and blood are contagious. In addition, the infectivity of the virus in the laboratory is proved beyond doubt.

Clinically, the illness begins insidiously after an incubation period of 1 to 24 days and is characterized by fever, chills, headaches, and myalgia that increase in the following days. In a local epidemiologic context, one would think of typhoid. The clinical picture, complete in about a week, includes chest and abdominal pains, vomiting, diarrhea, relative bradycardia, vesicular or ulcerative pharyngitis, maculopapular rash, and polyadenopathy. The hemorrhagic signs, petechiae and bleeding, warn of the disease, in general during the second week of the illness. Shock is likely to supervene rapidly, leading to a mortality rate of 8 to 52% of cases. Routine laboratory tests give the following picture: marked leukopenia ($< 4000/mm^3$) with neutrophilia and the presence of immature polymorphonuclear leukocytes, marked proteinuria, increased levels of transaminases (SGOT), creatinine phosphokinase (CPK), and lactose dehydrogenase (LDH), and occasionally, radiologic evidence of an atypical pneumonia and electrocardiographic signs of myocarditis. The Lassa virus can be specifically and rapidly identified by means of a fluorescent slide test from a conjunctival smear, with confirmation by viral culture (a dangerous procedure and only permitted in specific laboratories), or by complement fixation (not positive before about 2 weeks.)

No specific treatment exists, but supportive measures improve the prognosis. The importance of an exact etiologic diagnosis is tied to the epidemic risks of the disease. Isolating the patient, handling the blood samples with extreme caution, warning the laboratory of the risks, and alerting and occasionally isolating the patient's contacts are required preventive measures.

RICKETTSIA

The rickettsiae are small, obligatory, intracellular bacteria. The one exception to this definition, *Rochalimaea quintana*, the agent of trench fever, can grow outside a cell. For this reason, some authors have placed this bacterium outside of the rickettsiae. According to Bergey's *Manual of Determinative Bacteriology* (eighth edition), the family of Rickettsiaceae includes three genera: rickettsia, coxiella (Q fever), and rochalimaea. The rickettsia are gram-negative and carry a cell wall composed of multiple layers that gives them a rigid egg- or rod-shaped form. These bacteria survive in nature thanks to transmission cycles from animal hosts to bloodsucking insect vectors, such as ticks, fleas, and lice, and back again. Coxiella (Q fever) stands out because resistance to environmental conditions enables it to survive in air and fomites and hence to infect man by the respiratory route. In the laboratory, one obviously cannot isolate rickettsiae on acellular media, with the exception, once again, of rochalimaea, and thus it is usually necessary to inoculate laboratory animals such as guinea pigs, mice, and field mice. Because this procedure carries the risk of disseminating the disease, it is limited to specialized laboratories.

Serologic tests are the usual means of making the diagnosis. The Weil-Felix reaction rests on the immunologic analogies between some rickettsiae of the typhus and spotted fever groups and somatic antigens on nonmotile proteus, that is OX-19, OX-2, and OX-K. Although this simple test has only mediocre specificity and sensitivity, specific rickettseal antigens can be used in complement-fixation or indirect-immunofluorescent techniques, to demonstrate specific antibody in patients.

All species of rickettsia are sensitive to chloramphenicol and the tetracyclines.

States, but more than half the cases are reported from the southern part of the country, and the most are from the eastern half of the country. Contrary to the name of the disease, only a few cases arise in the Rocky Mountains (under 5%). Perhaps such has always been the case, but the disease was first recognized in the Rocky Mountains. The disease has also been described in Canada, Mexico (pinta), Panama, Colombia (Tobia fever), and Brazil (Sao Paulo fever). The endemic zones are unevenly distributed, with pockets from which the majority of cases are reported.

Finally, Rocky Mountain spotted fever is seasonal; ticks hibernate during the winter and do not become infectious until after their first blood meal. Thus, it is basically a springtime disease, although in recent years it has extended from April to September and even December, and the annual incidence appears to be increasing.

Routine laboratory tests show slight hypoalbuminemia and a normal white blood cell count and differential, with slight anemia and thrombocytopenia corresponding to the severity of the illness. Disseminated intravascular coagulopathy has been described in the most serious cases. The diagnosis is definitively confirmed by the serologic testing of properly spaced serum samples; that is, the Weil-Felix reaction, which depends on the agglutination of proteus OX-19, OX-2, and OX-K antigens, or the more specific and sensitive complement-fixation test. Isolation of the rickettsia is difficult and hazardous because of the danger of widespread laboratory transmission; however, one technique for early detection is direct immunofluorescence of a skin biopsy, which is positive from the third to fourth day of the illness.

Treatment reduces the mortality rate in a spectacular fashion. When the following antibiotic therapy is begun sufficiently early in the course of the disease, the mortality rate is practically nil: tetracycline, 25 to 50 mg/kg/day (2 to 4 g/day in adults), or chloramphenicol, 50 mg/kg/day (4 g/day), divided into 4 daily oral doses (unless intravenous therapy is necessary because of the gravity of the illness), administered for an average of 5 to 7 days.

Attempts at vaccine development have not yet resulted in a commercial product, and the only preventive measure available is to avoid tick bites. In an endemic area, regular personal inspection, including the hair and scalp, of the body and clothes limits the risk of infection. When a tick is found in the act of biting, it should not be smashed or pulled out, but made to release its hold by means of gasoline or alcohol, or with a lit cigarette.

Two other rickettsioses are also worth considering under the heading of infectious exanthems for which immediate appropriate therapy improves the prognosis: epidemic and scrub typhus. In these diseases, in contrast to Rocky Mountain spotted fever, the eruption starts on the trunk and extends centrifugally. No initial eschar is seen at the portal of entry in epidemic typhus, which is transmitted by louse excreta that the patient, on scratching, inoculates into the bite, but such a lesion may be seen in scrub typhus, in which it is valuable diagnostic evidence. The clinical picture is more severe than in Rocky Mountain spotted fever, with, in particular, a more elevated fever and more frequent encephalitic findings. The Weil-Felix reaction is positive with the proteus OX-19 antigen in epidemic typhus and with the OX-K antigen in scrub typhus; specific complement-fixation tests are also available. Treatment is similar to that recommended for Rocky Mountain spotted fever. Table 27-3 provides supplementary information on the epidemiologic features of these two forms of typhus, as well as a comparison with other rickettsioses.

GENERALIZED ERYTHEMA AND EXFOLIATIVE DERMATITIS OF PRESUMED STAPHYLOCOCCAL ORIGIN

Some disorders causing exfoliative dermatitis are definitely associated with exotoxigenic staphylococci: Ritter's disease, Lyell's syndrome, and toxic shock syndrome. Although the pathogenetic mechanisms of these syndromes may still be unknown, three important facts of interest to physicians are certain: (1) the mortality rates are high; (2) rapid diagnosis and immediate attention to fluid and electrolyte balance, compensation for protein loss through the skin, and treatment of shock improve the prognosis; and (3) administration of an antistaphylococcal antibiotic is recommended.

Ritter's Disease. This acute, generalized, exfoliative, bullous dermatitis occurs in the first to fifth week of life. The portal of entry varies from one patient to another, for example, an infected circumcision or an umbilical lesion. Sometimes, infection occurs in the context of a neonatal nursery outbreak. Along with the erythematous appearance of the patient's skin, one observes bullae and large fragments of skin that peel off spontaneously or with slight pressure and leave behind a denuded, red, and edematous dermal layer. High fever and a toxic appearance complete the clinical picture. The prognosis de-

Table 27-3. Rickettsial Infections

Disease	Agent	Vector	Principal Endemic Foci	Epidemic Circumstances	Incubation Period (days)	Mortality Rate Without Antibiotics
Typhus group						
Epidemic typhus	*Rickettsia prowazeki*	Louse	Historically worldwide	Wars, famines, prisons; louse feces inoculated into broken skin	7–15	High
Recrudescent typhus (Brill's disease)	*Rickettsia prowazeki*	Louse	Worldwide	Relapsing disease sometimes long after initial episode	Variable, sometimes years	Low
Murine or endemic typhus	*Rickettsia typhi*	Rat, flea	Worldwide	Contact with rats; flea feces transmitting the disease	6–14	Low
Scrub typhus (tsutsugamushi)	*Rickettsia tsutsugamushi*	Thrombiculid mite (mouse)	Southeast Asia, Far East, India, Australia, Pacific islands	In rural forests and brush, mites parasitize man and inoculating the rickettsia	6–20	High
Unnamed	*Rickettsia canada*	Tick	United States, Canada	Uncertain	Uncertain	Moderate
Group of Spotted Fevers						
Rocky Mountain spotted fever	*Rickettsia rickettsii*	Ixodid tick	United States, Canada, Mexico, Columbia, Brazil	Bite by brush or dog tick	2–14	High
African tick fever	*Rickettsia conori*	Ixodid tick	Mediterranean Basin, South Africa, Kenya, Ethiopia, Congo Pakistan, India	Tick bite	7–18	Low
North Asian or Siberian tick fever	*Rickettsia sibirica*	Tick	Siberia, Mongolia	Tick bite	7	Low
Queensland tick fever	*Rickettsia australis*	Tick	Australia	Tick bite	7–10	Low
Rickettsialpox (vesicular fever) (varicelliform rash)	*Rickettsia akari*	*Allodermanyssus sanguineus* (mouse mite)	United States, Soviet Union, equatorial and South Africa	Urban areas	10–24	Low
Other Rickettsial Infections						
Q Fever	*Coxiella burnetii*	Tick or aerosol or contact with infected material	Worldwide	Inhalation of contaminated dust	9–20	Low
Trench fever	*Rochalimea quintana*	Body louse (*Pediculus humanus*)	Europe, Africa, Japan, China, Mexico, Bolivia	Louse feces contaminating abraded skin	10–30	Low

pends on the vigor of the supportive efforts and on antistaphylococcal antibiotic therapy with a staphylococcal, penicillinase-resistant penicillin before test results are known. Without expert care, the mortality rate approaches 50%. Because of the risk of a nursery epidemic, strict isolation of the patient is necessary.

Lyell's Syndrome. This disorder is observed in older children, generally up to the age of 5 years, but it has also been seen in adults. Although it was initially observed following the ingestion of certain drugs, sulfonamides, in particular, a proportion of these cases seem to be linked to staphylococcal infection. In fact, two different entities can be distinguished: (1) scalded skin syndrome (Plate 8A and B), probably associated with *Staphylococcus aureus*; and (2) toxic epidermal necrolysis (Plate 9A and B and Table 27–4). The patient has a striking appearance, resembling someone with a severe scald burn characterized by generalized erythema, wide bullae ripped here and there, and exposed dermis. The lesions progressively develop over a week or so. The patient's general condition, initially good, eventually deteriorates. Those afflicted with scalded skin syndrome are treated as burn patients, an antistaphylococcal agent is added to the therapeutic regimen.

Toxic Shock Syndrome. The sudden appearance of erythroderma in a young woman until then in good health may indicate this unusual disease, only recently recognized.

Toxic shock syndrome occurs most often on the second to fifth day of menstruation, with an abrupt onslaught of fever over 39° C (102° F), severe headache, sore throat, obnubilation, episodes of confusion, nausea and vomiting, profuse and watery diarrhea, and hypotension extending into shock. The rash looks like a generalized sunburn and often involves the palms of the patient's hands. The erythema extends to the oropharyngeal, conjunctival, and vaginal mucosas, where small ulcerations without exudates can be noted. In 2 to 3 days, desquamation appears on the patient's hands and feet, at first fine and scaly, and then in large sheets. The results of several laboratory tests are altered: one sees moderate anemia, slight leukocytosis with immature granulocytes, initial thrombocytopenia followed by thrombocytosis, hypocalcemia and hypoproteinemia, limited signs of disseminated intravascular coagulation, and evidence of renal, hepatic, and muscular involvement.

Despite some uncertainty about the exact pathogenesis, two associations have been firmly established. The first is that many of these women have used tampons during their menstrual periods, and most commonly, before the association was publicized, "super-

Table 27–4. Scalded Skin Syndrome versus Toxic Epidermal Necrolysis

	Scalded Skin Syndrome	Toxic Epidermal Necrolysis
Origin	Exfoliation-producing *Staphylococcus aureus*	Drug reaction (sulfonamides); viral infections (?)
Cleavage plane in skin biopsies	Within the epidermal layer	Deep, beneath the prickle cell layer
Onset	Progressive	Rapid
Mucosa	Spared	Involved (mouth, pharynx)
Nikolsky's sign	Positive, even in apparently normal skin	Positive only in involved areas
Duration	Rapidly cured if properly treated	Long duration
Mortality rate	Low if properly treated	High (> 10%)
Treatment	Antistaphylococcal agents required, corticosteroids contraindicated	Corticosteroids indicated

absorbent" types of tampons. The second is the presence of an exotoxin-secreting *Staphylococcus aureus*, which appears to be the bacterial cause of the syndrome. Tampon usage appears to be a facilitating but not a necessary cause, because cases of the syndrome have occurred without their use and in women who were not menstruating, as well as in children, men, and the aged. The firmest association is with *S. aureus*, which can be isolated more than 75% of the time from the vagina or cervix of untreated patients; many of the isolated staphylococci produce an exotoxin C, which is thought to be responsible for the pathogenesis of the syndrome.

This serious disease has a mortality rate of 2 to 8%, depending on the series. Early and energetic measures against the hypotension and the use of a staphylococcal beta-lactamase-resistant penicillin, such as oxacillin, nafcillin, cloxacillin, or dicloxacillin, should improve the prognosis. Rapid diagnosis is essential.

In certain women, the disease recurs with subsequent menstrual periods. Not using tampons or changing them frequently can be recommended to all women who have had an initial episode of toxic shock syndrome. Specific antistaphylococcal treatment also seems to diminish the risk of recurrence.

ECTHYMA GANGRENOSUM

Ecthyma gangrenosum (see Plate 3C) is practically pathognomonic for gram-negative bacillary septicemia. This lesion was initially thought to be characteristic of infection with *Pseudomonas aeruginosa*, but it has also been associated with *Aeromonas hydrophilia*, *Escherichia coli*, klebsiella, enterobacter, and serratia. The lesion starts as one or more tender macules that enlarge, become slightly elevated, and most particularly, necrose in their centers. The lesion soon reaches palm size with clearly demarked, irregular borders, and the necrotic area takes on a blackish color. This typical appearance is easily recognizable and immediately suggests a specific cause.

Gram-negative bacilli swarming within the lesion are easily observed microscopically following aspiration or biopsy and grow on culture as well. The high mortality rate and the rapid progression of this entity, however, necessitate placing greater importance on the smear and Gram staining in confirming the diagnosis.

> **Objective 27–2. Identify the most probable cause of an infectious exanthem by means of the clinical signs.**

The diagnosis of an exanthem or rash has to be precise because these illnesses sometimes have serious consequences (1) for the patient, as in septic shock and purpura with meningococcemia, (2) for the contracts, as in congenital malformation due to rubella infection transmitted to a pregnant woman, and (3) for the community, as in severe varicella following the infection of immunosuppressed patients.

The clinical picture comprises a variety of signs and symptoms of infection, local or generalized, heralding or accompanying the appearance of the eruption, which consists of a mass of cutaneous lesions of a particular type. These lesions change the color (macules, petechiae) or the texture (papules, vesicles) of the skin, they appear suddenly and regress spontaneously in several days, and they involve various areas, depending on the nature and the evolution of the illness.

The infectious nature of these diseases accounts for their transmissibility, most often by direct contact, their immunizing potential (reinfections are possible but most often asymptomatic), their concentration in certain age groups by function of their local epidemiology, and their control by recourse to specific preventive measures such as vaccines and gamma globulin. The epidemiologic features of exanthems are given in Table 27–5.

TYPES OF LESIONS

Macules. One must analyze the type of lesions. Macules are flat lesions of a different

Table 27–5. Epidemiologic Features of Exanthems

Agent or Disease	Age of Predilection (years)	Incubation to First Symptoms (days)	Contagious Period (days)	Specific Prevention — At time of contact	Specific Prevention — Vaccination	Hospital Isolation
Adenovirus	<6	5–6	Acute phase to ?	None	Experimental	No
Erythema infectiosum	5–14	6–14	Unknown	None	None available	No
Roseola infantum	½–3	?	Unknown	None	None available	No
Hand-foot-mouth disease	1–9	3–7	Acute phase to ?	None	None available	No
Herpes simplex	type 1: ½–4; type 2: 15 and up	2–15 (4)*	Acute phase to ?	None	Experimental	Yes
Meningococcemia	<6	1–10 (3–5)*	Acute phase to ?	Chemoprophylaxis	Vaccine A-C	Yes
Infectious mononucleosis	10 and up	10–14	Acute phase to ?	None	None available	No
Rubeola (measles)	2–6	8–15	5 after contact; 5 after eruption	Immunoglobulin	Yes	Yes
Rubella (German measles)	3–9	14–21 (17)*	7 after contact; 5 after eruption	Immunoglobulin	Yes	No
Scarlet fever	6–9	2–5	3 before to 5 after eruption	Chemoprophylaxis	None available	Yes
Varicella	3–12 Sometimes adults	10–21 (14–16)*	2 before to 10 after eruption	Immunoglobulin	Experimental	Yes
Variola (smallpox)	Variable	7–12 (12)*	3 before eruption and until scabs fall	Chemoprophylaxis	Yes	Yes

*Numbers in parentheses indicate modal values

color than the skin. In the acute stage of illness, they represent a circumscribed hyperemia, during early convalescence, a hyperpigmentation (measles), and during late convalescence, a depigmented area (varicella).

Papules. These solid lesions are less than a centimeter in diameter and are raised by a coexisting cellular infiltrate and a localized exudate.

Vesicles. These circumscribed, raised lesions correspond to an accumulation of intra- or extracellular fluid situated in the layers of the epidermis. The word bulla or blister is applied to similar lesions of a diameter greater than 5 mm. Vesiculation may be perceptible only microscopically, as in measles and meningococcemia. The vesicular fluid may take on a cloudy purulent appearance (pustule) with a bacterial infection or with intense cellular necrosis, as in smallpox vaccination.

Petechiae. These hemorrhagic effusions occur in normal skin, result from vascular breaks in the superficial layers of the dermis, and do not blanch on pressure. Petechiae are seen in meningococcemia. Macules, papules, or vesicles can be the site of such lesions, as in measles, scarlet fever, infectious mononucleosis, or smallpox.

These basic lesions are not pathognomonic for any one exanthem. On a practical basis, exanthems are classified as maculopapular (Tables 27–6 and 27–7) or papulovesicular (Table 27–8). In a typical maculopapular lesion, the papule is due to localized cellular infiltrates and exudates, whereas in a typical papulovesicular lesion, the vesicle is due an accumulation of fluids in the epidermal layers. Petechial lesions may coexist with these two types, or it may be the only skin lesion (see Objective 27–1). Whichever type, the rash usually has a specific anatomic localization, such as on the limbs, in radicular distribution, or in skin folds; it can be either discrete or confluent.

DIAGNOSTIC CLUES

The following information from the patient's medical history and the physical examination is particularly useful in the diagnosis of exanthems:

1. History of a contact, which is easier to trace when the incubation period is short and the infection is symptomatic (see Table 27–5).
2. History of a prodrome, either diffuse, with fever, prostration, and irritability, or localized, with respiratory (cough, rhinitis, pharyngitis, conjunctivitis), gastrointestinal (vomiting, diarrhea), or lymphoreticular (adenopathy, splenomegaly) manifestations.
3. Presence of accompanying notable respiratory, gastrointestinal, or articular signs.
4. Specifics of the appearance, extension, and regression of the eruption.
5. Absence of a past history of that illness or of specific immunization.
6. Absence of exposure to medications known to cause secondary skin rashes: anticonvulsants, sulfonamides, barbiturates, antibiotics such as penicillin, cephalosporins and tetracyclines, antipyretics, antimetabolites, and antihistamines.

Objective 27–3. Diagnose measles in a febrile patient with a maculopapular rash on the basis of epidemiologic, clinical, and laboratory clinical evidence.

Measles is an extremely contagious illness whose well-characterized symptoms make it generally easy to recognize; however, modified and atypical measles are seen in partially immune individuals.

Measles rarely occurs in infants under 6 months of age because of the persistence of protective maternal antibody. Because immunity to measles is stable, individuals who have been vaccinated or those who have previously had the illness do not have symptomatic infections if exposed.

In identifying an infectious contact, one must remember that the incubation period is long, 10 days (contagious during the second

Table 27-6. Maculopapular Exanthems

Disease	Prodrome	Accompanying Signs	Rash
Maculopapular Exanthems Characteristically Accompanied by Fever			
Roseola infantum	Fever for 3 to 4 days, disappears with eruption; no change in general well-being	Exudative pharyngitis; nontender occipital lymphendenopathy; sometimes febrile convulsions	Discrete, chiefly on trunk, appears with drop in fever; no desquamation
Rubeola (measles)	Fever for 3 to 5 days and during eruption; oculonasal catarrh; Koplik's spots (2 to 3 days); marked changes in general state	Irritability; photophobia; paroxysmal cough	Spreading, initially in cervical and retroauricular areas, generalized on third to ninth days; regression at fifth to sixth day; dry desquamation
Scarlet fever	Fever with eruption for several hours to 2 days; abdominal pains, vomiting	Diffuse pharyngitis, possibly exudative; petechiae on soft palate; raspberry-strawberry tongue; submaxillary adenopathy	Punctate, accentuated in skin folds and pressure points, starting on trunk, generalized in 2 days, and lasting 5 to 7 days; palmar and plantar desquamation
Maculopapular Exanthems Occasionally Accompanied by Fever			
Rubella (German measles)	*Adults*: slight fever for 1 to 4 days; oculonasal dripping; adenopathy: occipital, postmastoid, or cervical 4 to 10 days before rash *Children*: variable	Persistent adenopathy; for several weeks, petechiae on soft palate; possible arthralgias or arthritis	First day: morbilliform; Second day: scarlatiniform; Third day: disappearing; lasting 3 days (children) to 7 days (adults) and sparing the axilla and popliteal fossa
Erythema infectiosum (fifth disease)	None	Enanthem; frequent pruritus; possible arthralgias or arthritis	First day: erythema on cheeks (slapped); Second day: extends to limbs, possible reticular appearance; Third day: extends to flexor surfaces, trunk, and buttocks; Tenth day: disappearing, reappearing occasionally if skin is irritated

Table 27-7. Infectious Diseases Occasionally Producing a Maculopapular Rash

Disease or Agent	Prodrome	Accompanying Signs	Rash
Adenoviridae			
Adenoviruses 1 to 4, 7 and 7a	Fever; oculonasal dripping	Conjunctivitis, pharyngitis	Principally on face and neck, upper part of trunk; lasting 1 to 5 days
Picornaviridae			
Coxsackievirus A 2, 4, 5, 7, 9, 10, and 16 Coxsackievirus B 1 to 5 Echoviruses 1 to 7, 9, 11, 13, 14, 16 to 19, 22, 25, 30, and 33	Fever and enanthem, possibly vesicular, gastrointestinal symptoms	Aseptic meningitis with echovirus 9 or coxsackievirus A 23	Of variable intensity, sometimes purpuric; localization distally or proximally; lasting 1 to 5 days
Boston (echovirus 16)	Fever, variable		Discrete, on face, shoulders, and trunk; no desquamation; rarely petechial; no relation to course of fever; lasting 2 to 8 days
Herpesviridae			
Infectious mononucleosis (Epstein-Barr virus)	Variable fever	Exudative tonsillitis, possibly with palatal petechiae; general adenopathy, splenomegaly	Confluent on trunk and buttocks; can involve palms and soles; duration variable, but around 7 days; sometimes purpuric, more often urticarial with administration of ampicillin
Cytomegalovirus	Fever	Lymphadenopathy; sometimes hepatitis; interstitial pneumonia	Discrete, mainly on trunk and proximal extremities; lasting 2 to 7 days
Other viruses			
Hepatitis B	Variable	Rash may occur during the prodromal period, before the icterus, along with headaches and arthritis	Often urticarial; lasting 4 to 7 days
Respiratory viruses (influenza A and B, parainfluenza 1 to 3, respiratory syncytial)	Variable	Variable upper respiratory tract symptoms	May occur in some patients; mainly on trunk and face, spreading to extremities; lasting 1 to 3 days
Mumps	Fever	Salivary gland swelling, headache, fever	Variable; lasting 2 to 5 days
Geographically important viruses (Lassa, Marburg, Chikungunya, Colorado tick fever, West Nile, Dengue, Kinjin)	Variable	Variable	Variable, often purpuric
Other Diseases			
Toxoplasmosis	8 days of variable fever; fatigue with possible pneumonia	Generalized adenopathy, possible hepatosplenomegaly	Generalized, spares palms and soles; variable progression
Rickettsiosis (see Table 27–3) Secondary syphilis (see Objective 23–1)			

Table 27-8. Exanthems with Vesicular Rashes*

Disease	Prodrome	Accompanying Signs	Rash
Rickettsialpox	Herald papule at point of inoculation evolving to scab	Fever, myalgia, vomiting for 4 to 5 days; Eschar at portal of entry, adenopathy and splenomegaly	Papules, vesicles, scabs generalized by 5 to 10 days; spares palms and soles
Varicella (chickenpox)	Children: brief fever; adults: fever and irritability for 1 to 2 days	Possible ulcerations on buccal mucosa, pharynx, eardrum; generalized adenopathy possible	Macules in groups, papules, vesicles, cysts in several hours; successive crops in the same area for 3 days; duration of 7 to 14 days; central distribution principally
Herpes zoster	Fever, pain in affected area (adults)	Pain in distribution of rash; occasional transient paralysis (can harm anterior spinal cord)	Vesicles grouped along sensory nerve distribution; spread from medial to distal areas; duration of 5 to 10 days
Variola (smallpox)	Marked pyrexia for 3 to 4 days; general prostration possible; fleeting rash on trunk	Gastrointestinal hemorrhages	Macules, papules, transformation to vesicles in several days, pustules with scabs in 5 to 25 days; in the same stage in same area; peripheral distribution principally

*Vesicular rashes have been also described with coxsackievirus A types 4, 5, 8, 10, and 16, with coxsackievirus B types 1 to 3, with echovirus types 6, 9, 11, and 17, with atypical measles in persons who received the killed virus vaccine, with mumps, and with secondary syphilis.

> **MEASLES VIRUS**
>
> Measles virus, antigenically unique, belongs to the family of the paramyxoviruses and shares with them their morphologic properties (see Table 2–1). Around the nucleocapsid or infecting particle that incorporates the RNA, the virus possesses an envelope composed of proteins and lipids, which probably derive from the membrane of the infected cell. This composition results in an antigenic linkage, which could, according to one hypothesis, be the basis for the demyelinating process in measles encephalopathy. On the virus envelope, as in influenza virus (a myxovirus also) (see Fig. 5–1), are located projections or spicules that contain several antigens, in particular, a hemolysin and a hemagglutinin. The hemolysin possesses the property of inducing cell membrane defects, and in the course of infecting a tissue culture, it gives rise to the formation of a multinucleated giant cell syncytium, which represent the basis for the laboratory diagnosis of the disease. In addition, the intracellular viral infection provokes the formation of eosinophilic cystoplasmic inclusion. The virus shows evidence of a particular affinity for the mucopolysaccharide receptors on epithelial and conjunctival cells. Measles is thus, first of all, a respiratory disease, in that the portal of entry is respiratory.
>
> In the first 48 hours following infection, a viremia allows the spread of the virus to the lymphatic tissue. This phase generally goes unnoticed, and the only possible clinical manifestations are limited to a transitory rash. From 3 to 8 days after infection, a secondary viremia appears; the propagation, this time, is by the circulating lymphocytes that carry the virus to the respiratory, intestinal, and cutaneous surfaces. Contagiousness begins during the secondary viremia. In the invaded tissues, the cellular changes produced by viral multiplication also begin. These changes are found in the gastrointestinal tract, especially on the buccal mucosa (Koplik's spots), the bronchial epithelium, the peribronchial and interalveolar spaces (interstitial pneumonia), and the covering and tissue of the central nervous system. Following a natural infection by measles virus, immunity is solid, both cellular and humoral, with, in particular, the secretion of IgA respiratory antibody. In case of a later pharyngeal reinfection, the illness remains strictly asymptomatic.

half), and that the rash appears around 14 days after the contact (the range is 10 to 19 days).

CLINICAL FEATURES

Clinically, the illness begins with a prodromal period of 3 to 5 days characterized by intense fever, malaise, coryza, conjunctivitis photophobia, a dry cough, and a hoarse voice. On examination of the mouth, small whitish spots, not detachable with the tongue blade, may be found on the mucosal surface in the region of the parotid duct (Koplik's spots). These lesions are practically pathognomonic, although certain adenoviral infections and hand-foot-mouth disease may also have similar manifestations. Several days later, the maculopapular rash appears. In the beginning, the rash is sparse and discrete upon the forehead, hairline, behind the ears, and on the upper neck; it later extends to the face (Plate 9C), the upper thorax, and the upper arms. Two days later it reaches the trunk (Plate 10A) and the lower limbs. By then the rash is confluent, occasionally purpuric, but leaves intervals of unaffected skin. At this point, the temperature curve drops in the absence of complications. On the sixth day of the rash, the macules take on a brown-pigmented appearance, and a flaky desquamation appears in the most intensely affected areas.

DIFFERENTIAL DIAGNOSIS

With such a clinical picture, little reason exists to consider rubella, which is generally much less febrile and less symptomatic. Roseola (exanthema subitum) is sufficiently well characterized in its course that one can distinguish it clinically (see Objective 27–5). Some rashes, seen in the course of infectious mononucleosis in the child, usually over 6 months of age, and other viral infections, closely simulate measles. The same is also true for drug rashes that occur from antibiotic therapy in a patient with influenza syndrome or infectious mononucleosis, as well as for certain rickettsial infections, such as Rocky Mountain spotted fever.

Modified measles is seen in children with residual maternal antibody or in those who received gamma globulins earlier in the incubation period. In this case, the incubation period is prolonged, the prodromal period is almost missing, and the rash is discrete. The lesions are not confluent. So-called atypical measles has been described in children previously immunized with killed measles virus vaccine. Clinical characteristics include fever, prostration, myalgia, edema of the extremities, and an atypical rash that is located primarily on the hands and feet. Frequently, vesicles and petechial lesions occur. Interstitial pneumonia is also common with atypical measles. The differential diagnosis includes Rocky Mountain spotted fever and even meningococcemia.

A doubtful clinical diagnosis can be confirmed by specific laboratory tests. The isolation of the virus from nasal secretions during the febrile phase or from the urine up to 4 days after the rash appears is simple, but it is not currently practical. Immunofluorescent microscopic examination permits a rapid diagnosis when the disease is suspected. The most commonly used tests, however, are the hemagglutination inhibition or the complement fixation antibody tests. Hemagglutination inhibition antibody appears between the first and third days following the rash and generally lasts for life, even in the absence of a new contact. Complement fixation antibody appears towards the tenth day after the eruption and persists for 5 to 10 years. The absence of both these types of antibodies indicates the susceptibility of the individual to the disease.

Antibody surveys are indicated in determining the acquisition rate of measles antibody in the population and in evaluating the usefulness of vaccination as a function of the degree of immunity, or lack of it, detected.

TREATMENT

Treatment is entirely symptomatic. One must take the following isolation precautions: in a hospital environment, from as soon as one suspects the disease to the fifth day of the rash; in a school setting, for a duration that varies according to local public health regulations. After contact with a patient with measles, 2 types of prevention can be prescribed: (1) intramuscular injection of standard gamma globulin during the 6 days following the contact (0.25 ml/kg); and (2) subcutaneous injection of further attenuated vaccine, in the absence of contraindications, during the 3 days following the contact. This second type of prevention is definitely more effective.

> **Objective 27–4. Define the circumstances that worsen the prognosis in measles.**

Factors related to the individual's past, his social group, or his environment can confer a special seriousness on this disease. First of all is the patient's age. In industrialized countries, the mortality rate is lowest between 5 and 9 years of age (0.7/1000), is higher under 1 year of age (1.1/1000), and is highest over 15 years of age. Next is the immune state of the individual. All situations that depress the level of immunity, especially cellular immunity, increase the risk, whether it be immunosuppressant drug therapy or a malignant disorder such as leukemia or lymphoma. The concern here is notably with a giant cell interstitial pneumonia due to the measles virus that may be fatal to infants and immunosuppressed patients even before the classic signs of rash appear. As for measles in patients with chronic neurologic or cardiorespiratory disease, the prognosis is equally doubtful. In industrial countries, such conditions can be responsible for 50% of the measles mortality rate.

Malnutrition, poor hygiene, and overcrowding are equally important considerations. At the beginning of the century in Glasgow, as in Paris, the mortality rate was 30 times higher than it is today. In tropical countries, the mortality rate can vary from 5 to 12% in the weeks following the illness.

The absence of regular or frequent contact of the population with the virus apparently also makes a difference. In areas where the disease is epidemic, as in Western countries, the infection is asymptomatic in 10 to 15% of cases, and the mortality rate is around 1/10,000 in Europe and North America. On the other hand, without periodic epidemic contact, in isolated populations such as the Eskimos and the inhabitants of seldom visited islands, measles was routinely a symptomatic disease before the introduction of immunization programs, and the mortality rate was said to be nearly 50%.

> **Objective 27–5. Demonstrate the importance of measles vaccination.**

Because so many people in Western countries have had measles, most often without any problem, the disease is considered benign. In reality, the disease overwhelms the child who has it and is followed by a high number of complications that may result in death. In 1979, deaths from measles in the third world were estimated at 900,000.

COMPLICATIONS OF MEASLES

The complications can be due to the measles virus itself or to bacterial superinfections; no easy way of separating them exists. The frequencies mentioned in the following section are appropriate for industrialized countries.

Bronchopneumonias. These illnesses, which complicate 3 to 5% of cases of measles, may be interstitial pneumonias beginning during the early invasive phase. The clinical manifestations range from simple, asymptomatic radiologic changes in more than 20% of the total of measles cases to more striking presentations with a rapid demise. The bacterial infections occur after the third day of the rash, chiefly in children under 18 months of age. In this instance, the bronchopneumonia is of an alveolar type. The prognosis is guarded, above all when it is a staphylococcal superinfection with the hazard of sudden pyopneumothorax. Other organisms often involved include *Haemophilus influenza* and *Streptococcus pneumoniae.*

Otitis Media. This disorder complicates 3 to 5% of cases. As with bronchopneumonia, one can distinguish between early infections that are properly viral and late infections that are bacterial.

Tracheolaryngitis. Among the respiratory complications of measles, severe tracheolaryngitis occurs most rarely. It produces a laryngeal subglottal obstruction in the small infants and allows dramatic bacterial superinfections in malnourished children.

Neurologic Complications. These are feared most. Febrile convulsions affect 7% of patients, chiefly the youngest children. Acute measles encephalitis complicates about 1 case in a thousand and results in death (15%), significant neurologic deficiencies including mental retardation and deafness (25%), or full recovery (60%). Subacute sclerosis panencephalitis, considered to be a central nervous system infection with a slow viral agent related antigenically to measles virus is even more rare, on the order of 5.2 to 9.7 per million cases (see Chap. 29).

Hemorrhages. Among the minor complications that can be cited in arguing for vaccination are oral, nasal, and gastrointestinal hemorrhages, which must be distinguished from the common purpuric appearance of the measles rash. A marked thrombocytopenia is seen in these hemorrhages, whereas the platelet count remains normal in uncomplicated measles.

The mortality rate associated with the complications, their sequelae, the morbidity, and the public cost have led scientists to search for a vaccine.

MEASLES VACCINE

At first, an inactivated vaccine was prepared, but because of its mediocre effectiveness, it was abandoned in 1972. Current materials are live vaccines attenuated by passage of the measles virus through avian tissue culture. The first strain, called Edmondston B, was highly reactive; vaccination produced attenuated measles in 10 to 20% of vaccinated subjects and required the simultaneous administration of gamma globulin, which led in turn to a loss of immunogenic potency. Further attenuated vaccines, the Schwartz type and its derivatives, were then developed. These vaccines are much less likely to produce reactions, and they give rise to acceptable levels of immunity, if the recommended conditions of preservation and administration are followed. A seroconversion indeed occurs in at least 95% of susceptible individuals over 15 months of age who are properly vaccinated. The levels of hemagglutination inhibition measles antibody following both natural infection and vaccination are comparable for at least 14 years. The percentage of individuals possessing detectable circulating antibody capable of protecting them 12 years after the vaccination varies from 62% to 91%. In addition, anamnestic responses are observed in vaccinated individuals who have become seronegative, when they come into contact with the virus again.

Epidemiologic Changes Associated with Measles Vaccine. Since 1963, more than 100 million doses of attenuated measles vaccine have been given in the United States and Canada. The number of reported cases and, similarly, the number of cases of encephalitis have been reduced by 90%. A decrease in the vaccinations in 1970 was balanced by an increased number of cases of measles and encephalitis in the months that followed. Immunity induced after vaccination does not seem to depend on the persistence of wild virus in the community, but this persistence does ensure high titers of measles antibody. Epidemics of measles in the United States today are attributable to the following:

1. An insufficient level of coverage; 35% of children between 1 and 4 years of age are not immunized.
2. Vaccination too early; seroconversion is only 85% when the vaccine is given before 12 months of age, probably because of the persistence of maternal antibody.
3. Attenuation of vaccine infective potency because of recent or simultaneous administration of gamma globulin.
4. Loss of infectious potency in the course of preservation or reconstitution of the vaccine.
5. Occasional disappearance of immunity after vaccination.

Side Effects. The side effects of vaccination are limited, as a general rule, to a few, minor febrile reactions, rarely accompanied by a rash, 5 to 12 days after vaccination. Some neurologic postvaccinal complications have been described. In the immediate period, acute encephalitis occurs in 1 case in a million, an incidence that is 1000 times less frequent than after natural measles. The potential risk of subacute sclerosing panencephalitis, which may occur in the 3.5 years following vaccination, is 0.48 per million. Thus, the advantages of vaccination largely outweigh the disadvantages.

Indications. We now have reason to hope that measles can be eradicated. Cheaper, more efficient, and more heat-stable vaccines are now available. The measles virus seems antigenically stable; no animal reservoir is known, nor does a chronic carrier state exist in man. Indications for systematic immunization are as follows:

1. Age of 15 months for the general population of industrialized countries.
2. Age of 6 to 12 months for the population of underdeveloped countries or for economically disadvantaged groups in industrialized countries. A booster injection 18 months later is absolutely necessary.

Vaccination is particularly indicated for institutionalized children and for those with mucoviscidosis, tuberculosis, cardiac disease, or chronic pulmonary disease. Contraindications include pregnancy, altered immune status (immune disease, corticosteroid therapy, irradiation, and therapy with alkylating agents or antimetabolites), and egg or chicken allergy (the source of the tissue culture for the virus). Active and untreated tuberculosis or a fever are temporary contraindications for vaccination. The vaccine is available alone or in combination with rubella or with rubella and mumps vaccines.

Objective 27–6. Distinguish, in a patient with a maculopapular rash, rubella from roseola (exanthema subitum) and from fifth disease (erythema infectiosum).

These three "minor" illnesses are easily distinguished from one another once they have taken on their characteristic clinical appearance. Because many patients with rubella have atypical features, however, the clinical diagnosis is often aleatory. These difficulties are important in view of the risks of fetal malformation if the disease occurs during the first 3 months of pregnancy (see Objective 24–2).

RUBELLA

Rubella is due to an RNA virus classified in the group of arboviruses, more precisely the togaviruses. In contrast to the other members of this group, rubella virus is not transmitted by arthropod vectors. Antigenically, the virus is unique, and only one serotype is known. It is particularly susceptible to variations of temperature, pH, and various chemical agents. Rubella has a worldwide distribution and appears principally in the late winter and spring. Occasionally, epidemic peaks are observed, as in the United States in 1935 and 1964. Rubella mainly affects children between the ages of 5 and 9, who are the reservoir of the infection. Far more frequently than either measles or varicella, however, rubella does strike adolescents and young adults.

The diagnosis depends, first of all, on a history of contact with a patient with rubella, usually 18 days before the rash appears. Because 20 to 50% of rubella infections occur without an evident rash, a history of contact is often inaccurate.

As for the clinical picture in the child, the prodrome is limited to a low-grade fever and to occipital, retroauricular and coracoid adenopathy 7 to 9 days after contact with the virus. The eruption follows, starting on the face and extending rapidly toward the neck, the trunk, the arms, and the legs. On the second day, it usually disappears from the face, and by the third day, it begins to fade elsewhere. The rash, which is discrete, maculopapular, and rose-colored, may be confluent on the trunk on the second day; it is brought out by heat, especially hot baths.

In children over 10 years, the prodrome is more marked; fever is higher, adenopathy can be generalized, painful, or tender, petechiae are seen on the soft palate, and a mild coryza and conjunctivitis can be observed. The maculopapular rash starts on the face, but is more evident on the trunk, where it has a morbilliform appearance (Plate 10B). The infection is often associated with joint complaints, in the form of arthralgias or even arthritis of the small and medium joints, chiefly in young women, in whom this symptom is observed in 15 to 30% of symptomatic patients with rubella. These arthralgias begin at the time of regression of the rash and persist for 1 to 2 weeks. On the whole, the disease is benign. It can be complicated, however, by encephalitis, with a frequency approximating 1 in 6000 cases.

Thrombocytopenia with increased capillary fragility may occur, but it remains mostly a biologic disease manifestation without clinical expression. When hemorrhages are observed, they begin abruptly 3 to 4 days after the start of the rash. These hemorrhages are generally localized on the skin and mucosa, but they may involve the gastrointestinal tract, the kidneys, and the central nervous system. The thrombocytopenia generally subsides in 1 to 2 weeks, but it may persist for several months. The mechanism appears complex; antiplatelet agglutinins are present, but platelet production is also depressed. The number of megakaryocytes in the bone marrow is normal or increased.

The transmission of this contagious virus can take place from an affected patient through the nasopharyngeal secretions, the urine, or the stools. The patient is infectious during the week preceding the rash and for at least 4 days after its appearance. In the absence of systematic vaccination, 10 to 25% of adolescents and young adults are susceptible either to symptomatic or asymptomatic rubella infection.

The laboratory diagnosis of rubella provides a degree of certainty that is important both for epidemiologic planning and for the individual woman. The isolation of the virus from nasal or pharyngeal secretions or from urine is not currently practical. One looks chiefly for the antibody, either the hemagglutination inhibition, which appears 3 to 5 days after the rash and lasts for life, or the complement fixation, which appears the tenth day after the rash and lasts 5 to 10 years). IgM-specific antibody appears with the rash and generally disappears rapidly, in several weeks to several months. These changes in antibody titer allow us, to a certain degree, to date the infection (see Objective 24–2 for discussion of rubella during pregnancy).

No specific treatment exists for rubella. Isolation is considered useless, partly because the infectivity starts 7 days before the rash and partly because of the frequency of asymptomatic but infectious forms of the illness.

ROSEOLA INFANTUM (EXANTHEMA SUBITUM)

A child under 3 years of age has a high fever, either level or hectic, of 3 to 4 days' duration, without signs of toxicity. Spontaneous defervescence is followed by a maculopapular rash similar to that of rubella. The rash appears on the trunk, and sometimes remains limited to it; otherwise, it spreads to the face and limbs. This rash lasts for 1 or 2 days, but it occasionally lasts only several hours. It can be accompanied by exudative pharyngitis, cervical and occipital adenopathy, and in the young infant, bulging of the fontanelle. The incubation period is about 10 days. This presumably viral infection is seen mainly in the spring and is frequently associated with febrile convulsions. A marked leukopenia (2000 cells/mm^3 or less) with a relative lymphocytosis observed during the febrile phase can become normal with the appearance of the exanthem. No prophylactic measures are yet known. Treatment is entirely symptomatic.

FIFTH DISEASE (ERYTHEMA INFECTIOSUM)

The patient's medical history often provides evidence of circumscribed family or school outbreaks. The clinical picture develops in 3 phases. During the first 3 days, erythema localizes to the face and becomes intense at the base of the nose and on the cheeks, with a perioral palor that gives the patient a "slapped cheek" appearance. From the third to the fifth day, the macules and papules extend from the original area to the extensor surfaces of the distal portion of the limbs. Later, they affect the flexor surface, the trunk, and the buttocks and take on a reticulated, urticarial, or marginated appearance with involvement of palmar and plantar surfaces that permits the distinction from measles, erythema multiforme, and scarlet fever. During the second or third week, the rash regresses, but it may reappear following skin irritation or heating, either mechanically or by radiation. The rash may be accompanied by myalgias and arthralgias.

The causative agent of this disorder is unknown. Prophylactic measures are not yet defined, and treatment is symptomatic.

> **Objective 27–7. Define the indications for rubella immunization.**

The available vaccines consist of strain of rubella virus attenuated by multiple passages in duck embryo cell lines, rabbit kidney cells or human diploid cells. The first two types are given by subcutaneous injections; the last one, by nasal instillation.

SUBCUTANEOUS INJECTION

The attenuated vaccines, administered by injection, are better known because they have been used for a longer time. The RA27/3 strain is the most extensively used and is the only one marketed in many countries because it provides better protection than previous vaccines (HPV 77 and Cendehill). Following immunization, a transitory viremia occurs; indeed, the vaccine should not be given to a possibly pregnant woman. Multiplication of the virus in the pharynx may also be observed for 1 or 2 weeks, without symptoms and apparently without possibility of transmission, even to close contacts. When one compares the levels of antibody, the peak is clearly higher after natural infection than after vaccination, but because the fall of antibodies is more pronounced after the natural disease, the 2 modes give comparable results in 7 years. About 8% of vaccinated individuals lack antibodies 5 years later. Immunization before the age of 12 months does not ensure a satisfactory level of seroconversion.

Reinfections after vaccination remain clinically inapparent, with no viremia and only minimal, transient pharyngeal virus shedding, but with a booster effect on rubella antibody levels.

The side effects of vaccination are of two different types. The teratogenic effect of the vaccine virus is probable, although still poorly known. Immunization of women of childbearing potential cannot be performed without assurance that they are not pregnant and will not conceive during the next 3 months. In adolescents and young adults, chiefly girls and women, some adenopathies are often observed during the week following vaccination. Athralgias, arthritis, and the presence of virus in the joint fluid complicate 2 to 18% of immunizations 2 to 4 weeks afterward, especially in women. It is possible to combine this vaccine with the attenuated vaccines for mumps and measles.

NASAL INSTILLATION

Attenuated vaccine administered by nasal instillation is more recent and, on the whole, better accepted. Immunization induces the production of specific IgA nasal secretory antibody, which gives adequate local protection against reinfection by the wild virus. The circulating antibodies elicited are comparable to those observed after natural infection in 97% of susceptible subjects, and it seems that they persist for at least 4 years. A possible drawback is that interhuman transmissibility cannot be excluded. Vaccination by nasal instillation carries great expectations, but deserves more investigations.

INDICATIONS FOR IMMUNIZATION

Indications for immunization by injection follow 2 different strategies. First, the so-called American program consists of mass vaccination of children of both sexes from 1 to 12 years and elective vaccination of women of child-bearing age presumed to be at professional or familial risk. Second, the so-called English program aims at systematically immunizing young girls 10 to 12 years old and selectively immunizing women of child-bearing age.

The American program led to a marked decrease in the incidence of rubella in the United States. The epidemic fluctuations of the disease, tabulated since 1940, would have indicated a probable recrudescence of rubella by the mid-1970s; however, it never occurred. More important, the number of reported cases of congenital rubella syndrome also declined. On the other hand, the incidence of congenital rubella has not yet changed in the United Kingdom. The British program would have required at least 90% of the girls to be immunized for curbing the statistics; actually, only 70% of them were vaccinated. After application of both programs for several years, rubella is still present. Because 10 to 15% of women with childbearing potential remain seronegative and unprotected, the physician should realize that congenital rubella remains a real threat.

> **Objective 27–8.** Tie together evidence of scarlet fever in a patient with a generalized maculopapular rash of recent origin.

The diagnosis of scarlet fever is often difficult because of the frequency of scarlatiniform rashes due to drug reactions, especially when a medication such as penicillin or ampicillin has been prescribed for a pharyngitis. Further, for reasons not yet understood, scarlet fever has been infrequent and mild in industrialized countries during the past 30 years. Finally, no laboratory tests can confirm the diagnosis with exactitude. In practical terms, when a patient has a generalized maculopapular eruption, one should investigate, both in the medical history and in the physical examination, those items that suggest scarlet fever. One must not attach much importance to a previous episode to exclude the diagnosis because the same individual can be affected several times in his life. The patient could also have had previous scarlatiniform eruptions of another origin that were mislabeled scarlet fever. Incidentally, immunity to scarlet fever is complex.

The disease is caused by group A streptococci, which give rise to a type-specific immunity (see Objective 3–2). These streptococci, however, secrete an erythrogenic toxin of which three distinct antigenic types are known. Secretion of this toxin depends on the infection of the streptococcus by a temperate bacteriophage that carries the necessary genetic information. The mechanism of toxin production is thus analogous to that of diphtheria toxin. The toxin induces the formation of antitoxin antibodies that protect the individual against future exposure to that toxin type.

A history of contact is found in only half the patients with scarlet fever because of the high incidence of asymptomatic and attenuated forms of the illness.

CLINICAL FEATURES

The duration of the invasive period is less than 48 hours. Typically, scarlet fever starts abruptly with a high fever, an extremely rapid pulse, vomiting, abdominal pains, and arthralgias.

The erythema is maculopapular, with a granular appearance and without an interval of normal skin, at least in the areas affected. It begins at the base of the neck and the upper parts of the limbs and becomes generalized in 1 or 2 days. The rash predominates on the trunk (Plate 10D), on the pelvis (Plate 11A), in the skin folds, but it is not found in the area around the mouth or on the palms or soles. It is associated with an enanthema. The changes on the tongue are well known. Although initially it is thick and coated, the tongue (Plate 10C) loses its coating in 2 to 4 days from the tip to base and then takes on a desquamated appearance, its papules uncovered, to resemble a strawberry or raspberry. Pharyngitis, theoretically of the streptococcal type, with noticeable dysphagia, tonsillar exudate, edema of the soft palate, and occasionally palatal petechiaes and submaxillary adenopathy, accompanies the erythema.

One may observe, at about the tenth day of illness, a cutaneous desquamation that is sometimes impressive on the patient's extremities (Plate 11B).

DIFFERENTIAL DIAGNOSIS

Unfortunately, the type of rash previously described is not restricted to scarlet fever; some drug eruptions mimic it perfectly. The oral and pharyngeal findings are the most reliable signs of scarlet fever, although similar features have been described in Kawasaki's syndrome (Plates 11C and D and 12A) (see also the boxed text at the end of this chapter). Toxic shock syndrome may also be part of the differential diagnosis in the most severe cases (see Objective 27–1).

Of course, group A streptococci are often recovered from the throat, but that finding does not permit a definitive diagnosis because many carriers are asymptomatic; besides, as stated before, some medications taken to treat pharyngitis can be responsible for the rash. The appearance of antistreptococcal antibody of the streptolysin type is variable.

TREATMENT

When scarlet fever is diagnosed or even only strongly suspected, one should treat it. Antibiotic therapy reduces the severity and duration of symptoms and it diminishes the suppurative complications, such as adenitis and otitis, and the risk of rheumatic fever; however, it does not seem to decrease the risk of developing poststreptococcal glomerulonephritis.

This 10-day course of treatment does not differ from that for ordinary streptococcal pharyngitis (see Chap. 3). It is also important to treat contacts who are possible carriers of this group A streptococcus when they have close familial contact, when they have a personal or familial history of rheumatic fever, or when their conditions of work create particular risks for themselves or for others. Such occupations include handling food and caring for children. Treatment is the same as for symptomatic infections.

> **Objective 27-9. Diagnose a vesicular rash as varicella.**

Varicella or chickenpox is a contagious disease most commonly seen in children. The causative virus belongs to the family Herpesviridae (see Chap. 3). Varicella represents a primary infection, whereas herpes zoster is a manifestation of the same virus in a patient already immunized. The diagnosis of varicella rests primarily on historical evidence. The contact occurs about 2 weeks before the illness, yet this evidence may be missing because mild forms of varicella may go unrecognized. The infection is easily transmitted, even indirectly, often in an erratic fashion and sometimes from a zoster. In fact, varicella is one of the most contagious illnesses. Because immunity is stable, the physician should always ask the patient about a previous episode.

CLINICAL FEATURES

Clinically, the prodrome often passes unnoticed, mainly in children. The typical lesion is first macular; then, in about 8 hours, it becomes vesicular (Plate 12B and C). A crust forms 24 to 48 hours later, and the lesion heals in 5 to 20 days. Lesions are scattered predominantly on the trunk, the face, and the scalp. They reach the mucosa, in particular, that of the mouth and the soft palate. In 2 to 7 days, 2 or more often 3 crops of vesicles follow each other so that, in the same anatomic region, lesions are found at different stages of development. The accompanying signs are moderate and include fever and some adenopathy for the first 3 to 4 days.

DIFFERENTIAL DIAGNOSIS

The differential diagnosis includes the following vesicular rashes: generalized herpes, which is rare (Plates 12D and 13A) smallpox, the last case of which was reported in 1977, vaccinia, in a patient with a history of vaccination of the individual or a contact, monkeypox, Kaposi's varicelliform eruption due to herpes or vaccinia, rickettsialpox, some forms of secondary syphilis, drug rashes, erythema multiforme, impetigo, and hand-foot-mouth syndrome.

To aid in the diagnosis, some laboratory tests can be used. Cytologic examination of the specific lesion demonstrates multinucleated giant cells on the floor of the vesicles and allows the detection of eosinophilic intranuclear inclusions in some cells. With the electron microscope, the type of herpes virus in the vesicular liquid can be identified. Isolation of the virus in tissue culture is possible but is uncommon. Serodiagnosis, to show a high titer or a rise in complement fixating or neutralizing antibody, is still the usual method.

TREATMENT AND COMPLICATIONS

Treatment is symptomatic, but because of the extreme contagiousness and grave risk of the disease in the immunosuppressed patient, isolation is recommended until the patient reaches the stage of scab formation for all lesions, a stage that takes up to 10 days. The course of varicella is generally favorable, except in patients at particular risk (see Objective 27-7). In exceptional circumstances, the disease can assume a hemorrhagic form that can be fatal, again, in those at particular risk. This form of varicella is characterized by a high fever, general debilitation, a generalized hemorrhagic rash manifested by hemorrhages within the vesicles and petechiae and ecchymotic plaques on the skin.

Another rare complication is encephalitis, which occurs around the eighth day after the rash and manifests as an acute illness with paralysis of the cranial nerves and limbs and cerebellar involvement; increased levels of protein and numbers of cells, mainly lymphocytes, are found in the cerebrospinal fluid. The prognosis is guarded; the mortality rate reaches 5 to 20%, and 15% of the survivors have psychomotor sequelae. This rare but serious complication must be distinguished from isolated cerebellar involvement, which carries a better prognosis and is characterized by a self-limited syndrome of acute ataxia. It is sometimes the only manifestation of the disease, if no vesicles indicate the diagnosis. Other exceptional complications are transverse myelitis peripheral neuritis, and optic neuritis, as well as nephritis, hepatitis, and arthritis.

> **Objective 27–10. Identify those at particular risk of having a severe varicella syndrome and take appropriate action.**

Varicella in a normal child generally has an uncomplicated course. On the other hand, the age of the patient and certain underlying conditions favor the development of serious, life-threatening forms. For example, adults, in contrast to children, may be at higher risk of varicella pneumonia. The beginning of the illness is marked by the sudden appearance of severe dyspnea and cyanosis. Hemoptysis is often seen. The chest roentgenogram shows a striking, atypical pneumonia, widespread and intense, consisting of nodular infiltrates that may become confluent. Despite modern techniques of pulmonary care, the prognosis is poor, and the mortality rate may reach 30% within the first 24 to 48 hours in severe forms.

Varicella acquired at the start of pregnancy can lead to fetal malformation (see Tables 24–1 and 24–2 and Objective 24–2). The disease can also affect the newborn when the mother develops the disease toward the end of pregnancy. If the rash appears on the woman 5 to 17 days before delivery, the infant may have varicella at birth or during the first 5 days of life; the prognosis is good. If the rash appears on the woman 5 days or less before delivery, the infant develops the disease later, during the second week of life. Then, varicella takes a serious form, with about a 25% mortality rate and visceral and pulmonary involvement.

Finally, another group at high risk consists of those persons with immunologic deficits, mainly cellular (see Chap. 33). Among the diseases most often responsible are leukemia and Hodgkin's disease, grades 3 and 4. Children undergoing antineoplastic or corticosteroid therapy are at higher risk of developing the severe forms of varicella. Such immunosuppressed patients can, clearly, have a normal disease course; however, they are at higher risk than other individuals of developing encephalomyelitis and other complications of varicella. In these patients, varicella may take a hemorrhagic form; on the second or third day of the rash, the patient's general condition suddenly deteriorates. Epistaxis, melena, hematuria, hemorrhagic gangrene in the extremities, hemorrhages, intravesicular or in normal skin, present a striking picture that may be associated with a disseminated intravascular coagulation syndrome. Other forms are simply an aggravation of the ordinary clinical picture with a particularly intense rash and clinical signs that are much more severe than usual (Plate 12C). This form of varicella includes disseminated visceral involvement; here, too, the prognosis is guarded.

PREVENTIVE MEASURES

The first action is mainly preventive. As soon as a case of varicella or zoster is diagnosed, one should search through the patient's possible contacts for individuals at high risk of a severe form of the disease in order to prevent their exposure, at least until the fourteenth day of the rash. One must also think of those who have not had varicella but who have been in contact with the patient and, consequently, could serve as intermediary carriers; this would be important between the seventh and the twenty-first day after contact. Once varicella is diagnosed in a hospital department of pediatrics, the hospitalization of children with neoplastic disease or receiving corticosteroid therapy should be avoided.

When a susceptible individual at risk has been in contact with a patient with varicella or zoster, passive immunization by means of specific immunoglobulin (varicella zoster immune globulin or VZIG) can be used to prevent or attenuate the illness. Standard immunoglobulin is of debatable efficacy. VZIG modifies the severity of the disease. Clinical studies have shown that, with this passive immunization of immunodepressed children, the observed frequencies of death (1%), pneumonia (6%), and widespread pox (27%) were less than 25% of those observed when hyperimmune globulin was not administered. Children who may be considered for VZIG include exposed patients with leukemia, lymphoma, immune deficiency, those receiving immunosuppressive therapy, and newborn infants whose mothers develop varicella 4 days before to 2 days after delivery. VZIG is more likely to be effective if given within 72 hours after exposure to varicella; after 96 hours, its value is uncertain. The duration of protection with VZIG is not well known.

OTHER MEASURES

If varicella does develop in an immunodepressed host receiving corticosteroid therapy, treatment should be maintained at 20 to 25 mg cortisone acetate/day. Besides nonspecific measures, various experimental approaches have been tried to counteract the disease. These measures include transfusion of HLA-compatible lymphocytes from donors who are immune to varicella and chemotherapy with vidarabine or acyclovir. It is too early to know the benefits or disadvantages of these regimens. The best long-term prevention is vaccination with live attenuated virus vaccine, which is in the process of development.

> **Objective 27–11. Distinguish a zoster from a herpes lesion in the case of a localized vesicular rash.**

Zoster and relapsing herpes infections have several points in common. First, both are caused by viruses belonging to the herpes group. Pathophysiologically, both diseases begin with a primary infection. In the case of zoster, this infection is a generalized varicella or chickenpox. In the case of herpes, the primary infection may be asymptomatic in 70 to 90% of the population. When a primary herpetic infection is symptomatic, it produces a generalized illness with fever, lasting several days, and a rash that depends on the type of virus. Herpes simplex virus 1 (HSV-1) is generally responsible for a gingivostomatitis, whereas herpes simplex virus 2 (HSV-2) causes a genital infection (see Chap. 22). Rarely, the primary infection occurs as a congenital infection, usually with HSV-2, or it appears as an encephalitis (usually HSV-1) or aseptic meningitis (HSV-2).

Following the primary infection, the virus of varicella-zoster or that of herpes simplex can persist for years or decades within the host. We know little of the inner mechanisms that permit this long latency, but the virus resides within cells, probably within nerve ganglia. In the case of zoster, it is believed that the virus remains latent within the posterior root ganglia of the spinal cord or in equivalent locations in the cranial nerves. In the case of herpes simplex, the virus is believed to remain latent within the geniculate ganglia (HSV-1) or the sacral plexic ganglia (HSV-2). Indeed, both infections express themselves in the form of localized vesicular eruptions. Vesicles, often grouped in small clusters, "flower" on an erythematous and painful base, which appears 24 to 48 hours previously. In the most characteristic case, the distinction between the 2 viruses is easy enough.

The patient's medical history is often the determining element because zoster generally occurs only once in a lifetime, whereas herpes, alas, relapses numerous times, under diverse circumstances such as menstruation, exposure to the sun, or fever.

A zoster usually (Plate 13B and C) has a precise distribution generally following the territory of a thoracic root or a trigeminal nerve or one of its branches (ophthalmic zoster). In contrast, the spread of herpes is much more limited, and although it is observed in the eye, the preferred sites are the upper lip or the periphery of the nostrils in the case of HSV-1 and the glans penis or the vulva for

HSV-2. Unfortunately, these topographic characteristics are not absolute.

Neither the histologic appearance nor the morphologic features of the virus under electron microscopy can settle the issue, but viral culture and serologic diagnosis do permit the distinction.

> **Objective 27–12. Gather the evidence of hand-foot-mouth disease in a patient with a vesicular rash.**

This infection, which is due to coxsackievirus A types 5, 10, or 16, occurs in children and sometimes in adults in small epidemics (Plates 13D, and 14A and B). The infection is frequently without rash and is asymptomatic. It can be seen, obviously, in patients who have previously had varicella.

Twenty-four to 48 hours after the start of the prodrome, which is characterized by sudden fever and gastrointestinal upset, the lesions appear and are limited to the buccal surface, buttocks, hands, and feet. These signs distinguish this disease from varicella. In the mouth, 1 to 10 lesions about 1 cm in size appear in the form of reddish macules or vesicles that may ulcerate. These lesions occur primarily on the lingual and buccal mucosa (distinguishing it from measles and herpangina) and do not extend to the lips (distinguishing it from herpes). The cutaneous lesions resemble the buccal ones, but are larger and consist of bullae; they are localized on the lateral surfaces of the fingers, toes, palms, and soles. Clinical variants are seen, such as a maculopapular rash on the buttocks that evolves into vesicles in a couple of hours, or even the absence of lesions on the lower limbs in infants of under 3 years of age, or dissociated forms with buccal lesions but without cutaneous ones and vice versa. Other clinical features may include malaise, anorexia, fever, submandibular or cervical adenitis, coryza, cough, diarrhea, nausea, and vomiting.

The differential diagnosis must include papuloerosive acrodermatitis of Gianotti and Crosti (due to hepatitis B virus), candidiasis, the cutaneous lesions of gonococcemia, and above all, secondary syphilis.

The virus can be isolated from saliva, stools, or cutaneous lesions. No routine di-

---

KAWASAKI'S SYNDROME

Kawasaki's syndrome (or mucocutaneous lymph node syndrome) was first described in Japan in 1967 and has been recognized worldwide. Eighty percent of patients are under 4 years of age, and few cases are seen in patients older than 10 years of age. The clinical course includes an acute febrile phase lasting from 7 to 14 days, a subacute phase that leads approximately to the twenty-fifth day, and a convalescent phase (high sedimentation rate) usually terminating 6 to 8 weeks after the onset of the illness.

The diagnosis rests upon clinical features, and 6 criteria have been described: (1) a high fever persisting for more than 5 days; (2) conjunctival injection; (3) changes in the mouth, including erythema and fissuring of the lips, diffuse erythema of the oropharynx, and a "strawberry" appearance of the tongue; (4) distinctive changes in the hands and feet, such as indurative edema, erythematous palms and soles, desquamation starting 2 to 3 weeks from the onset of illness (Plate 12A), and deep transverse grooves across the fingernails; (5) an erythematous rash (Plate 11C and D); and (6) enlarged lymph node masses more than 1.5 cm in diameter. To make the diagnosis, the child should meet 5 of the 6 criteria. Other systems may also be involved, as follows: urethritis with pyuria (70%); arthritis (40%); irritability (nearly 100%); aseptic meningitis (25%); diarrhea (25%); abdominal pain (25%); cardiac disease (20%), including congestive heart failure, pericardial effusion, mitral insufficiency, arrhythmias, and coronary thrombosis; obstructive jaundice; and hydrops of gallbladder (unusual).

Laboratory abnormalities remain nonspecific. The white blood cell count is over 20,000 in half the patients, with a predominance of polymorphonuclear leukocytes, a high sedimentation rate, and thrombocytosis. The disease is generally self-limited, with the exception of a fatal termination in 1.7% of the identified cases, mainly from heart disease. The cause is unknown, and no specific treatment is available. Because the syndrome has an inflammatory vasculitis as its major pathologic change, anti-inflammatory agents, especially aspirin, have been proposed as supportive therapy. A dose of 80 to 100 mg/kg/day shortens the mean duration of the fever. Once the patient's temperature is normal, a lower dose of aspirin (10 mg/kg/day) may prevent coronary thrombosis during the period of highest risk of mortality, from day 14 to day 35.

agnostic serologic test exists, nor are there specific recommendations for prevention, treatment, or isolation.

SUGGESTED READINGS

General

Cherry, J.D.: Viral exanthems. DM, 28:6, 1982.
Feigin, R.D., and Cherry, J.D. (eds.): Textbook of Pediatric Infectious Diseases. Philadelphia, W.B. Saunders, 1981.

Measles

Crawford, G.E., and Gremillion, D.H.: Epidemic measles and rubella in air force recruits: impact of immunization. J. Infect. Dis., 144:403, 1981.
Hall, W.J., and Breese Hall, C.: Atypical measles in adolescents: evaluation of clinical and pulmonary function. Ann. Intern. Med., 90:882, 1979.
Hinman, A.R., et al.: Progress in measles elimination. JAMA, 247:1592, 1982.
Hopkins, D.R., Hinman, A.R., Koplan, J.C., and Lane, J.M.: The case for global measles eradication. Lancet, 1:1396, 1982.
Martin, D.B., Weiner, L.B., Nieburg, P.I., and Blair, D.C.: Atypical measles in adolescents and young adults. Ann. Intern. Med., 90:877, 1979.
Yeager, A.S., Davis, J.H., Ross, L.A., and Harvey, B.: Measles immunization: successes and failures. JAMA, 237:347, 1977.
Zahradnik, J.M., Cherry, J.D., and Rachelefsky, G.: Atypical measles acquired abroad: foreign travel and pseudoexotic disease. JAMA, 241:1711, 1979.

Rubella

Cockburn, W.C.: World aspects of the epidemiology of rubella. Am. J. Dis. Child., 118:112, 1969.
Lamprecht, C., et al.: An outbreak of congenital rubella in Chicago. JAMA, 247:1129, 1982.
Orenstein, W.A., and Greaves, W.L.: Congenital rubella syndrome: a continuing problem. JAMA, 247:1174, 1982.
Preblud, S.R., et al.: Rubella vaccination in the United States: a ten-year review. Epidemiol. Rev., 2:171, 1980.
Schoenbaum, S.C., Hyde, J.N., Barthoshesky, L., and Crampton, K.: Benefit cost analysis of rubella vaccination policy. N. Engl. J. Med., 294:306, 1976.
Zealley, H., and Edmond, E.: Rubella screening and immunization of school girls: results six to seven years after vaccination. Br. Med. J., 284:382, 1982.

Varicella-Zoster

Anonymous: Varicella-zoster immune globulin. Med. Lett. Drugs Ther., 24:51, 1982.
Bean, B., Braun, C., and Balfour, H.H.: Acyclovir therapy for acute herpes zoster. Lancet, 2:118, 1982.
Evans, E.B., Pollock, T.M., Cradock-Watson, J.E., and Ridehalgh, M.K.S.: Human antichickenpox immunoglobulin in the prevention of chickenpox. Lancet, 1:354, 1980.
Gershon, A.A., Steinberg, S., and Brunell, P.A.: Zoster immune globulin: a further assessment. N. Engl. J. Med., 290:243, 1974.
Mazur, M.H., and Dolin, R.: Herpes zoster at the NIH: a 20-year experience. Am. J. Med., 65:738, 1978.
Oxman, M.N.: Varicella. Herpes zoster. In Medical Microbiology and Infectious Diseases. Edited by A.I. Braude. Philadelphia, W.B. Saunders, 1981.

Kawasaki Syndrome

Bell, D.M., et al.: Kawasaki syndrome: description of two outbreaks in the United States. N. Engl. J. Med., 304:1568, 1981.
Melish, M.E.: Kawasaki syndrome: the mucocutaneous lymph node syndrome. Annu. Rev. Med., 33:569, 1982.

Toxic Shock Syndrome

Anonymous: Elimination of indigenous measles: United States. Morbid. Mortal. Weekly Rep., 31:517, 1981.
Toxic Shock Syndrome (special issue). Ann. Intern. Med., 96:831, 1982.

CHAPTER 28

Bone and Joint Infections

F.A. Waldvogel

Objective 28–1. Distinguish acute hematogenous osteomyelitis from acute arthritis or an acute subcutaneous infection by the clinical characteristics.

When a patient has a fever and painful swelling localized just over an osseous or articular structure, three questions should be asked: (1) Is it an infection? (2) Does it involve the skeletal structures? (3) If so, is it arthritis, osteomyelitis, or both?

SIGNS OF INFECTION

The infectious origin of an inflammatory process is most often indicated by the presence of fever accompanied by the classic signs of pain, edema, heat, and erythema. These signs are not, however, specific to infection and are found in other inflammatory processes. Thus, similar, moderate clinical signs located around the ankle may be evidence of a deep thrombophlebitis; those located in the popliteal fossa or in the upper calf may indicate the rupture of a synovial cyst; and when several joints are affected, these signs may reflect polyarthritis caused by acute rheumatic fever, systemic lupus erythematosus, or serum sickness. In summary, particularly intense localized bone or joint pain, a high fever with toxicity, an otherwise normal venous system, and leukocytosis are evidence of an infectious cause, a diagnosis positively supported by direct puncture, aspiration, and bacteriologic examination of the bone tissue, joint, or adjacent tissue fluid.

DEPTH OF INFECTION

During the initial clinical examination, it is often difficult to determine the depth of the infection, or in other words, whether the process is superficial, subcutaneous, in the muscle and fascial planes, or deeper, in the bone or joint. Clinical experience has shown, paradoxically, that whereas prominent and extensive erythema is evidence of superficial, benign infection of moderate severity that may involve the periarticular bursas, the absence of erythema in conjunction with intense pain and tenderness is a serious sign indicating deep localization within the bone or joint. In case of doubt about the origin and depth of the infection, it is useful to draw a line along the border of the erythema with a marking pen and then observe the area again several hours later. Superficial infections expand their limits quickly, but in deep infections, the area of erythema, when present, remains well localized.

BONE VERSUS JOINT LESIONS

Finally, when the infection is clearly localized to the skeletal structures, it is still important to distinguish between bone and joint involvement. This distinction might be considered merely academic; this is certainly true for neonates, in whom the two entities are combined. On the other hand, in children and adults, each location has its own etiologic agents and its own therapeutic approaches.

How can these two types of infection be distinguished clinically? An infected joint, besides manifesting the signs of inflammation previously described, is exquisitely painful on movement. Any pressure on the articular surface is intolerable. Thus, when infection of the hip joint is suspected, pressure exerted along the axis of the femur toward the hip provokes a sharp and shooting pain. Although bone lesions may be equally painful at rest, the adjacent joints can nevertheless be slowly and delicately moved without provoking additional pain. When in doubt, puncture and aspiration are essential and remain the procedures of choice for localizing the infectious process.

The distinction between bone and articular lesions, so important clinically, can easily be understood on the basis of current knowledge of the pathophysiologic features of this type of infection. The multiple processes in the maturation of the skeleton have direct, logical repercussions on their clinical manifestations. Thus, the vascular connections between the metaphysis and the epiphysis, present in the neonate, easily allow the passage of infection from bone into the contiguous articular space and thereby render any distinction between osteomyelitis and arthritis impossible. In the older child or adolescent, the epiphyseal growth plate cartilage, a nonvascular structure, is impermeable to infection, which is then found just beneath this cartilage, in the richly vascular metaphysis. In the adult, the epiphyseal growth plate is no longer active, and the vascular network is much reduced; consequently, the metaphyseal localization of a septicemia becomes rare. On the contrary, hematogenous osteomyelitis in the adult occurs preferentially in the vertebral bodies and the adjacent intervertebral space. This particular location is perhaps explained by the high activity of the bone tissue around the hematopoietic bone marrow in the adult.

As discussed later in this chapter, however, not all forms of osteomyelitis are hematogenous in origin. Osteomyelitis is occasionally the result of a direct inoculation of the organism by a traumatic puncture wound, an adjacent soft tissue infection, or the insertion of a prosthesis, that is, osteomyelitis due to a contiguous infection. Osteomyelitis may also be the result of vascular insufficiency and ulceration of overlying tissues, as in the diabetic. Finally, it is unfortunately not rare for osteomyelitis, regardless of its pathogenicity, to become a chronic infection, creating special diagnostic and therapeutic problems. These three forms of the disease are discussed later in this chapter.

> **Objective 28–2. Confirm bone involvement by means of roentgenograms and scans.**

ROENTGENOGRAMS

We have seen that the diagnosis of osteomyelitis or septic arthritis puts the physician's clinical acumen to the test, as well as his patience; the radiologic confirmatory signs do not appear for a long time. Indeed, the density of bone must be reduced by close to 50% before it can be visualized as a rarefaction on a roentgenogram. Because of the slow lysis of bone in osteomyelitis, at least 2 to 3 weeks are required before the image of a bone defect appears on conventional radiographs. By the time the defect is finally visible, irregular and blurred enough to be best detected by tomography (Fig. 28–1), the roentgenogram no longer confirms the diagnosis, but is a source of new worry for the attending physician. Having undertaken to treat the patient at the first sign of the disease, with what was judged to be appropriate therapy, the physician observes the appearance and even worsening of the lytic lesion during the course of this treatment. The process of new bone apposition also takes several weeks to become manifest.

One must therefore allow this minimal waiting period of 2 to 3 weeks before radiologic visualization of the extent of the osteomyelitis permits one to evaluate the effectiveness of the therapy.

Apart from the lytic lesions previously described, periosteal reactions may be particularly violent around a focus of osteomyelitis caused by pyogenic organisms and may often represent the first radiologic indication of the infective process.

Without appropriate tomograms, the third type of radiologic lesion, sclerosis, is difficult to distinguish from compressive thickening of the bone or from a sequestrum and does not become obvious until 2 or 3 months into the course of the disease.

Even if radiographs are rarely of diagnostic aid at the beginning of the disease, they are indispensable in that they allow one to follow its evolution by comparison with later pictures; one must keep in mind the delays mentioned previously. Moreover, it is helpful to take roentgenograms of the patient's other bones at the onset of the illness, so as not to overlook a less-evident, secondary focus of infection.

BONE SCANS

Of all imaging techniques, bone scanning is most important in the early evaluation of bone lesions. Although the procedure is less specific than was originally hoped, it permits the detection of areas with a high uptake of radioactivity ("hot areas") during the initial, bacteremic phase of the illness (Fig. 28–2). This technique thus offers the clinician the possibility of focusing attention on unsuspected areas of infection, which may be almost or totally asymptomatic in this early phase. Indeed, unless bone lesions due to pyogenic organisms appear as purely lytic on routine roentgenograms, they show areas of increased uptake on the scan.

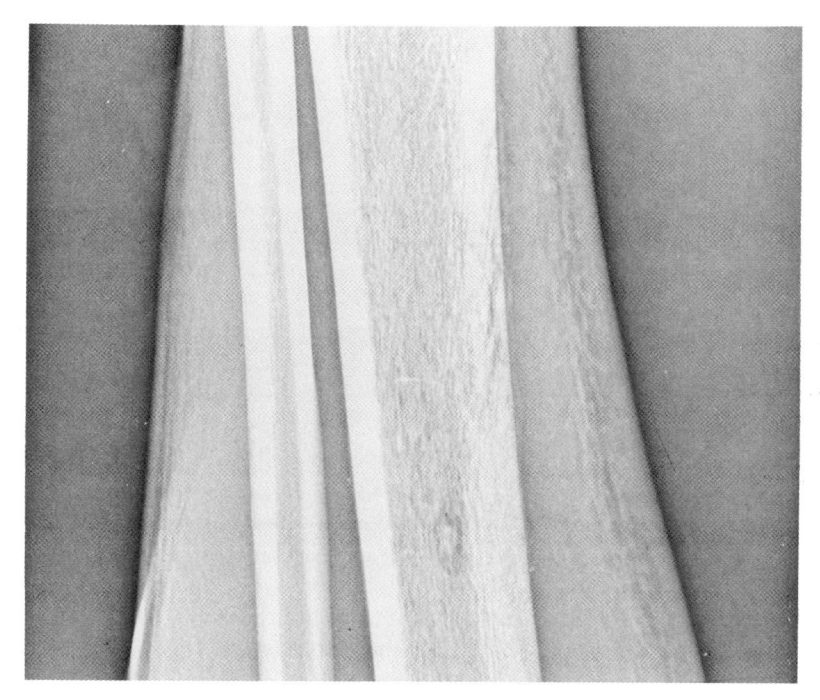

Fig. 28–1. Tomogram of a Brodie's abscess 3 months after the first appearance of symptoms. (Courtesy of the Radiology Institute, Cantonal University Hospital, Geneva.)

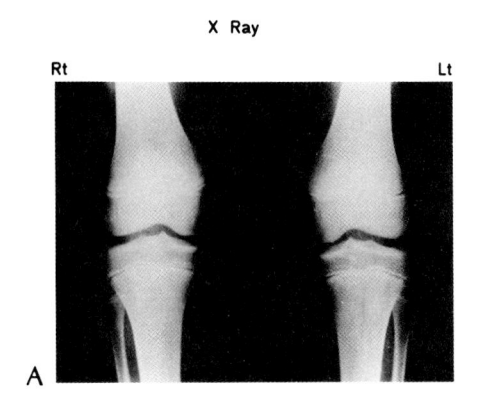

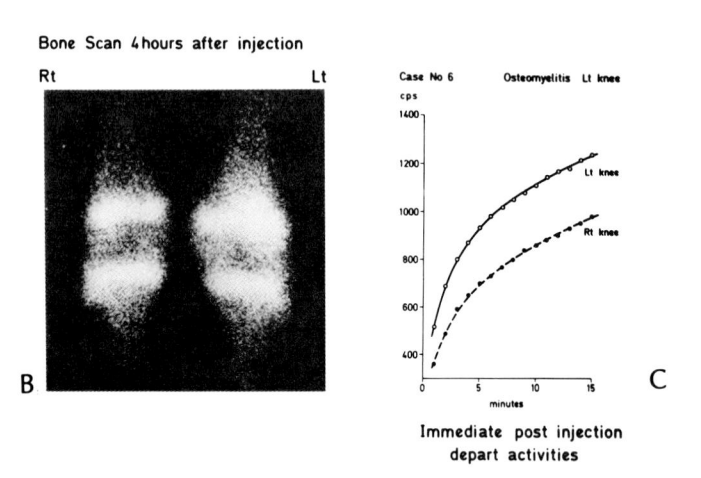

Fig. 28-2. Roentgenograms (A) and a technetium bone scan (B and C) in the early phase of hematogenous osteomyelitis. Note the normal appearance on the standard roentgenogram; the scan, taken on the same day, shows abnormal uptake on the left side. (Courtesy of A. Donath, Division of Nuclear Medicine, Cantonal University Hospital, Geneva.)

> **Objective 28-3.** Identify the organism responsible for a case of acute osteomyelitis by microbiologic examination.

GENERAL DIAGNOSTIC PRINCIPLES

Because hematogenous osteomyelitis is, by definition, associated with bacteremia, be it only transient, the organisms found in bone will be the same as those found in the blood. The septicemia-producing bacteria vary with the host's age, and the major causes of hematogenous osteomyelitis and their respective localizations therefore follow this age-related pattern. The most likely locations and causes according to age are summarized in Table 28-1. Two points are important: First, recent experience has shown that the vertebrae are a frequent secondary location in adults with septicemia. Thus, severe lumbar or back pain accompanied by septicemia or acute or subacute endocarditis may be the only indication of vertebral osteomyelitis, as discussed in detail later in this chapter. Second, these bone lesions are caused by the organisms found in the blood. In older patients, for instance, one frequently finds gram-negative rods. Vertebral infections often follow a transitory bacteremia or a migration of bacteria through the

Table 28–1. Age and Microbiologic Findings in Hematogenous Bone Infection

Age	Localization	Organisms Responsible
Neonates	Osteoarthritis (long bones, often multiple involvement)	Streptococci, groups A and B, *Haemophilus influenzae*, enteric bacteria, *Staphylococcus aureus*
Children and adolescents	Osteomyelitis (metaphysis of long bones)	*Staphylococcus aureus, Mycobacterium tuberculosis*
Adults	Osteomyelitis (rare)	*Staphylococcus epidermidis, S. aureus*, brucella, salmonella
	Spondylitis (frequent)	*Mycobacterium tuberculosis*, particular epidemiologic circumstances*
Elderly	Spondylitis	Gram-negative bacilli, *Staphylococcus aureus, Mycobacterium tuberculosis*, particular epidemiologic circumstances*

*See text

periprostatic veins of the pelvis into the perivertebral plexus. Most of the time, these infections have a urogenital origin, such as from the patient's bladder, kidney, or prostate.

The list of major organisms cited in Table 28–1 is not exhaustive, however. Indeed, the special infectious risks created by modern medical technology, such as arteriovenous shunts, endovenous catheters, and arterial monitors, and by drug addiction favor the development of septicemias and osteomyelitis caused by unusual pathogens often resistant to the majority of available antibiotics. In the rarer forms of osteomyelitis seen in patients with sickle cell disease, such as from infection with salmonella or pneumococci, the sites of infection in bone are difficult to distinguish from aseptic bone infarcts without appropriate bacteriologic testing, that is, aspiration and culture.

Finally, review of the microbiology of hematogenous osteomyelitis would be incomplete without mentioning tuberculosis of the bone, now a rare disease. It affects adults more frequently than children, and its primary symptom is localized, moderate pain. This type of tuberculosis most frequently involves the vertebral and, occasionally, the long bones. Radiologically, the disease produces an important lytic lesion. Tuberculosis is seldom diagnosed in this setting other than by biopsy.

PRACTICAL DIAGNOSTIC APPROACH

In view of the pathophysiologic and microbiologic aspects already discussed, the following approach to an etiologic diagnosis is proposed. First, blood cultures provide the necessary bacteriologic information in more than half the cases, particularly during the acute phase of the illness. Any suspect cutaneous lesions should be cultured with care, especially a lesion in contact with an intravascular foreign body such as a shunt, a pacemaker, or an intravenous or intra-arterial catheter. Then, if the clinical picture suggests a vertebral osteomyelitis, urine or prostatic fluid cultures should be obtained; they can often be of great help. A strongly positive serologic test for Brucella (1/1000) in the absence of recent immunization may allow one to diagnose this now unusual cause of spondylitis. In my experience, the serologic responses of salmonellae are too equivocal to allow prolonged therapy. Results of antistaphylococcal antibody testing are not yet dependable enough to be of diagnostic value.

If the various bacteriologic examinations proposed are performed carefully and as soon as the possibility of osteomyelitis is considered, they will often confirm the suspected bacteriologic diagnosis within a day or two. If these examinations do not confirm the diagnosis, then direct puncture of the focus of infection should be considered, especially when the focus is within practical reach and if general (age or associated illness) or local (localization in a cervical vertebra or risk of contamination of the cerebrospinal fluid) contraindications are absent. Histologic examination of the aspirate enables one to confirm the infectious nature of the lesion and to exclude the diagnosis of tuberculosis or a tumor; the microbiologic results determine the appropriate antibiotic therapy.

A spirit of collaboration should animate the medical and surgical teams once the decision is made to perform a bone biopsy. The surgeon must take a bone specimen of sufficient size from the appropriate area for adequate histologic and bacteriologic examinations. When a patient has already received antibiotic therapy, the conditions for a bacteriologic diagnosis are less than perfect; however, a diagnosis can still be established in the majority of cases if the following procedures are strictly followed: rapid transport to the laboratory, efficient homogenization of the fragment, and inoculation without delay on aerobic, anaerobic, mycobacterial, and fungal plates.

The decision for biopsy, assigned secondary importance when the results of the initial bacteriologic tests are unquestionable, takes on primary importance when the patient has a solitary, radiolucent bone lesion. Occasionally, medical help is sought for a child or adolescent who suffers from severe bone pain of recent onset, most often in the lower extremity. The physical examination is normal. Radiographs show a radiolucent lesion, generally localized in a metaphyseal area, that penetrates neither the periosteum nor the growth plate, and without an osteoblastic reaction in the surrounding area. The diagnoses suggested by such a picture range from subacute osteomyelitis (Brodie's abscess, Fig. 28–1) to osteoid osteoma (Jaffé-Lichtenstein tumor), or even a malignant tumor (Ewing's sarcoma). Whatever the physician's diagnostic skills may be, such a radiolucent lesion, just like a coin lesion in the lungs, requires surgical exploration. The diagnostic possibilities are diverse, and an error in judgment can have disastrous consequences.

> Objective 28–4. Plan the treatment and care of acute osteomyelitis in relation to the causative organism.

CHOICE OF ANTIBIOTIC

The choice of appropriate antibiotic therapy obviously depends, first of all, on the causative agent and its antibiotic sensitivities. Once again, the importance of the bacteriologic testing in the overall evaluation of the disease has to be underlined. The bacteriologic results, in general, indicate a limited choice of antibiotics active in vitro against the organism isolated; one must choose the particular agent indicated for the treatment of osteomyelitis.

In recent years, some reports have stressed the intraosseous penetration of certain antibiotics active against gram-positive cocci; these agents supposedly guarantee a cure by virtue of optimal tissue levels at the focus of infection. Such conclusions are based on experimental data flawed by technical problems, and it is difficult to interpret the clinical significance of these tissue levels at the present time. Thus, although it is logical to assume that some antibiotics with elevated tissue levels such as lincomycin or clindamycin may be indicated in staphylococcal osteomyelitis, it still remains to be proved that their clinical efficacy is superior to that of the beta-lactamase-resistant antistaphylococcal penicillins. In addition, hematogenous osteomyelitis is not the cause but rather the consequence of a bacteremia, and such a bacteremia, especially if it is due to *Staphylococcus aureus*, often causes septic lesions in the endocardium. The cure for these lesions lies in the use of bactericidal agents such as the beta-lactam antibiotics. Thus, in such situations, penicillin seems to be the antibiotic of choice.

General therapeutic recommendations for hematogenous osteomyelitis are summarized in Table 28–2. These recommendations take

Table 28–2. Treatment of Hematogenous Osteomyelitis in Adults

Causative Agent	Suggested Treatment	Alternate Treatment	Duration of Treatment
Group A streptococcus	Penicillin G, 24 million U/day IV	Erythromycin*, 2 g/day IV or Clindamycin*, 2–4 g/day IV†	4–6 weeks
Group B streptococcus	Penicillin G, 24 million U/day IV		
Staphylococcus aureus			
Penicillinase-negative	Vancomycin 1.2–2 g/day IV§		
Penicillinase-positive	Oxacillin or cloxacillin or nafcillin, 8–12 g/day IV	Cephalothin, 8 g/day IV, erythromycin*, 2 g/day IV, or clindamycin*, 24 g/day, IV†	6 weeks
Alpha-hemolytic streptococcus	(See Table 14–2)	Vancomycin 1.5–2 g/day IV	
Enterococcus	(See Objective 14–4)		
Gram-negative rod	Ampicillin, 12 g/day IV, cefoxitin or cefotaxime, 4–8 g/day IV, moxalactam, 4–8 g/day IV, or gentamicin 5 mg/kg/day, IV‡	According to antibiotic susceptibility tests	6 weeks

*To be avoided when an endocarditis possibly complicates the osteomyelitis
†Possible complications such as diarrhea and pseudomembranous colitis
‡Dose to be adjusted according to serum levels
§Penicillin G if sensitive
IV, Intravenously

for granted that all bacteriologic findings are available and that the causative agent has been isolated. Because early and correct treatment is a major guarantee of success, one must treat the patient as soon as adequate cultures are taken. The choice obviously falls on an antibiotic active against the most pathogenic suspected organism, although it may not necessarily be the most probable cause of the disorder. Thus, when gram-positive cocci are suspected, one should initiate treatment with a beta-lactamase-resistant penicillin; for suspected gram-negative organisms, the choice is gentamicin or one of the newer cephalosporins (Table 28–2). Later, the bacteriologic data permit definitive adjustment of the therapy.

When an infection due to *Staphylococcus aureus* is sensitive to penicillin G, the choice lies with this antibiotic, which has extraordinary activity against this bacterial strain and a history of confirmed efficacy. With infections due to strains of *S. aureus* resistant to penicillin G, and such is most often the case, one must resort to a beta-lactamase-resistant penicillin such as oxacillin, nafcillin, or cloxacillin, or even a cephalosporin, administered parenterally in doses of 8 to 12 g/day. Such early and agressive therapy generally limits and then cures the infection.

All the suggested therapeutic regimens should be administered parenterally, at least until clinical and radiologic evidence ensures that the disease is under control. This form of administration allows high dosage and solves the problems of absorption from the gastrointestinal tract and bioavailability of the drug. Parenteral therapy should be prolonged beyond 4 weeks. Best results are obtained with 6 weeks of parenteral therapy, but longer regimens do not increase the chances of success. Parenteral administration is another partial guarantee that the patient is receiving effective therapy. Oral therapy, if indicated, should be administered under strict medical control, with all doses recorded by the physician and with repeated determinations of the serum levels of the antibiotic.

MONITORING OF THERAPEUTIC EFFICACY

In osteomyelitis, the effectiveness of therapy should be monitored primarily by clinical criteria. Negative blood cultures are a necessary but insufficient criterion of effectiveness, and the other laboratory tests are of only limited value. Neither the sedimentation rate, which is altered by a multitude of factors including phlebitis, nor the white blood cell count and differential are of immediate diagnostic importance during the initial phase of therapy. The patient's alkaline phosphatase level is generally normal, and the roentgenographic changes are so slow that the usefulness of x-ray studies is limited during the course of treatment. Finally, although many authors have stressed the value of serum bacteriostatic and bactericidal levels of antibiotics, no study has yet demonstrated prospectively and definitely the value of these levels, either in the early or in the long-term evaluation of this disease.

On the other hand, clinical findings are useful in the evaluation of the effectiveness of treatment. The persistence of fever or of sharp pain at the site of infection beyond the first week of therapy raises the possibility of a therapeutic failure, which is not usually a consequence of any special properties of the infecting organism. If, after consultation with a specialist, the physician feels that the antibiotic therapy is well chosen and in accordance with the susceptibility test (antibiogram) of the organism isolated, he must search for other causes of an apparent failure in an undrained focus of infection. Examples of such causes are: a contiguous or distant septic arthritis; the presence of a bone sequestrum; an intramedullary abscess, with the bone painful on movement or percussion; or a paravertebral abscess in spondylitis manifested by persistent back pain or pyramidal tract signs, however minor. In all these cases, rapid decompression, surgical drainage, and curettage are imperative, including evacuation of the purulent material and, when present, of fragments of necrotic bone. Although infectious causes of persistent fever are the most frequent at the beginning of therapy, such is rarely the case when fever reappears after a transient improvement. One must look for so-called iatrogenic causes, such as drug fevers or thrombophlebitis.

CRITERIA FOR CURE

After 4 to 6 weeks of treatment, it is appropriate to evaluate the results of therapy. The significance of this evaluation depends on the extent to which one has followed the therapeutic approach. If the organism has been isolated either from blood culture or directly from the bone, if therapy in accordance with bacterial sensitivities has been administered parenterally for 6 weeks, and finally, if the infectious focus has been treated promptly after the appearance of symptoms, the infection is probably cured. This hypothetic conclusion must be substantiated in each patient by clinical observation. The patient should be afebrile and should not be in any pain, either spontaneously or on palpation of the bone. Furthermore, the patient who has been immobilized for a long period and is now anxious to resume physical activities should not experience any pain on movement of the affected limb.

The optimism of the physician, based on a normal clinical picture, is usually not confirmed at this stage by the radiologic results. Roentgenograms continue to show a lytic lesion, as well as fading osteoblastic and sclerotic reactions. Similarly, the laboratory signs of inflammation, such as anemia and a sedimentation rate, may take several weeks to return to normal. These data should be followed attentively, but in no case should more importance be attached to them than to the physical examination.

Therapeutic Failure. Treatment failure must be suspected when pain, edema, anemia and a high sedimentation rate persist, or in the presence of a lytic lesion with a possible sequestrum (Fig. 28–3). Etiologically, the possibilities are limited, if the therapy was administered logically. Most often, a persisting sequestrum acts as an avascular foreign body in maintaining the infection. Occasionally, the infection has spread to the medullary area, to form an abscess that should be widely drained; less frequently, a poorly controlled

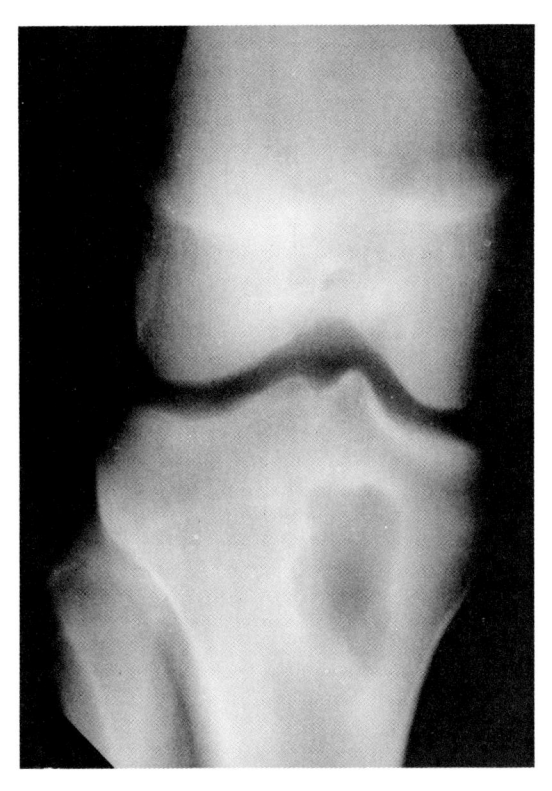

Fig. 28–3. Acute hematogenous osteomyelitis. Xerogram showing the formation of a lytic lesion within bone with a sequestrum. (Courtesy of W. Wettstein, Radiology Institute, Cantonal University Hospital, Geneva.)

underlying disease such as diabetes or a neutrophil deficit plays a role in the persistence of the infection. Finally, and exceptionally, the organism itself is responsible for the therapeutic failure; for example, development of antibiotic resistance, or an incorrect antibiogram.

If the failure of treatment is otherwise unexplained, either microbiologically or therapeutically, a new trial of antibiotic therapy should be initiated, combined with surgical exploration of the infected area to look for avascular foci of necrotic material. The same antibiotic therapy, repeated after surgical drainage, may then produce the expected response, provided it is administered parenterally for 4 to 6 weeks. The aggressive approach is especially appropriate in the young patient, in whom the social and psychologic repercussions of chronic osteomyelitis can be catastrophic.

> **Objective 28–5. Find a solution to the diagnostic and therapeutic problems inherent in an infection adjacent to bone or joint prosthetic material.**

In the diagnostic and therapeutic strategies described in the previous objectives, the model of acute hematogenous osteomyelitis was used. This simplified picture does not take into consideration the entire range of clinical presentations of osteomyelitis. Thus, a septic focus adjacent to a synthetic or prosthetic bone or joint implant poses special problems. Such infections are unfortunately common nowadays because of the frequency of trauma and the growing use of prosthetic material in orthopedic surgery.

DIAGNOSTIC PROBLEMS

The most frequent clinical presentation of this type of infection is that of fever following an orthopedic procedure for insertion of prosthetic material. The patient's detailed medical history is important because it permits one to evaluate the risk of infection. For example, the insertion of a simple femoral prosthesis under proper aseptic conditions is accompanied by a risk of infection of less than 5%, but the risk increases rapidly when the insertion is performed in the presence of multiple trauma (18%) or open fractures (35%). Even when the diagnosis of osteomyelitis is suspected, however, it is often difficult to confirm because these postoperative patients have many other reasons for fever and leukocytosis, as well as local pain, edema, and erythema at the operative site. Further, the roentgenograms are often rendered uninterpretable by the surgical intervention, which, in itself, provokes osteoblastic and osteolytic reactions. Finally, the development of reflex sympathetic dystrophy, not uncommon in such conditions, may have the same radiologic features as osteomyelitis, although the initial bone involvement is usually purely lytic and more mottled.

If the clinical signs and roentgenograms are often difficult to interpret in such patients, the same can be said about the bacteriologic data. Although the presence of pathogens in high concentrations, such as *Staphylococcus aureus*, generally indicates the presence of an infection, some microorganisms reputed to be nonpathogenic, such as *S. epidermidis* and corynebacteria, can be responsible for these infections. These less-pathogenic microorganisms can take several months to produce purulent drainage, and the only initial warning signs are a low-grade fever and slight pain on movement. The following clinical evidence should, however, alert the physician to the possibility of such a low-grade infection: persistent edema in the surgical scar, serous drainage from the operative wound, a low-grade fever starting several days after the procedure, and finally, the persistence of pain more than a week after the surgical procedure, or the reappearance of pain on mobilization of the affected area.

In such situations, it is sometimes possible to obtain bacteriologic confirmation of the infection by culturing the seropurulent drainage from the operative wound. Unfortunately, this material may be contaminated by commensal organisms from the skin, which may themselves be responsible for such infections. In doubtful cases, one should proceed directly to an exploration of the operative wound by fistulography and deep needle aspiration or biopsy. Gram staining and culture of the purulent material can confirm the etiologic diagnosis and define the degree and depth of the infection.

THERAPEUTIC PROBLEMS

Experience shows that early initiation of therapy, according to the same rules as for hematogenous osteomyelitis, can sometimes eliminate the infection and save the prosthesis. Considering the difficulties generally encountered with foreign bodies, one wonders whether this infection really is a case of osteomyelitis.

The fate of the prosthesis is difficult to determine at the beginning of therapy, and the decision to remove it should follow the evaluation of numerous factors, such as the rapidity of the diagnosis of osteomyelitis and its treatment, the necessity of maintaining the prosthesis in place, the pathogenicity of the organism isolated from the wound, the technical complexity of later reinsertion of synthetic material, and the age of the recipient, which may contraindicate reoperation. These different factors are arguments in favor of temporization and purely medical treatment. If, one the other hand, after 4 to 6 weeks of antibiotic therapy administered according to the regimen described for hematogenous osteomyelitis, no improvement at all is discerned, the chances of cure are practically eliminated, and one must remove the synthetic material, with immediate or delayed reimplantation.

> **Objective 28–6. Evaluate the clinical and bacteriologic evidence of vertebral osteomyelitis in a patient with back pain and fever, and determine the appropriate treatment.**

It is not uncommon for adults or aged patients to seek medical advice for back pain and fever. Even though such a complaint in the absence of fever is common and is generally due to posture problems and minor trauma, many patients with back pain and fever do have an infection. Nothing is more frustrating than to recognize one's own diagnostic error 3 months after an initial consultation for back pain, when a roentgenogram of the spine clearly shows spondylitis. Recent experience has taught us that this bone lesion is also frequently seen in a variety of septicemias. It is even possible to demonstrate, in some cases of subacute or acute endocarditis, spondylitis that is cured in the course of treatment of the endocarditis. Finally, spondylitis may develop only later, when the bacteremia has long since been controlled by a short course of treatment that cleared the septicemia, but did not sterilize the vertebral focus of infection, which then develops surreptitiously.

CLINICAL AND RADIOLOGIC SIGNS OF VERTEBRAL OSTEOMYELITIS

Such patients generally have a fever of variable degree and excruciating back pain localized in the infected vertebrae. Often, the pain is so sharp that the patient is almost incapable of moving from his bed. On physical examination, one notes fever, as well as the vertebral syndrome consisting of pain on pressure and spasm of the paravertebral musculature. Even light percussion of the spinal vertebral process is likely to be painful. Important aspects of the initial examination include a rectal examination to look for prostatitis, a microscopic urinalysis and culture, and finally, a close examination of the skin to detect possible portals of entry, past or present, for the bacteremia.

Neither the clinical picture nor the actual identification of an apparent primary infectious focus allows one to define the precise nature of the disorder in the vertebral body. Benign tumors, primary or secondary malignant tumors, or even multiple myeloma may share the described symptoms and signs.

Roentgenograms of the painful area may be of considerable help. Vertebral bone lesions due to pyogenic organisms have the following characteristics: they involve two adjacent vertebral bodies in an irregular fashion; the disc space is reduced; except in tuberculosis, these lesions cause a violent and rapid osteophytic reaction on the anterior faces of the vertebral bodies with a tendency toward fusion (Fig. 28-4); when the lesions extend to other vertebral bodies, they do so by contiguity.

BACTERIOLOGIC AND SURGICAL DIAGNOSIS

Although roentgenograms may be valuable in determining the probable infectious nature of the lesion, they cannot determine the precise bacterial origin. This information is obtained only from positive blood cultures or from a needle biopsy of the affected bone. The lower the vertebral lesion, the easier the biopsy is to perform. If needle biopsy fails, an open surgical biopsy is indicated to obtain an adequate specimen. Once the responsible organism has been identified, parenteral therapy is initiated according to the criteria previously described. Most organisms isolated from spinal lesions are cephalosporin-sensitive organisms; therefore, initial treatment with a second-generation compound is my usual approach. Treatment regimens are adjusted later, depending on the bacteriologic test results. Further surgical intervention for curettage and drainage should be undertaken only in two circumstances: the appearance of neurologic complications and the demonstration of an adjacent abscess.

> **Objective 28-7. Define a plan of action for a patient with chronic osteomyelitis.**

Unfortunately, the diagnostic and therapeutic guidelines presented in the preceding objectives are not infallible. Indeed, therapeutic failure is common in osteomyelitis, especially in the presence of a foreign body. Furthermore, the disease is often misdiagnosed or incompletely treated, resulting in a persistent infection and the creation of chronic suppurative foci. Whether spread by hematogenous means or by contiguity, or whether postsurgical in origin, these foci pose particularly difficult therapeutic problems; the osteomyelitis nearly inevitably recurs. One only has to look at a roentgenogram of a focus of chronic osteomyelitis with its multiple lytic and sclerotic areas and sequestra to be convinced of the inadequate penetration of antibiotics into these areas.

Because relapse is the rule in chronic osteomyelitis, one must first define the goal of treatment: to go all out to obtain a cure, or to undertake palliative therapy to permit the patient to resume an active life as soon as possible? In the latter case, prolonged oral antibiotic therapy often eliminates or reduces the purulent drainage and relieves the pain. In no instance can one expect the infection

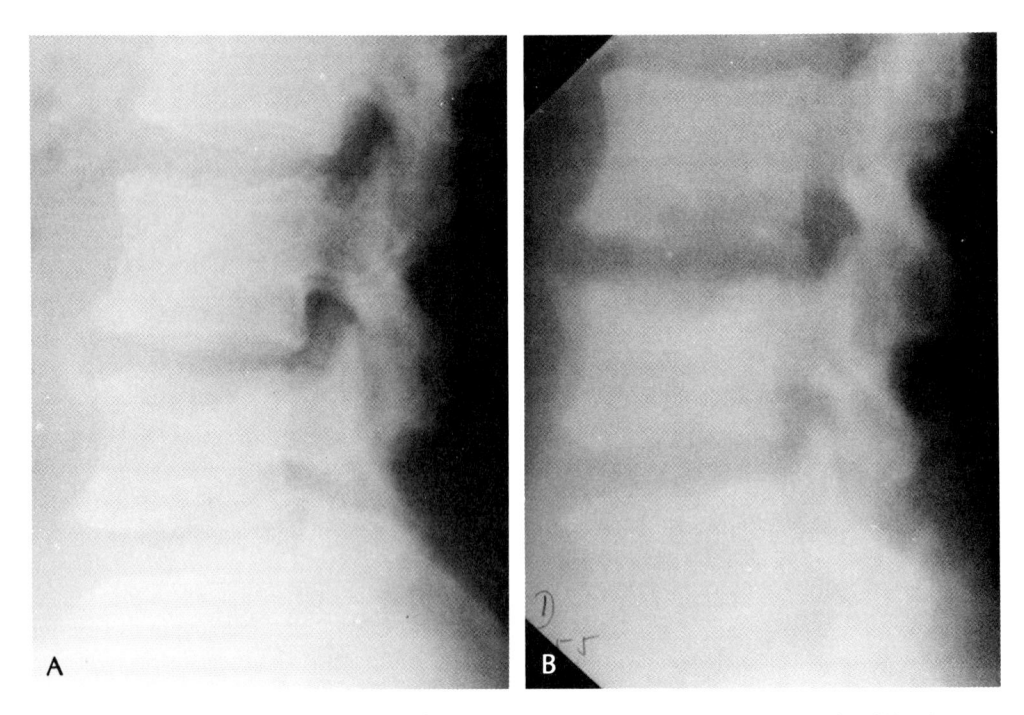

Fig. 28–4. *A* and *B*, Vertebral osteomyelitis L3 to L4 due to *Staphylococcus aureus*. Lateral view *(A)* and tomogram *(B)*. Note the lysis of the two adjacent vertebral bodies as well as the beginning of the formation of bone bridge between the two vertebrae. (Courtesy of the Radiology Institute, Cantonal University Hospital, Geneva.)

to be eliminated by this therapy. If, on the contrary, the physician and the patient decide on a more radical approach, the patient's problem must be re-evaluated in detail from the beginning. Because culture of the purulent drainage generally reveals many organisms, it is difficult to decide which one to treat. One must then investigate the bone lesion itself through various radiologic views and tomographic and fistulographic studies, to determine the extent of the infection. With a trocar or by means of open surgical intervention, one may obtain a specimen of material from the site of the infection to provide a reliable bacteriologic diagnosis, as well as antibiotic-sensitivity data that serve as a logical basis for chemotherapy. Long-term parenteral therapy is reinstituted, according to the guidelines for hematogenous osteomyelitis. Usually, as soon as treatment is begun, one should surgically debride and drain the lesions, as well as remove any foreign bodies (sequestra) and intervening connective tissue. Thus, such a combined medicosurgical approach can, if not cure the illness, at least stabilize it for many years.

> **Objective 28–8. Diagnose bacterial arthritis by means of the clinical signs and examination of the joint fluid.**

The appearance of a swollen, painful joint in a patient with fever raises questions similar to those raised in Objective 28–1, with regard to bone: (1) Is the inflammation superficial, or does it involve deeper structures? (2) Does the inflammatory process involve the joint or the adjacent bone? (3) Finally, is it of infectious origin?

Some of these issues are discussed in detail in Objective 28–1. Whether or not an infectious process is ongoing is often difficult to determine. Clinical examination does not allow for an easy differentiation between, for example, gouty arthritis and acute pyogenic septic arthritis. Both afflictions are abrupt in onset and are accompanied by violent pain on movement or at rest, with fever and occasional signs of periarticular lymphangitis. The same is true of an acute episode of chondrocalcinosis or, on rare occasions, rheumatic fever, in which the illness may have all the clinical characteristics of a septic process. The radiologic examination does not permit any such distinction either, because it is virtually normal. In this era of antibiotics, acute septic arthritis only rarely causes radiologically apparent destruction of cartilage or underlying bone. Exceptions are: poorly treated chronic infections; tuberculosis; infections in immunodepressed patients such as the newborn and those receiving immunosuppressants; and joint infections complicated by reflex sympathetic dystrophy. Therefore, the key to diagnosis lies in a close analysis of the fluid obtained from the joint by aspiration, on condition that the specimen is not contaminated and that the bacteriology laboratory is technically adequate. Consequently, this fluid analysis is of the greatest importance.

JOINT ASPIRATION

Even though intra-articular injections are difficult to perform under some circumstances, aspiration of a joint effusion for diagnostic purposes is, in principle, easy. Septic arthritis localizes preferentially in large joints and produces large effusions that enable one to determine their contours precisely. If only one or a few small joints are inflamed, it is better to ask for the assistance of a specialist, either a rheumatologist or an orthopedic surgeon. Even a small volume of synovial fluid obtained on a first attempt, without contamination with blood, may be sufficient for the diagnosis of gout, pseudogout, or septic arthritis, whereas a traumatic aspiration or uncertainty about the origin of the fluid may complicate and confuse further diagnostic efforts.

CHEMICAL ANALYSIS AND CELL COUNT OF SYNOVIAL FLUID

The principal characteristics of synovial fluid in different types of joint diseases are summarized in Table 28–3. Two important points should be emphasized. First, the patient should be fasting when the synovial aspiration is performed, to ensure a stable ratio of joint fluid to serum glucose. Second, the microscopic examination must be performed quickly because clots of mucin and fibrin may form and may entrap the leukocytes and thus alter the cell count of the synovial fluid. The urgent nature of bacteriologic examinations and inoculations is discussed at greater length later in this chapter.

MICROBIOLOGIC EXAMINATION OF SYNOVIAL FLUID

As we have already seen in the discussion of hematogenous osteomyelitis, septic arthritis is nearly always due to blood-borne dissemination of bacteria. This disorder is thus an osteoarticular manifestation of the bacteremia and has the same origin. The bacterial causes of septic arthritis therefore vary with age, as do those of septicemia or hematogenous osteomyelitis (Table 28–4). A new bacterial agent, the gonococcus, has been added to the list of possible causes of septic arthritis in adolescents and adults. Because the gonococcus is difficult to grow from synovial fluid, direct inoculation onto an appropriate medium, immediately after aspiration, and Gram staining are essential to obtain the most accurate bacteriologic diagnosis. Moreover, appropriate cultures from genital areas are indispensable when the diagnosis of gonococcal arthritis is suspected.

What culture media should be inoculated to cover all the multiple etiologic possibilities? First, basic media such as blood and MacConkey agar should be used; also recommended are chocolate agar and thioglycolate or cooked meat broth. A common error is direct inoculation of the agent onto Thayer-Martin plates or similar selective media, which are useful for the isolation of gonococci from specimens contaminated by normal resident bacterial flora; this flora, of course, does not exist within the joint. Finally, the inoculated plates must be transported as rapidly as possible to the laboratory for incubation

Table 28–3. Composition of the Synovial Fluid in Articular Disorders

Characteristics and Composition	Septic Arthritis (bacterial)	Metabolic Arthritis (gout, pseudogout)	Inflammatory Arthritis (rheumatoid)	Traumatic Effusion
Appearance	Cloudy to purulent	Clear to slightly cloudy	Clear to slightly cloudy	Clear to slightly cloudy
Color and mucin clot	Yellow to grayish green, friable	Yellow, compact, sometimes friable	Yellow, friable	Compact, clear to brownish
Leukocytes/mm^3	10^5 or more	$> 10^4$	10^4 to 5×10^4	$< 10^3$
Presence of polymorphonuclear leukocytes	Predominant	Predominant	Predominant	Some
Presence of urate and pyrophosphate crystals	Absent	Present	Absent	Absent
Glucose ratio*	< 0.6	0.6–0.8	0.6–0.8	0.6–0.8
Presence of bacteria	Present	Absent	Absent	Absent

*Glucose ratio = synovial fluid glucose to serum glucose; the specimens should be taken simultaneously while the patient is fasting

Table 28–4. Relative Frequency of Infecting Organisms in Septic Arthritis according to Age

	Group A Streptococci, Pneumococci, Haemophilus influenzae	Staphylococcus aureus	Gonococci	Enteric bacteria (Pseudomonas aeruginosa)
Newborn	+++ (+ group B Streptococci)	+++	0	+
Child or adolescent	+	+++	+	0
Adult	(+)	++	+++	0
Elderly	(+)	+++	0	++

+++, Common; ++, occasional; +, uncommon; (+), rare; 0, nonexistent.

under appropriate conditions including an atmosphere rich in carbon dioxide. Only by following these various directions scrupulously can the clinician promote the growth of the gonococcus.

Other Microbiologic Tests. The evaluation of a patient with arthritis does not end with culturing the joint fluid. A presumptive diagnosis of gonococcal arthritis, for example, is more often reached by the isolation of the organism from the urethra, rectum, or pharynx than from the joint fluid. These particular cultures should be inoculated onto Thayer-Martin medium, which selectively suppresses the growth of normal mucosal flora. It is equally important to obtain blood cultures, which may reveal the septicemic phase of an infection with septic arthritis as its sole clinical manifestation; for example, rare cases of staphylococcal and meningococcal septicemia, some cases of endocarditis (in which joint localization is indeed rare), and infections with *Streptobacillus moniliformis*.

Serologic diagnosis is of little help in the investigation of bacterial monoarthritis. At the most, serologic techniques are useful in diagnosing yersinia and brucella infections, diseases that produce polyarthralgias or polyarthritis rather than a simple joint involvement (see Objective 28–11). Viral infections that may produce febrile polyarthritis or even monoarthritis include rubella and rubella immunization in young women, unusual cases of varicella, and viral hepatitis, especially type B. In these cases, appropriate serologic tests and early identification of serum HB$_s$Ag sometimes allow rapid diagnosis. In the case of viral hepatitis, an assay of hemolytic complement activation often reveals the presence of circulating immune complexes.

> **Objective 28-9.** Determine the most likely cause of low-grade monoarthritis by means of clinical examination and laboratory tests.

Occasionally, monoarthritis does not manifest itself dramatically, but only by pain on movement and, perhaps, a faint periarticular erythema. The problem then extends beyond the realm of infectious diseases, and the physician must draw upon his general knowledge of internal medicine. These cases of low-grade monoarthritis can have several origins: infectious, as in tuberculosis; purely inflammatory, as in psoriatic arthritis; metabolic, as in chondrocalcinosis; degenerative, as in osteoarthritis; or even tumoral.

The importance of an in-depth physical examination cannot be overemphasized. This examination should include a search for such signs as patches of psoriasis on the scalp, adhesions in the anterior chamber of the eye due to previous iridocyclitis, or anal fissures and fistulas accompanying undiagnosed Crohn's disease.

The clinical examination is complemented by appropriate laboratory procedures. An abnormal urine sediment, the presence of HLA antigen B27, or the involvement of the calcaneus and the sacroiliac joint suggest the possibility of Reiter's syndrome; an active pulmonary lesion suggests tuberculosis or, in some clinical situations, fungal disease such as coccidioidomycosis or histoplasmosis. Several generalized illnesses such as gout, psoriasis, and dysenteric or inflammatory bowel disease, including Crohn's disease and ulcerative colitis, must be excluded by proper studies. Biopsies should be performed on all suspicious cutaneous lesions for histologic evidence of a vasculitis such as periarteritis nodosa or Behçet's disease. Finally, many specialized laboratories are now able to demonstrate a chlamydial origin for some of these cases of arthritis by the direct isolation of the organism from the genital tract or by serologic testing.

What information can be obtained from the involved joint itself? The location and clinical appearance may be characteristic of a specific cause; for example, involvement of the distal interphalangeal joints or appearance of swollen "sausage digits" in psoriasis. Sacroiliac involvement is particularly suggestive of Reiter's syndrome. The presence of cutaneous fistulas generally favors a diagnosis of tuberculosis or fungal disease. The radiologic features of the joint can be equally helpful. The presence of linear calcification in the joint cartilage suggests chondrocalcinosis. A significant lytic bone lesion involving the cartilage, with reduction of the joint space, enables one to suspect a tuberculous arthritis. Massive joint destruction without surrounding bone reaction is characteristic of Charcot's arthropathy, seen more often nowadays in roentgenographic museums than at the bedside.

Finally, examination of the synovial biopsy often resolves any difficulty in distinguishing among tuberculosis (caseation and granuloma), malignant disease (metastatic tumor from the kidney, the lung, or the pancreas or rarely, primary tumor), villonodular synovitis (pigmentation and presence of inflammatory granuloma), and the other less well defined joint diseases. The tissue obtained should be appropriately cultured for acid-fast organisms, brucella, and fungi. All these investigations usually guide a coherent therapeutic approach to the patient's problem.

> **Objective 28-10.** Plan the treatment and care of a patient with septic arthritis.

ANTIBIOTIC THERAPY

That the choice of antibiotic depends on the organism isolated and its antibiotic sensitivity cannot be overemphasized. With the exception of gonococcal arthritis, which can be treated with oral antibiotics when necessary, septic arthritis requires parenteral therapy because such a focus of infection can, if inadequately treated, lead to the destruction and permanent ankylosis of the joint. Many therapeutic guidelines have been proposed; some used in the treatment of adults are summarized in Table 28–5. The agents listed are not the only effective ones, but they seem to me to be particularly logical. Certain important aspects of the treatment of septic arthritis are not included in the table. For example, in septic arthritis in a child, organisms such as *Haemophilus influenzae* and pneumococci must be sought with special care; *Staphylococcus aureus*, in contrast to these others, is seldom difficult to isolate or to identify in the laboratory. If in doubt as to the etiologic agent of septic arthritis in a child, a combination of ampicillin and oxacillin or nafcillin, or one of the new cephalosporins such as cefotaxime, seems appropriate, considering the different possibilities within this age group. Finally, in the neonate and young infant, septic arthritis is occasionally due to enteric bacteria, including salmonella, for which antibiotic sensitivities vary, sometimes from one hospital to another.

OTHER THERAPEUTIC MEASURES

Surgical drainage of the joint, popular in its time, is no longer indicated in the treatment of septic arthritis. On the other hand, repeated aspiration of the joint fluid is an appropriate therapeutic measure because intrasynovial inflammation with local activation of leukocytes has deleterious effects on the articular cartilage. If synovial fluid reaccumulates despite an apparently adequate course of therapy, surgical exploration can be justified to reduce inflammation and pressure, which may impede the vascular flow in adjacent tissues. The penetration into the joint fluid of the antibiotics listed in Table 28–5 is sufficient to avoid local injection into the joint. Gram-negative septic arthritis, which is rare but has a poor prognosis, may be an exception to this rule and may require a daily

Table 28–5. Recommendations for Treatment of Septic Arthritis in Adults

Organism Responsible	Antibiotic of First Choice	Dose and Route of Administration	Duration of Treatment	Antibiotic of Second Choice
Group A streptococci	Penicillin G	12–24 million U/day IV	4 weeks*	Cephalothin† or erythromycin
Staphylococcus aureus Penicillinase-negative (10%)				Vancomycin
Penicillinase-positive (90%)	Oxacillin‡ or nafcillin	8–12 g/day IV	4–6 weeks	Cephalothin†
Neisseria gonorrhoeae	Penicillin G IV or IM, then ampicillin	10 million U/day IV	Until defervescence (5–10 days)	Ampicillin orally with probenecid§, tetracycline 2 g/day, or cefoxitin or cefotaxime 4 g/day#
Gram-negative rods	Gentamicin, possibly with ticarcillin	5 mg/kg/day IM∥ 16 g/day IV	4–6 weeks	Ampicillin IV, or cephalothin IV, cefoxitin or cefotaxime or other cephalosporins depending on susceptibility testing

*4–6 weeks for *Staphylococcus aureus* infection
†Or any of the first- or second-generation cephalosporins
‡Or any of the beta-lactamase-resistant penicillins
§2 g/day with 1 g probenicid in divided doses for 10 days
∥Dosage to be determined by serum levels
#For penicillin resistant strains
IV, Intravenously; IM, intramuscularly

injection of, for example, 1 to 2 mg gentamicin. Such treatment should be combined with a beta-lactam antibiotic, for example, carbenicillin, ticarcillin, or mezlocillin, for pseudomonas arthritis. In addition, the third-generation cephalosporins have further reduced the indications for both general and local uses of aminoglycosides. Recent studies indicate that gentamicin undergoes inactivation in such purulent collections, and these observations underline the importance of repeated aspiration of the pus and the utility of surgical drainage if needed.

MOBILIZATION

During the initial phase of septic arthritis, the pain is usually so intense that moving the limb is out of the question. One should therefore maintain the joint in a cradle splint to avoid contractures or pressure injuries. When the synovial effusion diminishes, the patient will regain motion of the affected joint. Although no study has reported on this aspect of therapy, it is generally recommended to avoid weight bearing until the end of the antibiotic regimen. Moreover, a recrudescence of joint inflammation is sometimes noted when physical activity resumes; this does not indicate a relapse of the disease, however, and usually subsides within a few days or weeks.

> Objective 28–11. Link a febrile polyarthritis to an infection treatable with antibiotics, and specify the mode of treatment.

We have seen that the clinical presentations of joint infections range from acute monoarthritis to low-grade monoarthritis and even to febrile polyarthritis. Earlier in this chapter, I have attempted to define the major etiologic possibilities for the first two types of presentation and have noted that the differential diagnosis largely transcends the field of infectious diseases. The same holds true for the diagnosis of febrile polyarthritis, a large group of diseases among which I shall try to sort out important syndromes requiring immediate antibiotic treatment.

GONOCOCCEMIA AND REITER'S SYNDROME

The combination of urethritis, polyarthritis or monoarthritis, and sometimes, conjunctivitis should evoke three diagnostic possibilities: disseminated gonococcemia, Reiter's syndrome, or a possible combination of the two. Table 28–6 summarizes the characteristic signs of these two types of polyarthritis.

The skin lesions of gonococcemia, in particular, show a predilection for the lateral surfaces of the hand and pulp of the fingers; these elevated and painless lesions evolve rapidly into nodules or necrotic plaques, or even into true bullae. Reiter's syndrome, on the other hand, is less likely to produce skin lesions, although one may observe a nummular hyperkeratosis of the palms and soles (keratoderma blennorrhagicum) as well as a circinate balanitis. With regard to mono- or polyarticular joint involvement, two distinctive clinical signs favor the diagnosis of one or the other syndrome: involvement of the sacroiliac joint is only seen in Reiter's syndrome and in the related ankylosing spondylitis; in contrast, tenosynovitis, either of the hand or of the Achilles tendon, is sufficiently characteristic of gonococcemia to warrant immediate specific therapy. Finally, although the presence of the histocompatibility antigen HLA B27 in a patient with a compatible clinical picture does not confirm the diagnosis of Reiter's syndrome, it allows one to identify patients who are at an increased risk of developing the illness when exposed to *Chlamydia trachomatis* or other possible pathogens.

ACUTE RHEUMATIC FEVER

In addition to the clinical features previously described, diagnosed either by isolation of the causative microorganism or by demonstration of the presence of a well-defined genetic marker, a large group of febrile polyarthritic disorders (so-called rheumatisms) have an indirect or even only hypothetic connection with an infectious agent. The best-

Table 28-6. Differential Diagnosis of Urethral and Arthritic Syndromes

Clinical and Laboratory Characteristics	Gonococcemia	Reiter's Syndrome
Male-to-female ratios	Men < women	Men > women
Cutaneous lesions		
Preferred localization	Lateral surface of fingers	Palms of hands
Macroscopic appearance	Evolution toward necrosis	Hyperkeratosis
Frequency	Frequent but not numerous (< 20)	Rare
Urethritis		
Appearance of exudate	Purulent	Less purulent
Gram staining characteristics	Intracellular gram-negative diplococci	Mixed flora
Conjunctivitis	Absent	Common
Articular involvement		
Clinical characteristics	Tenosynovitis present	Tenosynovitis absent
Typical localization	Large joints	Sacroiliac joints
Histocompatibility	No association with HLA B27	Usually associated with HLA B27

known example of a close association is that of acute rheumatic fever following a group A streptococcal pharyngitis. The pathogenic mechanism linking the two episodes of illness is not entirely known, although it probably involves an immunologic cross-reaction of either humoral or cellular type with certain streptococcal antigens and myocardial cell constituents. Other clinical and epidemiologic characteristics of acute rheumatic fever remain completely unexplained. Examples are: the increased frequency of this disease in childhood; the reasons for the frequent relapses and their decreased frequency with age; and the irreversibility of cardiac damage in contrast with the complete resolution of joint inflammation. Finally, we are currently witnessing the disappearance of acute rheumatic fever from North America and Europe without having a valid explanation for this phenomenon.

Should the clinician still consider the diagnosis of acute rheumatic fever? The question clearly arises only in the case of an initial episode of febrile polyarthritis in a child or adolescent in whom a scrupulous, in-depth clinical investigation has not yielded a diagnosis. Negative blood and joint fluid cultures suggest the possibility of this diagnosis, a hypothesis reinforced by the recovery of group A streptococci from the pharynx. The presence, although rare, of a skin rash on the trunk, lightly erythematous with sharp borders (erythema annularum rheumaticum), or cardiac involvement, as evidenced by arrhythmias, disturbances in atrioventricular conduction, and a systolic murmur of mitral insufficiency, are sufficient indications for immediate anti-inflammatory therapy and penicillin administration. The electrocardiogram furnishes objective evidence of carditis, as manifested by prolongation of the P–R interval and altered repolarization or by the demonstration of pericardial effusion. On the other hand, elevation of the antistreptolysin O titer is of limited importance and reflects merely a present or past group A streptococcal infection.

INFECTIONS WITH YERSINIA

Infections with *Yersinia pseudotuberculosis* and *Y. enterocolitica* are frequent causes of mesenteric lymphadenitis, which can simulate an acute appendicitis. These two related organisms sometimes also produce an acute polyarthritis accompanied by erythema nodosum. In contrast to acute rheumatic fever, this form of polyarthritis affects adults more frequently than children. It rarely affects the heart and usually resolves without specific treatment. This curious affliction may be suspected when yersinia is isolated from the pa-

LYME DISEASE

Lyme disease was named after the initially recognized outbreak, in 1972, which occurred in Lyme, Connecticut. This illness has been related to bites of certain ticks (the so-callled *Ixodes ricinus* complex); recent evidence suggests a treponemal origin. Cases have been reported from Massachusetts to Maryland on the northeastern coast of the United States, as well as from Minnesota, Wisconsin, Oregon, and California. A similar tick-borne disease, with the notable absence of reported joint and heart involvement, occurs in northern Europe.

Lyme disease usually begins in the summer and presents sequential clinical features. It generally starts 2 weeks after a tick bite (range: 4–20 days) with a skin eruption called erythema chronicum migrans (ECM). The initial lesion, usually on a proximal extremity or the trunk, begins as a red macule or papule that expands to form a large, annular lesion 6 to 52 cm in diameter. Subsequent lesions are usually smaller. The outer border of a lesion has a typically intense red color, whereas the center shows partial clearing. The lesions cause a burning sensation and are warm. Spontaneous ECM lasts approximately 10 days, with a range from 3 days to 18 months. Recurrent episodes are possible. ECM may be followed by neurologic symptoms, from 2 to 11 weeks after the tick bite. These symptoms may lead the physician to diagnose meningitis, encephalitis, chorea, or Bell's paralysis. By that time, ECM has often disappeared.

Migratory polyarthritis, intermittent attacks of arthritis, or chronic arthritis in the knee joints may occur 3 to 24 weeks after tick bites. At about the same time, myocardial conduction abnormalities may also be observed.

Some response to penicillin or tetracycline has been reported with regard to the initial skin lesion and the incidence of subsequent arthritis. Other late manifestations of this disease do not seem to be altered by antibiotic administration.

---

tient's stools, and the diagnosis can be confirmed by the appropriate serologic tests.

In conclusion, this chapter, which is essentially oriented toward treatable cases of acute polyarthritis due to bacteria or their antigenic products, would not be complete without two important comments. In the presence of acute febrile polyarthritis with intense myalgias, the physician should bear in mind the possibility of acute meningococcemia, one of the great masqueraders in infectious disease. Finally, one must consider other diseases that do not require antibiotic therapy, but that may be important from an epidemiologic standpoint, such as Lyme disease, rubella, and acute hepatitis.

SUGGESTED READINGS

Arnett, F.C., McClusky, P.E., Schacter, B.Z., and Lordon, R.E.: Incomplete Reiter's syndrome: discriminating features and HL-A W 27 in diagnosis. Ann. Intern. Med., 84:8, 1976.

Goldenberg, D.L., and Cohen, A.S.: Acute infectious arthritis: a review of patients with non-gonococcal joint infections (with emphasis on therapy and prognosis). Am. J. Med., 60:369, 1976.

Goldenberg, D.L., Brandt, K.D., Cohen, A.S., and Cathcart, E.S.: Treatment of septic arthritis. Comparison of needle aspiration and surgery as initial modes of joint drainage. Arthritis Rheum., 18:83, 1975.

Hedstrom, S.A.: The prognosis of chronic staphylococcal osteomyelitis after long-term antibiotic treatment. Scand. J. Infect. Dis., 6:33, 1974.

Hollander, J.L., Reginato, A., and Torralba, T.P.: Examination of synovial fluid as a diagnostic aid in arthritis. Med. Clin. North Am., 50:1281, 1966.

Holmes, K.K., and Stilwell, G.A.: Gonococcal infection. In Infectious Diseases. 2nd Ed. Edited by P.D. Hoeprich. Hagerstown, MD, Harper & Row, 1977.

Leino, R., and Kalliomäki, J.L.: Yersiniosis as an internal disease. Ann. Intern. Med., 81:458, 1974.

Musher, D.M., Thorsteinsson, S.B., Minuth, J.N., and Luchi, R.J. Vertebral osteomyelitis. Arch. Intern. Med., 136:105, 1976.

Nelson, J.D., Howard, J.B., and Shelton, S.: Oral antibiotic therapy for skeletal infections of children. Antibiotic concentration in suppurative synovial fluid. J. Pediatr., 92:131, 1978.

Newman, J.H.: Review of septic arthritis throughout antibiotic era. Ann. Rheum. Dis., 35:198, 1976.

Norden, C.W.: Experimental osteomyelitis. I.A. Description of the model. J. Infect. Dis., 122:410, 1970.

Polyarthritis and Yersinia enterocolitica infection. (Editorial.) Br. Med. J., 1:404, 1975.

Vaudaux, P., and Waldvogel, F.A.: Gentamicin inactivation in purulent exudates: role of cell lysis. J. Infect. Dis., 142:586, 1980.

Waldvogel, F.A., and Vasey, H.: Osteomyelitis: the past decade. N. Engl. J. Med., 303:360, 1980.

Lyme Disease

Schrock, C.G.: Lyme disease: additional evidence of widespread distribution. Recognition of a tick borne dermatitis-encephalitis, arthritis syndrome in an area of known Ixodes tick distribution. Am. J. Med., 72:700, 1982.

Steere, A.C., et al.: Erythema chronicum migrans and Lyme arthritis. Ann. Intern. Med., 86:685, 1977.

Steere, A.C., and Malawista, S.E.: Cases of Lyme disease in the United States. Locations correlated with distribution of Ixodes olammini. Ann. Intern. Med., 91:730, 1979.

CHAPTER 29

Encephalitis and Parameningeal Infections

M.F. Para and P. Gardner

> **Objective 29–1.** Indicate the approach to a patient with a recently altered mental status in whom an infection is suspected.

The differential diagnosis of a patient with a disturbance of consciousness is broad, especially because several conditions can occur together. A list of the most common causes is included in Table 29–1. The patient's medical history and the physical examination are keys to the diagnosis.

MEDICAL HISTORY

The physician must obtain as much information as possible concerning the patient's medical history and the circumstances surrounding the onset and progression of the mental changes. Particularly suggestive of an infectious cause is a history of headache, fever, concomitant infection in another organ system, and exposure to other sick people. The absence of these findings does not preclude an infectious origin, however. The epidemiologic history, including travel, pets, and occupational exposure, may provide additional important clues.

PHYSICAL EXAMINATION

A thorough physical examination, including a detailed neurologic evaluation, must be performed. The absence of fever should not exclude an infectious disorder because as many as half the patients with a brain abscess are afebrile, and hypothermia is seen in gram-negative sepsis. The patient's skin may yield important clues to central nervous system (CNS) infections due to bacteria, as evidenced by hemorrhagic macules or papules in meningococcal disease; viruses, as in vesicular exanthem in encephalitis due to pox virus; rickettsiae, as manifested by petechiae involving the extremities in Rocky Mountain spotted fever; and collagen vascular diseases. The funduscopic examination of the eye may reveal signs of increased intracranial pressure, metastatic infectious lesions such as tubercles, or evidence of vasculitis such as Roth's spots.

Because most parameningeal infections are secondary to infection of the sinuses, middle ears, or mastoids, careful evaluation of these sites is particularly important. Recurrent meningitis should suggest the possibility of anatomic defects, such as a midline dermal sinus, an occult meningomyelocele, or a cribriform plate defect with leakage of the cere-

Table 29–1. Common Causes of Disturbances of Consciousness

Metabolic Causes
    Electrolyte or glucose imbalances
    Hepatic or renal dysfunction
    Hypoxia or hypercapnia
    Hyper- or hypofunction of the endocrine organs
    Vitamin deficiencies
Vascular and Cardiac Causes
    Hypertensive encephalopathy
    Hemorrhage
    Stroke
    Decreased cardiac output
    Vasculitis, such as collagen vascular and immune complex diseases
Intoxications (or Withdrawal)
    Ethanol
    Drugs, including some antimicrobials
Trauma
Infectious Causes
    Systemic infection
    Primary central nervous system infection
        Focal infections, such as parameningeal infections including abscesses
        Diffuse processes such as meningitis, encephalitis
Tumor
Psychiatric Causes
Epilepsy, Encephalopathy, or Other Noninfectious Primary Central Nervous System Conditions

brospinal fluid (CSF). In evaluating meningismus, the presence of Kernig's and Brudzinski's signs are particularly suggestive of meningitis, but the characteristic nuchal rigidity may be absent, especially in neonates or the elderly.

INITIAL DIAGNOSTIC STUDIES

In general, the diagnostic studies indicated in the evaluation of the obtunded patient include the following:

1. Chemical: glucose, electrolytes, blood urea nitrogen, liver function, and arterial blood gases.
2. Hematologic: complete blood count with examination of the Wright-stained smear.
3. Microbiologic: thorough cultures of sites of inflammation and blood cultures.
4. Serologic: for suspected viral, rickettsial, or mycoplasma infection.
5. Radiologic: skull roentgenograms to detect anatomic abnormalities, evidence of mass effect, or increased intracranial pressure; mastoid and sinus roentgenograms when patient has a history of headache, sinus, or ear infections; chest roentgenogram; and radionuclide scan or computer-assisted tomography when a mass lesion is suspected.
6. Lumbar Puncture: timing is important; early examination of CSF is necessary when acute bacterial meningitis is suspected, but lumbar puncture may precipitate tentorial or foramen magnum herniation in localized parameningeal infections, which cause a mass effect (Table 29–2).

Lumbar Puncture Technique. If lumbar puncture is not contraindicated, the physician should proceed with caution, using a small, 22- or 24-gauge needle. Then, the physician should measure the opening pressure and observe the oscillations of pressure due to respiratory phase and venous pulsation. Jugular manometrics (Queckenstedt's sign) should not be performed in patients with suspected mass lesions or increased intracranial pressure. No more than 6 ml fluid should be removed. Dexamethasone, 10 mg intravenously and then 4 mg every 6 hours, and mannitol, 1 g/kg intravenously, should be given if cerebral edema is present and if the patient's condition deteriorates soon after the lumbar puncture.

Cerebrospinal Fluid (CSF) Examination.

Table 29–2. Considerations Prior to Performing Lumbar Puncture

Contraindications	Indications
1. Papilledema	1. History compatible with acute meningitis, such as infection of under 24 hours' duration in a child
2. Lateralizing signs, except ophthalmoplegia	
3. Radiologic studies suggesting mass, lesion, or increased intracranial pressure	
4. Presence of bacterial infections predisposing to brain abscess, such as cyanotic congenital heart disease or abscess elsewhere	2. Any alteration of mental status in which mass lesion, and local puncture site infection are excluded
5. Infection at the site of puncture	

Table 29–3. Processing of Cerebrospinal Fluid (CFS) Specimens in Patients with Central Nervous System Infections

Tube Number	CSF Volume	Diagnostic Tests
1	1.0–2.0 ml	Culture (use large inoculum on slants)
2	0.5 ml	Protein and glucose (compare with simultaneous blood glucose)

3	1.0 ml	Total white and red blood cell count
		Sediment for:
		  Wright's stain—differential white blood cell count
		  Gram-stained smear
		Other tests (as indicated):
		  Methylene blue smear
		  Wet mount (india ink, other)
		  Acid-fast stain (Ziehl-Neelsen)
		  Immunologic tests

(From Gardner, P., and Provine, H.T.: Manual of Acute Bacterial Infections. Boston, Little, Brown, 1975.)

After measuring the opening pressure, CSF should be collected in 3 tubes, to be sent for testing as outlined in Table 29–3. The CSF in patients with encephalitis or with parameningeal infections characteristically contains a modest number of white blood cells (fewer than 1000/mm^3 and usually fewer than 500/mm^3) with 25% or more mononuclear forms. The CSF glucose level is more than 50% of the simultaneous blood glucose level; the CSF protein level is usually elevated.

With aseptic meningitis, the CSF may show a transient predominance of polymorphonuclear leukocytes early in the infection. CSF glucose levels may be decreased (< 50% of simultaneous blood sugar) in some patients with encephalitis due to herpes simplex or mumps viruses. Herpes simplex viral encephalitis and naegleria meningoencephalitis commonly cause many red blood cells to be present in the CSF. Stained smears of the CSF may reveal bacteria, mycobacteria, fungi, or parasites. Specific CSF antibodies to the agents of syphilis, measles, or rubella are diagnostic if titers are elevated. In addition to the CSF culture, viral cultures of the stool, throat, and blood should be performed if encephalitis is suspected. Because most causes of CNS inflammation, except for bacterial or fungal meningitis, elicit similar alterations of the CSF formula, the observed abnormalities are usually not of great value in differentiating among various potential causes.

If the initial evaluation fails to yield a diagnosis, one should conduct a more detailed and directed search for the cause of the patient's altered mental status. In addition to focusing more intensely on clues in the patient's medical history and the physical examination, the following neurodiagnostic procedures should be considered:

1. Computerized axial tomographic (CT) scanning, if available, is the best noninvasive method for determining intracranial anatomic features. The enhanced uptake of infused dye by inflamed areas usually allows one to differentiate between infectious and noninflammatory processes.
2. The brain scan is a useful technique for demonstrating areas of inflammation in brain tissue, but it lacks the resolution and specificity of CT scans.
3. The electroencephalogram, although helpful in demonstrating diffuse processes and seizure activity, has limited usefulness in most CNS infections because of its poor localization and definition of underlying pathologic processes. In addition, parasellar and posterior fossa lesions are often silent.

If these studies rule out the presence of an intracranial mass, then a lumbar puncture should be performed, if it has not previously been done. If the patient's medical history, the physical examination, and the preliminary laboratory data suggest the presence of a bacterial CNS infection, one should then initiate antibiotic therapy prior to definitive studies. Penicillin G, 20 million U/day intravenously, and chloramphenicol, 50 to 75 mg/kg/day, is reasonable initial therapy. Metronidazole, 500 mg every 8 hours, is also useful in certain CNS infections in which anaerobic organisms are likely pathogens. Because its activity is limited to strict anaerobes, metronidazole is generally used in combination with other agents.

At this point, it is convenient to separate localized infectious processes, detected by physical examination and radiologic studies (see Objective 29–3), from processes with more diffuse CNS involvement (see Objective 29–2).

> **Objective 29–2. Recognize the treatable causes of encephalitis.**

Encephalitis is an inflammatory process involving the parenchymal brain tissue. Patients with encephalitis usually have fever, headache, occasionally seizures or meningeal signs, and cerebral dysfunction evidenced by an altered mental status with generalized (or sometimes localized) neurologic abnormalities.

Encephalitis can be the result of three distinct types of infectious processes. First, the infectious agent can invade the nervous tissue directly, as seen in herpes simplex or rabies viral infections. Second, the infection can reside primarily in the vascular endothelial cells and may give rise to CNS vasculitis, as in rickettsial diseases. Finally, the encephalitis can be caused by immunologic reactivity to nervous tissue with subsequent demyelination, as is occasionally seen following a systemic viral infection or immunization.

It is important to differentiate viral encephalitis, which is mostly untreatable, from the nonviral causes of encephalitis, which are generally treatable. Table 29–4 lists the major nonviral causes of encephalitis, including clinical clues, diagnostic tests, and specific therapy.

The specific diagnosis of viral encephalitis is usually made either by demonstrating a rise in antibody titers to the infecting agent or by a direct demonstration of the virus in culture or by immunofluorescence. The patient's medical history and a knowledge of the possible epidemiologic features are important in focusing the laboratory search for viruses on the most common possibilities. Herpes simplex viral encephalitis has a specific recommended therapy, and therefore the definitive diagnosis of viral encephalitis is therapeutically relevant. The clinical characteristics of common forms of viral encephalitis are reviewed in the following paragraphs.

HERPES SIMPLEX VIRUS

Herpes simplex virus, one of the most common causes of severe encephalitis, should be considered in the diagnosis of any acute encephalitis occurring in the absence of other systemic illness. In adults, the infection is primarily caused by herpes simplex virus 1. The encephalitis occurs sporadically, with no seasonal or epidemic pattern, and its pathogenesis is poorly understood. The clinical features of the illness are variable, although the onset is characteristically abrupt, with fever, focal signs, sensory hallucinations, and focal or generalized seizures. The CSF has a predominance of mononuclear cells, with some red blood cells, but recovery of the virus from CSF culture is rare. Serologic testing lacks specificity and therefore is not helpful. The definitive diagnosis requires identification of the virus by culture or immunofluorescent staining of material from a brain biopsy.

The necessity of performing a brain biopsy has been debated, but careful studies have verified the diagnostic usefulness and low risk of this procedure in patients with suspected herpes simplex encephalitis.

Prompt treatment with vidarabine, 15 mg/kg/day for 10 days, or acyclovir, 750 mg/m^2/day for 7 days, reduces the high mortality rate of herpes simplex encephalitis, although significant residual neurologic impairment is common. The use of these antiviral drugs as a therapeutic and diagnostic test for herpes simplex encephalitis is to be discouraged for several reasons. First, the current formulation of these drugs requires an instillation of large amounts of fluids that can worsen cerebral edema. Second, drug treatment of en-

Table 29–4. Infectious Nonviral Causes of Acute Encephalitis

Infection	Clinical and Epidemiologic Clues	Diagnostic Test	Treatment
Malaria	Travel to endemic area	Blood smear	Quinine hydrochloride
Syphilis (tertiary)	Positive serologic test, tabes dorsalis	CSF examination, Venereal Disease Research Laboratory	Penicillin
Relapsing fever	Tick or louse exposure	Blood smear	Tetracycline, chloramphenicol
Brucellosis	Domestic animal contact, unpasteurized milk ingestion	Positive blood culture, high agglutination titer	Tetracycline and streptomycin
Mycoplasma pneumonia	Associated respiratory symptoms	Complement-fixation	Tetracycline
Toxoplasmosis	Raw meat ingestion, mononucleosis syndrome	Serologic examination	Pyrimethamine and sulfonamide
Trypanosomiasis	Travel to central Africa	Blood smear or node aspirate	Suramin and melarsoprol
Naegleria infection	Freshwater swimming, hemorrhagic CSF	CSF smear and culture	Amphotericin B
Cryptococcosis	Immunosuppression, pulmonary involvement	CSF smear and culture, cryptococcal antigen in CSF	Amphotericin B and 5-fluorocytosine
Tuberculosis	Positive chest roentgenogram, low CSF glucose level, positive Mantoux reaction	CSF culture and smear	Isoniazid, ethambutol, rifampin
Rickettsiosis	Rash, tick, and louse exposure	Weil-Felix or complement-fixation	Tetracycline
Leptospirosis	Animal contact	CSF smear, slide agglutination	Tetracycline
Endocarditis	Cardiopathy, cutaneous signs	Blood culture	Objective 14–4
Listeriosis	Immunosuppression	CSF culture	Ampicillin
Trichinosis	Myositis, periorbital edema, eosinophilia	Serologic examination	Corticosteroids, thiabendazole
Schistosomiasis	Travel to endemic area with water contact	Eggs in stool or urine	Niridazole

CSF, Cerebrospinal fluid

cephalitis of unknown origin often delays the correct diagnosis of a potentially treatable disease. Third, brain biopsy may lead one to diagnose other treatable causes of encephalitis and also allows placement of pressure monitors for better control of cerebral edema.

OTHER HERPESVIRUSES

Herpes Varicella-Zoster Virus. Encephalitis can complicate both varicella and herpes zoster. The CNS findings usually have their onset after the characteristic rash, but they may precede it. A benign, acute cerebellitis is often found, although a rarer multifocal encephalitis can cause death or permanent neurologic sequelae. The value of antiviral drugs in this syndrome has not been determined.

Cytomegalovirus (CMV). This virus often causes encephalitis in the infant with congenital and possibly perinatal infection. In adults with a CMV mononucleosis syndrome or in immunocompromised patients with disseminated disease, encephalitis is a rare manifestation. The diagnosis is made from the clinical picture and from isolation of the virus from the throat, urine, or blood. Serologic testing is not particularly helpful unless seroconversion is observed in paired specimens. The use of vidarabine has not been carefully evaluated in CMV encephalitis. Some success has been reported in CMV retinitis in the immunocompromised patient, but the drug level administered, 20 mg/kg/day, caused significant toxicity.

Epstein-Barr virus (EBV). Infectious mononucleosis, which is caused by this virus, has neurologic complications in fewer than 1% of patients. Encephalitis, whether diffuse or localized to the cerebellum, may be an isolated manifestation of this infection. EBV must be considered even in the absence of a typical mononucleosis syndrome. The CSF may show atypical lymphocytes and EBV antibodies. Serologic diagnosis is based on rising titers of specific EBV antibodies. Recovery is usually complete, although serious illness and death may occur. In subjective clinical observations, corticosteroid therapy has been reported to be beneficial.

ARBOVIRUSES

The arboviruses were grouped together because they are all transmitted by arthropod vectors such as mosquitoes or ticks. This classification was subsequently replaced by one based upon physical and chemical properties. The arboviruses have been found to cross several families of viruses. The ratio of inapparent to clinical infection varies with the infectious agent and may be as high as 99 to 1 in St. Louis encephalitis. The clinical diagnosis of arboviral encephalitis requires an accurate exposure history and knowledge of the public health status of the affected area. The specific diagnosis is primarily made by serologic determinations, which become positive about 10 days into the illness. Viral isolation from blood or brain biopsy may also be helpful, particularly in tick-borne viruses. Table 29–5 lists the major causes of arboviral encephalitis, the age group primarily affected, and the geographic region in which the disease is prevalent.

PARAMYXOVIRUSES

Encephalitis can occur as an uncommon complication of systemic infections with mumps and measles viruses. Prior to the widespread use of mumps vaccine, mumps was a leading cause of viral encephalitis. Clinically, both mumps and measles viruses produce a nonfocal encephalitis that may be more the result of a hypersensitivity phenomenon than viral cellular destruction. Mumps encephalitis can occur in the absence of parotitis; the patient may have a low CSF glucose level. The diagnosis of mumps can be made serologically or by isolating the virus from the saliva, the urine, or occasionally, the CSF. Although measles virus can be isolated from saliva, serodiagnostic techniques such as hemagglutination inhibition are most frequently used. Both viral encephalitides can have serious neurologic sequelae.

ENTEROVIRUSES

The diagnosis of enteroviral encephalitis is suggested by the epidemiologic features of the infections. In temperate climates, infection is most common in summer and early fall. In addition, certain clinical syndromes, such as herpangina, pleurodynia, and pleuropericarditis, may occur among the patient's close contacts or immediate family and should suggest an enteroviral outbreak. CNS infections caused by echo- or coxsackieviruses most commonly cause aseptic meningitis; encephalitis is much less frequent. The encephalitis may appear as a focal process, occasionally with a flaccid motor paralysis resembling poliomyelitis. The diagnosis is made by viral isolation from saliva, CSF, or feces. Because of the multiple enteroviral immunotypes, serologic diagnosis is not usually practical, except for poliovirus. The prognosis of these diseases is generally good, but permanent neurologic damage may occur. Patients with agammaglobulinemia often have protracted enteroviral CNS infections.

ARENAVIRUSES

Lymphocytic choriomeningitis virus is an arenavirus that typically causes meningitis or encephalitis. The disease is most commonly contracted from mice, but pet and laboratory hamsters have also been implicated in outbreaks. A characteristic clinical feature of the illness is its biphasic nature. After an initial

Table 29–5. Arboviral Encephalitis

Virus	Geographic Distribution	Age Group Most Affected	Mortality Rate (%)	Sequelae
Mosquito-borne				
Eastern equine encephalitis	East coast of United States and Canada	Children	50–75	In all survivors
Western equine encephalitis	Western Hemisphere	All, especially children	< 10	Only in < 1-year-old children
Venezuelan equine encephalitis	Southern United States, Central America, northern South America	Children	<1	Few
St. Louis encephalitis	North, Central, and South America	Adults, increasing with age	< 10, increasing with age	—
Japanese B encephalitis	Southwestern and Eastern Asia, Pacific Islands	All	20–50, increasing with age in children	10–20%
Murray Valley encephalitis	Northern Australia and New Guinea	Children under 10 years	> 40	Frequent
West Nile	Africa, Middle East, southern Eurasia	Adults, increasing with age	Low except in elderly	—
California	United States	Children under 15 years	< 5	Few
Tick-borne				
Russian spring-summer encephalitis (also caused by raw milk ingestion)	Eurasia	Adults	30	20% with paralysis
Central Europe tick-borne	Eurasia	Adults	< 5	Few
Louping ill	Great Britian	Adults	< 5	Few
Colorado tick fever	United States	Children	< 5	Few
Powassan	Canada, northern United States	All	High	Frequent

phase characterized by fever, myalgia, respiratory symptoms, and occasionally parotitis or orchitis, the disease begins to resolve. The patient may then recover completely or may suffer a second phase characterized by the abrupt onset of headache and meningeal signs. As with enteroviral infections, aseptic meningitis is more common than encephalitis. Depressed CSF glucose levels are sometimes found. The diagnosis is based upon viral isolation from the blood or CSF, or by complement-fixing serologic testing, which becomes positive in the first 2 weeks of illness. Recovery is usually complete.

ENCEPHALOMYELITIS FOLLOWING INFECTION AND VACCINATION

Encephalitis or myelitis may follow a variety of infections and vaccinations (Table 29–6). The pathogenesis of this disorder may involve the sensitization of the patient to myelin antigens. Although such clearly appears to have been the case when rabies vaccination was prepared from animal brain tissue, a primary immune pathogenesis for other agents has not been proved, and it is often difficult to separate immune from infectious processes. Clinically, the onset of the disease is usually abrupt with fever, headache, altered consciousness, and seizures. Differentiating acute infections from postinfectious encephalitis may be impossible. Treatment in either case should be supportive and should try to reduce cerebral edema. Corticosteroid therapy should be reserved unless other measures, such as mannitol administration, are unsuccessful.

Table 29–6. Agents Associated with Postinfectious and Postvaccination Encephalitis

Viruses	Bacteria	Vaccines
Rubella	Mycoplasma	Rabies
Influenza	Bordetella	Influenza
Mumps	pertussis	Tetanus
Measles	Group A	Pertussis
Vaccinia	strepto-	Vaccinia
Herpes simplex	coccus	
Varicella-zoster		
Variola		
Epstein-Barr		
Other respiratory		

REYE'S SYNDROME

Reye's syndrome is an acute encephalopathy with fatty infiltration and dysfunction of the liver following viral infections. The pathogenesis of the disorder and relationships among the virus, the brain, and the liver are not known. The disease occurs in children 2 to 16 years old and commonly follows influenza B infections, although it may occur after influenza A, varicella, or other viral infections. Typically, 4 to 6 days after the viral infection, the patient has sudden and persistent nausea and vomiting, followed by changes in mental status, seizures, and sometimes coma. The CSF is normal, but laboratory findings reveal liver dysfunction with high blood ammonia and low blood glucose levels. Cerebral edema is marked, and therapy should be directed at lowering the intracranial pressure and maintaining the blood glucose levels. Because epidemiologic evidence suggests that Reye's syndrome is linked with aspirin usage, some recommend that salicylates be avoided during respiratory illnesses in childhood.

> **Objective 29–3.** Diagnose an infection in a patient with localized symptoms of the central nervous system.

Localized pyogenic infections (parameningeal infections) of the CNS generally result from the spread of infection from contiguous or distant foci, but they can be caused by direct, penetrating injuries to the head (see Fig. 29–1 for anatomic relationships). Because of the localized nature of these processes, which include brain abscess, subdural empyema, cerebral epidural abscess, and intracranial phlebitis, these diagnoses must be considered in patients with focal neurologic signs, especially if other foci of infection are present. As previously discussed, focal neurologic findings sometimes occur in encephalitis caused by herpes simplex or other neurotropic viruses. The clinical and epidemiologic features and the radiologic examinations usually allow one to distinguish bacterial from viral causes, however.

Parameningeal infections are diagnosed by finding a focal neurologic abnormality, such as hemiplegia, in the appropriate setting, such as in chronic otitis or mastoid disease; and by confirmatory radiologic studies. Where available, computerized axial tomography (CT) scanning offers the best definition of intracranial anatomic features, but early in the course of intracranial infection, the radionuclide brain scan may be more sensitive in detecting lesions that have not yet suppurated (Fig. 29–2). These techniques have diminished the need for angiography in the evaluation of parameningeal infection.

In all types of parameningeal infections, examination of the CSF characteristically reveals a mild pleocytosis (fewer than 500 cells), predominately mononuclear cells, and elevated protein and normal glucose levels. Because the CSF examination is of little differential value, and because lumbar puncture carries a significant risk of herniation due to mass effect, the physician should not perform a lumbar puncture without clinical and radiologic signs that the risk of herniation is low.

BRAIN ABSCESS

In adults, brain abscesses most commonly arise by direct extension or retrograde spread of infection through communicating veins from contiguous areas of suppuration in paranasal and otic sites. The abscesses associated with parasinus infections are usually single and are seen in the frontal and, less com-

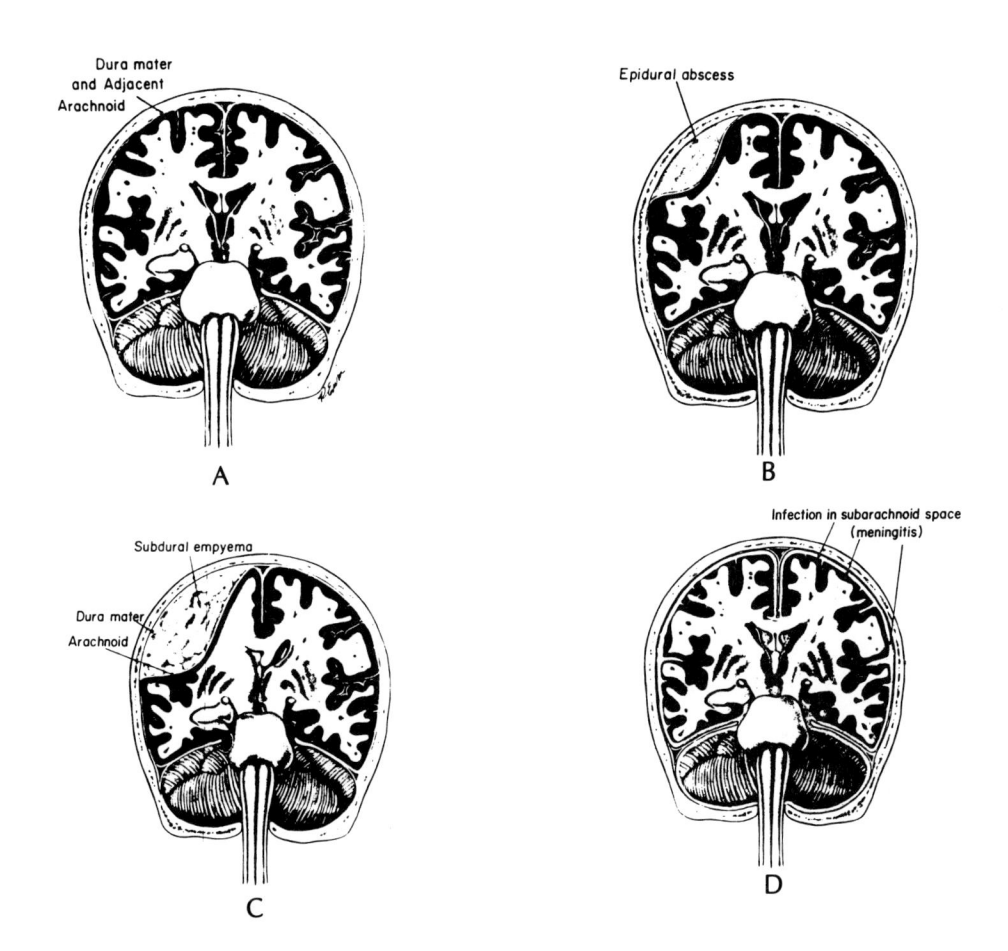

Fig. 29–1. The cranial meninges. *A*, Normal anatomic relationships; *B*, epidural abscess; *C*, subdural empyema; *D*, meningitis. (From Mandell, G.L., Douglas, R.G., Jr., and Bennett, J. (eds.): Principles and Practice of Infectious Disease. New York, John Wiley & Sons, 1979.)

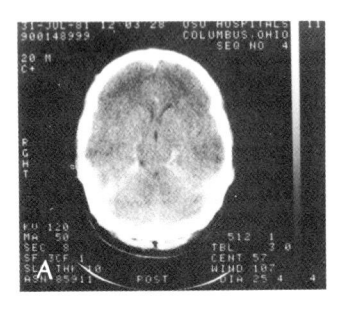

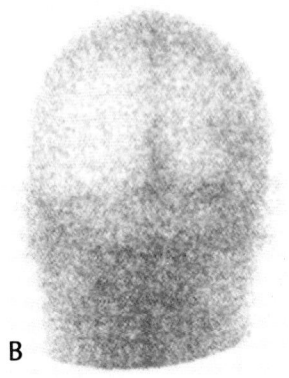

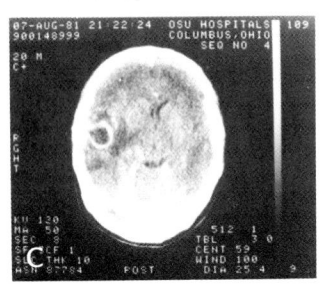

Fig. 29–2. Scans from a 30-year-old patient with chronic, right-sided otitis media and left hemianopia. Upon presentation the CT scan *(A)* was normal, but a brain scan *(B)* on the same day showed right-sided uptake (posterior view). One week later, the CT scan with enhancement *(C)* showed the developing brain abscess.

monly, temporal lobes. Otic infections mainly give rise to temporal lobe abscesses, although the cerebellum and, rarely, parietal lobe may be involved. Approximately one-third of brain abscesses arise from bacteremia from distant infections.

Congenital heart disease with right-to-left shunting is the most common setting for brain abscess in children. Abscesses resulting from bacteremia are often multiple and occur in the white matter of the brain in the distribution of the middle cerebral artery.

Clinical Features. Brain abscesses are intracranial masses that usually cause headache, altered consciousness, nausea, and vomiting. Fever is found in fewer than half of the patients. Specific neurologic findings reflect the location of the inflammatory mass; for example, cerebellar abscesses cause ataxia and nystagmus, whereas temporal lobe abscesses result in aphasia or visual-field defects.

Cause. The etiologic agents of brain abscesses are determined by the primary focus of infection. Otorhinogenic abscesses generally contain a mixture of organisms, with anaerobes predominating. Causative bacteria include aerobic and anaerobic streptococci, bacteroides, fusobacterium, Haemophilus, *Staphylococcus aureus*, and occasionally enteric pathogens or pseudomonas. Because the same organisms are often found in suppurative lung processes, these bacteria and nocardia must also be considered when brain abscesses occur in association with lung abscesses. Direct penetrating or surgically related abscesses are most commonly due to *Staphylococcus aureus. Entamoeba histolytica* and cerebral cysticercosis should be considered if the patient's dietary or travel history suggests exposure to the causative parasites.

Treatment. The initial management of brain abscesses involves the relief of increased intracranial pressure and the proper choice of antibiotics, followed by optimally timed surgical drainage or excision. Mannitol and corticosteroids may be indicated to control brain edema. The selection of antibiotics is determined by the primary source of infection. Penicillin, 20 million U/day, and chloramphenicol, 50 to 75 mg/kg/day, is appropriate initial therapy in most cases. Methicillin, 12 to 16 g/day, penetrates brain abscesses and is recommended when *Staphylococcus aureus* is the suspected cause. Intravenous metronidazole has excellent activity against many anaerobes, including *Bacteroides fragilis*, and it penetrates brain abscesses well. Several reports have confirmed the effectiveness of metronidazole against parameningeal infections. Because most infections are mixed, metronidazole should be used in combination with another agent effective against aerobes, such as penicillin G.

Certain patients with clinical and radiographic evidence of brain abscess are diagnosed at an early stage and are cured by prolonged antibiotic therapy alone. The majority of patients, however, require surgical drainage or excision of the abscess. Indications for surgical intervention include (1) evidence of an uncontrolled mass effect, (2) failure of the patient to show steady clinical and radiologic improvement, and (3) evidence of encapsulation of the abscess.

SUBDURAL EMPYEMA

Although subdural empyema is not as common as brain abscess, the characteristic and rapidly progressive course of this disorder presents an urgent need for diagnosis and neurosurgical drainage. In adults, the pathogenesis of subdural empyema is most commonly related to an extension of otorhinogenic infection through the valveless emissary veins into the potential space between the dura mater and arachnoidea. In the cranium, this space is bounded only at the midline by the falx cerebri and at the base by the tentorium cerebelli, so infection spreads widely over the surface of the brain. Subsequent cortical thrombophlebitis and infarction contribute to the clinical picture.

Clinical Features. The accelerated nature of the disease, the focal neurologic signs, and the nuchal rigidity seen in a patient with sinusitis distinguish subdural empyema from other intracranial disorders. Headache, vomiting, fever, and meningeal signs are generally followed within 1 to 2 days by localizing neurologic deficits and, occasionally, by seizures. Lumbar puncture is extremely hazardous and should be absolutely avoided.

Diagnosis. Because papilledema is seen in fewer than half the patients and radionuclide scans are not accurate, CT scans or angiograms are required to confirm the diagnosis.

Treatment. Initial medical therapy should be directed toward the management of intracranial hypertension as an emergency, as outlined previously. Penicillin, 20 million U/day, chloramphenicol 50 to 75 mg/kg/day, and a penicillinase-resistant penicillin should be administered. Surgical drainage of the empyema by bur holes or craniotomy should be performed on an emergency basis. Aerobic and anaerobic cultures, as well as Gram staining of smears from material obtained surgically may help one to choose the appropriate antibiotic. Recurrent collections of pus in the subdural space often require repeated drainage. Antimicrobial therapy should be continued for at least 3 weeks.

Association with Meningitis. Subdural empyema can complicate pyogenic meningitis in young children and is most frequently seen in *Haemophilus influenzae* infections. Lethargy, persistent fever, bulging fontanelles, and focal neurologic signs suggest the diagnosis, which can be confirmed by CT scanning. Subdural taps can be both diagnostic and therapeutic. Antibiotics directed against the pathogen responsible for the meningitis should be continued.

EPIDURAL ABSCESS

Like subdural empyema epidural abscesses arise from otorhinogenic or operative foci of infection and are almost always associated with osteomyelitis of the skull. These abscesses form by separation of the dura mater from the bone of the skull to which the meninges are bound. Because of this anatomic configuration, the infection is usually local, is limited in size, and consequently does not increase intracranial pressure. Thus, the clinical manifestations of epidural abscess may be subtle and may include persistent headache, fever, sinusitis, and local tenderness. The diagnosis can be made by angiography or CT scanning. The choice of antibiotics, as mentioned previously, should be guided by the primary source of infection. Because *Staphylococcus aureus* is frequently the cause, a penicillinase-resistant antibiotic such as nafcillin should be included in the drug regimen. Surgical drainage should be performed if the patient has an increase in intracranial pressure or coexisting subdural empyema. The abscess may resolve following prolonged antimicrobial therapy alone, however, if the primary source of infection is appropriately managed.

Spinal Epidural Abscess. In the spine, epidural abscesses are not confined because the dura mater is separated from the bone by loose, vascular, fatty tissues, and infection easily spreads longitudinally. These abscesses usually arise by hematogenous spread or by direct extension of vertebral osteomyelitis. The primary site of infection is often the skin, and *Staphylococcus aureus* is the pathogen in at least three-fourths of the cases. Streptococci and gram-negative rods are also found, and tuberculosis should be considered in chronic epidural infection. Clinically, the mass effect and inflammation cause symptoms to progress from localized back pain to radicular pain to signs of spinal cord compression with weakness and paralysis. In addition to the localized tenderness and pain, which can be severe, nuchal rigidity and signs of systemic infection with fever and leukocytosis are common. Once suspected, the diagnosis can be confirmed by myelographic study or CT scanning.

One must exercise extreme caution to avoid introducing bacteria into the subarachnoid space during the spinal tap. The puncture should be performed away from the site of tenderness, and the needle should be advanced slowly with suction. The CSF characteristically contains a moderate-to-high protein elevation, few inflammatory cells, and normal glucose levels. A penicillinase-resistant penicillin should be given, and an emergency laminectomy should be performed to prevent permanent loss of spinal cord function.

INTRACRANIAL THROMBOPHLEBITIS

Thrombophlebitis of the intracranial venous sinuses is a complication of either otorhinogenic or skin infection that has spread to the CNS or extension of other paramenigeal infections.

Clinical Features. The clinical manifestations of this disorder vary with the site of involvement, but high fevers, systemic toxicity, increased intracranial pressure, and bacteremia are characteristic. Thrombosis of the small cortical veins is seen in bacterial meningitis and is usually manifested by stupor, focal neurologic deficits, and seizures. The most commonly involved dural sinuses are the cavernous, lateral, and sagittal sinuses. The clinical manifestations of cavernous sinus thrombosis, which is usually associated with facial and paranasal sinus infections, reflect the passage of cranial nerves III, IV, V, and VII through the sinus and include diplopia, ophthalmoplegia, proptosis, conjunctival chemosis, and papilledema. The onset is usually rapid and initially involves only one eye, but an extension of the thrombosis may produce a bilateral disorder. Lateral sinus thrombosis follows otic infections, especially chronic mastoiditis, and is usually manifested by pain and swelling behind the ear, headache, and, in some cases, seizures. Septic thrombosis of the superior sagittal sinus can occur as an extension of lateral or cavernous sinus thrombophlebitis and can complicate meningitis and parameningeal infections. The condition is asymptomatic unless the cortical veins of the superior cerebrum are compromised; then unilateral or bilateral paresis occurs, especially in the legs. If the thrombosis is extensive, parenchymal infarction and abscess formation can result.

Diagnosis. The diagnosis of septic intracranial thrombophlebitis is confirmed by demonstrating diminished filling of the veins during the venous phase of carotid arteriography or infusion CT scanning. Parameningeal infections, which can cause or complicate thrombophlebitis, can be difficult to differentiate clinically from the thrombotic process, but control of infection is the primary consideration in both processes.

Treatment. Therapy should initially be directed toward control of intracranial hypertension and seizures. Antimicrobial therapy should include the administration of a penicillinase-resistant semisynthetic penicillin, as well as urgent surgical drainage of abscesses and, if necessary, debridement of other infected tissues. Because of the risk of hemorrhage in the infarcted areas, anticoagulants are not recommended.

SUGGESTED READINGS

Acha, P., and Szyfres, B.: Zoonoses and Communicable Diseases Common to Man and Animals. Scientific publication no. 354. Pan American Health Organization, 1980.

Brewer, N.S., MacCarty, C.S., and Wellman, W.E.: Brain abscess: a review of recent experience. Ann. Intern. Med., 82:571, 1975.

Gardner, P., and Provine, H.T.: Manual of Acute Bacterial Infections. Boston, Little, Brown, 1984.

Kaufman, D., et al.: Subdural empyema: analysis of 17 recent cases and review of the literature. Medicine, 54:485, 1975.

Weisberg, L.A.: Computed tomography in the diagnosis of intracranial disease. Ann. Intern. Med., 91:87, 1979.

Whitley, R., et al.: Herpes simplex encephalitis: vidarabine therapy and diagnostic problems. N. Engl. J. Med., 304:313, 1981.

CHAPTER 30

Acute Infectious Meningitis

M. Armengaud and C. Cherubin

> **Objective 30–1. Specify the clinical indications for a lumbar puncture.**

The prognosis of acute meningitis is so closely tied to its early diagnosis and prompt treatment that this objective is essential. Because the major means of diagnosis is the lumbar puncture (LP), one must recognize the early indications for this procedure. LP is immediately indicated in all patients who have fever in combination with any recent neurologic or psychiatric alteration. The indication for LP is also obvious when nuchal rigidity or Kernig's and Brudzinski's signs are present or when the patient complains of a severe, persistent, pathologic headache and vomiting. Other clear indications are encephalitic signs, coma, and acute delirium, even in the absence of actual meningeal signs. Some patients, however, require more clinical judgment. Typical symptoms are often lacking in alcoholic, elderly, debilitated, and immunosuppressed patients, in whom fever may not be present. Any recent alteration of consciousness should lead one to suspect the diagnosis of meningitis, even in absence of the classic signs. Newborns present an even more difficult diagnostic problem because their axial musculature is generally unable to produce neck rigidity. For this reason, LP is necessary in all neonates with: (1) fever or hypothermia; (2) apnea, respiratory distress, or cyanosis; (3) convulsions; (4) lethargy or failure to awaken.

> **Objective 30–2. Perform a lumbar puncture and direct examination of the cerebrospinal fluid.**

Preliminary examination of the fundus of the patient's eyes should be performed before the LP. Papilledema indicates increased intracranial pressure of several days' duration and is unusual in meningitis of recent onset. The LP may then be deferred until an emergency CT scan of the head has been taken. One should take the same precaution if focal signs suggest a possible intracranial mass. Otherwise, one should proceed to the LP. If an emergency CT scan cannot be obtained, the LP must be done, even with the assumed risk.

TECHNIQUE FOR LUMBAR PUNCTURE

Ideally, the physician should have one assistant to hold the patient in proper position and another to pass the necessary instruments. The procedure tray should contain several LP needles, a manometer tube, and several sterile, dry tubes for bacteriologic, cytologic, and biochemical analysis. Some trays contain chocolate and blood agar media for direct inoculation, although this method has no advantage over the immediate transport of the specimens to the laboratory.

The patient is held in either a seated or a recumbent position, bent forward to eliminate the lordotic lumbar curve. The needle is pushed anteriorly at the junction of the lines connecting the dorsal spinal processes and the line connecting the two posterior iliac crests, that is, the horizontal and vertical lines crossing at interspace L4 to L5 or L3 to L4. The needle is directed slightly superiorly in the direction of the navel. The obturator should be in place to avoid clogging the bore with skin or tissue fragments and pushing them into the spinal canal. A trained clinician feels the give of the needle when it passes through the dura mater and stops before passing into the anterior venous plexus. The flow of the cerebrospinal fluid (CSF) can be controlled with the obturator, to prevent sudden decompression of CSF and, perhaps, brain stem herniation when the fluid is under increased pressure.

EXAMINATION OF THE CEREBROSPINAL FLUID

The CSF should be delivered to the laboratory personally. Gross examination of the CSF yields important information at the patient's bedside. If the CSF appears crystal clear, fewer than 300 cells/ml are present. Shining a bright light across the tube of CSF may reveal a slight turbidity, even at this low concentration of cells. Naturally, this examination must be supplemented by an actual cell count in a blood cell counting chamber. Cloudy or turbid fluid that one can read through probably contains around 300 to 1000 cells/ml, and completely opaque fluid has more than a thousand (Table 30–1).

Gram staining of the centrifuged sediment should be performed immediately. If the CSF is grossly purulent, a drop of the uncentrifuged fluid will suffice. Because white blood cells cannot be easily identified by Gram staining, Wright's or Giemsa staining of the sediment is also necessary. When neurosyphilis is considered in the diagnosis, one should perform a serologic test for syphilis, such as the Venereal Disease Research Laboratory (VDRL) test. In a patient with chronic meningitis, a cryptococcal antigen and a culture for *Mycobacterium tuberculosis* and, in the American Southwest and California, a fungal culture for coccidioides are also indicated. The CSF samples cultured for meningeal pathogens are routinely inoculated onto blood and chocolate agar plates and, perhaps, onto a tube of thioglycolate broth and incubated in a 10% carbon dioxide atmosphere. Counterimmunoelectrophoresis or slide agglutination tests for the presence of bacterial capsular antigens in the CSF may be helpful, especially for *Haemophilus influenzae*, type B, but they do not replace properly performed cultures.

To be meaningful, the patient's CSF glucose level must be compared to the simultaneous serum glucose level. For greater accuracy, both should be obtained before an intravenous infusion of glucose is started or, if not, at least 30 minutes to 2 hours after a steady intravenous flow has been established. Abnormally low glucose levels, < 30 to 50% of the serum values, are seen in 60 to 75% of individuals with bacterial meningitis. The chloride determination, far less reliable, is a remnant of the early biochemical investigations of biologic fluids. This level is increased in purulent fluids (> 7 mg/L; > 120 mEq) but it may be decreased in tuberculous meningitis because it is tied to the serum sodium concentration, which is sometimes low in tuberculous meningitis, and to the protein level. One sees a decrease in pH, an increase in lactic acid, and a decrease in the P_{O_2} in both purulent and tuberculous meningitis (< 30 mmHg), as well as an elevation of the lactic dehydrogenase isoenzymes in pyogenic meningitis.

Table 30–1. Comparative Cerebrospinal Fluid (CSF) Findings in Meningitis

Type of Meningitis	CSF Pressure (mm H$_2$O)	Appearance of CSF	Numbers of Cells	Differential Cell Count	Protein Level (mg/100 ml)	Glucose Level (mg/100 ml)	Microscopic Findings
Pyogenic	Usually elevated, average 300	Slightly cloudy to purulent	Several hundred to thousands; may be low early in disease	80% polymorphonuclear leukocytes PMN*	100–500, sometimes >1000	<40 in 50% of cases	Organism on smear > 50%; organism grown ∼ 80%
Tuberculous	Usually elevated > 500, late in course of illness	Clear to slightly cloudy	25–100, may be ≥500	Lymphocytes predominate, except in early stages	100–200 (early), > 1 g† (late)	< 50 in 67% of cases	Organism seldom seen, grows ∼ 50%
Viral	Normal to slightly elevated, ∼ 100–150‡	Clear to slightly hazy	5–300, may be > 1000	Lymphocytes predominate after the first day	≤ 100	Usually normal	Require tissue culture for isolation of virus
None (normal)	80–150	Clear	<2	All lymphocytes	< 50	50–60% that of blood glucose level	No bacteria

*May be a lymphocyte predominance with listeriosis
†Particularly high if there is CSF block
‡High numbers of cells, polymorphonuclear leukocytes on the first day, with elevated protein levels and CSF pressure are seen in mumps, some coxsackievirus B, and other enterovirus aseptic meningitis cases; that is, they may imitate pyogenic meningitis successfully. In lymphocytic choriomeningitis, several thousand lymphocytes are generally present in the CSF.

> **Objective 30–3. Identify the bacteria causing the meningitis with the help of all available clinical and laboratory evidence.**

Many agents are capable of producing a purulent meningitis, and the cause must be known, or at least knowledgeably hypothesized, to prescribe appropriate therapy.

MENINGOCOCCAL MENINGITIS

This disease occurs all year round, but is more common during the colder months in the temperate zone. In North America as well as in Europe, this disease has an 8- to 11-year cycle, for reasons unknown, and therefore the yearly incidence varies. In addition, meningococcal meningitis occurs in sporadic outbreaks, as in Brazil several years ago, and seems to have a predilection for crowds, as in barracks, boarding schools, camps for displaced persons, and residential institutions.

Not all the meningococcal serogroups behave the same way or have the same distribution. *Neisseria meningitidis* serogroup A, which has a greater epidemic capacity, ravages subsaharan Africa and is the major serogroup in Europe. This strain left North America long ago, although some signs point to its return. On the other hand, serogroups B and C are the most common new groups in North America. Further, at least one-third of the cases of meningococcal meningitis are due to recently identified serogroups, especially Y and W135, but also X, Z, and 29E, although these serogroups produce septicemia more frequently than they do meningitis.

Clinical clues for the recognition of a meningococcal origin of meningitis include the epidemiologic context, the abrupt onset of the disease, a concomitant herpes labialis (also seen with pneumococci, however), and certain other manifestations besides the meningitis. In fact, in addition to purulent meningitis, meningococci may produce a variety of syndromes ranging from a fulminant septicemia with shock and ecchymotic or necrotic skin lesions (see Plate 5A and B) and visceral hemorrhages, particularly adrenal (Waterhouse-Friderichsen syndrome), to subacute or persistent septicemia with pustular or petechial skin lesions, to polyserositis, monoarthritis, or pericarditis. Although the disease mainly affects children, adolescents, and, to a lesser extent, young adults, it may occur in all age groups.

The definitive diagnosis depends both upon the observation of typical morphologic features on the Gram stain (Fig. 30–1) and upon growing the organism from the patient's CSF. Owing to the fragility of the organism, this culture is estimated to be successful less than two thirds of the time. One can also demonstrate the presence of capsular antigens in the CSF by counterimmunoelectrophoresis; however, because of the multiplicity of serogroups, this procedure is not widely used.

Thus far, all meningococci remain sensitive to penicillin G.

PNEUMOCOCCI

The pneumococci, organisms of the species *Streptococcus pneumoniae,* are the most common cause of bacterial meningitis in North America, affecting both children and middle-aged to elderly adults. This organism produces a sporadic, nonepidemic disease with a clearly demonstrable peak in the late winter in the temperate zones. Pneumococcal meningitis is probably the result of a hematogenous dissemination of the pathogen from the respiratory tract, and in perhaps one case out of four, a pulmonic infiltrate is present on the chest roentgenogram. On Gram staining, the organism appears as a gram-positive diplococcus; the so-called lancet shape refers to the common willow-blade lancet of the nineteenth century.

Certain groups of individuals are predisposed to pneumococcal meningitis (see boxed text). When a patient with meningitis belongs to one of these groups, a pneumococcal cause is probable.

Other clinical findings that suggest a pneumococcal etiology are the patient's age (pneumococci are the most common cause of men-

MENINGOCOCCI

Meningococci, or organisms of the species *Neisseria meningitidis,* are the most common cause of acute bacterial meningitis in continental Europe and the second or third most common cause, depending on the epidemic cycle, in North America. These organisms appear, on Gram staining, as gram-negative kidney- or coffee-bean-shaped diplococci, both intra- and extracellular (Fig. 30–1), and are identical in appearance to the gonococci.

Meningococci die rapidly on cooling and drying. Isolation requires rapid inoculation of chocolate agar plates immediately incubated at 37° C. The CSF specimen should be brought to the laboratory in the hand or at least the breast pocket of the physician because the organism dies when cooled to room temperature. If neither the laboratory nor the culture plate is available, the CSF specimen can be kept in an incubator at 37° C for several hours. Incubation should take place in a humid atmosphere enriched with carbon dioxide. In less than 24 hours, small, translucent, smooth colonies can be seen that, along with the biochemical reactions, differentiate the meningococci clearly from the nonpathogenic pharyngeal neisseria species, which are seen on nearly all throat cultures.

The serologic properties of the capsule distinguish the various serogroups, which are designated A, B, C, D, X, Y, Z, W135, and 29E (Z[1]). These serogroups, as well as the biotypes, lysotypes, and bacteriocinotypes are useful in epidemiologic studies. To some extent, the serogroups are also linked to their susceptibility to sulfonamides and to an apparently type-specific immunity, although to little else of importance, as far as we know at present. The reservoir is entirely in man. Transmission is from person to person, probably, considering the fragility of the organism, by respiratory droplets from asymptomatic carriers. All contacts may become carriers; the duration of the carrier state depends on the presence of antibody. For the most part, this carrier state is asymptomatic and may be related to mucosal adherence properties of the strain of meningococcus. Fewer than 1 in 500 or 1000 individuals develops a hematogenous dissemination resulting in septicemia or meningitis.

Nothing, in our current knowledge, can explain why so few individuals develop the disease and why most others become asymptomatic carriers in the course of an epidemic. Group-specific immunity clearly exists, as evidenced by the successful trials of serogroup A and C meningococcal vaccine. Immunization for serogroup B apparently presents a more complex problem.

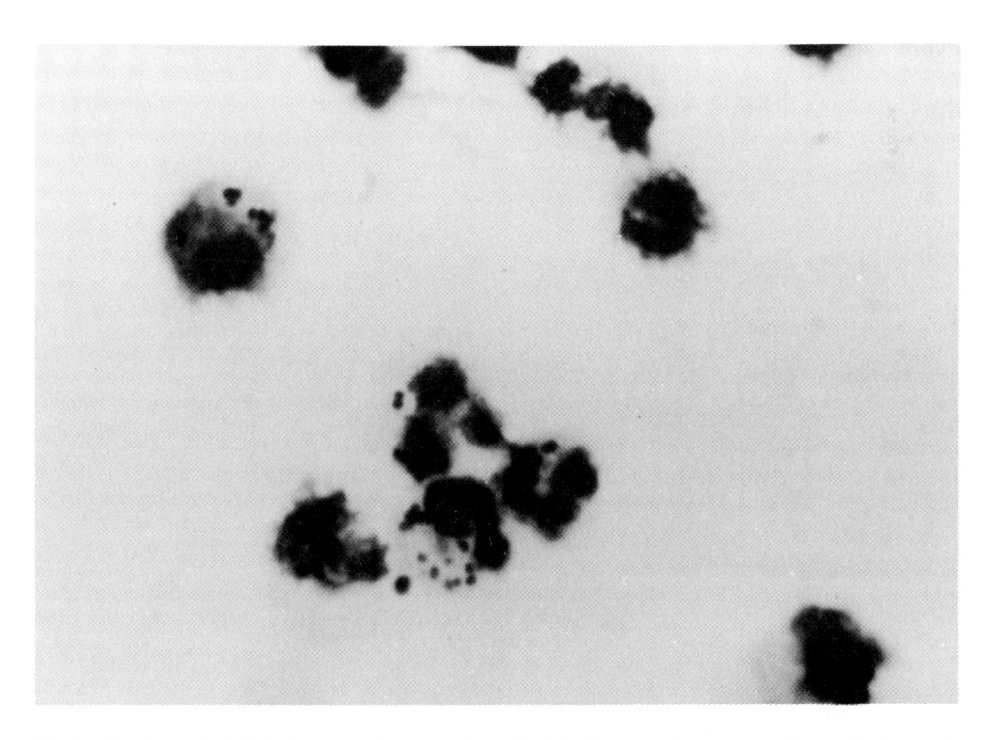

Fig. 30–1. Cerebrospinal fluid in a meningococcal meningitis. Polymorphonuclear cells and intra- and extracellular gram-negative cocci are visible. (Courtesy of Dr. J.C. Pechère.)

ingitis in North American adults, especially the elderly), the season of the year (late winter), a concomitant lobar pneumonia, coma (especially in alcoholics, the elderly, or in patients who have not sought prompt medical attention), and possibly, the presence of a herpesviral infection (more common in the literature than in clinical experience).

The pneumococci are generally exquisitely sensitive to penicillin G. Chloramphenicol is usually recommended for patients who are hypersensitive to penicillin, but it may not be as effective as penicillin against this disease. Further, strains of penicillin-resistant pneumococci have been isolated in South Africa and sporadically, although rarely, in other parts of the world. The only two agents effective, at least in the laboratory, against these strains and capable of providing effective CSF levels are vancomycin and cefotaxime.

HAEMOPHILUS INFLUENZAE

This bacterium is the second and third most common cause of bacterial meningitis in North America and Europe, respectively. It seems less common in continental Europe than in England and North America, where it is the most frequent cause of purulent meningitis between the ages of 6 months and 6 years. In the adult, it is nevertheless responsible for at least 2 to 3% of the diagnosed cases. Usually, no associated pulmonary infiltrate is seen, although preliminary respiratory symptoms are noted for 2 to 3 days. The infection most probably disseminates from the respiratory tract. Because it is an encapsulated organism, *H. influenzae* shares with the pneumococcus some of the same high-risk groups of patients. Six capsular polysaccharide antigenic groups have been identified, of which type b is the primary pathogen. The nonencapsulated and hence nontypable strains are important only in otitis in children and in bronchitis in adults. Because a single pathogenic capsular type is known, counterimmunoelectrophoresis or slide agglutination tests can be used to make the diagnosis from the soluble capsular antigen present in the CSF in patients with meningitis.

Haemophilus influenzae is as fragile an organism as the meningococcus or pneumococcus. Its growth requires hemin (X) and nicotinamide-adenine dinucleotide (NAD) (V) provided by chocolate agar, as well as a hu-

---

GROUPS AT RISK FOR PNEUMOCOCCAL MENINGITIS

Individuals with a variety of underlying diseases or physical states are at a high risk for pneumococcal septicemia and meningitis.

The first group of patients includes those with conditions that interfere with the capacity for clearing the blood of invading encapsulated organisms, such as the pneumococcus. An observable portal of entry is not usually seen in these patients, although the respiratory tract is the undoubted origin of the infection. Further, these patients are prone to a fulminant septicemia that is so rapidly fatal that the meningitis component may not have the chance to develop. This group includes individuals with primary or secondary hypogammaglobulinemia, those lacking a spleen, patients with severe neutropenia or phagocytic and leukotactic deficiencies (probably, patients with sickle cell anemia fall into this group), and those receiving immunosuppressant therapy.

The second and largest group includes severe alcoholics. No other group has as high a mortality rate, except for the aged, who are predisposed to pneumococcal pneumonia with overwhelming septicemia. The frequency of pneumococcal meningitis in alcoholics parallels the high incidence in these patients of pneumococcal pneumonias; the reasons for this phenomenon are not fully understood, but these diseases may be secondary to the following: (1) aspiration of upper pharyngeal secretions due to obtundation of the glottal reflex; (2) decreased tissue stores of neutrophils following bone marrow arrest due to alcohol toxicity or folic acid deficiency; (3) decreased leukotaxis resulting from metabolic acidosis; or (4) invasion of the lower respiratory tract by the pharyngeal flora in chronic bronchitis, present in most alcoholics. A radiologically evident pulmonary infiltrate is often seen in the alcoholic as well as in the aged patient.

In the third group of patients at risk, the infection has a nonpulmonary portal of entry. These patients have a CSF leak into a sinus space, either from a congenital malformation or from a fracture at the base of the skull. These patients often suffer repeated episodes of meningitis, in which the pneumococcus is the most frequent pathogen. Pneumococcal meningitis can also be secondary to pneumococcal sinusitis, whether frontal, ethmoid, or sphenoid, or to otitis and mastoiditis, classically described but rarely encountered today.

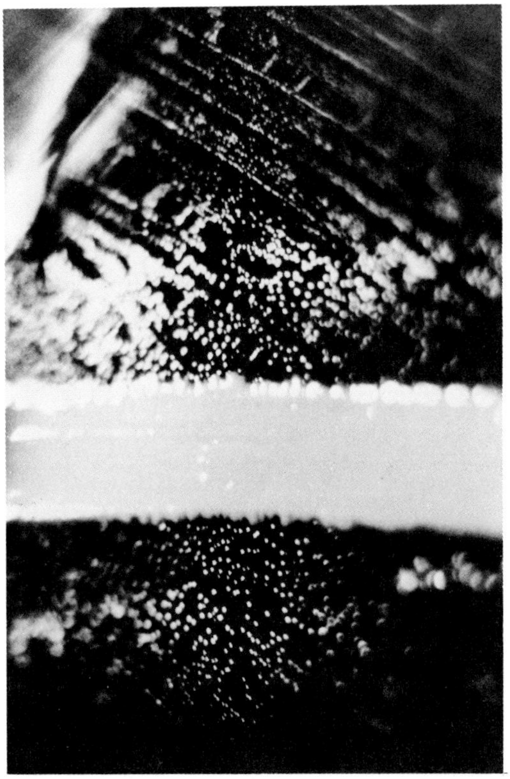

Fig. 30–2. Satellite phenomenon of *Haemophilus influenzae*. On regular agar, colonies appear on both sides of a streak of *Staphylococcus aureus*, which brings the X and V factors necessary to the growth of haemophilus. (Courtesy of Dr. J.C. Pechère.)

midified atmosphere rich in carbon dioxide. A satellite phenomenon accelerates the growth of the small, grayish colonies around streaks of staphylococci and streptococci that provide the needed NAD. This phenomenon is useful in the identification of the organism (Fig. 30–2). On Gram staining, *H. influenzae* appears as a pleomorphic gram-negative to gram-variable coccobacillus, often mistaken for a meningococcus. When in doubt, the slide agglutination test for the capsular polysaccharide mentioned previously aids in the rapid identification of the organism.

Several years ago, all strains of *Haemophilus influenzae* seemed sensitive to both ampicillin and chloramphenicol. Now, beta-lactamase-producing strains, resistant to ampicillin, have appeared and have spread widely; they now constitute 10 to 45% of the isolates in some areas. This change has made chloramphenicol, even with its disadvantages, the agent of choice from the time diagnosis is made until the determination of the organism's susceptibility to ampicillin.

It is more appropriate and more expedient to test for beta-lactamase production by means of a test strip containing a chromogenic cephalosporin directly from the bacterial colony than to wait 16 to 24 hours for the results of agar disc diffusion tests. Many pediatricians use ampicillin and chloramphenicol simultaneously as initial therapy in *Haemophilus influenzae* meningitis, but chloramphenicol-resistant strains, although still uncommon, have recently been reported. The new cephalosporins, such as cefotaxime and moxalactam, which are resistant to beta-lactamase, may soon become the drugs of choice.

GROUP B STREPTOCOCCI

This group, comprised of *Streptococcus agalactiae*, has become the commonest cause of neonatal sepsis and meningitis in recent years (see Objective 24–3).

These streptococci appear on the Gram stain as paired cocci in short chains; pneumococci in CSF may sometimes appear this way. The organism produces small, grayish white colonies on blood agar with a smaller zone of beta hemolysis than group A organisms. Group B streptococci are inhabitants of the vagina and the throat in about 25% of pregnant women in the United States. Transmitted to the neonate at birth, these pathogens may produce septicemia or meningitis during the first 2 weeks of life. This organism is ordinarily sensitive to penicillin (Objective 24–3). Group C and G streptococci rarely cause meningitis.

LISTERIA MONOCYTOGENES

This short, gram-positive organism can be mistaken, on Gram staining of the CSF, for diphtheroids or even pneumococci or isolated streptococci. It is not usually present in the CSF in large numbers, but as its name implies, it provokes a CSF pleocytosis with a high proportion of lymphocytes. *L. monocytogenes* forms small, grayish, slightly hemolytic colonies on sheep's blood agar. If sheep cells are not used in the agar, this means of identification is lost. A particularly characteristic spiraling mobility is seen on a wet mount of the culture, but the possibility of a listeria infection must first be considered. Because four serotypes are known, one may identify the organism by fluorescent antibody testing (see Chap. 24).

In Northern and Western continental Europe, listeria infections, usually septicemias, are found principally in the newborn and in pregnant women; with a few cases of septicemia or meningitis in the aged, the debilitated, and the immunosuppressed (classically those with Hodgkin's disease or those receiving immunosuppressants, corticosteroids, or on hemodialysis). In North America, neonatal and maternal infections are far less common, and the disease in debilitated or immunocompromised older adults is proportionately more common.

Only two drugs, ampicillin and chloramphenicol, are currently considered in the treatment of listeria meningitis. Clinical evidence suggests that ampicillin is far superior to chloramphenicol in therapeutic efficacy. Some laboratory data suggest that the concomitant use of streptomycin or other aminoglycosides may be useful, but these data have not yet been clinically confirmed. Cephalosporins have no place in the control of this organism.

GRAM-NEGATIVE BACILLI

Gram-negative bacillary meningitis is seen in neonates, in elderly, debilitated, alcoholic, or immunocompromised patients with gram-negative sepsis, or after skull fractures or neurosurgical procedures. *Escherichia coli* is the commonest pathogenic organism, followed by klebsiella, salmonella, serratia, proteus, enterobacter, and pseudomonas. Accumulating clinical evidence points to the inadequacy of chloramphenicol in this condition and the need for bactericidal beta-lactam antibiotics. For pseudomonas meningitis, the combination of an intrathecal aminoglycoside with parenteral carbenicillin, ticarcillin, mezlocillin, or piperacillin is recommended, but this difficult therapy may soon be supplanted by a third-generation cephalosporin with strong antipseudomonal activity, such as ceftazidime. For *E. coli*, salmonella, and proteus that are often sensitive to ampicillin, this is the agent of choice, whereas for the remaining resistant enteric bacteria, cefotaxime or moxalactam appear to be the best presently available agents.

OTHER CAUSES OF MENINGITIS

Staphylococcus aureus meningitis is seen in the course of staphylococcal endocarditis, such as occurs in drug addicts, but it may also be due to iatrogenic contamination following lumbar puncture or postcraniotomy osteomyelitis of the skull or a bone flap. The administration of oxacillin, nafcillin, or vancomycin is recommended.

Staphylococcus epidermidis (coagulase-negative) is usually associated with infections complicating intraventricular shunts. A combination of vancomycin and rifampin is reported to be effective, but a cure usually requires removal of the infected shunt and its replacement, at a later date, after a course of systemic antimicrobial therapy.

Enterococci cause an occasional case of meningitis in the neonate and in patients with enterococcal endocarditis. The treatment of this disease is the same as for endocarditis: ampicillin or vancomycin combined with streptomycin or an aminoglycoside.

Campylobacter fetus, once known as *Vibrio fetus*, produces an occasional case of septicemia or meningitis. The most effective treatment is reported to be tetracycline and erythromycin.

> Objective 30–4. Outline the immediate treatment of purulent meningitis.

In the majority of cases, the patient has a single, isolated problem, a life-threatening purulent meningitis. Usually, large doses of

> **DIFFERENTIAL DIAGNOSIS OF MENINGITIS AND SPECIAL PROBLEMS**
>
> Patients presenting with severe frontal headache preceding the apparent onset of meningitis may well have frontal sinusitis with subdural empyema rather than meningitis. Staphylococci, or mixed aerobic and anaerobic flora, are usually the organisms responsible for this condition, which is a medical emergency that requires prompt antibiotic therapy and immediate sinus drainage. In this condition, the organisms are seldom seen or grown from the CSF, probably because the infectious process is encapsulated. Similarly, in brain abscess, the organism does not appear in the CSF unless the abscess has ruptured, usually fatally, into the CSF. Sometimes, the pathogen leaks slowly into the CSF, and the appearance of a mixed flora on Gram staining or culture, especially the culture from the CSF of an anaerobe, such as bacteroides, anaerobic cocci, or fusobacterium, or gram-negative rods and gram-positive cocci seen on smear but not grown on culture should alert the physician to the possible presence of brain abscess or empyema.
>
> Focal signs representing the temporal lobe of the dominant side should suggest an acute herpes viral encephalitis. Oculomotor palsies are so frequent in tuberculous meningitis that their detection in any patient with meningitis should lead to a careful re-examination of the entire record and diagnosis.
>
> Any meningitis with an accompanying increase in CSF pressure enlarges the ventricles of the brain. Continuing mental obtundity of the patient should raise a question about the presence of a space-occupying lesion, subdural effusion, empyema, or internal hydrocephalus. Even CT scans do not clearly distinguish early cases of subarachnoid block. A steadily increasing CSF protein level, sometimes giving a golden color to the fluid, in the face of an apparent bacteriologic response of the infection, suggests this complication.
>
> Frank pyogenic bacterial meningitis involving common pathogens is seldom complicated by a focal collection in the arachnoid space or the brain; exceptions are an infrequent infection with *Listeria monocytogenes*, *Staphylococcus aureus* (epidural or subdural abscess, cerebritis, or endocarditis), and anaerobic organisms already mentioned. Alpha-hemolytic streptococci or enterococci in the CSF, when not due to contamination of the lumbar puncture, may be due to endocarditis with cerebral emboli, mycotic aneurysm, an infected intraventricular shunt, or in newborns, primary meningitis.

the appropriate antibiotic (Table 30–2), administered immediately upon recognition of the disease, and intravenous fluids are the only necessary therapy.

The level of consciousness in the course of meningitis varies, but it worsens with the duration of the infection. Stupor, coma, and grand mal or focal seizures are seen in the most seriously affected patients. Generally, in successfully treated cases, the patient wakes up in 24 to 48 hours, and the mental obtundity lifts totally by the fourth day. In some long-neglected comatose alcoholics with pneumococcal meningitis, the coma may persist for 8 to 10 days, and death may be due to persistent cerebral edema. In young children, especially those with *Haemophilus influenzae* meningitis, continued obtundity may result from a serous subdural effusion. Obviously, the longer the coma and the severe alteration of consciousness, the poorer the prognosis. Coma presents its own hazards, quite apart from the bacteriologic response.

After the start of antibiotic therapy, one should carefully monitor the patient's fluid and electrolyte balance and pulmonary function, preferably in an intensive care unit in the case of a comatose patient. Nasogastric tube feeding should be avoided because it produces an aspiration pneumonitis in obtunded patients. Nasogastric suction, on the other hand, can prevent the aspiration of stomach contents.

Maintenance of the airway is clearly of paramount importance; proper fluid and electrolyte balance comes next. One should control a high fever ($> 104°$ F or $40°$ C) by means of an ice blanket or a refrigerated mattress. Convulsions, more common in children, can be controlled with diazepam, phenytoin, or barbiturates; continued seizures must be avoided. Signs of cerebral edema with increased CSF pressures ($\simeq 500$ mm H_2O) were treated in the past with mannitol or corticosteroids, but no data substantiate the efficacy of this empiric approach. If the etiologic diagnosis of the meningitis is in error and the patient actually has a tuberculous meningitis, the administration of large doses of corticosteroids in the absence of adequate antituberculous therapy can be catastrophic.

Focal neurologic signs, hemiparesis, cranial nerve palsies, and focal seizures (Jack-

Table 30-2. Antibiotic Therapy of Purulent Meningitis

Age	Most Probable Cause	First Therapeutic Choice	Alternate Therapeutic Choice
I. Before the Identification of the Organism[1]			
Neonates (under 1 month old)	Group B streptococci, *Escherichia coli*, and other enteric bacteria, listeria, enterococci	Ampicillin[3] 400 mg/kg/day, IV, and gentamicin, 7.5 mg/kg/day, IV OR cefotaxime, 100–200 mg/kg/day, IV	Chloramphenicol,[4] 50 mg/kg/day, IV OR intrathecal gentamicin
Infants 1 to 6 months old	*Salmonella, Escherichia coli,* and other enteric bacteria	As above	As above
Young children 6 months to 6 years old	*Haemophilus influenzae* Pneumococci *Neisseria meningitidis*	Chloramphenicol, 100 mg/kg/day, IV, with ampicillin,[5] 200–400 mg/kg/day, IV	Cefotaxime, 100–200 mg/kg/day, IV
Children over age 6 and adults to age 35	Pneumococci *Neisseria meningitidis*[2]	Penicillin, 24 million U/day, IV	Chloramphenicol, 50–100 mg/kg/day, IV OR Cefotaxime, 200 mg/kg/day, IV
Adults age 35 and over	Pneumococci, *Neisseria meningitidis*, and rarely *Haemophilus influenzae* or gram-negative bacteria	Ampicillin, 200 mg/kg/day, IV	Cefotaxime, 100–200 mg/kg/day, IV (possibly the best choice) OR Chloramphenicol,[7] 50–100 mg/kg/day, IV

	First Therapeutic Choice	Alternate Therapeutic Choice
II. After the Identification of the Organism		
Neisseria meningitidis	Penicillin G	Chloramphenicol
Streptococcus pneumoniae	Penicillin G	Chloramphenicol[6]
Haemophilus influenzae	Chloramphenicol	Ampicillin (if a non-beta-lactamase-producing strain) or possibly cefotaxime or moxalactam or ceftriaxone

Acute Infectious Meningitis

Organism	Treatment
Enterococci	Ampicillin and aminoglycoside
Listeria	Ampicillin (with streptomycin?)
Staphylococcus aureus	Nafcillin and oxacillin (penicillin G if strain is sensitive) / Vancomycin / Chloramphenicol[7] / Vancomycin
Escherichia coli and other enteric bacteria	Cefotaxime and moxalactam / Ampicillin (if strain is sensitive) OR trimethoprim and sulfamethoxazole OR chloramphenicol[7]
Pseudomonas and resistant enteric bacteria	Intrathecal aminoglycoside with carbenicillin, 400–500 mg/kg/day, IV, or ticarcillin, 300–400 mg/kg/day, or mezlocillin, 200 mg/kg/day / Cefazidime[8]
Campylobacter fetus	Tetracycline / Chloramphenicol
Staphylococcus epidermidis	Vancomycin, 2 g/day, and rifampin 120 mg/day, and removal of ventricular shunt

IV, Intravenously.
1. The duration of therapy is usually up to 2 weeks for fragile organisms, such as pneumococci, meningococci, and *Haemophilus influenzae*, and up to 3 weeks for others.
2. If a patient is an addict, staphylococci should be suspected.
3. This is the conventional pediatric choice of drugs in this age group. It is effective against the majority of enteric organisms, as is cefotaxime, but it is not effective against listeria or enterococci.
4. Chloramphenicol must be used with caution in this age group. Intrathecal or intraventricular use is not without hazards of bleeding and iatrogenic contamination of the cerebrospinal fluid.
5. Some pediatricians start treatment with both agents and discontinue chloramphenicol if the organism is sensitive to ampicillin.
6. Some indications suggest that it is less effective here than penicillin G. Cefotaxime may be useful for this indication.
7. Serious doubts exist about its efficacy.
8. Only preliminary clinical data available.

sonian seizures) may all occur in purulent meningitis, most commonly in older patients. These signs, which are often fleeting and may shift from one side to another, usually clear by the fourth day. In some patients, again the elderly, hemiparesis may persist with slow resolution similar to a "stroke." In other patients, persistent or worsening CNS signs raise the ominous possibility of a brain abscess or subdural empyema. Nucleotide brain scans and, even more appropriately, CT scans are now mandatory in all patients in whom focal signs persist on repeated physical examination. Further, any patient with evidence of head trauma, and possibly all alcoholics, should be investigated for skull fracture or subdural hematoma because such patients are obviously at high risk for these complications.

> Objective 30-5. Identify the possible bacterial cause of a "clear fluid" meningitis.

DIAGNOSTIC GUIDELINES

Meningitis can still be bacterial in origin even when the CSF is not purulent or even clear. Such is the case in the initial stages of meningitis, when the disease has been adequately treated for 4 or more days, or when the infection is due to tuberculosis, leptospirosis, syphilis, listeriosis (sometimes), or brucellosis. In addition, the CSF is clear in bacterial meningitis when the patient is severely granulocytopenic and when a parameningeal bacterial focus, such as a subdural, epidural, or brain abscess, produces meningeal signs.

Clearly, the diagnosis of incipient meningitis does not apply if the meningeal signs are several days old. The diagnosis of a partially treated meningitis is popular in pediatrics, but is actually rarely seen. One or more oral doses of penicillin, tetracycline, or erythromycin in an infant should, at the most, have a minor and transient effect on the character of the CSF. It takes one or several large doses of oral amoxicillin or the trimethoprim-sulfamethoxazole combination to reduce the concentration of organisms in the CSF and to render cultures negative. Several days of frequent, repeated doses are required to decrease the number and change the nature of the inflammatory cells.

Tuberculous meningitis usually produces a lymphocytic pleocytosis suggesting a viral meningitis, but the origin is generally discernible because the inflammation persists and worsens in time, whereas viral meningitis is usually transitory. Sometimes, however, tuberculous meningitis does provoke a brief polymorphonuclear response that mimicks pyogenic meningitis. Only repeated and frequent lumbar punctures and examinations of the CSF are of practical use in making the diagnosis because *Mycobacterium tuberculosis* is seldom seen on CSF smears and takes up to 6 weeks to grow on the usual culture media.

Listeria grows readily on conventional media, although it is often initially mistaken for other organisms such as diphtheroids or gram-positive cocci. Syphilitic meningitis is most easily diagnosed by VDRL testing of the spinal fluid and by positive blood tests (see Objective 23-2). Similarly, leptospirosis and brucellosis are most easily detected by serologic tests, and the diagnosis is confirmed by supportive clinical signs and symptoms of the disease as well as by an appropriate exposure history, including farm, abbatoir, and sewer work.

Parameningeal foci are often associated with severe pain localized along the spine or in the skull, as well as with preceding endocarditis, septicemia, skull trauma, and purulent sinusitis. CT scans and other radiologic procedures are often helpful and are sometimes indispensable.

No individual spinal fluid examination is totally reliable. Neutrophils predominate transiently in viral meningitis, usually with severe inflammation, as well as in occasional cases of tuberculous meningitis. On the other hand, listeria often shows a lymphocytic predominance. Low spinal fluid glucose levels are seen in meningeal sarcoid, in severe inflammatory viral meningitis, and in cryptococcal and other fungal meningitis. The spinal fluid protein level, which usually distinguishes bacterial from viral meningitis, is low, almost normal, at the start of any form of the disease and becomes even more elevated with brain tumor, abscess, parameningeal foci, and brain necrosis due to trauma or ischemia. Only by a sequence of observations can one make the diagnosis in these cases.

The rapidly fatal course of bacterial meningitis demands presumptive treatment on the grounds of a strongly suspected diagnosis; the initial therapy may be continued or discontinued on the basis of later findings. Among the many concomitant findings that should suggest the diagnosis of bacterial meningitis to the physician are the following: (1) sudden onset of fever and alteration of consciousness in a child; (2) sudden onset of a syndrome of fever, vascular collapse, and petechial or ecchymotic rash; (3) endocarditis, particularly with certain pathogens, such as staphylococci and beta-hemolytic streptococci; (4) purulent sinusitis; (5) skull trauma with possible fracture; (6) neurosurgical procedures including myelography; (7) septicemia with alteration of consciousness in the alcoholic or elderly adult; (8) lumbar puncture during septicemia, with subsequent mental confusion or coma.

MENINGITIS DUE TO BRUCELLOSIS

Meningitis can complicate both acute and chronic brucellosis. In the acute disorder, brucella can be grown from blood or CSF cultures, provided they are kept for several weeks. The rest of the clinical picture and the exposure history, along with the positive serologic tests, aid in the diagnosis. In the meningoencephalitis of chronic brucellosis, the disease resembles tuberculous meningitis, with persistent, fluctuating fever, headache, signs of basilar meningitis, moderate lymphocytic pleocytosis, increased CSF protein levels, and decreased glucose levels.

The serum and, more important, the CSF serologic tests, such as complement-fixation, agglutination, immunofluorescent assay, and enzyme-linked immunosorbent assay, are positive for brucella. Because brucellosis is a zoonosis, a contact with infected animals or their contaminated food products is needed. In the United States, a resurgence of brucellosis in cattle and an endemic level of the disease in sheep have been reported, so abattoir workers, veterinarians, and farm workers are at risk. In southern Europe, Mexico and the Caribbean, the major reservoir is goats, and a common source of infection among travelers is the consumption of fresh, unpasteurized goat's milk or cheese.

Therapy consists of tetracycline with, as some authors suggest, rifampin for 6 weeks in meningitis or for up to 6 months in chronic meningoencephalitis.

MENINGITIS DUE TO LEPTOSPIROSIS

The diagnosis of Weil's disease or icterohemorrhagic fever is not difficult in a patient with a fully developed case. The accompanying meningeal inflammation is a minor part of a more impressive clinical picture and is most often ignored. In the initial phase (5 to 6 days), the disease may resemble a prolonged influenza with particularly severe muscle pains and facial and conjunctival suffusion often attributed to the fever. Headache is present, as well as polymorphonuclear CSF pleocytosis, which later becomes lymphocytic. Jaundice and signs of renal insufficiency start on the fifth to seventh day, and the fever classically decreases, only to rise again on the fourteenth day, producing a saddleback fever curve. The jaundice can readily be recognized; while the patient's bilirubin level is often greatly elevated, the transaminase and alkaline phosphatase level is only slightly increased.

The disease is serious, and penicillin, which is effective against leptospira, has little influence on the outcome of the illness.

Weil's disease is mainly caused by the *Leptospira icterohaemorrhagiae* serotype, which, although worldwide in its distribution, in the United States is found mainly in the northeastern part of the country. The so-called minor serotypes are more abundant and produce a far less severe illness. The clinical picture is often limited to a fever (recurrent or not) and signs of lymphocytic meningitis. One may see subicteric elevation of bilirubin levels and a small increase in blood urea nitrogen and creatinine levels with proteinuria. This form of leptospirosis is widespread in the southeastern and south central parts of the United States. Many authors have noted the particularly severe muscle pain and tenderness with this disease.

The diagnosis is generally made serologically, and the patient's medical history should point to exposure to infected animals or contaminated water.

Objective 30–6. Establish the diagnosis of tuberculous meningitis, using all the laboratory data, the patient's medical history, and the physical examination.

Tuberculous meningitis is found in the same groups of patients who suffer active tuberculosis of other organs: children, young adults 20 to 35 years of age, the elderly, immigrants, the poor, alcoholics, and, as described in the last century and only occasionally now, pregnant women. In a majority of cases, however, no clinical evidence of previous active infection exists.

CLINICAL FEATURES

Fever is constant, persistent, and unremitting. Persistent, unrelieved headache is another early sign that appears prior to the neck stiffness. Alteration of consciousness, from personality change and inability to concentrate to coma, is both frequent and progressive. Oculomotor palsies, another common sign, appear several weeks into the illness. Other focal neurologic signs may appear, and these signs may even be the major symptomatic manifestations of the disease. The infection can take the form of a localized cerebral lesion, such as a tuberculoma, with or without accompanying meningeal involvement. The most common diagnostic error is to concentrate on the focal or psychiatric signs and to ignore the significance of the fever.

LABORATORY AND OTHER DIAGNOSTIC TESTS

The pleocytosis is variable, but generally has a lymphocytic predominance and usually consists of only a few hundred cells, even while the protein content increases rapidly and often exceeds 1 g/L. Low glucose levels are consistent features late in the disease, and the low chloride level, classically described, is usually related to an inappropriate vasopressin secretion with lowered serum sodium concentrations. One cannot expect to see the

---

LEPTOSPIRA

Leptospira are spirochetes ranging in size from 6 to 25 µ. Ordinarily, 2 or 3 turns per cell are visible under a dark-field microscope or on silver staining. Serologically, a variety of types can be distinguished by agglutination or immunofluorescence. The classic type is *Leptospira icterohaemorrhagiae*, which produces the most severe and clinically identifiable disease. The "minor" serotypes, such as *L. canicola, L. pomona, L. bataviae, L. autumnalis, L. grippotyphosa*, produce a milder, clinically nondifferentiable disorder in which prolonged fever, severe myalgia (Fort Bragg fever) and, frequently, meningeal signs are the most prominent features.

The organism can be grown from blood, urine, or even the CSF during the early septicemic phase, but this procedure requires a special NNN medium or guinea pigs, which are not available in most laboratories. Moreover, presumption of the diagnosis when the symptoms are still nonspecific is improbable in sporadic cases. The organism can often be seen in the urinary sediment for several weeks or more on a dark-field examination, provided the patient has not received any of the many antibiotics to which the organism is sensitive. The serologic confirmation, that is, the demonstration of a rise in titer of antibody in samples taken 1 to 2 weeks apart, is the most common means of diagnosis.

The principal hosts of the organism are urban or rural rodents; large animals, dogs, horses, cattle, and man excrete the organism in the urine for a much shorter time and are less important epidemiologically. The bacterium is excreted in the urine and is transmitted by contact with contaminated freshwater or mud. The disease is an occupational hazard among hog farmers, rice growers, army personnel on maneuvers, janitors, and sewer and abattoir workers; people on summer vacation are also at risk.

organism often in the CSF, and growth on culture takes up to 6 weeks. Further, the tuberculin reaction is not always positive. The examination of the patient's eye rarely shows a retinal tubercle, but frequently reveals a papilledema or papillitis, a sign of prolonged increased intracranial pressure. CT scanning may indicate a tuberculoma, but more often it only gives nonspecific evidence of dilated ventricles and increased density in the subarachnoid fissures at the base of the patient's brain.

TREATMENT

Therapy must be based on a constellation of nonspecific signs and the patient's medical history. Because listeriosis, viral infections, cryptococcal and fungal meningitis, sarcoid, cerebral inflammation in endocarditis, or cerebral carcinomatosis can produce CSF manifestations similar to those of tuberculous meningitis, one can diagnose the disease only by repeated assays of the spinal fluid.

Again, the longer the disease goes untreated, the worse the prognosis. Conventionally, 3 drugs are recommended for this form of tuberculosis. The initial phase, with slow resolution of the inflammation, lasts about 4 months, and maintenance therapy lasts 18 months, for a total of almost 2 years. Isoniazid and rifampin penetrate well into the CSF, whereas streptomycin and ethambutol are present in adequate CSF concentrations only during the inflammatory phase of the disease. In retreatment cases in which resistant organisms are suspected, ethionamide, pyrizinamide, or low doses of cycloserine can be added. Although corticosteroids can relieve CSF hypertension and may spectacularly lighten coma or mental obtundity, no effect on the overall mortality rate or on sequelae has been demonstrated in controlled studies.

> **Objective 30–7.** Assemble the evidence for a nonbacterial cause of nonpurulent or "aseptic" meningitis.

VIRUSES

Viruses are the most common cause of clinically apparent meningitis. Primarily, viral meningitis is a disease of children, as is bacterial meningitis. Because most, with some rare but notable exceptions, are brief and benign illnesses, the majority of cases are probably not clinically diagnosed and, for the most part, are not seen by a physician. For example, a large proportion of cases of the childhood exanthems show a spinal fluid pleocytosis seldom expressed clinically. In addition, viral meningitis blends symptomatically into the large pool of arthropod-borne viral encephalitides, which necessarily carry a component of meningeal inflammation themselves. The degree of cerebral dysfunction, as evidenced by cerebellar ataxia, nystagmus, and obtundity, determines whether the disease is called encephalitis, meningitis, or meningoencephalitis. Indeed, in few cases of meningitis is there no disturbance of consciousness or thought processes. Added to this huge number of viral CNS infections are disorders caused by leptospira, mycoplasma (producing both meningitis and meningoencephalitis), and rickettsia (the agent of Rocky Mountain spotted fever) that have spinal fluid manifestations similar to those of viral meningitis.

Because the variety of agents in "aseptic meningitis" is enormous, the number of viral serologic types is even greater. The majority of cases, again with notable exceptions, are not accompanied by specific identifying clinical signs; therefore, most cases are not specifically diagnosed. A rise in antibody titer to the specific viral agent or, more precisely, to its serotype suggests the diagnosis. Isolation of the agent from body fluids, most typically from pharyngeal washings or a rectal swab, where it is fleetingly present, further supports this diagnosis, although concomitant infections are always possible. Because screening of the many viral agents is not economically feasible and because clinical virology laboratories are still uncommon, however, the specific etiologic diagnosis becomes possible in practice only under epidemic conditions. The principal reason for making the diagnosis of aseptic or viral meningitis or meningoencephalitis is to distinguish it from meningitis or meningoencephalitis due to acute pyogenic bacterial infection (not too difficult), chronic tuberculosis or cryptococcosis (much more difficult), or leptospira, rickettsial, or mycoplasma infection. Furthermore, it is important to identify those forms of viral meningitis that either have special clinical features or prognosis or demand specific therapy; examples are meningitis caused by mumps, lymphocytic choriomeningitis, and herpes simplex viruses.

Enteroviruses. In one well-known study, enteroviruses were responsible for 30% of all cases of meningitis. In view of the numerous serologic types of these viruses, it is likely that the incidence was underestimated. Transmitted by fecal-oral passage, enteroviruses are marked by a summer peak in fecal excretion as well as in clinical cases in the northern hemisphere. Clinically, this disease, which represents the archetype of what should be called clear fluid meningitis rather than aseptic meningitis, is characterized by fever, seldom as high as 40° C (104° F), myalgias, backache, variable stiffness of the neck, and often some photophobia. The CSF shows a lymphocytic pleocytosis, usually several hundreds per milliliter. Protein levels are generally ≤100 mg/100 ml (seldom more than 150 mg/100 ml), and glucose levels are unchanged. The illness is short; the meningeal symptoms last from 3 to 5 days, although the pleocytosis decreases slowly over a period of several weeks. Echovirus and coxsackieviruses A and B are currently the major causes of this form of meningitis, which is occasionally accompanied by a morbilliform or papulovascular rash (Table 27–7). Coxsackieviruses B occasionally produce a clinically severe disease resembling poliomyelitis, a fulminating disease in the newborn, pleurodynia (Bornholm disease), or even a severe meningeal inflammation with thousands of cells, initially neutrophils, and elevated protein and low glucose levels, that frankly mimics bacterial meningitis.

Before the introduction of the Salk and Sabin vaccines, the most important clinical form of enteroviral meningitis was due to the three polioviruses. In contrast to the other enteroviruses, poliovirus has a sudden rather than an insidious onset and generally causes a higher fever, severe myalgias, and about the fourth day of illness, an irregular, ascending, flaccid paralysis extending up to and including, in severe cases, the respiratory muscles, or in still more severe cases in young adults, a descending bulbar paralysis. Unfortunately, this disease may still be seen, even in Europe and North America, in unvaccinated groups in the population.

Mumps Virus. According to one study, meningoencephalitis caused by mumps virus comprises 7% of all cases of aseptic meningitis in children. This disorder is usually not difficult to diagnose because it is generally preceded, is occasionally accompanied, and in about 7% of the cases, is followed by the acute parotitis characteristic of mumps. In adolescents or in young adults, orchitis or oophoritis may occur. The disease is characteristically sudden in onset and severe, with confusion, delirium and subsequent coma, and high fever, with hundreds to more than a thousand lymphocytes in the CSF and an elevated protein level. Probably, no benign illness looks more severe. Although the parotitis generally evolves over a 16-day course, the meningoencephalitis stops abruptly with resolution of fever and awakening on the fourth or fifth day. The only major sequela, which is infrequent, is unilateral nerve deafness. The diagnosis can be further confirmed, if desired, by demonstrating a rise in hemagglutinating or complement-fixation antibody, but such confirmation is usually possible only after resolution of the illness.

Lymphocytic Choriomeningitis Virus. The North American zoonotic disease caused by this virus is carried by field mice and is transmitted to man, in general, at the onset of winter, when the rodents seek to enter houses or other inhabited structures. Clinically, it is unlike any of the other forms of viral meningitis in that it is often preceded by a respiratory illness and usually has a progressive onset, over several days, eventually leading to severe constitutional symptoms, including throbbing headache, photophobia, stiff neck, and high fever. The CSF shows thousands, sometimes tens of thousands, of lymphocytes; initially, the CSF contains a sizable proportion of neutrophils. The CSF protein level is usually > 100 mg/100 ml, and the glucose level is borderline or slightly depressed. In the beginning, it is difficult to distinguish this disease from acute bacterial meningitis, and most patients do receive a few days of antibiotic therapy. In 4 to 5 days, the symptoms begin to abate, although they persist with decreasing intensity for 3 to 6 weeks. The pleocytosis also slowly resolves. Cure is generally complete and is without sequelae. The diagnosis of lymphocytic choriomeningitis can be serologically confirmed, but usually when the patient is already recovering.

Mycoplasma. Meningitis and meningoencephalitis caused by mycoplasma are discussed here because they resemble clear fluid viral meningitis. Although simple meningitis have been described, meningoencephalitis is more commonly seen. The disease may not be accompanied by pulmonary findings, such as an infiltrate, and indeed may not be preceded by pulmonary symptoms suggestive of the diagnosis. The CSF pleocytosis is lymphocytic. The protein level may be over 100 mg/100 ml, but the glucose level is usually normal. Because the onset of the illness is generally gradual, it is not difficult to distinguish it from acute bacterial meningitis. The difficulty arises in differentiating it from tuberculous or cryptococcal meningitis, especially because the clinical picture resolves in several weeks rather than days. Probably, the majority of patients return to normal without having had an etiologic diagnosis, unless an alert physician notices an incredibly rapid sedimentation rate due to high titers of cold agglutinins or asks directly for a cold agglutinin titer or, more specifically, for mycoplasma complement fixation (usually > 1/64 high in extrapulmonary mycoplasma infections). The importance of the diagnosis lies first in the elimination of more serious causes and subsequently in what appears to be effective therapy for the extrapulmonary complications with 2 g/day tetracycline or erythromycin.

Herpes Simplex Virus. This virus is of two types and has two sites of predilection and two forms of CNS involvement. Type 2 produces herpes genitalis, is sexually transmitted, and is the occasional cause of a pure viral meningitis. This unusual form of meningitis, (mainly in young adults), either accompanies a primary infection, or occurs a short time afterwards, apparently by retrograde spread from the sacral ganglia where the virus subsequently becomes latent. More severe than enteroviral meningitis, herpes simplex 2 meningitis causes severe throbbing headache, photophobia, and back and neck pain, which are the subjective complaints in meningitis, as opposed to the objective sign of a stiff neck, but usually, no marked alteration of consciousness occurs. Unlike the enterovirusal disease, this illness lasts more than a week but is benign. The benign character of the disease contrasts with that of the disease produced by type 1 herpes simplex virus. This variant, which prefers the buccal mucosa and produces herpes labialis, is probably transmitted by oral secretions and is nearly a universal infection in most populations.

Whereas some of the viral CNS infections already mentioned have a frightening appearance but are benign, the meningoencephalitis caused by type 1 herpes simplex virus is a disease that looks and is dreadful. Because currently available treatment appears to be effective if administered early in the disease, prompt diagnosis is of paramount importance.

Whereas the other forms of viral encephalitis are diffuse and inflammatory, herpetic encephalitis is focal and necrotic. The only similar viral encephalitis is that due to varicella virus, which infrequently complicates, and all too often terminates, a herpes zoster infection of the ophthalmic branch of the trigeminal nerve in aged or immunosuppressed patients. After several days of fever and headache, the patient becomes confused, then progressively stuporous and comatose. The patient's temperature may fall toward normal, but focal signs indicate the involvement of temporal or adjacent areas on the dominant side of the brain. Focal or generalized seizures may occur. The CSF shows a moderate lymphocytic pleocytosis of up to several hundred cells with an admixture of neutrophils. Large numbers of red blood cells are frequently present, probably from the necrotic tissue. The CSF pressure is usually almost normal, but the protein concentration increases slowly and progressively and contains locally produced antibody. The antiherpesvirus titers in the serum and CSF are usually elevated, although too late in the course of the illness to be of diagnostic value. Indeed, because antibody is present in a majority of adults and is elevated in recurrent herpes labialis infections, and because any severe CNS inflammation allows the entry of serum protein into the CSF, antibody determinations probably have diagnostic significance only when they are absent.

The electroencephalogram may show diffuse or focal temporal abnormalities. The CT scan reveals unilateral or bilateral temporal lesions of decreased density (necrosis), with or without a space-occupying mass, which is difficult to distinguish from infarction, glioma, or focal cerebritis. The brain scan or arteriogram may be helpful, but the major means of confirming the diagnosis is by temporal brain biopsy, with the finding of a necrotic inflammatory lesion and the demonstration of the virus on cell culture, electron-microscopic examination, or immunofluorescent stain. Infarction, tuberculoma, parasitic cyst, cryptococcoma, tumor, and leukoencephalopathy, all possible diagnoses, can only be confirmed or eliminated by brain biopsy. Even with a morbidity rate of 2% for brain biopsy, this procedure is essential to the diagnosis of this rare but fatal encephalitis.

Vidarabine, 15 mg/kg/day for 10 days, that is, 400 mg in a liter of glucose over 12 hours, is too toxic an agent to be given blindly to a large number of patients on the mere presumption of the diagnosis. Studies on this agent show a therapeutic indication only in the first 5 days of illness. In practice, the drug is often started on strong presumptive evidence and is terminated in a few days if the diagnosis is not confirmed by biopsy or if evidence implicates another cause. Continuing the drug without further diagnostic intervention, as a trial of therapy, simply ensures that the other diagnostic possibilities will be ignored until too late to help the patient. The role of another agent, acyclovir 750 mg/m^2/day for 7 days, looks promising, and is less toxic (see Chap. 29).

As mentioned previously, most cases of viral meningitis are self-limiting illnesses that generally require only symptomatic therapy. These symptoms improve by the third to fifth day and clear by the seventh to tenth day. If a particular patient does not follow this pattern, then, in addition to the causes already discussed, several others should be considered, including parasitic or fungal agents and several syndromes of unknown origin. Before turning to these diseases, however, the physician should review the case; the term "aseptic meningitis" refers to the failure to grow a bacterial pathogen from the CSF on conventional media. There are far more failures to grow fragile organisms such as the pneumococci, meningococci, and *Haemophilus influenzae* because the CSF was not promptly and properly cultured than there are cases of meningitis due to the etiologies that follow. The same is true for tuberculous meningitis.

PARASITES

Nonpurulent, clear fluid parasitic meningitis comprises, in tropical areas, cerebral involvement in malignant falciparum malaria (cerebral malaria), African trypanosomiasis (sleeping sickness), and, on rare occasions, filariasis. In Southeast Asia and Hawaii, an eosinophilic meningitis due to *Angiostrongylus cantonensis* is seen.

Amebas. In North America, an amebic meningoencephalitis is caused by free-living amoeba of the naegleria and acanthamoeba groups, which are acquired by swimming in small, warm, freshwater lakes in the southeastern United States. The diagnosis is made by direct examination of the centrifuged sediment of a CSF sample, best realized with a phase-contrast microscope, or a brain biopsy. The prognosis is poor. The major current therapy is amphotericin B, but the nitrimidazoles show promise.

FUNGI

Among the fungal etiologies of meningitis, cryptococcosis is most important. Although histoplasma meningitis occurs occasionally wherever the histoplasma infection is endemic, and although meningeal coccidioidomycosis, which is difficult to treat, is seen in the southwestern United States and southern California, cryptococcosis is more common and has a broader geographic range. The clinical picture can be extraordinarily varied, but an insidious onset with headaches, personality changes, and low-grade fever is most common in the nonimmunosuppressed host; however, in patients with Hodgkin's disease or in those requiring prolonged corticosteroid or immunosuppressant therapy, the disease takes a more acute course. The best means of rapid diagnosis at present is the detection of cryptococcal antigen in the CSF. Current therapy consists of several months of parenteral amphotericin B and oral 5-flurocytosine, in reduced doses to avoid the bone marrow toxicity precipitated by accumulation of the drug following the decreased renal function by amphotericin B (see Chap. 33).

OTHER CAUSES

Among the other causes of meningitis with a clear, nonpurulent CSF are: secondary syphilis, for which one should obtain a CSF VDRL test; meningeal carcinomatosis, for which one should obtain a cytologic examination of the CSF; pyogenic brain abscess, for which a CT scan is indicated; nocardia abscess, for which a CT scan is indicated; and finally, Behçet's syndrome (uveitis and meningitis) and Mollaret's syndrome, in which one sees recurrent episodes with unusual reticuloendothelial cells in the CSF. These last two are mentioned in all texts, but the physician is more likely to see all the other diseases several times before finding one of these syndromes. Certainly, much more frequent, and one of the most underdiagnosed causes of aseptic meningitis, is leptospirosis.

> **Objective 30–8. Follow the course of a patient with acute meningitis.**

PURULENT MENINGITIS

First 24 Hours of Treatment. The prognosis is strongly and universally tied to the severity of the disease at the time therapy is initiated. In the course of the first 24 hours, no improvement may be apparent, even in the mildest cases. Indeed, in the most severe cases, the clinical picture often worsens and includes generalized seizures, deepening of coma, and respiratory arrest. Further, disease mechanisms already set in motion, such as vasculitis, cutaneous and visceral hemorrhages, and shock in meningococcemia, do not abruptly halt with the start of antibiotic therapy.

Focal neurologic signs are particularly difficult to interpret at this stage. They may well be transient, but the risk of waiting and watching without investigation is almost impossible to underestimate. Focal signs may represent a subdural hematoma in an alcoholic or an elderly patient, a purulent sinusitis with epidural abscess, a brain abscess, or a serous subdural effusion in a child, or even a cerebral venous sinus thrombosis. Unilateral exophthalmos may indicate rhinocerebral phycomycosis, whereas bilateral exophthalmos may represent a cavernous sinus thrombosis. Probably, the safest approach is to take a CT scan or another appropriate radiologic examination if doubt exists about the localization of the infection.

The best rule during the first 24 hours is as follows: if the results of the spinal fluid examination do not seem consistent with the diagnosis, for example, if the CSF has too many lymphocytes, too high a protein level, or a glucose level too high or, conversely, too

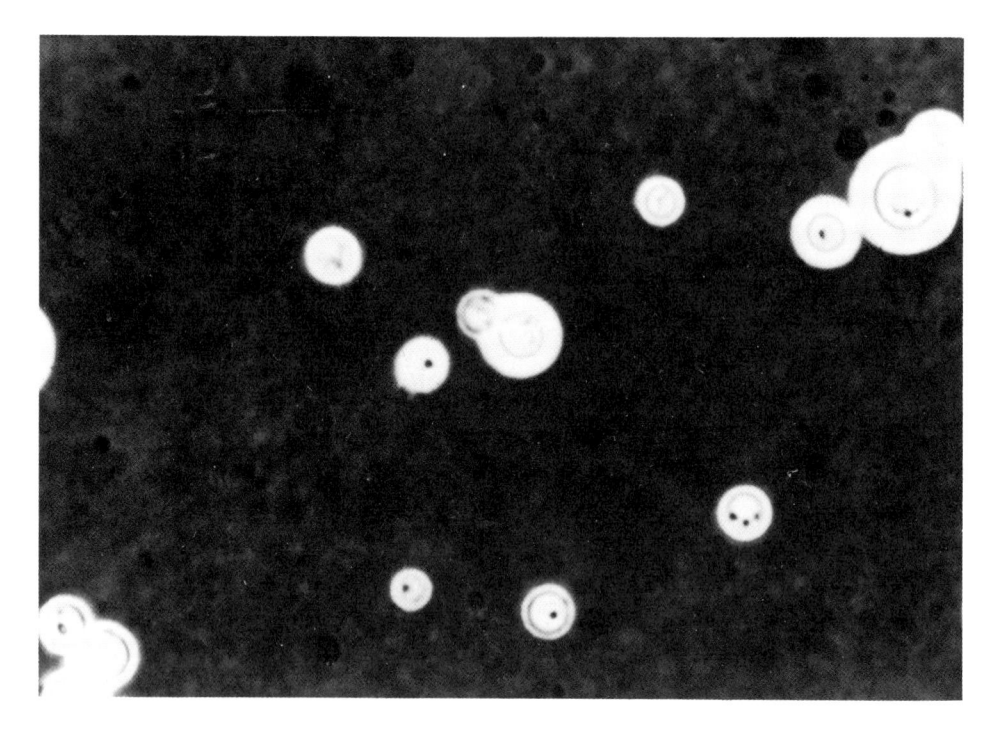

Fig. 30–3. *Cryptococcus neoformans* in CSF (india ink staining). (Courtesy of Dr. J.C. Pechère.)

CRYPTOCOCCUS NEOFORMANS

Cryptococcus neoformans (Fig. 30–3) is a yeast-like organism that can easily be mistaken for a white blood cell (lymphocyte) on smear or during the cell count of the CSF. The large capsule helps to differentiate the pathogen from a white blood cell on an india ink preparation; however, visualization of the capsule requires a high concentration of organisms in the CSF usually seen only in the immunosuppressed patient. Because the organism is peculiarly variable in its growth on Sabouraud agar and often requires the inoculation of repeated samples and of large quantities of CSF (again, *C. neoformans* is easier to culture in the immunosuppressed), the best rapid diagnostic method is the test for cryptococcal antigen. The polysaccharide capsule is partially soluble; therefore, a slide agglutination test is currently commercially available for its detection and appears to be reliable.

---

low when all the other findings are normal, the test should be repeated. If repeated samples of CSF continue to vary and remain inconsistent with any particular type of meningitis, then a brain abscess may be considered because it typically produces inconsistent findings, such as neutrophils or lymphocytes in any number, high or almost normal protein levels, and normal or elevated pressure.

Second to the Fourth Day of Treatment. The clinical picture dramatically improves during this period, with a rapid lightening of the patient's mental obtundity, a return of temperature to nearly normal, and a marked clearing of the CSF. After 24 hours of therapy, pneumococci, meningococci, and *Haemophilus influenzae* should no longer be seen in the CSF if penicillin or ampicillin is administered. These organisms may be present in reduced numbers, however, if chloramphenicol is administered. Gram-negative organisms take longer to clear and should be inapparent on the Gram stain by the third day of treatment. A spinal tap on the fourth day should show mainly lymphocytes in much reduced numbers, a normal glucose level, and an almost normal protein level (usually $\sim$ 100 mg/100 ml).

The persistence of fever may be unrelated to the meningitis itself and may be due to the following:

1. Poor hydration of the patient.

2. Infected intravenous site (common).
3. Drug fever, particularly with penicillins and cephalosporins.
4. Pneumonitis, especially when the patient has been intubated or fed through a nasogastric tube.
5. Inappropriate schedule of administration, such as penicillin G every 6 hours; in some cases, the prescribed antibiotic may not even have been administered.

Persistent fever may also be due to inappropriate therapy, either because a resistant organism is not anticipated or, more often, because a strain is resistant to the prescribed antibiotic, such as ampicillin-resistant strains of *Haemophilus influenzae* or the treatment of gram-negative bacilli with chloramphenicol. Persistent growth of the organism from repeated lumbar punctures should suggest this possibility.

Finally, in an infant 2 years old or under, serous subdural effusions are seen, especially with *Haemophilus influenzae* meningitis. These effusions may be asymptomatic, or they may lead to persistent fever, elevated CSF protein and pressure levels, and continued obtundity. Transillumination of the skull in the infant, CT scanning, or echography can easily identify the effusion.

Occasionally, alcoholics with pneumococcal meningitis who are comatose for some time prior to hospital admission and who have several thousand cells in the CSF, with elevated protein levels and CSF pressure, respond slowly and do not regain consciousness until the sixth to tenth day; sometimes, these patients even worsen and die during this period. The sole postmortem finding is usually cerebral edema, although a subdural hematoma is sometimes present. Such deaths are due not to a bacteriologic failure to kill the pneumococcus, but rather to the difficulty of reversing pre-existing cerebral injury. Measures to reduce CSF pressure, corticosteroids, and mannitol have been proposed, but are of uncertain efficacy.

Tenth to the Fourteenth Day and After. By this time, most properly treated patients with meningitis caused by the three major pathogens are long since fully alert and are fretting about the intravenous lines. Their CSF is almost normal; a few lymphocytes may remain. Because, for the most part with the major 3 meningeal pathogens, the CSF reaches this condition by the fourth day of therapy, some experienced clinicians have wondered whether 4 to 7 days of therapy might not be adequate. A 7- to 10-day course produces excellent results, whereas therapy beyond 2 weeks is unnecessary.

With meningitis due to gram-negative bacilli and some cases of infection with *Listeria monocytogenes*, the CSF findings take longer to return to normal; most patients with meningitis due to gram-negative rods have more grossly abnormal CSF to start with. Therefore, such patients are usually treated for at least 2 weeks, and therapy is extended to 3 weeks or more if the CSF contains more than 50 cells and more than 100 mg/100 ml protein on the fourteenth day. Persistent focal neurologic signs should be investigated long before this point. A continued elevation of CSF protein levels suggests hydrocephalus or parameningeal abscess.

Immediate relapses are rare and suggest a parameningeal focus of infection. Repeated episodes of infection with meningococci are seen in individuals with a complement cascade defect, and repeated episodes of pneumococcal meningitis occur in cases of a dural fistula with leakage of CSF into a sinus, a condition that is surgically correctable.

OTHER FORMS OF MENINGITIS

In enteroviral meningitis, the patient is much improved by the third to fifth day and feels completely well by the tenth day. Patients with mumps meningoencephalitis wake up by the third or fifth day, and patients with lymphocytic choriomeningitis are much better by the seventh to tenth day, although they still have headache and some photophobia. The patient with herpes meningoencephalitis is beyond hope by the seventh day.

The patient with leptospirosis spontaneously improves by the tenth to fifteenth day, much before the serologic results are available. The patient with tuberculous meningitis, however, does not begin to improve until after the third week of treatment, and the patient's condition may well deteriorate during that time. The lymphocytosis in the CSF lasts 2 to 4 months, the fever at least a month, and the culture takes usually 6 weeks to be reported. The usual duration of therapy for tuberculous meningitis is 18 to 24 months.

Objective 30–9. Prescribe intrathecal therapy when indicated.

The purpose of intrathecal injection is to obtain adequate CSF antibiotic concentrations, that is, presumably well over the minimal bactericidal concentration, when parenteral administration is inadequate. On the whole, this route of administration is only necessary for the aminoglycosides, such as gentamicin and amikacin. The introduction of the newer cephalosporins, such as cefotaxime, moxalactam, and ceftazidime, has reduced the scope of this indication. At the present time, the intrathecal administration of aminoglycosides, for example, gentamicin, 4 to 12 mg every 24 to 48 hours for an adult, is appropriate only for meningitis due either to *Pseudomonas aeruginosa* or to those strains of serratia and enterobacter that are not highly susceptible to the newer cephalosporins.

The risks of intrathecal use of antibiotics include infection, bleeding, and, for the penicillins and cephalosporins, arachnoiditis. The use of intraventricular injection seems largely restricted to patients with coccidioidal meningitis who respond poorly to parenteral amphotericin B, when renal function is threatened by the continued parenteral administration of this drug, and in patients with persistent infections caused by gram-negative bacteria resistant to parenteral therapy.

Objective 30–10. Take proper prophylactic measures when bacterial meningitis is recognized.

Nothing definite can be said about prophylaxis. It seems reasonable to use types A and C meningococcal vaccine for army recruits and for individuals traveling to endemic or especially epidemic zones. In particular, type A vaccine is appropriate for travelers to the Subsaharan zones of Africa. Interestingly, European airlines recommend it, but American carriers remain silent on the subject. Similarly, the vaccine appears useful in quelling an epidemic; 6 days are required for the appearance of protective antibody.

Pneumococcal vaccine should be given to children with sickle cell (and probably SC, SD) anemia, as well as to patients who have undergone splenectomy. The vaccine is less effective in children under 2 years of age, and the efficacy of the varieties of type 6 antigen is questionable. Moreover, many capsular types, important in childhood, are not contained in the vaccine. These reasons have prompted the suggestion of administering continuous penicillin coverage to these children. In addition, asplenic adults should receive the vaccine, although their response is not normal.

Haemophilus influenzae type B vaccine, currently under development, is likely to be recommended for all children and probably for older adults lacking specific antibody. Streptococcal group B vaccine is intended for pregnant women, to protect their infants by passively transferred antibody.

Chemoprophylaxis probably relieves the anxieties of the patient's contacts more than it protects those at risk. When the meningococci, which cause the cyclical-epidemic type of bacterial meningitis, as contrasted with the seasonal but sporadic pneumococcal and *Haemophilus influenzae* meningitis, were uniformly sensitive to the sulfonamide agents, large amounts of inexpensive sulfadiazine tablets were handed out to anyone with the remotest contact with an index case, and thus one could quell anxiety and suppress the carrier rate in the community. Because a significant proportion of strains are now resistant to the sulfonamides, only minocycline, 200 mg twice a day for 2 days, or rifampin, 600 mg twice a day for 4 days, can be recommended. Both drugs are expensive. Further, minocycline can produce severe vertigo, particularly in young women, and is therefore an extraordinary medication for nurses, whereas rifampin simply allows resistant strains to emerge rapidly, a property that renders this agent inappropriate for wide-scale use.

Moreover, it is not likely that either drug is used properly in actual practice because the risk of dissemination of the infection to the CNS is greatest in the first few days of acquisition of the carrier state. Because the etiologic identification of the organism usually takes 3 days, it is probable that the greatest risk has already passed when the prescriptions are written. Dr. Harry Feldman claimed that no evidence suggested that any physician had ever acquired meningococcal meningitis from a patient; some nurses, however, may have. It seems reasonable to administer prophylactic agents to intimate contacts of the patient and to individual hospital personnel who intubate a patient or give mouth-to-mouth resuscitation, because this fragile organism can only be transmitted by close respiratory contact. Even better is close medical surveillance of the family and contacts, with throat culture and immediate penicillin therapy upon the appearance of fever, pharyngitis, or headache.

Patients with a skull fracture and rhinocerebral leakage should receive penicillin therapy until the defect is corrected.

SUGGESTED READINGS

Feigin, R.D., and Dodge, P.R.: Bacterial meningitis: newer concepts of pathophysiology and neurologic sequelae. Pediatr. Clin. North Am., 23:541, 1976.

Fraser, D.W., et al.: Risk factors in bacterial meningitis: Charleston County, South Carolina. J. Infect. Dis., 127:271, 1973.

Gotschlich, E.C.: Bacterial meningitis: the beginning of the end. Am. J. Med., 65:719, 1978.

Johnson, R.T., and Mims, C.A.: Pathogenesis of viral infections of the nervous system. N. Engl. J. Med., 278:23, 84, 1968.

Landesman, S.H., et al.: Past and current roles for cephalosporin antibiotics in treatment of meningitis. Emphasis on use in Gram-negative bacillary meningitis. Am. J. Med., 71:693, 1981.

Levine, D.P., Lauter, C.B., and Lerner, A.M.: Simultaneous serum and CSF antibodies in herpes simplex virus encephalitis. JAMA, 240:356, 1978.

Sande, M.A.: Antibiotic therapy of bacterial meningitis: lessons we've learned. Am. J. Med., 71:507, 1981.

Schaad, U.B., et al.: Clinical evaluation of a new broad-spectrum oxa-beta-lactam antibiotic, moxalactam, in neonates and infants. J. Pediatr., 98:129, 1981.

CHAPTER 31

Infections Affecting the Peripheral Nervous System

J. Drucker

> **Objective 31–1. Delineate the clinical characteristics of the principal neurologic presentations of peripheral nervous system infections.**

Whether or not it is of infectious origin, peripheral nervous system involvement is manifested by acute muscular weakness at varying sites. Schematically, four major clinical situations can be described.

Acute Paralysis of the Limbs. In this situation, the peripheral motor deficit is asymmetric, without any objective sensory disorder when the lesion involves the neurons of the anterior horn of the spinal cord, as in acute anterior poliomyelitis. The clinical picture is that of a symmetric peripheral motor deficit associated with objective and subjective sensory disorders if the site of the lesion is in the roots, spinal ganglia, or trunk of peripheral nerves, as in Guillain-Barré syndrome. Finally, peripheral palsies may be localized, associated with often predominant parasympathetic autonomic disorders, when the neurologic lesion involves the motor plates and blocks the cholinergic motor system; this type of lesion is observed in botulism.

Peripheral Facial Palsies. These disorders have well-known characteristics that distinguish them from central palsies, and in particular the involvement of the upper part of the face. In some cases, peripheral facial palsies of infectious origin are bilateral.

Ocular Palsies. These palsies are manifested essentially by diplopia. Paralysis of accommodation and an involvement of the extrinsic musculature of the eye may also occur.

Alimentary Disorders. In infants, a particular clinical entity is constituted by alimentary disorders that may be the first or even the only symptoms of a peripheral neuropathy, such as poliomyelitis or diphtheria.

These four localizations may be variously combined in a given patient.

> **Objective 31–2. Collect clinical, epidemiologic, and laboratory evidence of neurologic involvement due to botulism.**

CLINICAL EVIDENCE

Gastrointestinal Signs. In nearly one case out of two, the disease begins with nausea and vomiting, but dysphagia, especially when combined with dryness of the mouth, is more characteristic. Other patients complain mainly of constipation, sometimes with signs of intestinal obstruction. Severe abdominal pain may also be observed.

Paralysis. Diplopia is a frequent and early occurrence and is sometimes accompanied by paralysis of accommodation, mydriasis, ptosis, and divergent strabismus. These ocular involvements worsen progressively and affect both eyes. Paralysis of the facial, pharyngeal, respiratory, and sphincteral muscles may produce dysarthria, acute urinary retention, and paralysis of the diaphragm with progressive asphyxia. An ascending or descending symmetric paralysis of the extremities may also appear. The tendon reflexes are preserved, except in cases of unusually significant paralysis. No sensory disorders occur, and the patient's temperature and degree of consciousness remain normal.

Infant Botulism. This form of botulism is a special case. The disease usually remains benign and is limited to constipation and transitory apathy. In rare cases, infants may have more severe signs, such as difficulty in swallowing, paralytic strabismus, and hypotonia of the trunk and limbs, which regress spontaneously without sequelae. This clinical form of botulism is a result of the colonization of the infant's intestinal tract by *Clostridium botulinum* to produce a sufficient quantity of toxin in situ to give these clinical signs. When this phenomenon occurs, the toxin may be found in the infant's stools.

EPIDEMIOLOGIC EVIDENCE

Botulism often occurs in family "microepidemics" following the ingestion of foods contaminated with botulin. The contaminated foodstuffs are mostly home-canned goods, and dried, salted, or smoked fish or meat, but rarely commercially canned goods. Frozen foods do not cause botulism.

The particular epidemiologic characteristics of Canada, France, and the United States are shown in Table 31–1. In young children, honey has been incriminated as a cause of botulism. In rare instances, the intoxication is not related to the ingestion of food, but is a complication of a wound infected by *Clostridium botulinum.*

LABORATORY CONFIRMATION OF THE DIAGNOSIS

To distinguish botulism definitively from other neurologic intoxications caused by food such as mussels and certain fish, the botulin has to be isolated. Therefore, the diagnosis of botulism is based on the characterization of the toxin. A seroprotection test is performed by inoculating an extract of the suspected food, the patient's serum, and his gastric fluid to mice or guinea pigs prepared by antibodies to the different types of botulin. If the toxin is present, the animals will develop botulism and will die within 24 hours, except those animals protected by the antiserum corresponding to the type of toxin.

Clostridium botulinum can also be isolated by means of rapid immunofluorescence techniques from foods and from the patient's stools. The presence of the organism in the stools is not itself diagnostic, however.

The patient's cerebrospinal fluid (CSF) is normal.

TREATMENT

If it appears that botulin poisoning may have occurred, the patient must be hospitalized immediately because the signs may become aggravated in a matter of hours. The principal danger is respiratory paralysis. In addition, the suspected foods are collected, all persons who may have ingested the foods are identified, and an epidemiologic investigation is launched.

The value of administering antitoxin is uncertain. It is doubtful that the antitoxin can act on the toxin that is already fixed to neurofibrils. Therefore, the indications for specific serotherapy are not well codified. In severe forms of botulism, it is customary to inject 50,000 U type-specific antitoxin when the type is known, or 100,000 U trivalent ABE antitoxin in other cases. Individual sensitivity to the antitoxin must first be tested;

Table 31–1. Botulism in Canada, France, and the United States

	Canada	France	United States
Predominant Serotypes	E	B	C, A
Foods most often Responsible for Intoxication	Fish (preserved)	Ham (raw or smoked)	Vegetables (home-canned)
Mortality Rate	30%	3%	35%

one should bear in mind that 20% of patients manifest an immediate hypersensitivity reaction.

For persons who have ingested foods containing the toxin, but have not yet manifested clinical signs, the prophylactic administration of antitoxin must be discussed in each individual case by weighing the risk of a hypersensitivity reaction.

The value of the oral administration of penicillin has not been established, but the drug may reduce the multiplication of *Clostridium botulinum* in the gastrointestinal tract and thus may prevent further elaboration of the toxin.

Ventilatory assistance may be necessary in patients with respiratory disorders. Guanidine hydrochloride may be administered orally, 15 to 50 mg/kg/day. This drug appears to improve certain patients, although unfortunately it is not effective in the most severe cases and does not alter the mortality rate, which is about 10%.

Prevention depends on the proper preparation of home-canned goods and adequate cooking of preserved foodstuffs. Anatoxin vaccination can be proposed for laboratory personnel handling botulin. Because botulism is not a contagious disease, isolation of the patients is unnecessary.

Objective 31–3. Differentiate between acute anterior poliomyelitis and Guillain-Barré syndrome in a patient with acute peripheral nervous system involvement.

Acute anterior poliomyelitis (AAP) and Guillain-Barré (GB) syndrome can be differ-

---

PATHOGENESIS OF BOTULISM

Botulism is an infection with a toxin caused by *Clostridium botulinum*, a strictly anaerobic gram-positive rod. *C. botulinum* releases a potent, heat-labile exotoxin (destroyed by heating to 80° C for 30 minutes or to 100° C for 10 minutes), of which 6 antigenically different types, A through F, are known.

Until 1976, it was thought that botulism in man was a pure intoxication rather than an infection with a toxin because *Clostridium botulinum* did not appear to be able to multiply in living tissues after its ingestion by humans. The toxin responsible for the disease was thought to be elaborated prior to ingestion or excreted during bacterial lysis. Recently, colonization by this organism and the spontaneous production of toxin in the intestine have been demonstrated in infant botulism. Therefore, the infectious origin of botulism, previously suggested by animal experiments, is now recognized in man.

After its release into and passage in the blood, the toxin acts at the myoneural junction, more precisely on the cholinergic fibers, to prevent the release, although not the synthesis, of acetylcholine (ACh). This release of ACh is inhibited by a disturbance of conduction in the terminal unmyelinated nerve fibrils. At this level, the mode of action of the toxin is biochemical. The muscle fibers themselves continue to react normally to a direct electrical stimulus, and nervous conduction is not affected.

All cranial nerves may be involved, except the olfactory and optic nerves. The nerves of the limbs and the diaphragmatic and intercostal nerves may also be affected by the toxin.

---

entiated on the basis of clinical, epidemiologic, and laboratory findings, as summarized in Table 31–2.

CLINICAL MANIFESTATIONS

The onset of AAP is usually marked by a febrile syndrome with sore throat or rhinopharyngitis, nausea, vomiting, and meningeal signs. This picture precedes by some days the sudden appearance of paralysis, which is immediately most severe in the territory of the lesions and is accompanied by frank myalgia

Table 31–2. Differential Diagnosis of Acute Anterior Poliomyelitis and Guillain-Barré Syndrome

Features	Poliomyelitis	Guillain-Barré Syndrome
Fever	Usually present	Moderate or absent
Motor deficit	Asymmetric	Symmetric
Nuchal Rigidity	Present	Absent
Objective Sensory Disorders	Absent	Present (usually)
History of Adequate Poliomyelitis Vaccination	Absent	Present (usually)
CSF		
Protein Level	Normal	Elevated
Leukocytes/mm^3	20–500	20

(disturbances of subjective sensation) and early muscular atrophy. No objective sensory disorders are present; polioviruses specifically attack the anterior horn of the spinal cord and spare the sensory pathways. The anarchic distribution of paralysis affects a muscle group, a muscle, or a muscle bundle in various areas. All skeletal muscles may be involved. The paralysis has an asymmetric topography, but this remarkable feature may be difficult to delineate when the involvement is severe and extensive. The phase of extension of paralysis lasts approximately 3 to 5 days and then gives way to a phase of subsidence, which is at first frank, rapid, and reflective of the reversibility of the inflammatory lesions, and then is slow and prolonged. In 2 years, the sequelae of the irreversible neuronal destruction can be ascertained.

In GB syndrome, the onset of the motor deficit is generally less sudden and does not occur in the context of a recent febrile episode. Sensory disorders are always present, sometimes in the forefront, with paresthesias of the extremities, myalgia, and disturbance of the sense of position of the extremities and of the sense of vibration (tuning fork test). Vasomotor disorders of the extremities are frequent. Deep tendon reflexes are already absent before paralysis is complete. Muscular atrophy, not found in all cases, is moderate when it does exist. The distribution of paralysis is symmetric, but its extension is unpredictable, usually progressively ascending, and may involve the cranial nerves, with facial paralysis in 85% of patients.

The disease advances over a period of a few days to several weeks and then subsides over a long time span. A complete recovery free of residua is seen in 80% of the cases. The most serious consequence of GB syndrome is an impairment of respiration, which occurs in 20% of patients and may cause cardiopulmonary failure.

EPIDEMIOLOGIC CONSIDERATIONS

AAP is a complication of infection by a poliomyelitis virus, of which 3 antigenic types, 1, 2, and 3, are known. Prior to the introduction of attenuated live vaccine, poliomyelitis viral infections were prevalent, but were complicated by paralysis in only 1 case out of 100. Inapparent infection or minor illness confers solid and lasting natural immunity to the antigenic type of the virus. Man appears to be the natural host of the virus, which is spread by fecal-oral or by oral-oral transmission. The introduction of vaccination transformed the epidemiologic profile of the disease and reduced its annual incidence to a few cases in areas where mass vaccination is practiced. AAP is still endemic in Africa, Asia, and Latin America, however. In countries where vaccination is administered routinely, AAP is found in individuals who have not been vaccinated, usually children. Other cases occur in individuals vaccinated within 30 days or in persons close to an individual vaccinated with live oral vaccine within 60 days.

In contrast, the origin of GB syndrome remains unknown in 50 to 70% of cases. The illness may occur as the patient recovers from a viral or bacterial infection or an intoxication, or following a vaccination (see Objective 31–5). Exceptionally, this syndrome is epidemic in character.

LABORATORY FINDINGS

Examination of the CSF is basic to the diagnosis of peripheral nervous system involvement. If the CSF is normal, a toxic neuropathy is most likely, such as fish or shellfish poisoning, or the patient has botulism. In an infectious neuropathy, the CSF is abnormal and suggests GB syndrome, AAP, epidural abscess, or postinfectious transverse myelitis.

In all cases of AAP, the CSF reveals meningitis (clear liquid), with 20 to 500 lymphocytes/mm^3, normal or moderately elevated protein levels, and normal glucose levels. In GB syndrome, the CSF has a protein level of about 1 g/L or sometimes even higher, but the number of cells remains normal or moderately elevated (under 20/mm^2).

In AAP, isolation of the causative virus can be performed rapidly from cell cultures of pharyngeal secretions or stool specimens. The serotype of the poliovirus isolated can be identified by serologic neutralization tests. Rarely, the virus can be demonstrated from a CSF culture.

The detection of specific neutralizing antibody against the causative poliovirus, with a significant elevation in antibody titer in 2 samples of serum taken at an interval of 10 to 15 days, confirms the diagnosis of AAP. When the AAP is associated with the live vaccine viruses, as in an exceptional 55 cases after 193 million doses, a simultaneous elevation in all 3 types of specific antibodies is observed.

Because of the many infectious causes to be considered in GB syndrome, specific microbiologic investigations should be guided by the clinical context of the paralysis. The various infectious agents associated with about 50% of the cases of this syndrome are listed in Table 31–3.

Table 31–3. Infectious Causes to Consider in a Patient with Guillain-Barré Syndrome

Viruses	Bacteria
Herpes viruses	Mycoplasma pneumoniae
Epstein-Barr virus	Corynebacterium diphtheriae
Cytomegalovirus	
Herpes simplex virus	
Varicella-zoster virus	
Hepatitis B virus	
Orthomyxoviruses	
Influenza A virus	
Influenza B virus	
Paramyxoviruses	
Measles virus	
Mumps virus	

> **Objective 31–4.** Plan collective and individual preventive measures against acute anterior poliomyelitis.

VACCINATION

Because man appears to be the only natural host of poliovirus, the goal of active immunization against AAP is to eradicate the virus. Actually, it is more realistic to expect to reduce the number of infected persons and thus to diminish the likelihood of transmitting the disease. When the vaccination reaches a sufficient percentage in a given population, the spread of the virus is interrupted, and AAP disappears in that population; this phenomenon is known as the herd effect.

The three antigenically distinct types of poliomyelitis virus, 1, 2, and 3, demonstrate great stability. To induce adequate immunity, the vaccine must contain the three antigenic types of poliovirus. Two types of vaccine are available: an injectable, inactivated vaccine introduced in 1955 (Salk) and, since 1960, an attenuated live vaccine for oral administration (Sabin).

Inactivated Vaccine. The inactivated vaccine induces the formation of antibodies against the three types of poliovirus. These antibodies neutralize viremia and the transmission of the virus to the nervous system. Furthermore, that the inactivated vaccine appears to interrupt pharyngeal transmission of the virus may explain the herd effect observed in regions where the vaccine is used extensively. Replication of the poliovirus in the intestinal tract and its elimination in the feces may continue in persons who have been vaccinated, however.

Intramuscular injection of 2 doses of vaccine (1 ml) at an interval of 1 month induces a humoral response in 95% of the subjects for type 1, 100% for type 2, and 98% for type 3. When followed a year later by a booster dose, this vaccination makes possible a lasting immunity, and neutralizing antibodies are detected for 6 to 12 years.

Attenuated Live Vaccine. The oral administration of this vaccine makes it possible to induce intestinal immunity through the production of secretory IgA and thereby to prevent the implantation or to interrupt the intestinal replication of the wild virus. This method of vaccination rapidly halts an epidemic of AAP through a mechanism of interference between the vaccinal strains and the wild strains and thus blocks fecal-oral transmission of the wild virus. The quality and duration of the individual and collective immunity induced by the live vaccine seem no better than when inactivated vaccine is employed, however. Furthermore, the potential neurologic virulence of the attenuated vaccinal strain appears to have been responsible for 27 of the 30 cases of paralytic AAP recorded in the United States between January 1973 and September 1976 and for 6 of the 26 cases reported in England in 1976. This risk means that, notwithstanding its ease of administration, oral vaccination with the attenuated live strain should be used only in epidemics or where mass immunization is necessary.

The introduction of poliomyelitis vaccination in 1955 was followed by a spectacular decline in the incidence of this disease in affected countries. In the United States, the incidence of the disease was 20 to 40 cases per 100,000 annually prior to 1955, whereas at present, only a few cases are reported yearly. In Sweden and Finland, where only the inactivated vaccine has been used, no case of poliomyelitis has been registered since 1964. A systematic search for poliomyelitis virus in stool specimens of school-age children in these countries has failed to demonstrate the virus. This finding suggests that vaccination could eradicate the wild viral strain.

PREVENTIVE MEASURES WHEN A CASE OF POLIOMYELITIS IS IDENTIFIED

The period during which patients with AAP remain contagious is poorly known. It seems to depend on the duration of excretion of the virus in pharyngeal secretions and stools. This virulent excretion begins a few days before the onset of the clinical manifestations and may persist for 4 to 6 weeks in the stools. Prophylactic measures include isolation of the patient, disinfection of feces with chemical agents, and separate cleaning of the patient's linen and dishes. The patient's contacts must be vaccinated or revaccinated with trivalent attenuated vaccine. The only contraindication to vaccination with attenuated vaccine is in immune deficiency states such as in thymus dysplasia, anomaly of B-lymphocyte function, and treatment with immunodepressants. In these persons, inactivated vaccine must be used.

In industrialized countries, an epidemic of AAP is defined by the identification of at least two cases caused by the same poliovirus serotype within the same month in a well-defined population. In this event, all individuals aged over 6 weeks who have not been previously vaccinated or have only been partially vaccinated must receive an emergency vaccination with trivalent oral vaccine. The schedule of administration of the vaccine includes primary vaccination and revaccination.

Primary Vaccination. In infants, one should administer 2 doses of attenuated vaccine at an interval of 2 months starting at 2 months of age (a third dose is given in countries where the disease is endemic), with a booster dose a year later. This same primary series schedule is adopted for older children or adolescents who have never received the vaccine.

This vaccination schedule is now controversial, however, and the trend is to avoid the use of attenuated live vaccine in infants under 6 months of age and to give inactivated vaccine instead.

Revaccination. In school-age children, revaccination consists of administering a booster dose of trivalent oral vaccine. Subsequently, the immunity-maintenance schedule depends on individual epidemiologic conditions. Adults who have no detectable immunity against poliomyelitis and who risk infection may receive the inactivated vaccine according to the primary series schedule.

> **Objective 31–5. Relate Guillain-Barré syndrome to its most probable cause.**

Histologic peripheral nerve lesions characterized by infiltration of lymphocytes and destruction of myelin, observed in GB syndrome, suggest an autoimmune response mechanism. In 50% of patients, a particular cause can be considered. A toxic, chemical, or drug-related factor is sometimes implicated in the development of GB syndrome. This discussion is limited to postinfectious and postimmunization causes. In 30 to 40% of patients, a significant association exists between this syndrome and certain infectious diseases. Thus, an influenza-like febrile syndrome has frequently been described in the weeks preceding the onset of paralysis in patients with GB syndrome. Various possible causes are listed in Table 31–3.

HERPESVIRUS

In the series reported by Wahren and Link,[1] 60% of patients with GB syndrome had a significant rise in antibodies to Epstein-Barr virus in the course of the illness. In all these cases, however, tests for IgM-type heterophil antibodies were negative. In this same series and in that of Klemola and associates,[2] 30 to 50% of patients with GB syndrome showed a frank rise in antibodies to cytomegalovirus (CMV). Specific IgM antibodies against CMV has recently been demonstrated in GB syndrome. Herpes simplex virus or varicella-zoster viral infection has been proved serologically in GB syndrome. The significance of these observations is not clear. Either GB syndrome is actually caused by these different viral infections or the syndrome secondarily reactivates a latent infection with these various viruses through immune disorders.

HEPATITIS B VIRUS

The appearance of GB syndrome has been observed during the preicteric stage of hepatitis B. The mechanism of this association is unknown. An immune response with immune complex deposits, often mentioned in connection with the pathogenesis of the extrahepatic manifestations of hepatitis B, could account for this disorder.

A similar mechanism has been proposed in GB syndrome occurring after vaccinations against rabies, measles, and swine influenza, as well as after revaccination against smallpox.

MYCOPLASMA PNEUMONIAE

Mycoplasma pneumoniae has been isolated in the sputum of several patients with GB syndrome. This observation is comparable to the autoallergy phenomena caused by mycoplasmal infections; 70% of these infections are accompanied by the appearance of antibodies to lung, and 50% are associated with the presence of cold agglutinins (antibodies against erythrocytes).

In conclusion, although numerous infectious causes have been associated with GB syndrome, none have definitely been proved responsible for this disease.

> **Objective 31–6. Diagnose tick paralysis.**

Tick paralysis is manifested by the sudden onset of ascending flaccid paralysis, acute ataxia, or both. The patients are often agitated and irritable, but have no fever. Usually, no associated sensory disorders are present. Results of routine laboratory tests, electroencephalograms, and CSF examinations are normal. Electrodiagnostic tests sometimes reveal a reduction in nerve conduction velocity.

The etiologic diagnosis depends on the discovery of a tick on the patient's body or scalp. The tick is usually present for 4 to 7 days before symptoms appear, and its removal is the only treatment. Removal of the tick is followed by rapid improvement and by full recovery in 48 hours. Failure to discover the cause and to apply treatment can be serious. If the tick is not removed, the paralysis may progress and may result in bulbar involvement, respiratory paralysis, and death within a few days. The overall mortality rate is 10%; fatalities are observed only in children.

Most cases of tick-bite paralysis occur in the spring and summer in children and adolescents, usually girls. Adult cases are rare and involve men more often than women.

This disease is believed to be caused by a toxin secreted in tick saliva. This toxin has a marked affinity for the central nervous system, the peripheral nervous system, and the motor end plate. In the United States, 43 species of ticks are known to cause this type of paralysis in humans, in other mammals, and in birds. In man, most cases are due to ticks belonging to the genus dermacentor.

Because this disease is rapidly reversible and is potentially severe if unrecognized, one must consider the diagnosis in any patient who manifests ascending flaccid paralysis or acute ataxia.

> **Objective 31–7. Consider the diagnosis of leprosy in peripheral neuropathy.**

Leprosy is still common worldwide. At present, some 2 million cases are known. This disease is associated with economic underdevelopment, malnutrition, and overpopulation. Thus, only a few hundred cases are known in the Western world, whereas leprosy is endemic in India.

Leprosy is an infection caused by *Mycobacterium leprae*, which has a particular tropism for tissues of ectodermal origin. The skin and cutaneous nerves are the essential targets of this organism (Fig. 31–1). Schwann nerve cells with unmyelinated fibers are attacked most often.

TYPES OF LEPROSY

Depending on the immunologic resistance to infection of the individual, the expression of the disease varies greatly. At opposite ends of the clinical spectrum are the following polar forms:

Lepromatous Leprosy. This form of the disease is characterized by immunologic tolerance to *Mycobacterium leprae* (low resistance) and is expressed by a moderate inflammatory response, the presence of large numbers of bacilli, and the existence of extensive and severe cutaneous nerve lesions.

Tuberculoid Leprosy. This type of leprosy is defined by a high immunologic competence with respect to the infection (high resistance), with an intense, delayed hypersensitivity type of inflammatory response, few bacilli, and localized and circumscribed skin lesions.

In addition, borderline or intermediate forms of leprosy exist.

CARDINAL NEUROLOGIC MANIFESTATIONS

Loss of cutaneous sensibility, first to temperature and then to touch and pressure, is the first manifestation of neurogenic involvement, which culminates in total cutaneous anesthesia. The areas of skin most exposed to cold are particularly affected, such as the ears, nose, cheeks, forearms, and legs. In untreated patients, the anesthesia extends inexorably, but always spares the scalp and skin folds. Traumas in anesthetic areas often lead to trophic changes such as ulcers and deformations.

The motor involvement affects nerve trunks along their most superficial course: the ulnar nerve at the elbow, the median nerve at the wrist, and the peroneal nerve at the ankle, as well as the superficial branch of the facial nerve.

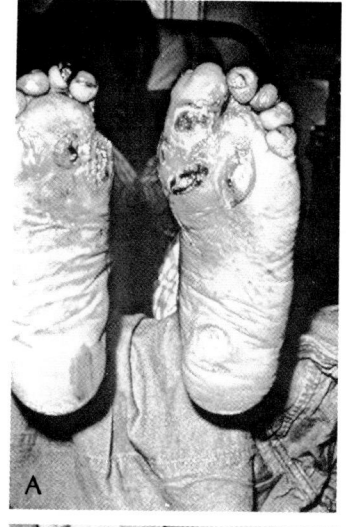

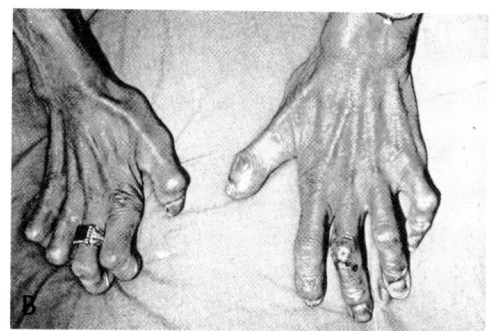

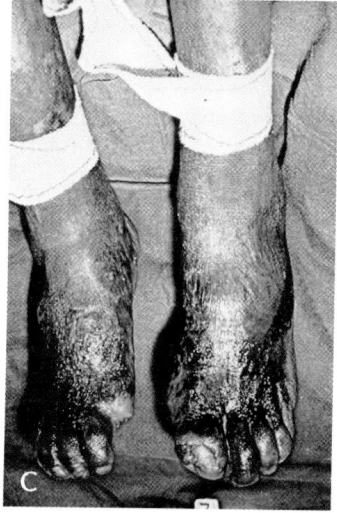

Infections Affecting the Peripheral Nervous System

Fig. 31–1. *A* to *C*, Leprosy.

The deep tendon reflexes and proprioceptive sensations remain normal because they receive their impulses from deeper-lying nerves. Pathologic examination reveals the destruction of intracutaneous nerve endings, with an intense, granulomatous, inflammatory reaction in the tuberculoid form of the disease. In the lepromatous form, the predominant lesions are fibrosis within and around the nerves and alternating demyelination and remyelination.

OTHER CLINICAL MANIFESTATIONS

In the tuberculoid form of leprosy, one often sees hypopigmented macules that have lost their capacity to produce sweat. In addition to these cutaneous signs, lepromatous leprosy has many more signs and symptoms, including subcutaneous nodules (lepromas), which may produce facial deformities, rhinitis, pharyngitis, laryngitis, hepatomegaly, involvement of the testes, bone pain, and eye disorders. Confirmation of the diagnosis of leprosy is based on histologic findings in the tuberculoid form of the disease. In lepromatous leprosy, large numbers of acid- and alcohol-resistant bacilli are readily observed in various specimens, nasal in particular.

TREATMENT

Treatment must be continued for 3 years in the tuberculoid form of leprosy and longer in the lepromatous form. Sulfones, initially 25 mg/day orally, increasing to 100 mg/day in 3 to 4 months, but contraindicated in glucose-6-phosphate dehydrogenase deficiency, are inexpensive and are widely administered in endemic areas. Long-acting sulfonamides are administered on a 2-day (125 to 500 mg) or a weekly basis (sulfadoxine, 1500 mg), also in progressive increments; unfortunately, these drugs are expensive and may produce adverse reactions such as rash and toxic epidermolysis. Rifampin, 600 mg/day orally, is effective but expensive for patients in third-world countries. Clofazimine, 100 mg/day, is an alternative to sulfones.

> **Objective 31–8.** Obtain clinical evidence of diphtheritic paralysis.

During or after diphtheria, three types of neurologic disorders may be observed. They are listed by order of frequency.

1. Paralysis of the soft palate, evidenced by nasal speech, regurgitation of fluids through the nose, false passage of food, and dysphagia. Examination shows a flaccid, inert soft palate, and the pharyngeal (gag) reflex is often abolished.
2. Paralysis of accommodation, resulting in diplopia.
3. Polyradiculoneuritis of the limbs, predominantly the lower limbs. Symptoms are either purely sensory or are associated with a motor deficit. This paralysis may be extensive and may affect the abdominal muscles and the diaphragm and other respiratory muscles.

Relating these neurologic disorders to a diphtheritic origin may be simple if the paralysis is of recent onset, as is usual with paralysis of the soft palate and of accommodation. A known recent or concomitant pharyngitis with a membrane is suggestive of the diagnosis and is an indication for a throat swab to search for *Corynebacterium diphtheriae*. Therefore, when considering the cause of a polyradiculoneuritis, diphtheria must be included in the differential diagnosis, even in countries where this infection has been uncommon since the introduction of diphtheria vaccination. Even in countries where vaccination is otherwise properly administered, adults usually fail to receive booster injections, and most of them are no longer immunized. Furthermore, a mild and undetected infection may occur in children who have been properly vaccinated and are immune.

The prognosis of diphtheritic neuropathies is favorable because the disease nearly always resolves completely without sequelae. The polyradiculoneuritis may persist for several months before receding, however.

The preventive treatment of the neurologic complications of diphtheria is based on early administration of antitoxin (10 to 80,000 U, depending on the clinical severity of the initial infection), after testing the sensitivity of the patient to antitoxin serum. The diphtheria toxin is responsible for these demyelinating neuropathies. Vaccination is the best way to prevent diphtheritic infection. The present vaccines make it possible to immunize children and adults without serious adverse reactions. Immunity against diphtheria in the adult should be provided or extended by this method.

REFERENCES

1. Wahren, B., and Link, H.: Antibodies to Epstein-Barr virus and cytomegalovirus in Guillain-Barré syndrome. J. Neurol. Sci., 28:129, 1976.
2. Klemola, E., Weckman, N., Haltia, K., and Kaariainen, L.: The Guillain-Barré syndrome associated with acquired cytomegalovirus infection. Acta Med. Scand., 181:603, 1967.

SUGGESTED READINGS

Anonymous: Tick-paralysis. Morbid. Mortal. Weekly Rep., 30:217, 1981.

Arnason, B.G.: Inflammatory polyradiculopathies. *In* Peripheral Neuropathy. Vol. II. Edited by P.J. Dyck, P.L. Thomas, and E.L. Lambert. Philadelphia, W.B. Saunders, 1975.

Cherington, M.: Botulism: ten years' experience. Arch. Neurol., *30*:432, 1974.

Collingham, K.E., Pollock, T.M., and Roebuck, M.O.: Paralytic poliomyelitis in England and Wales, 1976–1977. Lancet, *1*:976, 1978.

Freemon, F.R.: Toxin polyneuropathy. *In* Causes of polyneuropathy. Acta Neurol. Scand., *59, 51* (Suppl.):16, 1975.

Klemola, E., Weckman, N., Haltia, K., and Kaariainen, L.: The Guillain-Barré syndrome associated with acquired cytomegalovirus infection. Acta Med. Scand., *181*:603, 1967.

Krugman, B.D., et al.: Antibody persistence after primary immunization with trivalent oral poliovirus vaccine. Pediatrics, *60*:80, 1977.

Krugman, S., Ward, R., and Katz, S.L.: Enteroviral infections. *In* Infectious Diseases of Children. 7th Ed. St. Louis, C.V. Mosby, 1981.

Lupton, M.D., and Klawans, H.: Neurologic complications of diphtheria. *In* Handbook of Clinical Neurology: Infections of the Nervous System. Edited by P. Vinken, and G. Bruyn. New York, Elsevier North-Holland, 1978.

McLeod, J.C., Walsh, J.C., Prineas, J.W., and Polland, J.D.: Acute idiopathic polyneuritis. J. Neurol. Sci., *27*:145, 1976.

Openshaw, H., and Lieberman, J.S.: Vaccine-related poliomyelitis. Arch. Intern. Med., *142*:1617, 1982.

Salk, J., and Salk, D.: Control of influenza and poliomyelitis with killed virus vaccines. Science, *195*:834, 1977.

Shepard, C.C.: Leprosy today. N. Engl. J. Med., *307*:1640, 1982.

Smith, L.D.: Botulism: The Organism, Its Toxin, the Disease. Springfield, IL, Charles C Thomas, 1977.

Turner, H.D., Brett, E.M., Gilbert, R.J., and Ghosh, A.C.: Infant botulism in England. Lancet, *1*:1277, 1978.

Wahren, B., and Link, H.: Antibodies to Epstein-Barr virus and cytomegalovirus in Guillain-Barré syndrome. J. Neurol. Sci., *28*:129, 1976.

CHAPTER 32

Eye Infections

R. Michaud and A. Rousseau

Objective 32–1. Evaluate a probable eye infection clinically and microbiologically.

Bacteria, fungi, viruses, and parasites may infect the eye (Table 32–1). The infections may be limited to the eye or its adnexa, or they may represent a specific localization of a systemic disease. Nearly all organisms pathogenic for man can produce an eye infection. Furthermore, certain organisms such as *Haemophilus aegypticus* and *Moraxella lacunata* are found almost exclusively in ocular infections. Certain saprophytes, such as *Staphylococcus epidermidis*, *Corynebacterium xerosis*, and *Branhamella catarrhalis*, may become pathogenic when they grow in the eye.

When dealing with a severe eye infection, the physician should keep in mind the following guidelines: (1) if the essential means of diagnosis is not available locally, do nothing, administer no treatment, and immediately refer the patient to a specialized center; no topical treatment should be prescribed before specimens are obtained; a single local application of antibiotics is of no value in severe infections and may complicate the future selection of an adequate treatment; (2) avoid diluting the patient's tears through the unnecessary use of commercial "eye drops;" tears contain lysozymes, antibacterial biochemical factors, and leukocytes that provide natural protection; and (3) except when absolutely necessary, no local dressing should be applied; the temperature at the surface of the eye, 34° C, limits the growth of bacterial pathogens.

CLINICAL EVALUATION

The patient's medical history and the clinical examination may permit one to identify the etiologic factor. The clinical picture of an eye infection depends on the causative organism, the host, and the structure of the infected tissues. Thus, the conjunctival reaction differs with the nature of the infectious agent: a lymphoid reaction with viruses, chlamydiae, and a few other bacteria, including moraxella; a papillary reaction with most bacterial infections. In contrast, neonates, who have no conjunctival lymphoid tissue, respond uniformly to any kind of infection by a papillary reaction. Debilitated persons or those who receive immunosuppressive treatment may develop a severe infection with an infectious agent that would show little virulence otherwise. The structure of the infected tissues also determines a particular type of response.

Vascularized Tissue. Such tissue, including the conjunctiva, reacts classically with redness, pain, heat, edema (called chemosis

Table 32-1. Principal Bacterial Infections of the Eye

Bacterium	Infection
Staphylococcus	Blepharitis, acute or chronic conjunctivitis, punctate keratitis, corneal ulcer, orbital cellulitis
Streptococcus	Pseudomembranous conjunctivitis, corneal ulcer, phlegmon of eyelids, orbital cellulitis
Moraxella	Angular blepharoconjunctivitis, corneal ulcer
Chlamydia	Inclusion conjunctivitis, trachoma
Haemophilus aegypticus and *H. influenzae*	Conjunctivitis, orbital cellulitis
Neisseria gonorrhoeae	Purulent conjunctivitis of the adult and the newborn, corneal ulcer, endophthalmitis, uveitis
Neisseria meningitidis	Conjunctivitis with petechiae, bilateral endophthalmitis
Mycobacterium tuberculosis	Phlyctenular conjunctivitis, uveitis, retinitis
Pseudomonas aeruginosa	Blepharitis, conjunctivitis, corneal ulcer, endophthalmitis

Table 32-2. Conjunctival Flora in 7461 Normal Eyes in the United States

Bacterium	Percentage Affected (%)
Staphylococcus epidermidis	68.5
Staphylococcus aureus	42.0
Diphtheroids (*Corynebacterium xerosis*)	28.7
Alpha-hemolytic streptococcus	5.0
Streptococcus pneumoniae	3.2
Gram-negative bacilli	2.6
Gram-negative diplococci (*Branhamella*)	2.5
Gram-positive bacilli	0.7
Micrococcus tetragenus	0.3

(Modified from Locatcher-Khorazo, D., and Seegal, B.: Microbiology of the Eye. St. Louis, C.V. Mosby, 1972.)

when it occurs in the bulbar conjunctiva), and an exudate whose consistency may be serous, mucopurulent, purulent, or hemorrhagic. See Table 32-2 for a list of conjunctival flora.

Nonvascularized Tissue. The cornea, vitreum, and lens may develop opacities or necrosis with wasting of the tissues. The sclera, an already opaque structure, can become necrotic.

Nervous Tissue. The optic nerve and the retina, can develop edema, necrosis, and finally gliosis at the cicatricial phase.

Tissue Fluid. Fluids such as the aqueous humor may become fibrinous with large quantities of inflammatory cells that sometimes form a solid level called a hypopyon. The hypopyon results from an intraocular infection, or it may be aseptic when it accompanies a severe external infection.

Types of Infection. Acute infection with causative organisms present in large numbers locally may be caused by pneumococcus, haemophilus, and staphylococcus. Mild infection with maceration of the surface epithelium may be produced by the exotoxin of some bacteria, such as staphylococcus and moraxella, whose numbers are often too few to be found in culture. Opportunistic invasion may follow a local trauma, especially in infections with pseudomonas and pneumococcus. Epithelial parasitism may occur without breach of the surface membrane, as in infections with *Corynebacterium diphtheriae*, *Haemophilus aegyptius*, *Neisseria gonorrhoeae*, and *Corynebacterium xerosis* in dead cells of keratitis sicca. Surface proliferation may be promoted by abundant oily secretions in the host in moraxella and pseudomonas infections. In addition, allergies may exist to infectious products; examples are allergic microbial conjunctivitis caused by hypersensitivity to staphylococcus, phlyctenular conjunctivitis from infection with *Mycobacterium tuberculosis* and *Staphylococcus aureus*, and eczematoid blepharitis caused by staphylococcus and moraxella.

ADENOVIRUSES

Adenoviruses contain double-stranded DNA and have 252 capsomers forming an icosahedron of 70 to 90 nm in diameter. These viruses penetrate the cells of the host and form nuclear inclusions that can be observed at high magnification.

Adenoviruses, which have a predilection for mucous membranes, produce acute respiratory diseases including colds and pharyngitis, as well as conjunctivitis sometimes associated with keratitis. They may remain in the host's stools for up to 2 months after the acute infection.

The principal adenoviruses in human eye infections are: type 3, which is responsible for epidemic pharyngoconjunctivitis, a disease that may also be caused by other viral types such as 1, 4, 5, 6, 7, and 14; and type 8, which is responsible for epidemic keratoconjunctivitis, a disorder capable of producing residual keratitis lasting for up to 2 years. Types 2, 4, 7, 9, 10, 14, 16, 19, and 29 may also be isolated from patients with epidemic keratoconjunctivitis.

Adenovirus infections are diagnosed by studying smears of cells that show a great preponderance of mononuclear cells, as well as cells with nuclear inclusions. In cell culture on HeLa cells, the cytopathic effect is diagnostic of adenovirus infections. Moreover, in these cultures, nuclear inclusions are more easily demonstrated. By means of serologic studies such as complement-fixation, neutralization, and hemagglutination-inhibition tests, the adenoviruses can also be typed.

No specific treatment exists for adenovirus infections. Instead, treatment is purely symptomatic and is aimed at reducing the systemic and local malaise. The use of corticosteroids should be avoided in all patients with adenovirus infections. These viruses are contagious, and persons affected should stay away from their place of employment if they have contact with the public, to prevent an epidemic. This absence from work should last for 10 days after the onset of the clinical signs because patients are infective for this length of time. The incubation period is from 8 to 10 days. In cases of adenovirus infection, the hands must be washed frequently because contamination occurs from hand to hand, directly, or through the use of shared objects.

MORAXELLA

Organisms belonging to the genus moraxella are large, thick, gram-negative bacilli with rounded or rectangular ends. They stain easily. These organisms are often found in pairs or in short chains and sometimes take Gram's stain, so that gram-negative and gram-positive organisms can be seen on the same slide. This nonmotile, non-spore-forming bacillus is usually implicated only in eye infections.

Moraxella lacunata, encountered most often in ophthalmology, proliferates in abundant sebaceous secretions or on desquamated epithelial cells. It causes blepharoconjunctivitis and peripheral keratitis that can progress to serpiginous corneal ulcer. *Moraxella lacunata* subspecies *liquefaciens* is responsible for central corneal ulcers with hypopyon that can eventually perforate the eye. This subspecies is generally more virulent than *Moraxella lacunata* and often infects debilitated persons, particularly alcoholics.

The diagnosis of moraxella infection is based primarily on examination of a smear containing the typical organisms. The culture of moraxella is difficult because the morphologic features of the bacillus change on different culture media. Moraxella does not grow on chocolate agar, whereas on blood agar, growth is slow, and the bacterial colonies are small, semitransparent, and can easily go unnoticed. The best culture medium is Loeffler medium, in which the bacillus forms excavations by liquefaction but in which no colony can be seen.

Moraxella is sensitive to products containing zinc. Patients with blepharoconjunctivitis respond well to treatment with zinc sulfate in a solution of 0.25% to 0.5%, 4 times daily. In more severe infections, moraxella usually responds to sulfonamides, tetracycline, streptomycin, erythromycin, and chloramphenicol. This organism is also sensitive to heat.

MICROBIOLOGIC DIAGNOSIS

Bacteriologic culture is necessary in all cases of hyperacute, membranous, chronic, severe, or relapsing conjunctivitis, in Parinaud's oculoglandular syndrome, in ophthalmia neonatorum, in corneal ulcer, and in endophthalmitis.

Specimen Collection. For specimen collection, a platinum loop is usually inadequate because it frequently collects only tears. Secretions on the edge of the eyelids should be collected with a sterile, cotton-tipped swab, passing over the line of the eyelashes, whereas conjunctival secretions are collected with a sterile, cotton-tipped swab stick in the upper or lower cul-de-sac. In either case, the product is inoculated immediately on both blood agar and chocolate agar. Lacrimal secretions are pooled at the lacrimal point by digital pressure on the lacrimal sac, in the oculonasal angle, and are collected with a sterile, cotton-tipped swab as they leave the punctum lacrimale. Before these secretions

CHLAMYDIAE

Chlamydiae are gram-negative bacteria that, because of their inability to produce their own metabolic energy, are obligate intracellular parasites. These bacteria differ from viruses in the following ways:
1. Their molecular structure includes both DNA and RNA.
2. They reproduce by binary fission.
3. They have ribosomes.
4. They have bacterial walls containing glycoproteins in which muramic acid is found.
5. They are sensitive to several antimicrobial agents including sulfonamides and tetracycline; these bacteria do not grow on the usual culture media, however.

Chlamydiae have a growth cycle that lasts 24 to 48 hours. The infectious particle, called the elementary body, whose diameter is approximately 0.3 μ, is phagocytized in the cytoplasm of the host cell. There the particle gradually turns into an initial body, which is larger (0.5 to 1 μ) and is surrounded only by a vacuole. The vacuole gradually becomes filled with the growth and binary fission of the initial bodies. A vacuole filled with initial bodies forms a cytoplasmic inclusion in the host cell. The particles in this inclusion body are then released and infect other host cells, so the cycle starts anew.

Chlamydiae are commonly classified into groups A and B. Group A chlamydiae are generally inhibited by sulfonamides and have inclusions containing glycogen. These are the trachoma inclusion conjunctivitis (TRIC) agents, responsible for trachoma, inclusion conjunctivitis, urethritis and cervicitis, and lymphogranuloma venereum. All these agents of group A constitute the species *Chlamydia trachomatis*.

Group B chlamydiae are usually resistant to sulfonamides, and their inclusions do not contain glycogen. Organisms of this group comprise the species *Chlamydia psittaci,* responsible for psittacosis and an isolated form of conjunctivitis.

The diagnosis of a chlamydial infection is established by the following:
1. The search for inclusion bodies in the cytoplasm of epithelial cells spread on a smear. The inclusion bodies stain purple with Giemsa stain. The inclusions of group A agents stain brown by Lugol's solution because of the glycogen matrix found in this group.
2. Growth on yolk sacs of chick embryos. The embryos are killed in 5 to 7 days by the chlamydial infection.
3. Cell culture on a single layer of irradiated McCoy cells.
4. Indirect immunofluorescence. A microimmunofluorescence technique allows the identification of species and groups on a specimen of tears and serum from an individual in whom a chlamydial infection is suspected.

Chlamydiae are easily inactivated by prolonged storage at room temperature or by heat, but they retain their infectivity for years when they are preserved at $-50°$ C or $-70°$ C. Any specimen taken for laboratory examination must be kept on ice or, better yet, frozen immediately after collection.

Chlamydiae are inhibited by several antibiotics, of which the most widely used is still tetracycline. For individuals suffering from inclusion conjunctivitis, systemic treatment must be given because this disease is sexually transmitted. Sulfonamides are also effective against group A chlamydiae.

Despite intensive research in this area, no vaccine has yet been developed against chlamydiae. The infections themselves produce no lasting immunity in affected individuals.

---

come into contact with the other stuctures, they should be inoculated directly on chocolate agar, thioglycolate medium, and Sabouraud medium. Corneal secretions must be taken delicately with a Kimura-type spatula or, if not available, with the dull edge of a Bard-Parker No. 15 knife blade, under direct microscopic observation.

Smears. For all severe or chronic infections, one should prepare smears for direct bacteriologic examination (Gram's stain) or cytologic study and examination for cell inclusions (Giemsa stain).

A viral infection should be suspected if one observes a preponderance of lymphocytes, and sometimes cellular inclusion bodies or multinuclear cells on the smear. An acute bacterial infection is characterized by a preponderance of polymorphonuclear leukocytes, except in infections due to moraxella or to *Branhamella catarrhalis*. Fungal or chlamydial infections also produce large numbers of polymorphonuclear leukocytes, except chronic cases in which, as in chronic bacterial infections, the cytologic features are mixed. Eosinophils are found in allergic diseases, including vernal keratoconjunctivitis, or in parasitic infestations. Plasma cells are found in chlamydial infections, particularly in trachoma.

Special Cases. Specimens to be examined for viruses or chlamydiae are collected with a sterile swab stick and are placed in a special transport medium for either agent; one should leave the swab in the medium and break the stick over the edge of the container. The specimens should be kept on ice or frozen until they arrive at the virology laboratory. These specimens are then inoculated on the appropriate cell cultures.

The purpose of serologic studies is to determine the humoral immunologic response against a given infectious agent. The diagnosis is based on 2 examinations performed at 3-week intervals. The test is positive if the specific serum antibodies increase during this period. In ophthalmology, the most commonly requested serologic studies are for the following agents: histoplasma, toxoplasma, herpes simplex and zoster viruses, cytomegalovirus, adenovirus, and syphilis (fluorescent treponemal antibody absorption test).

Some skin tests can help to demonstrate hypersensitivity to antigens of the infecting agent. Most commonly used in ophthalmology are candidin tests, to which most normal individuals respond positively, and tuberculin tests (purified protein derivative). These tests must be administered with great caution because they can trigger a severe uveal reaction if the results are positive.

As soon as specimens have been taken, treatment may be started, based on the immediate examination of smears and the clinical appearance: this tentative treatment will have to be modified as soon as the laboratory results are available.

> Objective 32-2. Identify the major eye infections on the basis of their localization and suggest an appropriate course of action.

INFECTIONS OF THE EYEBROWS AND EYELIDS

Table 32-3 gives the clinical manifestations (Fig. 32-1), microbiologic causes, and suggested therapy of infections of the eyebrows and eyelids.

INTRAORBITAL INFECTIONS

Table 32-4 describes intraorbital infections, which are serious, potentially lethal problems that require immediate attention. The orbit is nearly surrounded by sinuses and this anatomic feature increases its vulnerability. The ethmoid sinus, separated from the orbit only by the thin lamina papyracea, is often infected in children, whereas the frontal sinus is generally involved in adults. The infection can follow an injury, entry of a foreign body, a systemic infection, or an infection of the eyelids.

LACRIMAL APPARATUS INFECTIONS

Dacryoadenitis, infection of the lacrimal gland, is rare nowadays. The differential diagnosis should include inflammations such as sarcoidosis, lymphoepithelial lesions, as in Sjögren's syndrome, and lymphomas. Infection of the canaliculi, often associated with conjunctivitis or acute dacryocystitis, may result in chronic or unilateral relapsing conjunctivitis.

Dacryocystitis, infection of the lacrimal sac (Fig. 32-2), is usually secondary to stenosis of the nasolacrimal duct. In adults, chronic dacryocystitis reflects an obstruction of the lacrimal sac or nasolacrimal ducts; the acute disorder occurs when the lacrimal passages are totally or partially obstructed and infected material is retained in the lacrimal sac. These disorders are the subject of Table 32-5.

CONJUNCTIVITIS

Acute bacterial conjunctivitis is often unilateral initially but spreads rapidly to the contralateral eye. This disorder is often associated with blepharitis or keratis because the surface epithelium of these structures is continuous with that of the conjunctiva.

Some forms of conjunctivitis occur a few weeks after sexual contact. One such disorder, inclusion conjunctivitis, passes spontaneously from an acute phase to a chronic phase refractory to all usual treatments. It also relapses relapsing periodically for several years. Gonorrheal conjunctivitis is mani-

Table 32–3. Infections of Eyebrows and Eyelids

	Clinical Appearance	Etiologic Agent	Recommended Therapy
Eyebrows			
Local infection	Folliculitis, abscess, phlegmon	Staphylococcus, streptococcus	Topical or systemic antibiotic rarely necessary
Systemic infection	Complete or partial alopecia of eyebrows or eyelashes	*Treponema pallidum, Mycobacterium leprae*	Specific therapy
	Simulation by basal cell carcinoma of chronic ulcerative dermatitis of the eyebrow	Unknown	Biopsy
Eyelids (blepharitis)	Burning, pruritus, tearing, local irritation, photophobia, crust formation in the cilia and nasal angle, vasodilatation of free edge of the eyelids, edema, ulceration, or necrosis at the base of the cilia and in the palpebral angles, eczematiform lesions	*Staphylococcus aureus* mostly, but also *Staphylococcus epidermidis*, streptococcus, pneumococcus, pseudomonas	Mechanical debridement of the base of the eyelashes and washing of the cilia with mild shampoo Topical sulfacetamide In severe cases only, systemic antibiotic according to sensitivity testing In hypersensitive patients, addition of a weak topical corticosteroid, if certain that herpes simplex virus not involved
Special Cases			
Acute infection of the eyelid margin	Possible abscess or phlegmon formation	Same as blepharitis	Surgical drainage sometimes necessary
Ulceration of the angles of the eyelids	Possible ulceration of the base of the cilia	Moraxella or staphylococcus	
Pediculosis palpebrarum	Severe pruritus with redness of eyelids and follicular conjunctivitis	*Phthirus pubis* or *Pediculus humanus capitis*	Local debridement, benzene hexachloride shampoo
Molluscum contagiosum	Umbilicated lesion on the edge of the eyelids with blepharitis and follicular conjunctivitis	Virus (eosinophilic viral inclusion bodies visible on biopsy)	Curettage, surgical removal, or local cryotherapy
Ulcerative or necrotic vesicular blepharitis of free edge of eyelid	Follicular conjunctivitis or specific keratitis associated	Herpes simplex virus, herpes zoster virus (differential diagnosis with *Bacillus anthracis* or vaccinia virus)	Treatment depends on cause (see Table 32–6)

Table 32-4. Intraorbital Infections

Type of Infection	Clinical Appearance	Etiologic Agent	Recommended Therapy
Orbital cellulitis	Seen in patients with a "bad cold" with sinusitis; local pain, redness, and heat, chemosis, proptosis, limited ocular motility, reduced vision, or even total loss of sight accompanied by high fever Pus in sinal orifices Possible complications: thrombosis of sinus cavernosus, meningeal signs, loss of visual acuity, mydriasis, paresis of the extraocular muscles (cranial nerves III and VI), ophthalmoplegia, papilledema, retinal venous congestion, spread to the other eye	*Staphylococcus aureus, Streptococcus pyogenes, Streptococcus pneumoniae, Haemophilus influenzae*, fungi (mucormycosis in debilitated or diabetic patients)	Intensive initial treatment with penicillinase-resistant penicillin or third-generation cephalosporin (*H. influenzae* suspected) Collection of a specimen at site of infection Possible surgical drainage
Parasitic infestation	Pain, redness, local heat, edema, and chemosis, slow development of exophthalmia, optic nerve atrophy, reduced ocular motility Intraocular involvement possible Differential diagnosis with purely inflammatory lesions, granulomas of various origin (sarcoidosis), and tumors	*Echinococcus granulosus, Taenia solium, Onchocerca volvulus, Toxocara canis*	Specific antiparasitic drugs (destruction of parasites may induce violent inflammatory reaction and possible anaphylactic shock), possible corticosteroid therapy, possible surgical exploration of orbit
Extraocular muscular infection	Rarely, a complication of a local infection or a parasitic infestation of the orbit Involvement of the extraocular muscles related to severe systemic disease, with paralysis or paresis of the extraocular muscles	*Mycobacterium tuberculosis, Trichinella spiralis*, bacterial toxins (botulism or diphtheria), neurotropic viruses (Guillain-Barré syndrome)	Etiologic systemic treatment

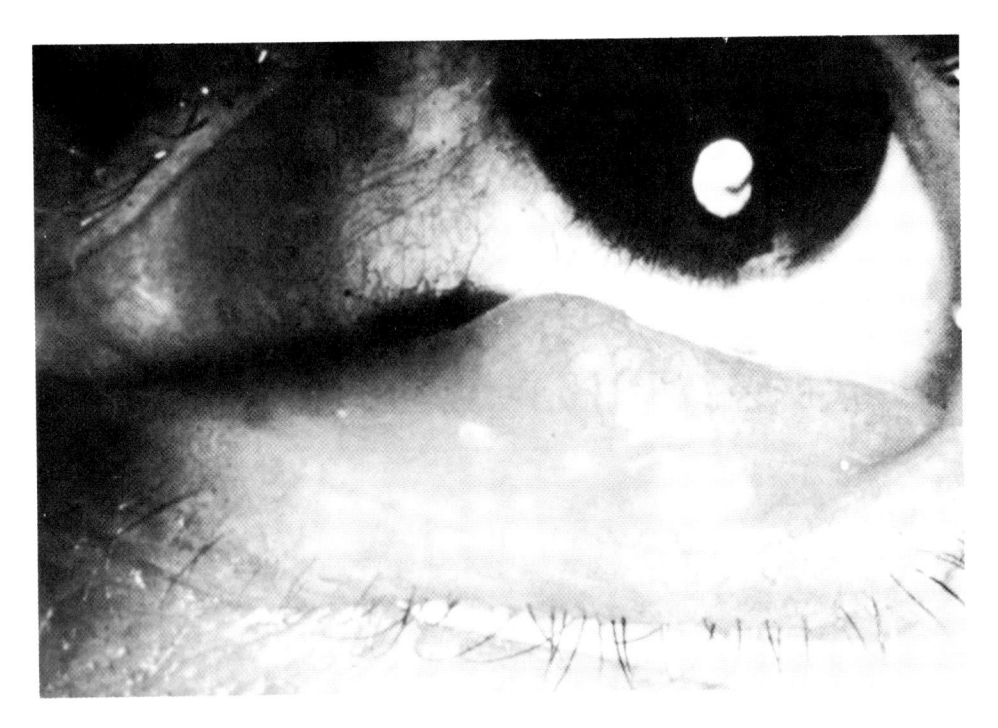

Fig. 32–1. Chalazion. By everting the lower lid, a swelling, generally localized in the tarsus, becomes evident. It is caused by the obstruction and secondary infection of a meibomian gland.

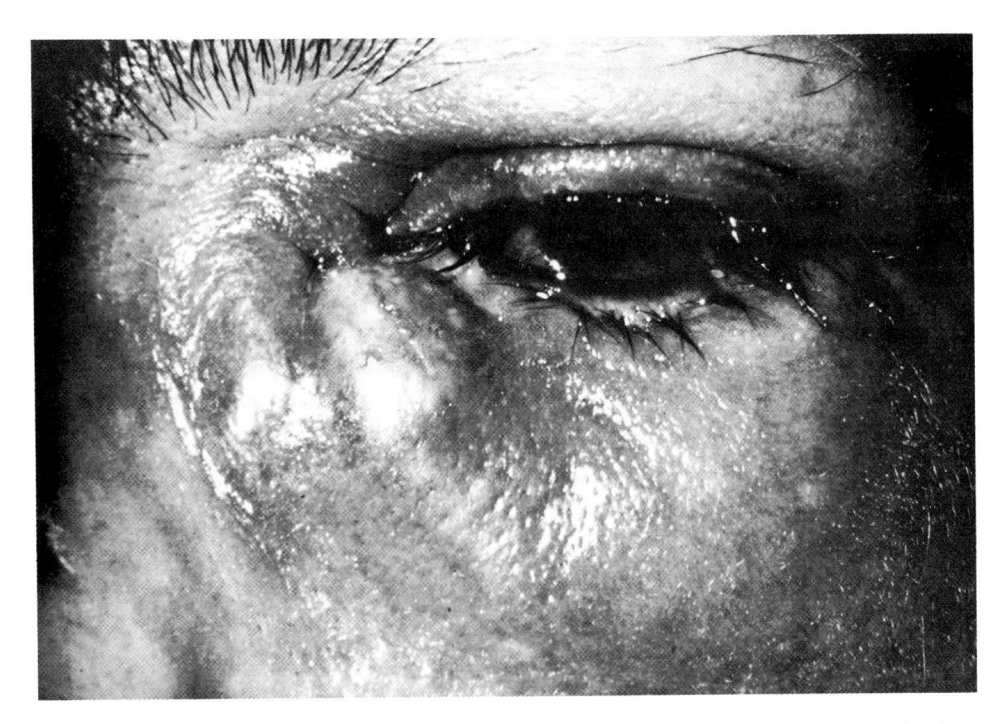

Fig. 32–2. Purulent dacryocystitis. Stasis of tear circulation in the lacrimal sac may cause secondary infection of the sac with the formation of an abscess. This infection, generally caused by *Staphylococcus aureus*, usually responds well to systemic antibiotic treatment, but later requires excision of the lacrimal sac.

Table 32–5. Infections of the Lacrimal Apparatus

Infection	Clinical Manifestation	Etiologic Agent	Recommended Therapy
Dacryoadenitis	Pain in upper external quadrant of orbit, redness, swelling, and pain in gland, tenderness of periosteum of orbital margin, preauricular adenopathy	*Acute bacterial infections*: *Staphylococcus aureus*, streptococcus *Chronic bacterial infections*: *Actinomyces israelii*, nocardia, *Mycobacterium tuberculosis*, *M. leprae*, *Treponema pallidum* *Viral infections*: Mumps virus, herpes zoster virus, Epstein-Barr virus *Mycotic infections*: blastomyces, histoplasma, sporothricosis Possibly *Actinomyces israelii*	Etiologic treatment Topical bacitracin or sulfacetamide
Dacryocystitis	In children: unilateral tearing with purulent secretions In adults: chronic dacryocystitis: tearing on the affected side and a small amount of secretion, especially in the morning acute dacryocystitis: pain, redness, swelling of lacrimal sac and underlying skin (cellulitis), sometimes spreading to contiguous structures, fever in severe cases	Pneumococcus, *Haemophilus influenzae*, *Pseudomonas aeruginosa* Pneumococcus, Staphylococcus, sometimes *Pseudomonas aeruginosa* or *Candida albicans* Pneumococcus in most cases, *Actinomyces israelii*, Staphylococcus, streptococcus, *Pseudomonas aeruginosa*, *Klebsiella pneumoniae*, *Haemophilus influenzae*, *Branhamella catarrhalis*, *Candida albicans*, aspergillus	Conservative treatment until 1 year old, except in uncontrollable and complicated infection; lacrimal sac massage 3 times daily and topical antibiotic selected by sensitivity tests; systemic antibiotic therapy in persistent infections, and lacrimal probing to remove obstruction after controlling the acute episode; surgical drainage possibly necessary Topical antibiotic, based on sensitivity tests; removal of obstruction; dacryocystorhinostomy possibly necessary Systemic and topical antibiotics to control acute phase; then, lacrimal probing to ascertain presence of obstruction; surgical removal of permanent obstruction (dacryocystorhinostomy) *Note*: Lacrimal probing should not be done during acute infection because of risk of injury to lacrimal passages

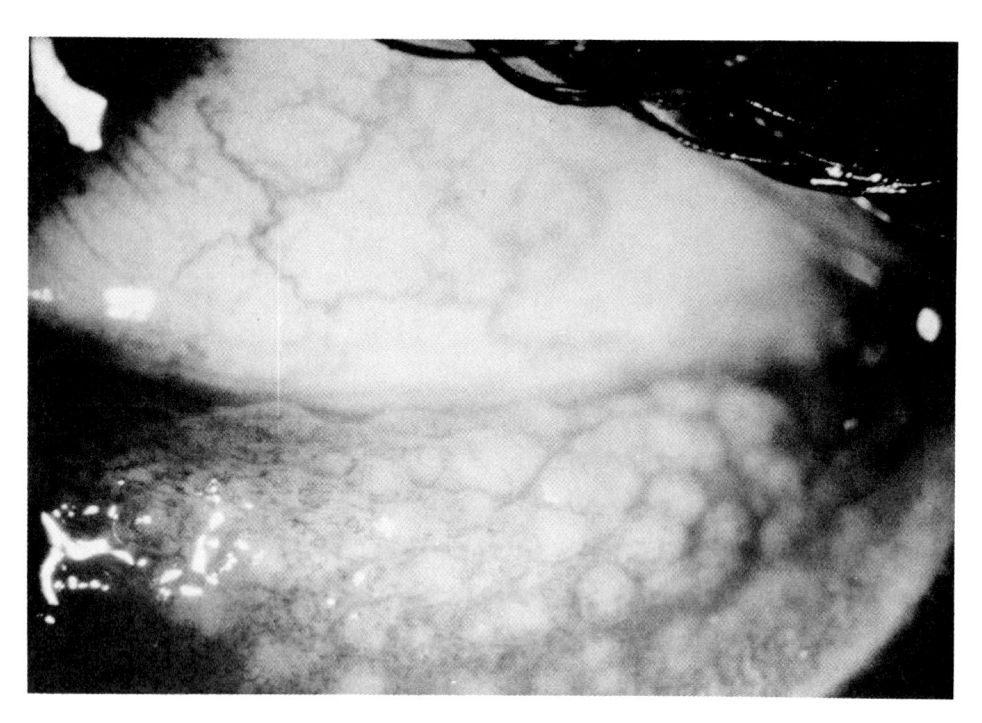

Fig. 32—3. Follicular conjunctivitis in a 13-year-old girl who had complained of bilateral redness of the eyes for 3 days. The upper and the lower conjunctiva are covered with follicles. This form of conjunctivitis is associated with herpes simplex virus primary infection.

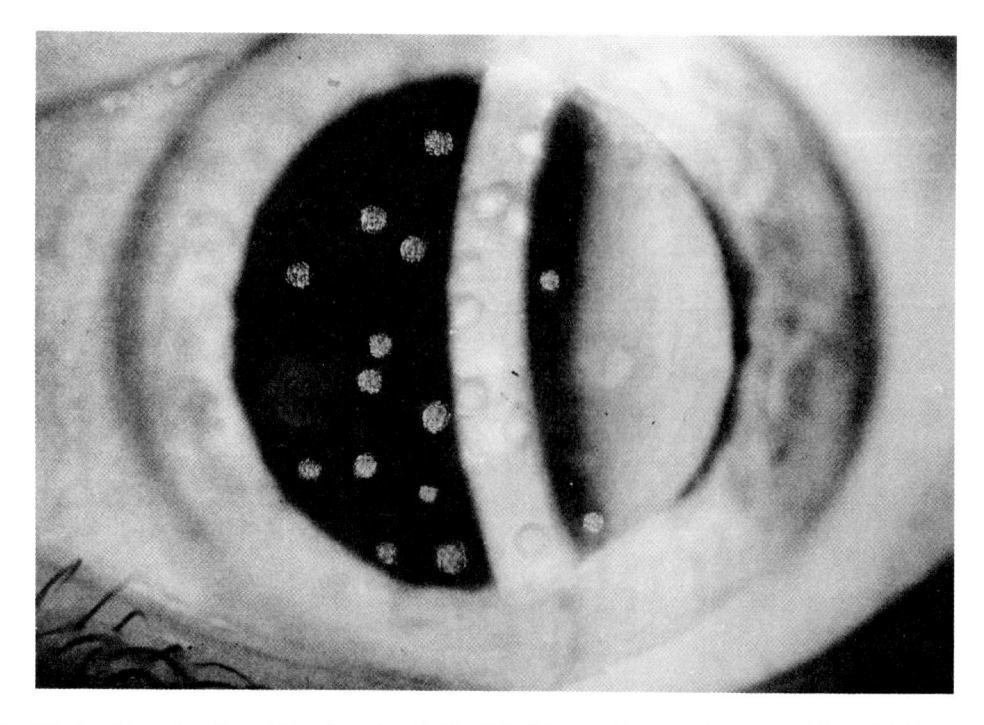

Fig. 32—4. Adenovirus (type 8) keratoconjunctivitis. This 23-year-old woman had severe bilateral follicular conjunctivitis with false membranes and preauricular adenopathies. After a course of 10 days, photophobia increased, and the cornea showed multiple subepithelial microinfiltrations.

fested by an exacerbation of all signs observed in acute forms and can be complicated by severe keratitis leading to corneal perforation in a matter of hours. It must always be considered a severe systemic infection and be treated as such.

Viral conjunctivitis is usually less purulent than bacterial conjunctivitis but often produces pseudomembranes and preauricular adenopathies tender to palpation. This conjunctivitis is of the follicular type (Figs. 32–3 and 32–4).

Parasites can also produce irritative conjunctivitis, with the possibility of bacterial superinfection accompanied by eosinophilia.

Numerous cases of chronic conjunctivitis are iatrogenic. Any patient who has a resistant conjunctivitis for 2 or 3 months should be reevaluated completely and referred to a specialized center if necessary. The differential diagnosis includes drug poisoning, vernal or allergic conjunctivitis, benign folliculosis of children, neoplasms, keratitis sicca, Stevens-Johnson syndrome, and benign mucous membrane pemphigoid.

Ophthalmia neonatorum includes all forms of conjunctivitis in the first month of life. It is usually bilateral; unilateral involvement suggests dacryostenosis. The time of appearance is an important indication, but is not absolutely diagnostic.

For specific causes and treatment of these forms of conjunctivitis, see Table 32–6.

KERATITIS

Table 32–7 discusses infections of the cornea, or keratitis. Keratitis, may be mild and punctate when associated with blepharoconjunctivitis, usually of staphylococcal origin, and may disappear with the treatment of blepharoconjunctivitis. Similarly, chlamydial or viral infections (adenovirus, measles, rubella, or infectious mononucleosis) are nearly always accompanied by a diffuse punctate keratitis that gradually changes to subepithelial infiltrates (Figs. 32–4 to 32–6); this hypersensitivity reaction to the infectious agent eventually disappears when the cause has been eliminated. This reaction should be differentiated from drug or other poisoning, however, as well as from Thygeson's superficial punctate keratitis.

ENDOPHTHALMITIS

Endophthalmitis (Table 32–8) is an infection of the contents of the eyeball including the aqueous humor and the vitreous humor, whereas panophthalmitis is an infection of all the structures of the eyeball, internal and external. The infection may be secondary to surgical or other trauma that creates a portal of entry for the infectious agents, or it may be endogenous. Patients who have undergone a filtration operation for glaucoma are at risk because a simple conjunctivitis can degenerate into endophthalmitis. Early treatment of the slightest infection in the ocular region is important in preventing severe infection.

Principles of Evaluation. Any intraocular infection is a high-priority emergency in ophthalmology. An intraocular specimen collected by the ophthalmologist is necessary for an etiologic diagnosis prior to the administration of any medication. A single dose of systemic or topical antibiotic can render cultures negative without altering the clinical course.

When an intraocular infection is present, bacteriologic studies at the surface of the eye are of no clinical value. The infectious agent inside the eye is nearly always different from the one found at the surface.

The intraocular specimen for the bacteriologic studies is taken by puncture of the anterior chamber and vitreous humor under a microscope. The intraocular fluids are aspirated in a syringe and are used to prepare smears (at least 4 for cytologic study and Gram staining) to inoculate different culture media, such as chocolate agar, blood agar, thioglycolate for cultivation at 37° C, and Sabouraud agar for cultivation at 23° C.

Immediate Treatment after Reading the Smear. If a gram-positive bacterium is seen or if no organism is found, one should administer penicillinase-resistant penicillin in addition to an aminoglycoside. Treatment may be systemic, subconjunctival, topical, or

Table 32-6. Conjunctivitis

Type of Conjunctivitis	Clinical Manifestations	Etiologic Agent	Recommended Therapy
Acute bacterial	Irritation of the eye, redness with or without chemosis, secretion of variable consistency and abundance, formation of pseudomembranes, bulbar or palpebral petechiae	*Staphylococcus aureus* or *S. epidermidis* (75% to 80% of cases), pneumococci (second most common, especially in winter when they cause small epidemics; petechiae in the bulbar conjunctiva reflect the hypersensitivity of the eye to the infectious agent), *Haemophilus influenzae*, *H. aegyptius*, group A streptococci	Removal of purulent secretions from eyelids; topical antimicrobials based on culture and sensitivity testing (preference to antimicrobials not usually employed systemically); sulfacetamide for infections cause by staphylococcus, pneumococcus, streptococcus, and Haemophilus; bacitracin and erythromycin for pneumococcal and streptococcal infections; tetracycline for haemophilus infections; sulfacetamide for infections of unknown origin; combined antibiotic or antibiotic-corticosteroid therapy contraindicated; topical penicillin and neomycin contraindicated
Sexually transmitted inclusion		*Chlamydia trachomatis*	Systemic tetracycline and topical sulfonamide for 3 weeks; simultaneous treatment of patient's sex partner; tetracycline contraindicated in pregnant women and the newborn
gonorrheal	Exacerbation of signs of acute bacterial conjunctivitis	*Neisseria gonorrhoeae*, possibly *Neisseria meningitidis*	Debridement of cilia and cul-de-sacs to dislodge abundant purulent secretions; topical antibiotics: bacitracin, sulfonamides, erythromycin, or tetracycline; systemic antibiotics: penicillin, ampicillin, or tetracycline
Viral	Formation of pseudomembranes and preauricular adenopathies tender to palpation	Herpes simplex virus, adenoviruses (especially types 3 and 8), influenza type A virus, varicella virus	Specific treatment for herpes simplex with idoxuridine, vidarabine, and trifluorothymidine; acyclovir seems promising; corticosteroids contraindicated (risk of corneal perforation with herpes simplex virus)
Chronic	Sensation of foreign body, worse in the morning, redness and moderate irritation; cosmetics, particularly mascara, may constitute culture media and means of repeated reinoculation of infection	Staphylococcus (most cases), *Actinomyces israelii* (unilateral conjunctivitis of nasal angle) moraxella (diagnosis easier on smear than culture); *Branhamella catarrhalis*, gram-negative rods including Proteus, Pseudomonas *Streptococcus pneumoniae*, *Escherichia coli*, *Serratia marcescens*	Sulfonamides for initial treatment, later modification according to antibiotic sensitivity test results; for refractory or relapsing chronic conjunctivitis, suspension of all treatment for a few days (noninfectious conjunctivitis often improves; underlying infection may be temporarily exacerbated, but suspension of antibiotic therapy permits bacterial identification)

Other			
Chronic associated with keratitis and avitaminosis	Occurrence in patients with keratitis sicca or vitamin A deficiency	*Corynebacterium xerosis* (proliferates in dead epithelial cells)	Correct deficiencies and heat keratitis (see Table 32–7)
Refractory	Persistence of infection for months or years	*Chlamydia trachomatis* (inclusion conjunctivitis or trachoma)	Systemic tetracycline
Unilateral granulomatous	Ipsilateral preauricular or submandibular adenopathies, (Parinaud's oculoglandular syndrome)	*Francisella tularensis, Mycobacterium tuberculosis, Treponema pallidum,* actinomyces, brucella, mumps virus, Epstein-Barr virus	According to cause
Parasitic	Conjunctival irritation, possible bacterial superinfection accompanied by eosinophilia	Fly larvae, filariae including *Onchocerca volvulus* and Loa, ascarides	According to cause
Chronic iatrogenic	Resistance to treatment for 2 or 3 months	Misdiagnosis of cause of original infection	Complete re-evaluation, including likely differential diagnoses
Ophthalmia neonatorum	Usually bilateral; unilateral involvement suggestive of dacryostenosis		Traditionally, 1% silver nitrate, with a success rate of about 98% (Credé's prophylaxis); topical application of antibiotics and sulfonamides as an alternative
Day			
0 to 2	Chemical conjunctivitis secondary to application of silver nitrate at birth; bilateral and disappears spontaneously in 24 to 36 hours; not severe	Silver nitrate	Observation
2 or 3	Moderate to hyperacute gonococcal conjunctivitis by contamination during passage in the birth canal ranges; risk of keratitis with loss of corneal substance, perforation, and panophthalmitis	*Neisseria gonorrhoeae*	Collection of specimen for culture, antibiotic sensitivity testing, and cytologic study; isolation and intensive topical (bacitracin and erythromycin) and systemic (penicillin) treatment; simultaneous treatment of patient's mother and her sex partner
5 to 12	Inclusion conjunctivitis, sometimes unilateral, by contamination in the infected birth canal; papillary conjunctival reaction with abundant purulent secretion; apparent spontaneous recovery conceals the risk of chronic infection that may lead to pannus formation and conjunctival scarring	*Chlamydia trachomatis*	Child: topical sulfonamides; mother and her sex partner: systemic tetracycline
15 to 30	Bacterial or viral infectious conjunctivitis; in the newborn, herpes infection acute and manifested by vesicular blepharokeratoconjunctivitis	Staphylococcus, pneumococcus, *Haemophilus influenzae,* streptococcus; less frequently, proteus, klebsiella, pseudomonas, *Escherichia coli,* meningococcus, or herpes simplex virus 2	Etiologic treatment
After 15 days	Possible dacryostenosis in unilateral infections		

Table 32–7. Infections of the Cornea (Keratitis)

Type of Infection	Clinical Manifestations	Etiologic Agent	Recommended Therapy
Ulcerative Infections			For both types of ulcerative infections: emergency referral of the patient to an ophthalmologist; adequate specimen for direct examination (smear), culture, and antibiotic sensitivity testing; topical or other antibiotics contraindicated before specimens are taken; topical anesthetics also best avoided; immediate smears for cytologic examination (Giemsa stain) and direct examination (Gram's stain); two additional slides prepared for immediate staining and microscopic examination by the specialist; initial treatment based on the tentative etiologic diagnosis, established after the smears; for bacterial ulcerations, treatment with topical and subconjunctival antibiotics; for gram-positive organisms or for no identifiable organism: combination of an aminoglycoside and a penicilli nase-resistant penicillin; for gram-negative organisms, combination of an aminoglycoside and carbenicillin or ticarcillin; therapeutic regimen modified if necessary on receipt of culture and sensitivity results; the treatment supplemented by cycloplegia, usually with topical atropine; topical corticosteroids contraindicated in bacterial or viral ulcers in which infectious agent persists locally (risk of loss of corneal substance and perforation); in mycotic ulcers, treatment on the basis of the presence of yeasts or filaments on gram-stained smear; amphotericin B or 5-fluorocytosine indicated primarily; surgical treatment possibly necessary.
Marginal	Infiltration of peripheral superficial portion of cornea, usually with a clear zone between the periphery and the infiltration; in chronic infections, phlyctenular keratitis reflecting chronic hypersensitivity to bacterial proteins, and development of fibrous nodules on the cornea (Salzmann's nodular degeneration); differential diagnosis; collagen diseases that produce a peripheral loss of corneal substance (Mooren's ulcer) and noninfectious peripheral degeneration	Staphylococcus, *Mycobacterium tuberculosis*; gonococcus (marginal ulcerations by combined action of bacterial toxins and pressure of tense eyelids in acute phase of infection)	
Central or paracentral	Bacterial or mycotic ulcers usually occurring after traumatic epithelial lesion of cornea; possible development on intact corneal surface; marked corneal and periorbital pain, impression of foreign body under eyelid, reduced vision, tearing, significant perilimbic redness with chemosis, palpebral edema, abundant secretions, corneal opacities, inflammatory reaction of anterior chamber, sometimes with hypopyon; course varying with virulence of infecting agent, precise site of the infection, and host resistance; differential diagnosis: viral keratitis due to herpes simplex or herpes zoster viruses	Opportunistic: pneumococcus, pseudomonas, moraxella, streptococcus, staphylococcus; invasive on intact corneal surface: *Neisseria gonorrhoeae*, *Haemophilus aegyptius*, *Corynebacterium diphtheriae*; most frequent fungi: *Candida albicans*, aspergillus, fusarium, cephalosporium, coccidioides	

Herpes simplex keratitis	To be suspected in patient with past history of herpetic keratitis or in conjunctivitis with a cold sore (herpes labialis) or influenza; epithelial lesion classically dendritic or sometimes simply ulcerative (geographic ulcer), resembling dendritic lesions caused by varicella virus; immunologic response of host to virus possibly causing keratouveitis or disciform keratitis that can relapse many times for several years	Herpes simplex virus	Specific antiviral agents for herpes simplex: idoxuridine, vidarabine, trifluorothymidine and acyclovir; topical corticosteroids contraindicated (major risk of corneal perforation)
Stromal keratitis without superficial ulcerative lesion (interstitial keratitis)	Corneal opacities, edema, deep vascularization; usually an immunologic phenomenon reflecting systemic infection in which the pathogen may not be present in the cornea	*Mycobacterium tuberculosis, Treponema pallidum*, chronic staphylococcal infection, herpes simplex virus and all viruses that can affect the epithelium of the eye	Nonherpetic interstitial keratitis: corticosteroids; herpetic disciform keratitis without epithelial ulcer: corticosteroids in combination with antiviral agents, under close ophthalmologic supervision
Corneal pannus	Fibrovascular membrane covering superficial corneal layers following severe chronic infection of conjunctiva and the cornea	*Chlamydia trachomatis* (trachoma and sometimes inclusion conjunctivitis), staphylococcus, *Mycobacterium leprae*	
Parasitic invasion of the cornea	Inflammatory reaction with opacities at various sites; possible penetration of anterior chamber by larvae	*Onchocerca volvulus, Loa loa, Trichinella spiralis*	Antiparasitic agents with great caution, corticosteroids

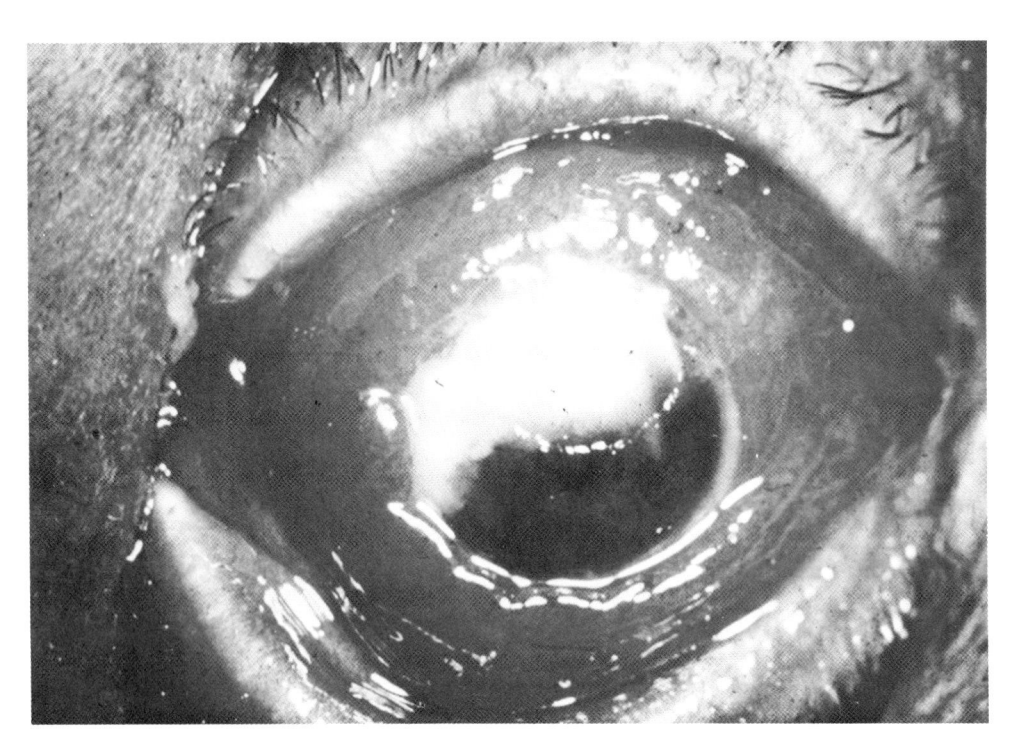

Fig. 32—5. Staphylococcal corneal ulcer. This 35-year-old patient had had a history of redness of the eye for 2 weeks. For the previous 2 days, the eye had been painful. The patient was unable to sleep, and vision was reduced. In addition to redness of the eye with edema of the conjunctiva and lid, examination revealed a pus-filled crater at the upper part of the cornea. Purulent secretions were abundant. Culture and bacteriologic examination of this corneal abscess revealed the presence of *Staphylococcus aureus*.

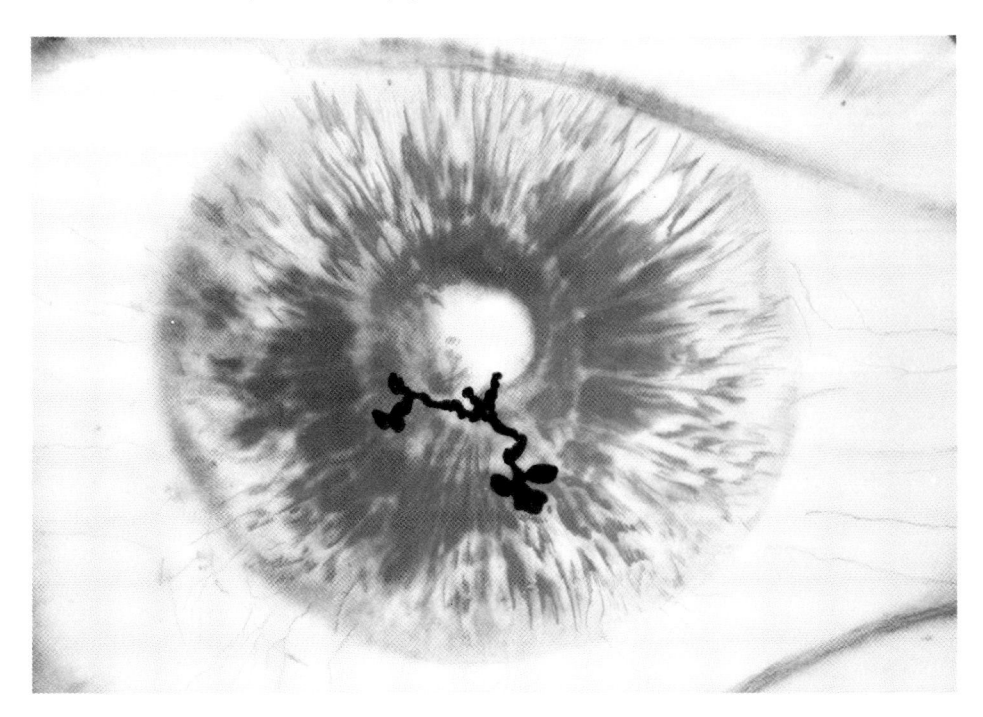

Fig. 32—6. This dendritic ulcer caused foreign-body and burning sensations of the right eye for 3 days in a 30-year-old man who had had a cold sore for a week.

Table 32-8. Endophthalmitis

Type of Infection	Clinical Manifestations	Etiologic Agents	Recommended Therapy
Bacterial	Development following surgical intervention or perforation of the eye; usually severe, aggravated within hours; lowered visual acuity, severe redness of eye, ocular and periorbital pain, palpebral edema and chemosis, corneal edema, fibrinous and cellular inflammatory reaction in anterior chamber shortly after onset, loss of red reflection in fundus; some cases appearing later, especially when infectious agent is not virulent or when antibiotics are administered prophylactically in insufficient doses	*Staphylococcus aureus*, streptococcus, pneumococcus, pseudomonas, proteus, klebsiella, anaerobes including *Clostridium perfringens*, *Actinomyces israelii*, and peptostreptococcus; *Haemophilus* and *Escherichia coli*; saprophytes or agents with low virulence include mainly *Staphylococcus epidermidis* and *Bacillus subtilis*	High doses of parenteral antibiotics, according to susceptibility, AND local injections of antibiotics. Differential diagnosis: aseptic uveitis, common in severe anterior segment injury
Mycotic	Development several days or weeks after surgical or other trauma; minimal eye irritation, moderate redness, little or no pain, slow reduction of visual acuity, moderate anterior chamber reaction, hazy appearance of vitreous humor, slow development of hypopyon (not all hypopyons are of infectious origin)	Aspergillus, fusarium, mucor, and other fungi not usually pathogenic	Amphotericin B
Endogenous	Occurrence during systemic disease or in debilitated patients	Bacterial: gonococcus, meningococcus, streptococcus; mycotic: *Candida albicans*, *Aspergillus flavus*, mucor, *Cryptococcus neoformans*, coccidioides	Systemic antibiotics or antimycotic drugs, according to cause of infection
Parasitic	Fulminant endophthalmitis from intraocular migration of parasites, particularly if these parasites die and release antigens	All filariae including *Onchocerca volvulus*, *Toxocara canis*, *Trichinella spiralis*	Antiparasitic drugs possibly harmful by releasing antigens; systemic corticosteroids indicated for reducing inflammatory reaction and limiting intraocular damage

Table 32–9. Infections of the Optic Nerve

Clinical Manifestations	Etiologic Agent	Recommended Therapy
Slight to severe loss of vision, often limited to loss of central vision or of color discrimination; tenderness on palpation of the eyeball or pain during eyeball movements; edema of optic papilla, but often no ocular sign if infection is behind the eyeball	Viruses of measles, chickenpox, mumps, smallpox, influenza, poliomyelitis, vaccinia, infectious mononucleosis, herpes simplex	Etiologic treatment, local and systemic anti-inflammatories to limit damage to nerve structures

even intraocular. If a gram-negative organism is found, one should prescribe an aminoglycoside combined with carbenicillin or ticarcillin. Treatment may be systemic, subconjunctival, topical, or even intraocular. If fungi are observed, treatment is begun immediately with systemic amphotericin B and, in some cases, with 5-fluorocytosine. Treatment is modified subsequently on the basis of the results of cultures and antibiotic sensitivity tests and according to the clinical response.

In the presence of an abscess of the vitreous humor or an uncontrollable infection, a vitrectomy should be performed, and intraocular antibiotics should be administered at the same time. Because a violent inflammatory reaction causes irreparable damage to the internal structures of the eye, systemic, subconjunctival, or even intraocular corticosteroids are sometimes added to reduce fibrosis, which itself produces loss of vision, once the infection has been treated with antibiotics for 24 hours.

The final prognosis for endophthalmitis or panophthalmitis is always guarded, even if, theoretically, the infectious agent is not virulent. In parasitic infections of the macula, the prognosis for visual function is poor.

INFECTIONS OF THE SCLERA AND EPISCLERA

Most cases of scleritis and episcleritis are associated with a collagen or immunologic disease, and their infectious nature has not been demonstrated. Systemic infections or infections near the orbit have long been suspected as possible causes of scleritis, but this association is unproved. The only clinical relation that appears to exist between scleritis, episcleritis, and infection is with herpes zoster; scleritis may precede, accompany, or follow the viral infection.

No specific treatment exists for herpes zoster. Topical anti-inflammatory agents are ineffective in scleritis whereas systemic anti-inflammatory agents may control the inflammatory reaction and stop the progress of the disease. For severe cases that do not respond to this treatment, the use of systemic corticosteroids can be considered if no contraindication exists.

INFECTIONS OF THE OPTIC NERVE

Optic neuritis may be associated with any type of systemic or local infection (Table 32–9). Purulent involvement of the optic nerve is rare and occurs only with the spread of an infection in the vicinity, either from meningitis, orbital cellulitis, or endophthalmitis. Treatment is systemic.

Most cases result from an extension of the inflammation from adjacent structures to the optic nerve, without purulent involvement, as in retinitis, choroiditis, sinusitis, and orbital inflammations. These diseases must be identified and treated, so the optic nerve edema can be controlled before damage becomes irreversible. In these patients, reduction of the inflammatory reaction may bring about recovery of visual function in a few weeks.

Viral diseases are often associated with unilateral or bilateral optic neuritis with severe loss of vision. Generally, visual recovery is good, often complete, but occasionally the disease progresses to demyelination with permanent loss of sight.

Table 32-10. Infections of the Uveal Tract and Retina

Infection	Clinical Appearance	Etiologic Agent	Recommended Therapy
Anterior uveitis, iritis, iridocyclitis	Pain, photophobia, tearing; reduced visual acuity; iritis may be nearly asymptomatic; red, infected eye with pericorneal vascular congestion; biomicroscopic turbidity of aqueous due to elevated protein level in anterior chambers; inflammatory cells in anterior chamber, perhaps on posterior corneal surface (keratic precipitates); dilatation of surface vessels of iris; adhesions between iris and lens or corneal periphery; cataracts from recurrent iritis with posterior subcapsular opacities; inflammatory cells in anterior vitreous body	Herpes simplex, herpes zoster, *Mycobacterium tuberculosis, Treponema pallidum*	Systemic treatment according to etiology
Posterior uveitis: chorioretinitis	Little or no reduction in visual acuity, unless lesion is central; floating specks from inflammatory cell debris; cells and cell membranes in vitreous body		Systemic treatment according to etiology
Retinitis	Edema, exudates giving retina a cloudy, fluffy, white appearance; possible hemorrhaging around lesions; scarred retinas have more distinct borders and uneven pigmentation; white atrophy with accumulation of pigments; cell debris from vitreous body	*Toxoplasma gondii* usually, but also viruses (measles, smallpox, rubella, influenza, herpes, chickenpox, cytomegalovirus), candida	Systemic treatment according to etiology
Choroiditis	Pale lesion (yellow, white, or gray) with well-defined borders if retina is intact; borders hazy when retina is affected; vessels cover inflammatory lesion; scarring characterized by white atrophy of choroid with well-defined borders revealing underlying pearly sclera; pigment accumulation, especially on edges; large vessels visible at bottom of scar; persistent residual and secondary opacities of vitreous; persistent vitreous floating bodies	*Brucella, T. pallidum, M. tuberculosis,* leptospira, *M. leprae,* herpes virus	Systemic treatment according to etiology
	Diffuse: fundal lesions, possibly contiguous	*T. pallidum, M. tuberculosis*	
	Disseminated: several lesions with disseminated foci; retina edematous and hazy	*T. pallidum* (congenital syphilis)	
	Exudative: circumscribed lesions (most frequent variety)	*T. pallidum, T. gondii*	
	Central: single lesion, often at posterior pole	*T. gondii*	

Table 32–10. Infections of the Uveal Tract and Retina (cont'd)

Infection	Clinical Appearance	Etiologic Agent	Recommended Therapy
Associated anterior and posterior uveitis	Symptoms varying in intensity	*M. tuberculosis, T. pallidum, T. gondii* Alpha-hemolytic streptococcus, other causes of endocarditis	Systemic treatment according to etiology
	Subacute infectives retinitis of Roth: occurring with severe bacteremia and subacute bacterial endocarditis; hazy retina; round, flame-shaped hemorrhages and punctate foci; isolated, round white spots in center of hemorrhagic focus (Roth's spots); symptoms may be few or absent		
	Uveitis secondary to remote center of infection: immunologic reaction to bacterial toxins; generally anterior; possible posterior segment manifestations; often associated with sinusitis, dental abscess, osteitis	Bacterial toxins	X-ray examination of mouth, sinuses, lungs; treatment of focus of infection
Tuberculous uveitis	*Anterior uveitis:* granulomatous disorder; small nodules on iris and keratic precipitates; if non-granulomatous, exudates from ciliary body (floating specks)	*M. tuberculosis*	Usual antituberculosis treatment, starting with isoniazid; for localized disease, corticosteroids (if mechanism is immunologic) (N.B.: Tuberculin tests may exacerbate condition)
	Posterior uveitis: polymorphous choroiditis; possibly immunologic hypersensitivity disorder; acute miliary lesions secondary to massive bacteremia; diffuse allergic inflammation in patients who previously had tuberculosis		
	Fundus: yellowish white nodules in choroid with retinal edema; lesions measuring ⅙ to ½ disc diameter, hazy edges; possible confluence of lesions, leading to dissemination; white nodules seen especially in miliary tuberculosis; granulomas of ciliary body or choroid with possible rupture of eyeball; immunologic reactions of choroid seen at median periphery of fundus; some lesions associated with allergy and infection combined		
Syphilitic uveitis	*Congenital:* bilateral salt and pepper appearance of retina at periphery or posterior pole or involving up to 3 quadrants; bluish dots surrounded by yellow, depigmented areas; vision not always affected; lesions not progressive	*T. pallidum*	Usual treatment for syphilis; usual serologic tests
	Acquired: acute iritis with secondary syphilis; small, dilated capillaries, vascularized papules, or yellowish red nodules on surface of iris		
	Posterior pole: lesions seen in late secondary or tertiary syphilis; bilateral lesions in 50% of cases; choroiditis manifested by grayish zones toward equator, sometimes at posterior pole or periphery;		

Uveitis of leprosy	hazy vitreous body; flame-shaped retinal hemorrhages; lesions progress to retinal gliosis and chorioretinal atrophy *Diffuse neuroretinitis:* occurring with or without papillitis; retinal edema; venous tortuosity; arterial occlusion; migration and proliferation of pigment resembling pigmentary retinopathy; localized chorioretinitis Anterior and granulomatous disorder; leprotic "pearls" on surface of iris; possible focal choroiditis, then proliferation of pigment at cicatricial stage	*M. leprae*	Usual treatment of leprosy
Uveitis with lymphogranuloma venereum	Anterior uveitis with hypopyon	Chlamydia	Frei test, sulfonamides
Viral uveitis	Anterior uveitis with corneal lesions (herpes simplex); pain, turbidity of aqueous humor; hyphema; retinitis and chorioretinitis with edema and vitreous exudate, primarily focal retinitis; retinal necrosis progressing toward choroid and neonatal chorioretinitis (herpes simplex); retinal necrosis progressing toward pigment epithelium and sensory part, by direct infestation (herpes zoster)	Herpes simplex and herpes zoster viruses	5 IDV acyclovir or virarabine (herpes simplex); steroids (herpes zoster)
	Juvenile iridocyclitis; focal retinitis with lesion often resembling multiple venous branch occlusion with zones of retinal atrophy (white to pale gray); affected zones dispersed between retinal hemorrhages; precipitates on posterior surface of vitreous; retinal lesions initially punctiform and white and later confluent and hemorrhagic with vasculitis simulating venous occlusion; possible central chorioretinitis as in toxoplasmosis N.B.: Common in patients with impaired defense mechanisms, especially those receiving immunosuppressants or chemotherapy or those with lymphoma, renal transplants, or neoplasms	Cytomegalovirus	Reduction of immunosuppressive therapy
	Anterior uveitis accompanying corneal lesions	Adenovirus	
	Multifocal pigmentary acute placoid epitheliopathy with rapidly progressive bilateral diminution of vision; fundal lesions multifocal, pale, situated in pigment epithelium or choriocapillaris; young adults affected; associated with inflammation of vitreous, iritis, episcleritis, papillitis, retinal vasculitis	Adenovirus type 5	Corticosteroids

Eye Infections   521

Table 32–10. Infections of the Uveal Tract and Retina (cont'd)

Infection	Clinical Appearance	Etiologic Agent	Recommended Therapy
	Congenital: secondary to maternal infection in first trimester of pregnancy; fetal ocular complications including cataract; infection of posterior pole possibly leading to proliferative retinitis of fine pigmentary changes extending to periphery; peripheral changes including borne corpuscles as in pigmentary retinopathy	Rubella virus	Antibody tests in mother and child; no specific treatment
	Acquired: anterior uveitis; retinitis in 25 to 50% of children with rubella; hazy vitreous with retinal pigmentary changes; fine pigmented spots over posterior pole		
	Congenital: as in rubella-associated uveitis	Measles virus	Clinical and serologic diagnosis
	Acquired: iritis associated with corneal ulcer; acute blindness following retinal involvement including retinal edema, retinal vascular stenosis, and exudative star figure at the macula		No specific treatment
	Iridocyclitis appearing 4 to 14 days after onset of mumps	Mumps virus	No specific treatment
	Clear media; disseminated spots ("histo spots"); atrophic change around optic disc; pigmented ring around macula with detachment of overlying sensory retina; detachment possibly serous, with or without bleeding; hemorrhage around macular lesion; detachment of associated pigment epithelium; originating from benign systemic histoplasmosis in childhood, with spots appearing in adolescence; macular disease developing at age 20 to 40; histoplasma scar areas of healed chorioditis with depigmentation of pigment epithelium; no pathogen present during development of macular lesion; bedridden patients, those receiving parenteral hyperalimentation, and drug addicts especially at risk	Histoplasma	Corticosteroids initially; amphotericin B of little value; photocoagulation; complement fixation of little value; histoplasmin skin test may reactivate lesions
Mycotic uveitis	Anterior uveitis, including exudative iridocyclitis; posterior uveitis, including focal retinitis as in toxoplasmosis; chorioretinitis at posterior pole with pale lesions with hazy borders; vitreous exudates; floating specks, reduced vision	*Candida albicans*	Blood cultures; antibiotics such as intravenous and intravitreous amphotericin B, 5-fluorocytosine; then, reduction of immunosuppressants
	Anterior iritis	Blastomyces	Topical corticosteroids, atropine, amphotericin B

		Coccidioides	Amphotericin B
		Sporothrix	Amphotericin B
Parasitic uveitis	Iridocyclitis, chorioretinitis Iridocyclitis	*Toxoplasma gondii*	Serologic tests of aqueous humor (low but significant titers); pyrimethamine, 75 mg/day initially and 50 mg/day subsequently for 6 weeks; weekly blood cell count; folinic acid, 3 mg 3 times weekly; spiramycin (Europe); corticosteroids with caution; close observation of contralateral eye
	Exudative focal retinitis; 30 to 50% of all cases of posterior uveitis; vision affected if macula involved; otherwise, vision initially good; floating specks due to vitreous inflammatory opacities; retinal lesion pale, elevated; hazy retina; lesion of posterior pole, sometimes near optic disc; *T. gondii* in retina; differential diagnosis; syphilis, cytomegalovirus, mycosis, tuberculosis		
	Course: retinal lesion heals in 3 weeks to 6 months, with atrophy of pigment epithelium; choroid atrophy, lesion becomes white, with proliferation of pigment on edges and at center of lesion; frequent recurrences with satellite lesions secondary to rupture of parasitic cysts; cysts contain hundreds of "dormant" parasites; rupture releases viable organisms and antigen and produces a hypersensitivity reaction, then an exudative reaction; recurrences accompanied by anterior chamber of inflammation		
	Congenital: secondary to fetal infection; cicatricial lesion with healed area of chorioretinitis at posterior pole, usually with macular involvement; heavily pigmented scar with white zones of atrophy and well-defined edges; frequent recurrences in first 3 decades		
	Chorioretinitis appearing at ages 4 to 16; macular granuloma at posterior pole	Toxocara	Puncture of anterior chamber: cytologic evidence of eosinophils in aqueous humor; 3 to 12% eosinophilia; ELISA test: positive is dilution of ⅛; corticosteroids with or without thiabendazole
	Chronic endophthalmitis: massive unilateral chronic uveitis with hazy vitreous and vascularized membrane in ciliary body that covers posterior surface of lens (cyclitic membrane)		
	Localized granuloma: white, solitary macular lesion, raised in the retina, with dark dot in center that indicates the location of the larva; size varying from 1 to 2 disc diameters; little inflammation		
	Peripheral granuloma: Hemispheric masses with fibrous tissues in vitreous		
	Anterior iridocyclitis; focal choroiditis with cutaneous nodules	Onchocerca	Biopsy (microfilariae in anterior chamber); serologic tests; diethylcarbamazine citrate (Hetrazan)

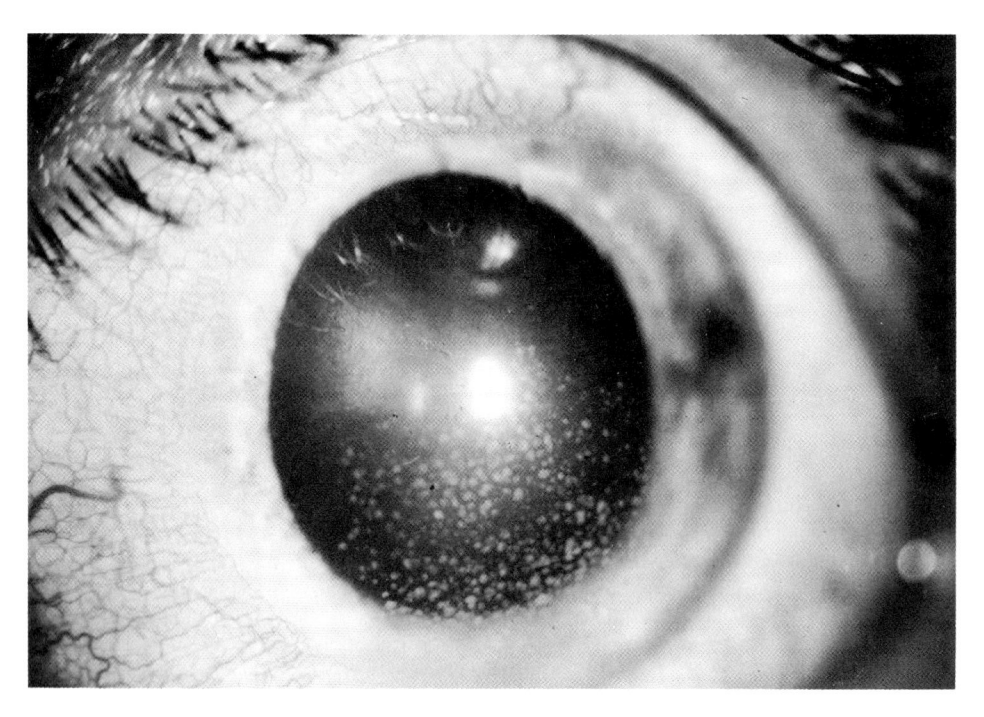

Fig. 32–7. In anterior uveitis, the cell deposits form keratic precipitates on the posterior surface of the cornea.

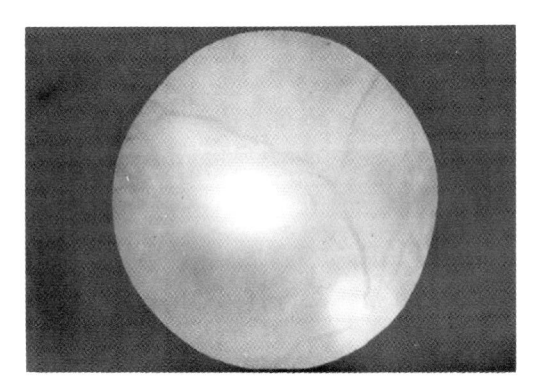

Fig. 32–8. Acute chorioretinitis. Chorioretinitis reflects the inflammation of the retina, the choroid, and, to some extent, the underlying vitreous. The lesion in the fundus is white with a hazy border and is edematous. The adjacent structures are masked.

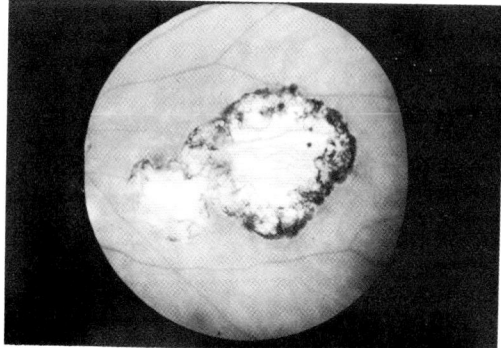

Fig. 32–9. Cicatricial chorioretinitis caused by toxoplasmosis. This 12-year-old patient was referred for defective vision in the left eye. Right at the posterior pole, involving the macular region, funduscopy revealed a white, cicatricial lesion surrounded by pigment, with the persistence of some large choroid vessels in the center. Note the presence of a small satellite lesion at the lower left. This is a typical picture of toxoplasmosis of the eye, which when congenital, is often accompanied by intracranial calcifications and convulsions.

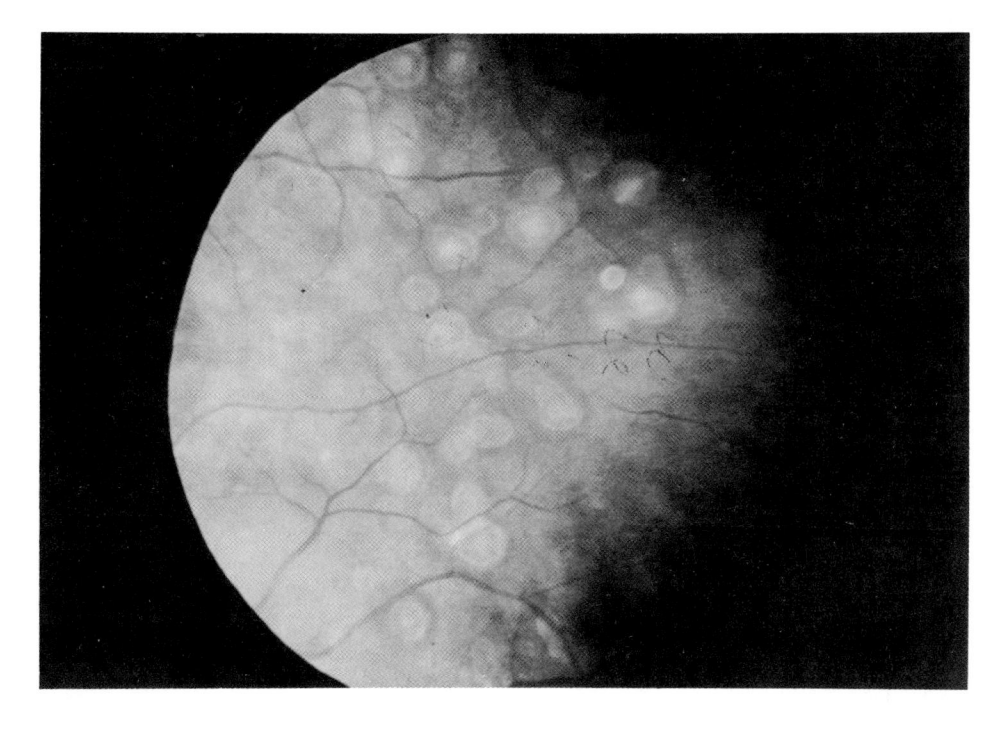

Fig. 32–10. The multifocal lesions of this placoid epithelial disorder are situated in the pigment epithelium. Because the posterior pole is particularly affected, a rapidly progressive visual impairment occurs.

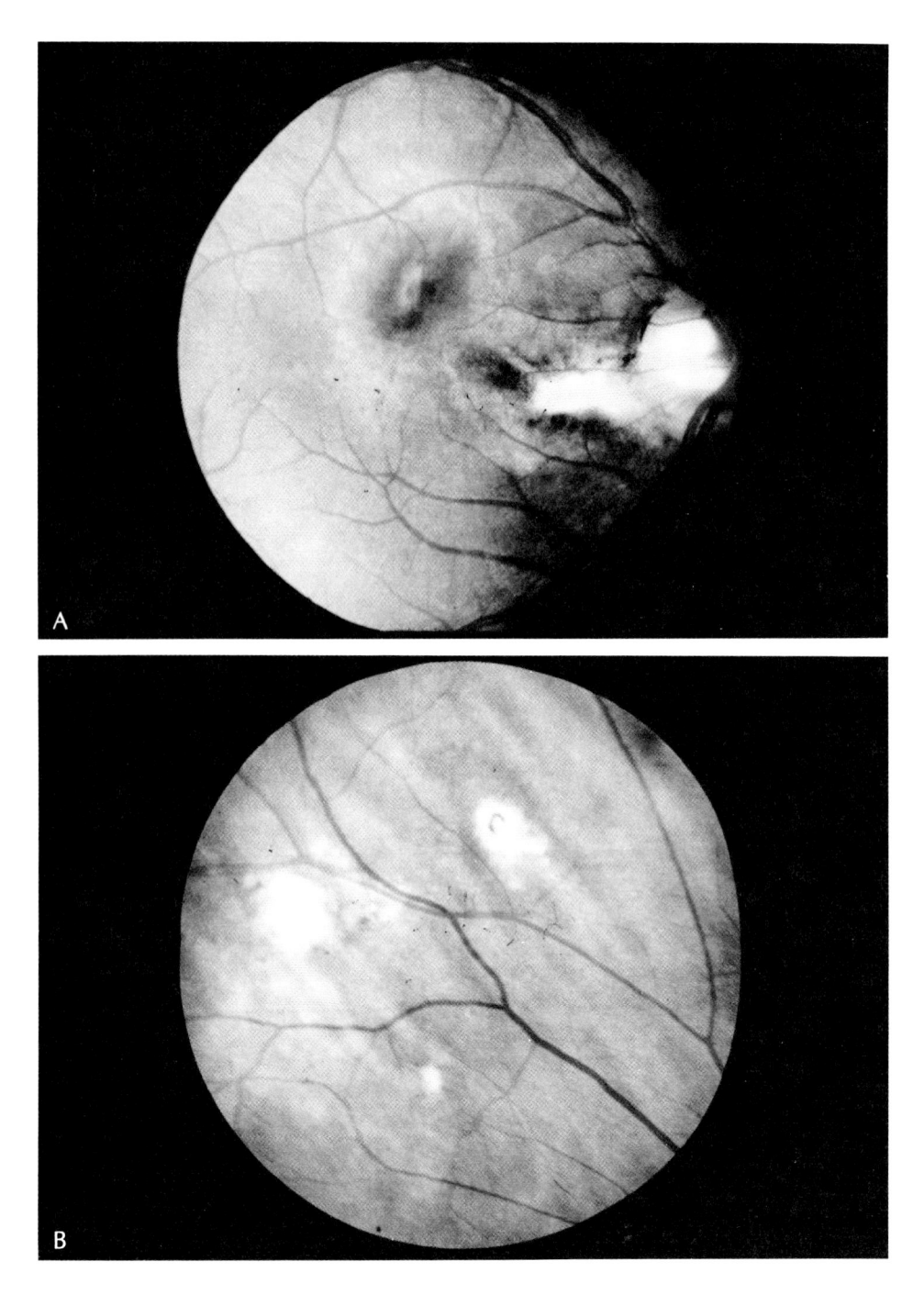

Fig. 32–11. *A* and *B,* Presumed syndrome of ocular histoplasmosis. This 35-year-old man had a rapid reduction in vision in the right eye, but he was otherwise healthy. The macular region is raised by a hemorrhagic detachment of the pigment epithelium. A subretinal hemorrhage is seen, and the entire lesion has a disciform appearance. A white atrophic lesion also is present near the disk. *(A).* The medial part of the retina, at the periphery, shows white, punched-out lesions *(B).*

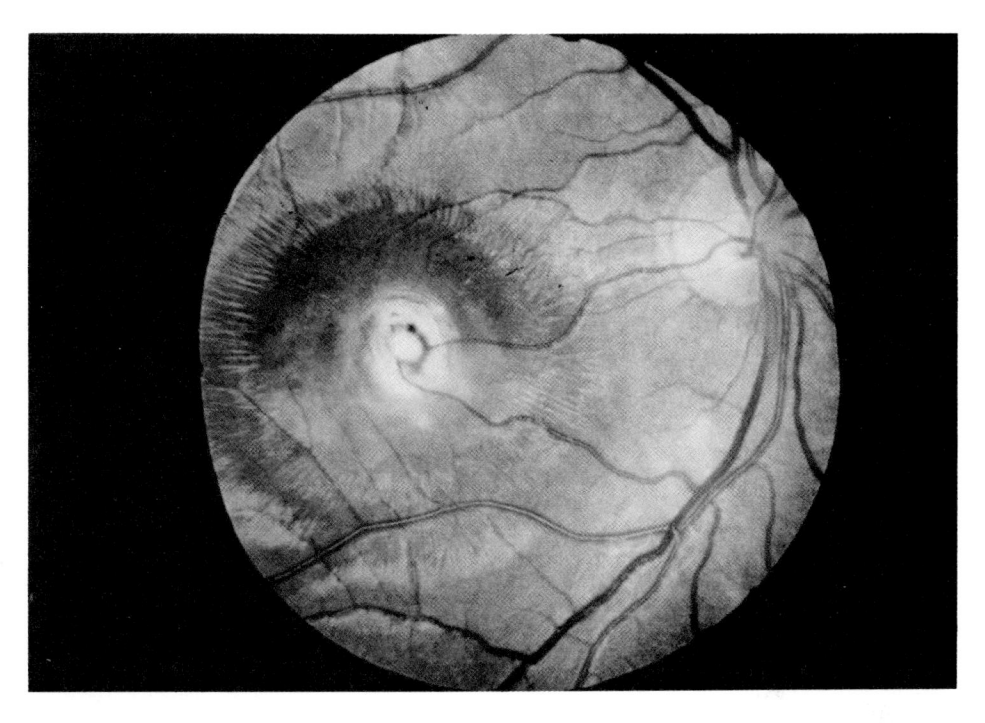

Fig. 32–12. This 7-year-old child was found by the school nurse to have poor vision in the right eye (vision was limited to finger counting). The ELISA test was positive. In the right macular region, one sees a raised, white, granulomatous lesion compatible with a diagnosis of *Toxocara canis* infection.

INFECTIONS OF THE UVEAL TRACT AND RETINA

The uveal tract (Table 32–10) includes the iris, ciliary body, and choroid. Involvement of the iris, iritis and anterior uveitis (Fig. 32–7), and of the ciliary body, iridocyclitis, are considered as an entity, whereas the choroid and retina (Figs. 32–8 to 32–12) can be studied together. The terms iritis and iridocyclitis generally suggest anterior uveitis; posterior uveitis generally refers to involvement of the choroid, with or without retinal manifestation. In addition, anterior segment infection may also spread to the posterior segment, and vice versa.

The inflammatory involvement of small retinal vessels often accompanies inflammation of the posterior pole and produces retinal exudates. Macular edema often accompanies peripheral chorioretinitis. It is characterized by a grayish appearance of the macular region and reduces vision significantly. Papillary or even retrobulbar optic neuritis may also be accompanied by inflammation of the choroid and retina and is characterized most often by a central scotoma or by atypical forms of contraction of the field of vision.

SUGGESTED READINGS

Aguilar, G.L., Blumenkrantz, M.S., Egbert, P.R., and McCulley, J.P.: Candida endophthalmitis after intravenous drug abuse. Arch. Ophthalmol., 97:96, 1979.

Broughton, W.L., Cupples, H.P., and Xarver, L.M.: Bilateral retinal detachment following cytomegalovirus retinitis. Arch. Ophthalmol., 96:618, 1978.

Cibis, G.W.: Neonatal herpes simplex retinitis. Albrecht Von Graefes Arch. Klin. Exp. Ophthalmol., 196:39, 1975.

Duke-Elder, S.S., and Dobree, J.H. (eds.): System of Ophthalmology. London, Henry Kimpton, 1969.

Fedukowicz, H.B.: External Infections of the Eye. 2nd Ed. New York, Appleton-Century-Crofts, 1978.

Gass, J.D.M.: Acute posterior multifocal placoid pigment epitheliopathy. Arch. Ophthalmol., 80:177, 1986.

Grayson, M.: Diseases of the Cornea. St. Louis, C.V. Mosby, 1979.

Jones, I.S., and Jakobiec, F.A.: Diseases of the Orbit. Hagerstown, MD, Harper & Row, 1979.

Korting, G.W., et al.: The Skin and Eye. Philadelphia, W.B. Saunders, 1973.

Locatcher-Knorazo, D., and Seegal, B.: Microbiology of the Eye. St. Louis, C.V. Mosby, 1972.

O'Connor, G.R.: Ocular toxoplasmosis. Jpn. J. Ophthalmol., 19:1, 1975.

O'Connor, G.R.: Manifestations and management of ocular toxoplasmosis. Bull. NY Acad. Med., 50:192, 1974.

O'Connor, G.R., and Frenkel, J.K.: Dangers of steroid treatment in toxoplasmosis. Periocular infections and systemic therapy. Arch. Ophthalmol., 94:213, 1976.

Perkins, W.S.: Ocular toxoplasmosis. Br. J. Ophthalmol., 57:1, 1973.

Sawelson, H., Golberg, R.E., Annesley, W.H., and Tomer, T.L.: Presumed ocular histoplasmosis syndrome. Arch. Ophthalmol., 94:221, 1976.

Schlaegel, T.F., Jr.: Ocular Histoplasmosis. New York, Grune and Stratton, 1977.

Schlaegel, T.F., Jr. (ed.): Ocular Histoplasmosis. Int. Ophthalmol. Clin., 15:3, 1975.

Thatcher, R.W., and Pettit, T.H.: Gonorrheal conjunctivitis. JAMA, 215:1494, 1971.

Thygeson, P.: Complications of staphylococcic blepharitis. Am. J. Ophthalmol., 68:446, 1969.

Thygeson, P., Diaz-Bonnet, V., and Okumoto, M.: Phlyctenulosis: attempts to produce an experimental model with B.C. G. Invest. Ophthalmol., 1:262, 1962.

Thylefors, B.: Ocular onchocerciasis. Bull. WHO, 56:63, 1978.

Valenton, M.J., and Okumoto, M.: Toxin-producing strains of Staphylococcus epidermidis. Arch. Ophthalmol., 89:187, 1973.

Watson, P., and Hazelman, B.: The Sclera and Systemic Diseases. Philadelphia, W.B. Saunders, 1976.

Wilson, L.A.: External Diseases of the Eye. Hagerstown, MD, Harper & Row, 1979.

CHAPTER 33

Infections in the Immunocompromised Host

S.H. Zinner

> Objective 33-1. Outline the normal mechanisms responsible for defense against infection.

The ability to maintain health and to recover from infection requires the normal function of a number of cells, including polymorphonuclear leukocytes, lymphocytes, plasma cells, and macrophages. The functions of these cells and of specialized immunologic organs, such as the spleen and lymphoid tissue as well as the bone marrow, result in immunity at the cellular or humoral level. Resistance to infection, which involves the operation of several systems, may be impaired by a variety of disorders, diseases, and drugs.

CELLULAR DEFENSE MECHANISMS

Neutrophilic polymorphonuclear leukocytes. These cells are key defense mechanisms against overwhelming infection by bacteria, fungi, and other single- and multicelled organisms. When stimulated by a variety of factors, including lymphokines, complement components, proteins, microbial products, enzymes, and other chemoattractants, neutrophils have the capacity to leave the circulation or their marginated position along blood vessel walls by migrating through the endothelium between cells. These cells become oriented to the attractant, and their migration is then determined by means of actin-and myosin-directed contraction, which produces locomotion.

The phagocytic cells must then recognize their attractants and must prepare to ingest the foreign material. Antibody and complement are involved in the opsonization or coating of the microorganisms that renders them suitable for ingestion. Certain immunoglobulin antibody molecules, notably IgG_1 and IgG_3, bind to Fc receptors on the phagocytic cell membrane. The complement component C3, activated by IgM, IgG or the alternate pathway, also has opsonic activity.

Once the pathogen is recognized, the cell ingests it by means of an energy-dependent mechanism that results in pseudopod formation and enclosure of the ingested particle in a membrane-bound vacuole. During chemotaxis, the neutrophils' intracellular granules, which contain a variety of enzymes, become organized at the advancing end of the cell and secrete their contents into the phagocytic vacuole or phagosome. These enzymes include collagenases, cathepsins, glucuronidases, galactosidases, glycosidases, lysozyme, myeloperoxidase, and others. Hydrogen peroxide is produced rapidly by superoxide anions formed by the reduction of molecular oxygen. In the presence of myeloperoxidase, halide, and low pH, hydrogen peroxide is lethal to bacteria. The other enzymes in the phagocytic vacuole also contribute to the elimination of bacteria.

Macrophages. These phagocytic cells may be found lining sinusoids in the spleen, liver, lymph nodes, bone marrow, lung, brain, and other tissues. These cells are useful in removing debris associated with infection and also in phagocytosing microbial pathogens. Macrophages have some of the microbicidal enzymes found in neutrophils and, when activated, can be useful in killing foreign invaders, although their microbial efficiency is less than that of the neutrophil. Moreover, the macrophage interacts with lymphocytes in the immune response. The macrophage is intimately involved with antigen processing, stimulates the proliferation of T cells, and is an important cooperating cell in immunoglobulin antibody production.

Lymphocytes. These cells are critical to the maintenance of normal immunity. Two broad populations of lymphocytes exist, and both are important in the mediation of the immune response. When stimulated by appropriate antigens, B cells or bursal-dependent lymphocytes develop into plasma cells that actively synthesize and secrete immunoglobulin antibody, which is responsible for humoral immunity. T cells or thymus-associated cells function in cell-mediated immunity, including tumor resistance and resistance to infections with viruses, fungi, and other intracellular microbial pathogens. When sensitized to specific pathogens or antigens, T lymphocytes are responsible for lymphokine production and may act as helper cells (TH, recognized by OKT8 antibody) to augment B-cell antibody production, or they may act as suppressor or cytotoxic cells (T_s, recognized by OKT8 antibody) that interact with other lymphocytes and inhibit their function.

HUMORAL DEFENSE MECHANISMS

Antibody activity resides in protein immunoglobulins secreted by activated B cells (plasma cells) in response to antigen stimulation, with the cooperation of activated macrophages and T lymphocytes. Each plasma cell secretes only one type of immunoglobulin, either IgA, IgD, IgE, IgG, or IgM. An antibody may mediate the host's defense against infection in the following ways: by its opsonic role in phagocytosis; by its bactericidal activity (with complement) against a variety of gram-negative bacilli; by agglutination, which may reduce the number of infectious particles; by blockade of the cellular attachment of bacteria; by neutralization of exotoxins and endotoxins produced by bacteria; by neutralization of viruses, to prevent attachment or absorption of virus to cells; and by mediation of the inflammatory response through activation of complement.

Complement System. The complement system is a complex group of serum proteins that mediates several functions in the immune response. Antigen-antibody complexing activates the classic complement pathway. The alternate complement pathway can be activated by endotoxin or immunoglobulin, but specific antibody is not required. Complement activation augments certain of the immune mechanisms already described, including bacterial attachment and opsonization, as well as ingestion by phagocytic cells. Activated terminal complement components may directly damage bacteria and viruses.

STRUCTURAL AND FUNCTIONAL DEFENSE MECHANISMS

Human skin and mucous membranes provide a physical barrier to infection by invasive organisms. Maintenance of the integrity of these organs is the key to preventing infection, especially in patients with defects in any of the immune functions previously outlined.

Normal gastrointestinal function is useful in the physical removal, by vomiting or diarrhea, of invading organisms or their products. The physical activity of normal ciliary function is critical to the removal of bacteria and other particles from the respiratory tract. Normal urinary bladder function removes small numbers of bacteria introduced through the urethra and protects against urinary tract infections.

> Objective 33–2. Indicate the common specific defects in the immune system that increase the risk of infection, and summarize the infections that typically occur with each defect.

NEUTROPENIA

Neutropenia enhances the risk of many infections (Table 33–1). The number of circulating mature granulocytes may fall below 1000 cells/mm^3 under a variety of circumstances. One particular form of congenital neutropenia may be chronic or cyclic. Other diseases associated with neutropenia are aplastic anemia, Schwachman-Diamond syndrome, which includes malabsorption and pancreatic exocrine insufficiency with metaphyseal dysostosis, Chediak-Higashi syndrome, and lazy leukocyte syndrome. More common causes of neutropenia include acute and chronic leukemias, cytotoxic chemotherapy, metastatic carcinoma to the bone marrow, infections associated with bone marrow arrest, such as tuberculosis, immune neutropenia, as seen in some thymic tumors, and systemic lupus erythematosus. Rheumatoid arthritis may be associated with hypersplenism and neutropenia (Felty's syndrome).

Chemotactic Defects. Patients may have normal numbers of circulating neutrophils, but these cells may not function normally. Chemotactic defects may occur in association with diabetic acidosis, glucocorticoid, indomethacin, or phenylbutazone therapy, excessive alcohol intake, and malnutrition, as well as during parenteral hyperalimentation. Patients with liver cirrhosis, myeloma, severe uremia, hypophosphatemia, Hodgkin's disease, lepromatous leprosy, and sarcoidosis

Table 33–1. Defects in Host Defense Mechanisms and Associated Infections

Defect	Disease or Drug	Type of Infection or Pathogen
Neutropenia	Leukemia, cytotoxic therapy, metastatic carcinoma to bone marrow	*Escherichia coli, Klebsiella pneumoniae, Pseudomonas aeruginosa, Staphylococcus aureus,* other gram-negative bacilli and gram-positive cocci, aspergillus, candida
Chemotactic defects	Diabetes, alcoholism, Hodgkin's disease, Job's syndrome, corticosteroids	Frequent bacterial infections
Impaired neutrophil killing	Chronic granulomatous disease of childhood, myeloperoxidase deficiency	Pyogenic infections with catalase-positive bacteria
B-cell deficiency states	Congenital agammaglobulinemias, nephrotic syndrome, burns, protein-losing enteropathies, multiple myeloma, lymphocytic leukemia	Pyogenic infections, especially with *Streptococcus pneumoniae, Haemophilus influenzae, Neisseria meningitidis*
T-cell defects	Congenital thymic aplasia, combined immunodeficiency, Swiss-type aggammaglobulinemia (also has B-cell defects), systemic lupus erythematosus, sarcoidosis, Hodgkin's disease, chemotherapy, antilymphocyte serum, viral infections, acquired immune deficiency syndrome (AIDS)	*Mycobacterium tuberculosis, Listeria monocytogenes,* salmonella, brucella, cytomegalovirus, herpes simplex virus, herpes varicella-zoster virus, other viral infections, cryptococcus, candida, mucor, *Pneumocystis carinii, Toxoplasma gondii, Nocardia asteroides*
Complement deficiencies	Congenital disorders	Recurrent bacterial infection (e.g., *Neisseria meningitidis*)

also have chemotactic defects. In some of these clinical settings chemotaxis may be affected by serum inhibitors, which bind activated complement chemotaxins. Other inhibitors of chemotaxis have been described; for example, plasma from children with Wiskott-Aldrich syndrome may contain inhibitors that affect macrophage chemotaxis in vitro. Specific deficiencies of the chemotactic factors C3a or C5a may result in defective chemotaxis. The neutrophils of newborn infants may be less deformable and less mobile than those of older children and adults. Moreover, patients with Job's syndrome, characterized by recurrent subcutaneous and cutaneous cold abscesses and lymphadenitis, may have chemotactic defects.

Impaired Opsonization. The recognition and ingestion phase of phagocytosis, opsonization, may be impaired in several conditions, such as the congenital and acquired hypogammaglobulinopathies and disorders associated with decreased immunoglobulin production or increased loss such as glomerulonephritis, lupus erythematosus, or gastroenteropathies. Chediak-Higashi syndrome consists of oculocutaneous albinism, nystagmus, photophobia, intermittent fevers, and abnormally large neutrophilic granules. Pyogenic infections are common and probably result from impaired degranulation and impaired chemotaxis, both secondary to presumed membrane defects.

Bacteria-Killing Defects. Impairment of the killing ability of neutrophils has been described in several genetic disorders associated with increased infections. Chronic granulomatous disease of childhood is the prototype of these disorders, but its occurrence is limited. This disease is characterized by frequent pyogenic infections with catalase-positive bacteria, such as *Staphylococcus aureus*, klebsiella and enterobacter, *Serratia marcescens*, acinetobacter, and proteus, as well as infections with candida and aspergillus, owing to the failure of the patient's granulocytes to produce hydrogen peroxide, singlet oxygen, or superoxides. The nitroblue tetrazolium dye test (NBT) can be used to identify this defect in affected patients or asymptomatic carriers. Other specific defects in the metabolic pathway for killing bacteria include myeloperoxidase deficiency and severe deficiency of glucose-6-phosphate dehydrogenase. Bacteria-killing defects may also occur in leukemias and following cranial or spinal radiation therapy.

LYMPHOCYTE DISORDERS

Because the T and B lymphocytes together are responsible for the development and maintenance of immunity, abnormalities or defects in their structure and function produce a variety of specific immunodeficiency syndromes or conditions. These may occur as congenital defects, or they may be acquired or associated with other diseases. The reader is referred to more definitive immunology texts for a thorough review of these disorders.

B-Cell Immune Deficiency. The disorders affecting B-cell immune function include the congenital agammaglobulinemias, such as infantile X-linked agammaglobulinemia (Bruton's), which may occur with low levels of IgG and in the absence of other immunoglobulin classes or with low IgG and high IgM levels. Selective immunodeficiencies of IgM, IgG, IgA, and IgE have been described. Thymomas decrease the number of B lymphocytes, with associated hypogammaglobulinemia.

Immune deficiency B-cell states may also be acquired, as seen in disorders associated with the abnormal loss of proteins, for example, the nephrotic syndrome, severe burns, and protein-losing enteropathies such as intestinal lymphangiectasia, sprue, regional enteritis with or without fistulas, and Menetrier's disease, as well as in severe malnutrition. In these conditions, serum immunoglobulin levels are reduced, but the response to antigenic stimulation is usually normal. In multiple myeloma, lymphocytic leukemia, and other malignant diseases, there may be selective suppression of B-cell activity with decreased immunoglobulin production. Decreased immunoglobulin levels also may be found in myotonic dystrophy and other hypercatabolic conditions, whereas increased levels are seen in the rheumatoid diseases, in sarcoidosis, and in some congenital infections. Patients who have had a splenectomy are at an increased risk of overwhelming sepsis with encapsulated bacteria; they also have diminished antibody responses to whole bacterial vaccines.

T-Cell Immune Deficiency. Congenital defects also may produce specific T-cell abnormalities or combined B- and T-lymphocyte deficiencies. The pharyngeal pouch syndrome of thymic aplasia (DiGeorge syndrome) is associated with a scarcity of, or the absence of, T lymphocytes. These cells may be repopulated after thymic implants. Chronic mucocutaneous candidiasis is associated with abnormal cell-mediated immunity, possibly because of a dysfunction of T lymphocytes, and usually responds transiently to transfer factor infusions if given with antifungal agents. Transfer factor, a substance of low molecular weight derived from sensitized lymphocytes, can transfer cell-mediated immune responses to unsensitized or nonresponsive individuals.

Defects in T-lymphocyte activity may be seen in the rheumatic diseases, including systemic lupus erythematosus, as well as in Hodgkin's disease and sarcoidosis. Other malignant disorders, x-irradiation, chemotherapy, and treatment with antilymphocyte serum may also affect T-cell function.

Within the past few years, hundreds of patients with an acquired immunodeficiency syndrome (AIDS) have been documented in the United States and elsewhere. Most of these patients are young, homosexually active men or intravenous drug abusers. The origin of this syndrome is unknown, but it is associated with the development of Kaposi's sarcoma and opportunistic infections.

Combined B- and T-Cell Immune Deficiency. Both B- and T-lymphocyte activities are decreased in severe combined immunodeficiency or Swiss-type agammaglobulinemia or its variant, with some B-lymphocyte activity and normal or near normal immunoglobulin levels (Nezelof's syndrome). The Wiscott-Aldrich syndrome is an X-linked inherited disease with thrombocytopenia, recurrent bacterial infections, and severe eczema. It is associated with an unclear immune defect in both humoral and cell-mediated immunity. Combined immunodeficiency may occur with ataxia telangiectasia and with adenosine deaminase deficiency. Variable immunodeficiencies have also been described.

Acquired combined defects may occur in toxin-produced aplastic anemia, malignant diseases including leukemia and lymphoma, and severe malnutrition; they also may follow immunosuppressive or cytotoxic therapy. Azathioprine (Imuran), used in immunosuppressive therapy in transplant recipients and for other conditions, may decrease the pri-

---

ACQUIRED IMMUNE DEFICIENCY SYNDROME (AIDS)

Definition: An acquired disorder of T-cell-mediated immunity associated with the occurrence of Kaposi's sarcoma and opportunistic infections in previously healthy patients with no known underlying immunosuppressive disease.

Etiology: Unknown.

Epidemiology: Almost 90% of these cases occur in homosexually or bisexually active men and intravenous drug abusers 20 to 45 years old. Haitian men (heterosexual) living in the United States and a few older men with hemophilia are also affected. Most patients reside in New York City, San Francisco, Los Angeles, and Miami, but scattered cases have been reported from other locations in the United States and from Canada, Haiti, and Europe. Over 2,400 cases were documented between July 1981 and September 1983.

Immunology: Lymphopenia, decreased ratios of helper to suppressor T cells; defective skin test response to recall antigens, diminished in vitro lymphocyte response to mitogens; normal polymorphonuclear leukocyte counts and function; polyclonal B-cell activation; elevated serum immunoglobulins.

Clinical Presentation: Kaposi's sarcoma occurring on any area of the body in young men. Febrile illness with malaise, weight loss, lymphadenopathy, and a variety of infections may occur, including *Pneumocystis carinii* pneumonia, cryptococcal meningitis, cytomegaloviral pneumonia, perianal herpes simplex infection, cerebral toxoplasmosis, disseminated infection with *Mycobacterium avium intracellulare*, and cryptosporidiosis.

Treatment: X-irradiation and chemotherapy for Kaposi's sarcoma; specific anti-infective therapy for opportunistic infections.

Case Fatality Rate: Averages 40%, but may be higher in cases diagnosed prior to 1979.

mary and secondary immune responses, may diminish cell-mediated immunity, and may decrease the number of circulating neutrophils.

A variety of defects in or deficiencies of the complement system have been reported. Deficiencies in complement components, especially C3 and C3b inactivator, are associated with serious recurrent bacterial infections, such as meningitis, pneumonia otitis, and bacteremia. Patients with deficient C5, C6, C7, and C8 are at heightened risk of neisseria infections.

> Objective 33–3. Give examples of recurrent infections that do not require detailed investigation of the patient's host defense mechanisms.

RECURRENT BACTERIAL INFECTIONS

Such infections (Table 33–2) occur commonly in many patients who are not suffering from any immune defects, as outlined in Objective 33–2. Patients with recurrent urinary tract infections due to relapse with the same organism or, more frequently, due to reinfections with new strains usually do not have a major defect in host defense. Similarly, the common syndrome of recurrent staphylococcal furunculosis, which often occurs in several family members, is rarely associated with an immune defect, except perhaps in patients with diabetes mellitus. Recurrent episodes of otitis media or streptococcal pharyngitis occur frequently in normal hosts and need not precipitate an extensive immunologic evaluation.

Patients with recurrent pneumococcal meningitis following head trauma or neurosurgical procedures may have structural, but not necessarily immunologic, defects. The presence of chronic osteomyelitis, chronic bronchitis, recurrent or chronic sinusitis, recurrent idiopathic pericarditis, chronic prostatitis, recurrent urethritis or cervicitis, wound infections following surgery or trauma, or self-inflicted recurrent skin infections does not imply a primary defect in host defense.

RECURRENT VIRAL INFECTIONS

Recurrent viral infections such as herpes labialis or herpes genitalis usually do not require extensive immunologic study. Young children usually experience frequent viral upper respiratory tract infections in their first decade, and these patients are not inherently immunosuppressed. A careful medical history should distinguish patients with recurrent infections due to re-exposure to infecting organisms and those with surgical or structural conditions that predispose them to frequent infections from those with specific immune defects, who require detailed immunologic study, diagnosis, and possibly specific therapy.

OTHER TYPES OF RECURRENT INFECTION

Patients with any surgically implanted foreign object, including shunts, valves, and catheters, are at an increased risk of repeated infections. Patients with obstructive urinary or respiratory tracts, including patients with asthma and cystic fibrosis, frequently have recurring infections with no underlying im-

Table 33–2. Organisms that Frequently Cause Infections in the Immunocompromised Host

Bacteria
   Enterobacteriaceae, especially *Escherichia coli*, klebsiella, salmonella
   Staphylococcus aureus
   Pseudomonas aeruginosa
   Listeria monocytogenes
   Mycobacterium tuberculosis
   Nocardia asteroides
Fungi
   Candida albicans and other species of candida
   Cryptococcus neoformans
   Aspergillus fumigatus
   Mucor, rhizopus
Viruses
   Cytomegalovirus
   Herpes simplex
   Herpes varicella-zoster
Other organisms
   Pneumocystis carinii
   Toxoplasma gondii
   Strongyloides stercoralis

mune defect. Many skin disorders predispose patients to repeated systemic infections with staphylococci; careful examination of the integument is important in evaluating these patients. Patients with cardiac valvular disease and those with microvascular disorders, such as diabetes or sickle cell anemia, may be at increased risk of infections without specific immune deficits.

> Objective 33–4. Describe some infections that require detailed investigation of the defect in the patient's host defense mechanism.

Overwhelming bacteremia due to *Staphylococcus aureus* or gram-negative rods, or recurrent serious invasive disease due to encapsulated bacteria, such as *Streptococcus pneumoniae, Haemophilus influenzae,* or *Neisseria meningitidis,* should prompt an immunologic evaluation. Moreover, frequent or recurrent episodes of pneumonia, soft tissue abscesses, septic arthritis, osteomyelitis, or meningitis should cause one to question the integrity of the host defense mechanisms. The occurrence of fungal infection at any site, other than contained, deep-tissue fungal infections in endemic areas, and the occurrence of infections with other opportunistic pathogens, such as *Pneumocystis carinii,* nocardia species, *Mycobacterium avium intracellulare* disseminated varicella-zoster, and cytomegalovirus, in the absence of known underlying disease, should stimulate a search for such disorders and an investigation of the patient's host defenses as outlined in the following paragraphs.

SCREENING STUDIES

Blood Count. The first steps in the immunologic evaluation of a patient with recurrent infections are to take a complete blood count and to evaluate the peripheral blood smear. The smear should include a total lymphocyte count, which is calculated by multiplying the total white blood cell count by the percentage of lymphocytes on the differential count (normal is 3000 to 6000 lymphocytes/mm^3). The presence of neutropenia is readily detectable, as is lymphopenia, which may be present in some immunodeficiencies, especially if few small lymphocytes are present. Howell-Jolly bodies, suggestive of asplenia, may be seen, and morphologic abnormalities of granulocytes should be obvious.

Quantitation of Immunoglobulin Levels. Immunoglobulin levels should be quantitated using radial immunodiffusion plates for IgG, IgM, and IgA. Normal values for these levels vary with age. For example, mean ± standard deviation IgG, IgM, and IgA levels are, respectively: for newborns, 1031 plus or minus 200, 11 plus or minus 5, and 1 plus or minus 2 mg/100 ml; for 3- to 5-year-old children, 929 plus or minus 228, 56 plus or minus 18, and 71 plus or minus 37 mg/100 ml; for adults, 1158 plus or minus 305, 99 plus or minus 27, and 200 plus or minus 61 mg/100 ml. A total immunoglobulin level under 400 mg/100 ml or an IgG concentration of less than 200 mg/100 ml is evidence of antibody deficiency. Immunoelectrophoresis is not useful for these determinations because it does not provide information about quantitation of individual immunoglobulins.

Antibody Function Testing. Some estimate of antibody function should be part of the screening study. The presence of serum antibody to antigens administered in routine immunization, such as immunization against poliovirus, rubella, or rubeola, suggests a normal IgG responsiveness that may be lacking in antibody deficiency syndromes. Alternatively, a positive Schick test in previously immunized individuals indicates a functional IgG deficiency. Isoagglutinins to blood group antigens may also be abnormal in patients with antibody deficiencies.

Skin Testing. Skin tests are useful screening procedures for cell-mediated immunity. Tests usually included are mumps, candida, streptokinase and streptodornase, trichophyton, purified protein derivative of tuberculin, and tetanus toxoid. Cellular immunodeficiency is suspected in patients over age 10 who do not react to any of these tests. Sensitization to dinitrochlorobenzene (DNCB) can be attempted, but this material may scar the skin of young children. In infants and young children, one should attempt to localize the thymus by means of chest roentgenograms, including posteroanterior and lateral views. Absence of this shadow suggests thymic hypoplasia.

Neutrophil Function Testing. Screening tests for suspected neutrophil dysfunction should include the nitroblue tetrazolium (NBT) dye test in addition to the quantitative and qualitative studies previously outlined. Neutrophils from patients with chronic granulomatous disease do not reduce NBT normally. Moreover, serum IgE levels should be measured because elevated values are found in some diseases with disordered chemotaxis.

Measurement of Complement Activity. Screening tests for complement activity include measurements of total hemolytic complement (CH_{50}) and levels of C3 and C4 in serum. Because the range of normal responses to these tests is wide, only unusually low or absent levels suggest complement deficiencies.

FURTHER TESTS

Most of the aforementioned tests are available in hospitals or in centralized laboratories that have access to medical centers. Tests capable of evaluating specific abnormalities of immune function in greater detail are available in reference centers. These evaluations, which are best coordinated by an immunologist, should include specific antibody response studies, determination of serum IgD and IgE levels, immunoglobulin subclass determinations, and enumeration of B lymphocytes, among other antibody studies. Some additional tests of cellular immune function are enumeration of T lymphocytes, lymphocyte proliferation studies in response to antigens or mitogens, assays of lymphokines, adenosine deaminase, and nucleoside phosphorylase, lymph node biopsy, and determination of the ratio of suppressor to helper T cells. More detailed tests of neutrophil function include in vitro chemotaxis and motility studies, Rebuck skin window technique, bactericidal assays, chemiluminescence, assays of myeloperoxidase, and the quantitative NBT test. Detailed investigation of the complement system includes functional assays of each component, activation studies, opsonic activity determinations, and chemotactic activity studies. The reader is referred to larger immunology texts for a more complete discussion of these and other tests.

TREATMENT

In general, the treatment of immune defects requires careful nutrition, prevention of infection, and avoidance of live vaccines. Continuous prophylactic antibiotics can be administered in some antibody deficiencies or in chronic granulomatous disease but this is not always recommended. Gamma globulin or immune serum globulin is useful in antibody deficiency syndromes, and leukocyte transfusions may be useful in some neutropenic patients, especially during a serious bacterial infection. Other specific therapies, including thymus or bone marrow transplantation and transfer factor may be effective in some immunodeficiency disorders.

Common examples of infection in patients with specific immunocompromised states are discussed in the following sections.

> Objective 33–5. Outline a clinical approach to the diagnosis and treatment of a patient with acute myelocytic leukemia, neutropenia, and fever to 39° C.

A patient with acute myelocytic leukemia and neutropenia (less than 500 circulating granulocytes/mm^3) develops a fever to 39° C. Clinical and laboratory evaluations fail to reveal an apparent site of infection.

CLINICAL EXAMINATION

A careful and complete physical examination is essential to discover any subtle clues that might aid in establishing a microbiologically documented source of fever. Because leukemic patients are often made profoundly neutropenic by their induction chemotherapy, neutropenia becomes the major risk factor for infection. The risk of bacterial infection increases with the duration and extent of neutropenia, and most patients with fewer than 100 circulating granulocytes/mm^3 develop a bacterial infection by the third neutropenic week.

The diagnosis of bacterial infection in severe neutropenia may be limited by the patient's decreased ability to form pus and to produce the usual signs of inflammation: pain, swelling, redness, and heat. In neutropenic patients with pneumonia, sputum may be lacking in pus cells, and the diagnosis must be suspected on careful clinical examination and frequent radiologic study. Infections may be poorly localized, and some typical signs and symptoms may be absent.

The physical examination may reveal small skin abrasions or lacerations or a single pustule, which would not be of concern in a normal host. Pustules or crusted erosions in the nasal mucosa can be the source of bacteremia. Oral and pharyngeal mucosal lesions should not be overlooked. Ocular and ophthalmic examinations may reveal fluffy exudates suggestive of candidemia. Axillary and inguinal lymph nodes should be examined carefully for even minimal signs of fluctuant lymphadenopathy, and the perirectal area should be searched for fissures and early abscess formation. The webs of the patient's toes should be examined because extensive dermatophytosis may be the only entry point for an invasive staphylococcus.

OTHER INVESTIGATIONS

Frequent blood cultures (a minimum of three) should be obtained from different venipuncture sites. Blood cultures should be processed for anaerobic as well as aerobic organisms. Cultures also should be obtained from the pharynx, urine, stool, and cerebrospinal fluid if the patient has any neurologic signs or symptoms. If necrotizing skin lesions are present, these should be aspirated, smeared, and cultured. Chest roentgenograms should be obtained daily or on alternate days, even in absence of specific signs of pneumonia.

In tropical areas, the presence of parasites should be determined prior to the initiation of immunosuppressive or cytotoxic therapy. Indwelling catheters in venous or urethral sites are potential sources of infection and should be removed and appropriately cultured. It is often useful to obtain and store a sample of serum at the onset of any febrile illness in these patients, to compare with convalescent or subsequent specimens as an aid to specific serologic diagnosis. When vigorous diagnostic attempts have been made, one should consider administering lifesaving anti-infective drugs empirically, based on the most likely causes of infection.

USUAL CAUSES OF FEVER IN NEUTROPENIC PATIENTS

Approximately 20% of febrile neutropenic patients have bacteremia responsible for their fever; another 20% have microbiologically documented infections at various body sites, whereas another 20% have infections that are clinically documented but microbiologically unprovable. Although bacteremia in the neutropenic patient can be caused by many organisms, the four most frequently isolated are *Staphylococcus aureus*, *Escherichia coli*, *Klebsiella pneumoniae*, and *Pseudomonas aeruginosa*. Bacteremic episodes in these patients are more frequent when associated with fewer than 100 circulating neutrophils/mm^3, with severely depressed peripheral platelet counts, and in the presence of fevers higher than 39° C. Fungemia and viremia may occur, but are less frequently the initial cause of fever in a neutropenic patient.

TREATMENT

Patients with neutropenia and fever should receive prompt antibiotic therapy as soon as cultures are obtained (Table 33–3). Antibiotics should be directed against gram-negative rods and staphylococci, the major pathogens expected in these patients. Although many new beta-lactam antibiotics have been introduced recently, experience with their single use in these patients is extremely limited. Most studies have shown that synergistic combinations of antibiotics afford better clinical results in neutropenic patients than combinations without synergistic activity in vitro against the infecting organism.

No antibiotic combination is optimal (Table 33–3), but a broad-spectrum beta-lactam agent in addition to an aminoglycoside should be given as initial empiric therapy. The choice of agents from this group depends on local patterns of antibiotic resistance and the frequency of isolation of organisms. If and when the offending organism is isolated, the antibiotic combination can be adjusted based on susceptibility studies. Aminoglycosides may be inactivated by beta-lactam agents in vitro and, to a lesser degree, in vivo. These drugs should not be mixed and administered together, but rather should be given sequentially.

If a patient with a proven infection responds to treatment promptly, antibiotics should be continued for at least 10 days, although one study suggests they should continue until the patient's granulocyte count rises above 500/mm^3. If a patient with a proven bacterial infection fails to respond to treatment, a careful search must be made for any drainable collections of pus or necrotic material. Antibiotics may be changed if susceptibility tests indicate that this is necessary. Granulocyte transfusions should be considered and may improve the response rate. Lithium carbonate has been shown to increase the release of granulocytes from the bone marrow; however, the number of clinical studies of its adjunctive role in sepsis is limited. The use of passive transfusion of antibodies to cross-reacting bacterial cell wall components (endotoxin) is promising, but remains experimental.

If the patient fails to respond to empiric antibiotics by the fourth febrile day and if no bacterial infection has been documented but such an infection remains likely, empiric administration of amphotericin B (rapidly approaching 1 mg/kg/day intravenously, given over 6 to 8 hours once daily) has been suggested and is currently under investigation. If evidence of possible infection no longer exists, antibiotics can be discontinued, and the fever can be attributed to a noninfective cause. Frequent cultures and careful observation of these patients are extremely important.

> **Objective 33–6.** Outline an approach to the diagnosis and treatment of the same neutropenic patient who initially responded to empiric antibiotic therapy, but who subsequently developed fever and pulmonary infection.

DIAGNOSIS

Numerous organisms can be responsible for pulmonary infection in a hospitalized neu-

Table 33–3. Empiric Treatment of Fever in a Neutropenic Patient

Initial Therapy
Beta-lactam antibiotic such as carbenicillin, ticarcillin, azlocillin, piperacillin, mezlocillin, moxalactam, cefotaxime, cefoperazone, ceftriaxone, ceftizoxime, or ceftazidime
Plus
Aminoglycoside such as amikacin, gentamicin, tobramycin, or netilmicin
Evaluation on Day 4

Patient improved, defervesced, infection was probable	Patient not improved		
	Definite bacterial infection	Infection likely, not proved	No infection
Continue antibiotics for 9 or 10 days or until granulocyte count rises to over 500/µL (not established fully)	Change antibiotics, drain abscess, add granulocyte transfusion, consider lithium, antiendotoxin serum	Continue antibiotics and add amphotericin B (suggested by preliminary studies)	Discontinue antibiotics

tropenic patient receiving chemotherapy and corticosteroids. Among these are gram-negative rods, such as *Pseudomonas aeruginosa, Klebsiella pneumoniae,* acinetobacter, and *Legionella pneumophila;* opportunistic bacteria such as *Nocardia asteroides;* mycobacteria; fungi, such as *Candida albicans, Aspergillus fumigatus,* mucor, and *Cryptococcus neoformans;* viruses, such as cytomegalovirus, herpes varicella-zoster, and herpes simplex; protozoa or similar organisms, such as *Toxoplasma gondii* or *Pneumocystis carinii;* and parasites, such as *Strongyloides stercoralis.* More common organisms, such as *Streptococcus pneumoniae, Haemophilus influenzae,* and *Staphylococcus aureus,* may also cause pneumonia in these patients. More than one infecting agent may be present in any given infection.

The specific diagnosis of pulmonary infection is often difficult in the immunocompromised patient. Few reliable clinical or radiologic clues exist. Pulmonary infections with pyogenic bacteria, nocardia, and fungi often produce dense alveolar infiltrates that may extend beyond a single pulmonary lobe. Viruses and *Pneumocystis carinii* are more likely to cause interstitial infiltrates. In severely neutropenic patients, however, interstitial infiltration may be the earliest radiologic abnormality, even in bacterial pneumonia.

Pneumocystis carinii pneumonia (Fig. 33–1) may cause a bilateral interstitial infiltrate spreading from the hilar areas in a febrile, hypoxic patient with leukemia or lymphoma. Wedge-shaped infiltrates, diffuse interstitial pneumonia, and invasive fungus balls have all been seen in neutropenic patients infected with aspergillus or mucor, and these agents as well as *Pseudomonas aeruginosa* may cause invasive vascular infarction in the lung.

Laboratory Techniques. The physician should attempt to isolate the organism or organisms responsible for infection. Coughed sputum or sputum obtained by transtracheal or endotracheal aspiration may be helpful in the diagnosis if the gram-stained smear or fungus preparation contains a single microorganism in abundance. Many organisms are likely to be present, however. In addition, transtracheal aspiration may cause serious or fatal bleeding in these patients, who often are severely thrombocytopenic. Organisms such as *Pneumocystis carinii,* which require silver stains to demonstrate its cysts, are rarely diagnosed on sputum smears and usually require more invasive diagnostic procedures to be identified in tissue secretions.

Endoscopic Study and Biopsy. Fiberoptic bronchoscopy with washings and transbronchoscopic biopsy may yield diagnostic material, but bleeding cannot be controlled directly. Percutaneous needle aspiration of the affected lung may allow diagnosis if the infiltrate is near the posterior chest wall, but pneumothorax and hemorrhage are complications.

Open lung biopsy is likely to yield the proper diagnosis. With the aid of platelet transfusions, the surgeon can obtain sufficient material from the involved area, and bleeding usually can be controlled directly. The tissue can be processed microbiologically and pathologically, and the diagnosis of specific infection or neoplasia can be made. This last approach usually requires a team comprising an oncologist, a surgeon, an infectious disease specialist, a microbiologist, and a pathologist to ensure that the procedure is performed rapidly and that maximal information is obtained.

Problems in Diagnosis. The diagnosis of lung infection in the immunosuppressed patient is difficult even with an optimal diagnostic approach. More than one organism is often present. The infection may also be due to an organism usually thought to be a harmless commensal, especially aspergillus, which is frequently isolated from the secretions of noninfected patients. Surveillance cultures of various body sites have been suggested as a means of predicting future infection with a given organism. One group has reported that the presence of *Aspergillus flavus* or possibly *A. fumigatus* on nose cultures may predict subsequent invasive aspergillosis.

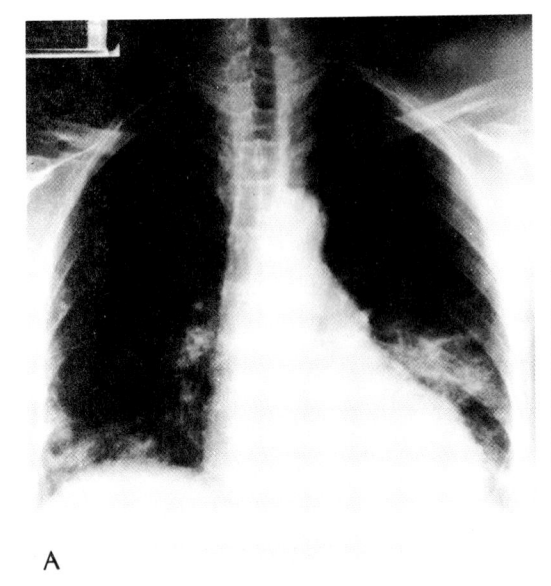

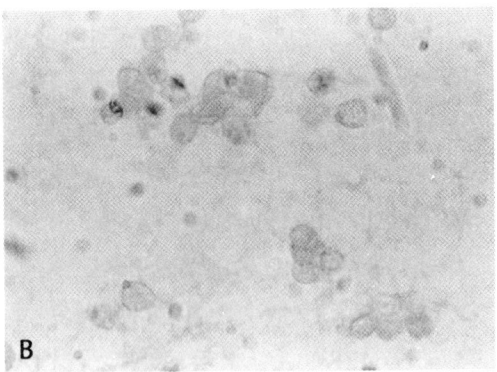

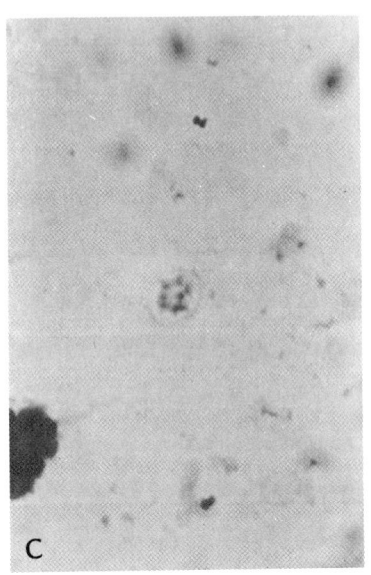

540 Infections: Recognition, Understanding, Treatment

Fig. 33–1. A, Pneumonia due to *Pneumocystis carinii* in a febrile, hypoxic, immunocompromised patient, 60 days after a renal graft. Note the bilateral interstitial infiltrates. B, Cyst-like structures in a lung biopsy (toluidine blue stain, 1000 X). C, Cyst-like structure containing light parasites (Giemsa stain, 4000 X).

Serologic Studies. Serologic techniques are available for some of the opportunistic pathogens, but many of these procedures remain experimental. Aspergillus antibodies can be detected by passive hemagglutination or immunodiffusion assays. Although the use of antibody detection tests in immunodepressed patients may be questioned, one group has recently shown that seroconversion to the immunodiffusion test can lead to early diagnosis and subsequent early therapy with improved survival rates in invasive aspergillosis. In the future, with improving technology, aspergillus antigenemia may be detectable by radioimmunoassay.

Invasive candidiasis is more difficult to diagnose than aspergillosis on serologic grounds, but many techniques have been studied. Candida antigenemia has been detected with serum precipitins, passive hemagglutination inhibition, countercurrent immunoelectrophoresis (CIE), and gas liquid

> **SOME OPPORTUNISTIC PATHOGENS IN THE IMMUNOCOMPROMISED HOST**
>
> *NOCARDIA ASTEROIDES*
>
> This gram-positive branching rod is weakly acid fast when decolorized with 1% sulfuric acid. It is nonmotile and has slow-growing, orange-red, wrinkled, and dry colonies. *N. asteroides* grows in 2 to 4 days on most aerobic culture media and is sensitive to sulfonamides, minocycline, cycloserine, and trimethoprim-sulfamethoxazole.
>
> *PNEUMOCYSTIS CARINII*
>
> This protozoa-like organism was only recently propagated in vitro in several cell lines. It exists in tissue as oval or spherical thick-walled cysts, containing eight sporozoites, or as trophozoites. Methenamine silver stain identifies the cyst in tissue; trophozoites are stained with Giemsa, Gram-Weigert, Wright's, and other polychrome stains. Infected patients may respond to treatment with pentamidine isethionate or high doses of trimethoprim-sulfamethoxazole.
>
> *STRONGYLOIDES STERCORALIS*
>
> This nematode or roundworm parasitizes the upper intestinal tract of man and can live freely in soil. Adult females may reach 2.2 mm in length. Larvae may penetrate skin or intestinal mucosa and may reach the lungs through the blood. They are subsequently brought to the posterior pharynx, where they are swallowed, and thereby establish themselves in the intestine. Autoinfection may result in an enormous worm burden. Thiabendazole administration is the treatment of choice.

chromatography. The enzyme-linked immunosorbent assay also may be useful in detecting candida (mannan) antigenemia. Antibody titer rises, less useful in these patients, can be detected with passive hemagglutination, slide agglutination, CIE, and latex agglutination techniques.

Noninfectious Disorders. Pulmonary interstitial infiltrates may be noninfectious in the immunosuppressed patient. Certain chemotherapeutic agents such as bleomycin, busulfan, methotrexate, and, occasionally, cyclophosphamide produce interstitial infiltrates indistinguishable radiographically from those caused by some invasive pathogens. In addition, these infiltrates may be caused by metastatic spread of the tumor or infiltration with leukemic cells. Ultimately, the lung may react with a similar pattern several months, or even years, after radiation therapy.

TREATMENT OF PNEUMONIA IN IMMUNOSUPPRESSED PATIENTS

To be effective, the therapy of pulmonary infection in immunosuppressed patients is best directed against the specific pathogen (Table 33–4). When the specific diagnosis cannot be established, however, one must use a combination of agents directed against a variety of organisms. Because the usual gram-negative bacilli or staphylococci may be implicated, the therapeutic regimen should contain antibiotics effective against these organisms, such as a semisynthetic penicillin or a cephalosporin in addition to an aminoglycoside in maximal doses. If the infection develops while the patient is receiving these antibiotics, then one should administer the following: erythromycin, 0.5 g every 6 hours intravenously, for legionella; and trimethoprim-sulfamethoxazole, 20/100 mg/kg/day, in 4 divided doses, orally or intravenously, for *Pneumocystis carinii* and nocardia, in addition to amphotericin B, 0.5 to 1.2 mg/kg/ every other day infused over 6 to 8 hours.

> **Objective 33–7.** Describe other common types of clinically documented infections in febrile neutropenic patients, and outline appropriate therapy.

Any common infection may occur in an immunosuppressed, neutropenic patient, but these infections are usually more severe and life-threatening than in other patients.

ORAL INFECTIONS

Oral ulceration, which may be severe in these patients, may be due to chemotherapeutic agents as well as to viruses such as *Herpesvirus hominis* (herpes simplex virus). Candida infection of the mouth and oropharynx appears as white plaques overlying shallow ulcers possibly extending to the esophagus. Both herpesvirus and candida may produce ulcerative esophagitis, which is sus-

Table 33–4. Treatment of Pneumonia in the Immunosuppressed Patient

Infecting Organism	Effective Agents*
Bacteria	
Pseudomonas aeruginosa	Carbenicillin, ticarcillin, piperacillin, or azlocillin† plus tobramycin, gentamicin, or amikacin
Klebsiella pneumoniae	Cefazolin, cefotaxime, moxalactam, cefoperazone, mezlocillin, ceftriaxone, or ceftazidime plus tobramycin, gentamicin, or amikacin
Legionella pneumophila	Erythromycin or rifampin
Nocardia asteroides	Sulfonamides, minocycline, or cycloserine
Mycobacterium tuberculosis	Isoniazid, ethambutol, rifampin, or streptomycin
Nontuberculous (atypical) mycobacteria	Pending susceptibility tests
Fungi	
Candida albicans and other species of candida	Amphotericin B (ketoconazole not fully evaluated in these patients)
Aspergillus fumigatus	Amphotericin B
Cryptococcus neoformans	Amphotericin B plus flucytosine
Viruses	
Cytomegalovirus	No proved therapy
Herpes simplex virus	Possibly acyclovir
Herpes varicella-zoster virus	Vidarabine or acyclovir
Parasites	
Toxoplasma gondii	Pyrimethamine plus sulfonamides
Other	
Pneumocystis carinii	Trimethoprim-sulfamethoxazole or pentamidine isethionate

*The drug of choice varies with local susceptibility patterns.
†New third-generation beta-lactams antibiotics, such as moxalactam, cefoperazone, cefotaxime, or ceftazidime, may be useful with an aminoglycoside.

pected by severe dysphagia and is proved by esophagoscopy and biopsy. Treatment of oropharyngeal herpes infection is symptomatic and includes the administration of oral analgesics and lubricants such as topical viscous lidocaine. Acyclovir is under active study for this infection. Treatment of oral candidiasis is with nystatin mouthwash, 1 ml of a suspension of 100,000 U/ml, every 6 to 8 hours. For more invasive candidiasis, amphotericin B, 0.1 to 0.5 mg/kg once daily for 10 days, may suffice. Ketoconazole, 400 to 1000 mg/day once daily, is an oral antifungal agent effective against local but not disseminated candida infections.

Streptococcal pharyngitis may manifest itself as severe tonsilitis with peritonsillar abscess formation. Obstruction of the trachea may result. Treatment is directed at maintaining the patient's airway and includes the administration of penicillin or erythromycin.

INTRAVENOUS CATHETER INFECTIONS

Suppurative thrombophlebitis may occur secondary to plastic intravenous catheters. These sites, as well as other needle puncture sites, are also portals of entry for bacteremia. Therefore, these devices should be maintained with utmost care, and plastic catheters should not be used in these patients unless absolutely necessary. Suppurative phlebitis usually responds to removal of the cannula, heat, and specific antibiotics. Excision of the vein may be necessary.

DISSEMINATED MYCOBACTERIAL DISEASE

Tuberculosis may occur in neutropenic patients, especially if they have undergone immunosuppressive and corticosteroid therapy. The diagnosis is often overlooked because symptoms of cough and fever may be partially suppressed by the corticosteroids. Tuberculosis may first appear as a pulmonary infection or in its miliary or disseminated form. The diagnosis is usually made on culture of sputum or tissue specimens from involved organs.

Atypical or nontuberculous mycobacteria

also cause infection in immunosuppressed patients. Overwhelming, fatal infection with *Mycobacterium intracellulare* or *M. kansasii* may occur in patients with leukemia, including hairy-cell leukemia or aplastic anemia, as well as in patients with renal transplants. Because these organisms are often resistant to isoniazid, ethambutol, and streptomycin, these infections should be treated with multiple antituberculous drugs based on susceptibility tests.

Patients whose underlying disease is likely to require the use of immunosuppressive drugs should receive a tuberculin test and a chest roentgenogram prior to chemotherapy. If the skin test is positive or if the roentgenogram reveals calcification of a node or lung area, isoniazid prophylaxis, at 300 mg/day, should be given for the duration of the immunosuppression. Standard antituberculous therapy should be administered if any evidence of active tuberculosis exists.

PERIANAL AND RECTAL INFECTIONS

Patients with prolonged, severe neutropenia may develop subtle or overt abscesses in the perianal or perirectal areas. These abscesses may begin with an anal fissure or an area of induration that may or may not be tender. Normal amounts of anal or rectal trauma, as in the course of a bowel movement, may cause small mucosal tears that allow the entry of fecal flora. Because of the dearth of polymorphonuclear leukocytes, these organisms multiply locally and lead to tissue necrosis and abscess formation. Careful examination of the anus and surrounding area should be repeatedly performed in severely neutropenic patients. Rectal thermometers should be avoided in these patients.

Treatment should include sitz baths in warm water and antibiotics directed against fecal flora; examples are clindamycin, 450 to 600 mg every 6 to 8 hours intravenously, in addition to amikacin, 15 mg/kg/day in 2 divided intravenous doses, or another combination of an aminoglycoside and a broad-spectrum beta-lactam agent (see Table 33–3). Surgical drainage is indicated when a recognizable collection is present. *Pseudomonas aeruginosa* is often isolated in neutropenia leukemic patients and appropriate antibiotics are needed (see Table 33–4).

STRONGYLOIDIASIS

Although normal hosts may harbor the parasite *Strongyloides stercoralis* without symptoms or with mild abdominal cramps or diarrhea, the compromised host, especially the patient with defective cell-mediated immunity, may develop overwhelming strongyloidiasis. This infection may cause crampy abdominal pain, bloating and abdominal distension, vomiting, diarrhea or constipation, fever, hypotension, pneumonia, abnormal liver function tests, and a variety of neurologic defects such as confusion, delirium, stupor, and coma. The diagnosis is made by identifying larval forms on aspirates from the patient's duodenum, blind loops, or stool.

This diagnosis should be suspected in the appropriate patient in the presence of eosinophilia, persistent bacteremia with one or more enteric organisms, and gastrointestinal complaints. Treatment is with thiabendazole, 25 mg/kg twice daily for 5 to 7 days. Repeat courses are often necessary.

Objective 33–8. Outline the likely causes of infection and the optimal treatment for a patient with multiple myeloma who develops fever, sepsis, and shock.

Patients with multiple myeloma have defective antibody synthesis and depressed levels of serum IgM. Infections in this disease occur at a frequency of 1.5 per patient-year. The risk of infection is greatest in the 2 months following the initiation of chemotherapy.

CAUSES OF INFECTION

The most frequent causes of septicemia in these patients are the polysaccharide encapsulated organisms, *Streptococcus pneumoniae*, *Haemophilus influenzae*, and *Neisseria meningitidis*. Because antibody is important in the opsonization of these organisms, the defective antibody production in multiple myeloma patients may play a role in the increased susceptibility of these persons to lethal, overwhelming septicemic infection. Other organisms, notably *Staphylococcus aureus* and gram-negative bacilli, have been isolated from bacteremic patients with multiple myeloma more frequently in recent years. These infections may be nosocomially acquired, and their increased incidence may reflect more frequent and prolonged hospitalization of these patients. Repeated episodes of pneumococcal pneumonia and bacteremia have been described in the literature. Clinical and radiologic evidence of pneumonia is often present in multiple myeloma patients with sepsis.

TREATMENT OF FEVER AND SEPSIS

The treatment of fever and sepsis in patients with multiple myeloma should be instituted promptly after obtaining cultures of blood, sputum, urine, and cerebrospinal fluid (CSF), if indicated. High doses of penicillin G, such as 2 million U every 4 hours intravenously, should be given to treat pneumococcal sepsis in these patients, although lower doses may be successful. If urinary or gastrointestinal foci are present, or if culture results are still awaited, an aminoglycoside in addition to a broad-spectrum beta-lactam antibiotic (see Table 33–3) should be given in maximal doses.

Prevention of infection in these patients is difficult. Pneumococcal vaccine may not increase the protection from infection with *Streptococcus pneumoniae* in these patients. Careful hygiene and a gut-decontaminating regimen might be useful (see Objective 33–11).

> **Objective 33–9.** Describe the probable infecting organisms and their appropriate management in a patient with advanced Hodgkin's disease with headache and mild nuchal rigidity.

The development of meningitis in the immunocompromised host, such as a patient with lymphoma, may be due to common pathogens, including *Streptococcus pneumoniae* and *Neisseria meningitidis*, but meningitis may also be caused by three other organisms to which these patients are particularly susceptible: *Cryptococcus neoformans*, *Listeria monocytogenes*, and *Toxoplasma gondii*.

CRYPTOCOCCUS NEOFORMANS

Signs and Symptoms. Meningitis due to cryptococcus is generally less aggressive clinically than meningitis caused by pyogenic bacteria. Headache is almost always present, but it may be mild. Fever is present in 50 to 80% of patients, but the temperature may not rise much above 101° F (38.3° C). Cranial nerve signs are common and may be subtle. Diplopia, pupillary abnormalities, blurred vision, mild hearing loss, facial paralysis, or abnormal taste sensation may be the only clues to an infection involving the central nervous system. Nuchal rigidity is present in up to 60% of patients, but is usually mild. Varying degrees of altered mental status, including confusion, disorientation, personality change, and, rarely, stupor or coma, may occur. Central localizing neurologic signs are not frequent, but abnormal deep tendon reflexes may be found.

The onset of cryptococcal meningitis is insidious, and symptoms may be present intermittently over several weeks to months. Cryptococci may cause lesions at other body sites, notably on the skin and in the lung. These lesions may occur in the absence of meningeal involvement, but their presence should prompt a search for cryptococcosis of the central nervous system.

Diagnosis. A lumbar puncture to obtain CSF is essential to establish the diagnosis of cryptococcal meningitis. The opening CSF pressure is mildly elevated (180 to 350 mm H_2O), and a lymphocytic pleocytosis is present. Usually, 10 to 500 lymphocytes/cu mm are present, but some patients may have up to 1000 cells/mm³. India ink smears of CSF may yield a presumptive diagnosis of cryptococcosis in about 50% of specimens, but this diagnosis must be confirmed by culture. CSF glucose levels are usually low, and protein concentrations are elevated.

Because any given milliliter of lumbar CSF may contain few organisms, a large volume of CSF (5 to 10 ml) should be obtained. Filtration through a millipore filter, which is then cultured, may increase the yield. Multiple samples may be necessary to confirm the presence of cryptococci. Culture media should not contain cycloheximide, which inhibits cryptococcal growth. The plates should be incubated at 30° C because these organisms grow more rapidly at this temperature than at 37° C. Sputum and urine cultures may yield *Cryptococcus neoformans*, but positive blood cultures, a poor prognostic sign, are rare.

Latex agglutination tests for the presence of cryptococcal polysaccharide antigen should be performed on CSF and serum, with a control test for rheumatoid factor. Antigen may be detected in up to 90% of CSF specimens, but this finding must be confirmed by positive culture. CSF anticryptococcal antibody is not diagnostic, although high titers may be associated with a good prognosis.

Treatment. The treatment of choice of cryptococcal meningitis is a combined regimen for 6 weeks with amphotericin B, 0.3 mg/kg/day intravenously over 6 hours or twice the dose every other day, in addition to flucytosine, 37.5 mg/kg orally every 6 hours. If renal function deteriorates with amphotericin B, the dose of flucytosine should be reduced. If flucytosine cannot be used or is discontinued because of bone marrow suppression, higher doses of amphotericin B must be given, 0.8 to 1.2 mg/kg/day intravenously once daily.

LISTERIA MONOCYTOGENES

Signs and Symptoms. In a patient with lymphoma, leukemia, multiple myeloma, or a solid tumor, or in a patient immunosuppressed by treatment for organ transplantation, collagen vascular disease, or other conditions, the onset of meningitis due to *Listeria monocytogenes* is abrupt and acute. High fever is usually present, and nuchal rigidity occurs in 80 to 90% of patients. Neurologic signs include drowsiness, confusion, stupor, coma, seizures, tremors, and dyskinetic movements.

Diagnosis. A lumbar puncture should be performed. It usually reveals a pleocytosis with 1,000 to 10,000 cells/mm^3 and a predominance of polymorphonuclear leukocytes (mean 60 to 70%). Some patients have a low CSF cell count. CSF glucose levels are often depressed, and CSF protein levels are elevated. Gram-stained CSF sediment reveals gram-positive rods in about one-third of patients. Cultures of CSF are often positive, and blood cultures should be drawn; they are positive in about 75% of cases.

Treatment. Ampicillin, 1 to 2 g every 4 hours intravenously, is probably the drug of choice, but high doses of penicillin, erythromycin, chloramphenicol, cephalothin, and tetracycline have been successful. Recent in vitro data and studies of experimental listerial meningitis in rabbits suggest that ampicillin and other broad-spectrum penicillins, in combination with aminoglycosides, are synergistic for these organisms and may prove to be the clinical regimen of choice.

TOXOPLASMA GONDII

Signs and Symptoms. This intracellular protozoan parasite actually produces a necrotizing meningoencephalitis in the immunocompromised host, often as a result of reactivation of latent infection. Fever and altered consciousness, headache, seizures, reflex abnormalities, and motor impairment may occur.

Diagnosis. The diagnosis is best made serologically, although trophozoites may be seen in biopsy specimens of the brain. Serologic documentation is by means of Sabin-Feldman dye, indirect hemagglutination antibody, complement-fixing antibody, and IgM fluorescent antibody tests. High titers of antibody may be formed even in immunodeficient persons, but it is difficult to distinguish active from chronic infection. It is useful to store serum prior to immunosuppressive therapy, to detect a change in CF or IgM fluorescent antibody if acute toxoplasmosis develops. Toxoplasmosis may coexist with other infections.

Treatment. The treatment of toxoplasmosis is with pyrimethamine, first with an oral loading dose of 100 to 200 mg in divided doses, followed by oral maintenance doses of 1 to 2 mg/kg to a maximum of 50 mg/kg/day, in combination with an oral sulfadiazine or triple sulfonamide mixture, 75 to 100 mg/kg/day in 4 divided doses following a loading dose of 50 to 75 mg/kg. The optimal duration of therapy has not been determined, but treatment should probably continue for at least 4 to 6 weeks. Folinic acid, up to 10 mg/day, may prevent the bone marrow suppression induced by pyrimethamine.

OTHER INFECTIONS

Tuberculous meningitis and histoplasma, coccidioidal, or candidal meningitis may also occur. Viral meningoencephalitis may be present alone or with other infections. These conditions are discussed elsewhere in this text.

> Objective 33–10. Describe the causes and possible therapy in a patient with stage IV-B Hodgkin's disease with pox-like skin lesions.

CAUSES OF INFECTION

Patients with lymphoma and leukemia, as well as other patients who receive immunosuppressive therapy, are subject to disseminated varicella-zoster or herpes simplex infection. Typically, zoster begins as pain in the distribution of a primary dermatome in the distribution of cervical, thoracic, or lumbar nerve roots. More rarely, a cranial nerve is involved. Vesicular lesions on an erythematous base form in clusters within the dermatome and progress to pustules that eventually become encrusted and heal, although some skin discoloration or hyperpigmentation and postherpetic neuralgia may remain. The lesions may disseminate in crops to all areas of the skin. Less commonly, visceral involvement of liver, spleen, lungs, and brain may occur.

Herpes simplex virus may cause a similar but less common picture with widespread vesicular lesions (Kaposi's varicelliform eruption). The diagnosis of either varicella-zoster or herpes simplex infection can be suggested by a Tzanck smear of scrapings from the base of an unroofed vesicle. Characteristic eosinophilic intranuclear inclusions and giant cells may be seen with Giemsa or Wright's stains. These findings are nonspecific for herpesviruses and are useful mainly in distinguishing these lesions from those of variola.

Culture of vesicles yields varicella-zoster virus for 7 to 10 days after the onset of the eruption in immunosuppressed patients. Serologic techniques, including the complement-fixation test, demonstrate a rise in antibody, but this method may require 3 to 4 weeks in severely immunodeficient patients.

TREATMENT

Vidarabine may decrease viral excretion and pain and is given in doses of 10 mg/kg/day infused intravenously over 12 hours for 5 days. Acyclovir (acycloguanisine) shows promise for treatment of these infections.

PREVENTION

Zoster immune globulin, convalescent serum from normal hosts recovering from zoster, is available to protect children at high risk, such as those with leukemia, under the age of 15 who have been exposed to active cases of chickenpox. It is effective in preventing or modifying this illness in recipients.

> Objective 33–11. Describe a reasonable approach to the prevention of opportunistic infections in the immunocompromised host.

The optimal approach to the prevention of infection in the compromised host has not been determined. Several investigators have suggested different programs, many of which are currently under intensive study.

GENERAL PREVENTIVE MEASURES

Most careful attention should be paid to general measures of hygiene and cleanliness, including vigorous handwashing when approaching any immunocompromised host. Patients undergoing prolonged episodes of neutropenia are usually placed in some form of isolation. A recent report failed to show any improvement in the incidence of infection by routine protective isolation, in the form of a single bedroom, a private toilet, and the wearing of mask, gown, and gloves when entering the patient's room.

LAMINAR AIR FLOW ISOLATION

The use of laminar air flow isolation, which removes particulate matter from the air by means of high-efficiency filters, reduces infections in neutropenic patients undergoing cancer and leukemia chemotherapy. Because of the expense of installing and maintaining these sterile air flow systems, their use is often limited to major cancer centers, and alternate forms of protection have been devised for use in other hospitals. The use of laminar air flow isolation rooms requires intensive nursing care, cooked or sterile food for the patient, and usually some method of oral antimicrobial decontamination.

CATHETER MAINTENANCE

Whether or not any isolation procedure is instituted, strict attention must be paid to maintaining intravenous needles and cannulas properly; the use of cannulas should be severely limited in these patients. Intensive care of indwelling urinary catheters is critical, but these catheters should be placed only when clearly indicated and should be removed as soon as possible. Respiratory access sites and respiratory therapy apparatus must be kept as clean as possible, and guidelines for their maintenance must be strict.

ORAL GUT DECONTAMINATION

The effectiveness of oral gut decontamination as a means of reducing bacterial infection in neutropenic patients has been thoroughly researched. Reduced infection rates have been demonstrated in controlled and uncontrolled studies of oral, nonabsorbable antibiotic combinations such as vancomycin, gentamicin, nystatin or neomycin B (framycetin), colistin and nystatin, and gentamicin and nystatin. Despite the efficacy of these regimens, they are distasteful, and compliance of the patient is far from optimal. The discontinuance of these nonabsorbable antibiotics during profound neutropenia is associated with rapid repopulation of the gut flora with gram-negative rods; these patients may then be even more susceptible to bacteremia due to these organisms. In one center, the incidence of infection with aminoglycoside-resistant gram-negative bacteria and fungi was increased in patients who discontinued oral antimicrobial agents while still neutropenic.

The combined use of laminar air flow with gut sterilization regimens has reduced infection in neutropenic patients hospitalized for long periods. Unfortunately, the outcome of the underlying disease is not improved by the use of laminar air flow rooms despite the longer remission achieved by reducing infection.

Alternatives to total gut decontamination have been introduced. Some have proposed partial decontamination of the gastrointestinal tract with the selective use of antibiotics that reduce the aerobic flora but leave the anaerobic flora intact. This method is based on the concept that colonization of the gastrointestinal tract with potentially pathogenic aerobic gram-negative rods requires higher inocula when the anaerobic flora are allowed to remain. Many fewer aerobic organisms can colonize the gut when decontamination procedures remove the anaerobic flora. Combinations of agents, such as trimethoprim-sulfamethoxazole with nalidixic acid, and some cephalosporins may remove the potential pathogens, but may leave intact the anaerobic flora, with its presumed resistant effect on bacterial colonization.

MISCELLANEOUS TECHNIQUES

The use of trimethoprim-sulfamethoxazole by itself to reduce infection in neutropenic patients has been suggested, and several studies are in progress to test its efficacy. Patients who are treated in laminar air flow units are also bathed with antiseptic solutions. Various orificial regimens with antibiotics and disinfectants have been recommended.

Although white blood cell transfusions may be effective in the treatment of severely neutropenic patients who are also bacteremic, preliminary studies of prophylactic white blood cell transfusions to prevent gram-negative rod and other bacteremias have not been encouraging.

Various attempts have been made to improve host defects in patients with cancer. Pneumococcal vaccine is useful in preventing infections due to the vaccine types of *Streptococcus pneumoniae*, but patients with Hodgkin's disease who are scheduled for splenectomy are best vaccinated prior to this procedure. Some data, obtained with a multivalent *Pseudomonas aeruginosa* vaccine, suggest that patients are able to mount a short-lived antibody response.

Passive immunization with antibodies to bacterial core glycolipids may minimize gram-negative bacteremia in neutropenic patients. Trimethoprim-sulfamethoxazole is effective in preventing infections due to *Pneumocystis carinii* in leukemic children.

SUGGESTED READINGS

General

Allen, J.C.: Infection and the Compromised Host. 2nd Ed. Baltimore, Williams & Wilkins, 1981.
Barrett, J.T.: Basic Immunology and Its Medical Application. 2nd Ed. St. Louis, C.V. Mosby, 1980.
Eisen, H.N.: Immunology: An Introduction to Molecular and Cellular Principles of the Immune Response. 2nd Ed. Hagerstown, MD, Harper & Row, 1980.
Rubin, R.H., and Young, L.S.: Clinical Approach to Infection in the Compromised Host. New York, Plenum Publishing, 1981.
Stiehm, E.R., and Fulginiti, V.A.: Immunologic Disorders in Infants and Children. Philadelphia, W.B. Saunders, 1980.

Laboratory Testing and Immune Defects

Alper, J.C., et al.: Increased susceptibility to infection associated with abnormalities of complement-mediated function and of the third component of complement C3. N. Engl. J. Med., 282:349, 1970.
Ammann, H.J., and Wara, D.W.: Evaluation of infants and children with recurrent infection. Curr. Prob. Pediatr., 4:1, 1975.
Baehner, R.L., and Nathan, D.G.: Quantitative nitroblue tetrazolium test in chronic granulomatous disease. N. Engl. J. Med., 278:971, 1968.
Blume, R.S., Bennett, J.M., Yankee, R.A., and Wolff, S.M.: Defective granulocyte regulation in the Chediak-Higashi syndrome. N. Engl. J. Med., 279:1009, 1968.
Cooper, M.R., et al.: Complete deficiency of leukocyte glucose-6-phosphate dehydrogenase with defective bactericidal activity. J. Clin. Invest., 51:769, 1972.
Fudenberg, H.H., et al.: Primary immunodeficiencies. Report of a World Health Organization committee. Pediatrics, 47:927, 1971.
Hill, H.R.: Laboratory aspects of immune deficiency in children. Pediatr. Clin. North Am., 27:805, 1980.
Hitzig, W.H., and Grob, P.J.: Therapeutic uses of transfer factor. Prog. Clin. Immunol., 2:69, 1976.
Johnston, R.B., Jr., and Stroud, R.M.: Complement and host defense against infection. J. Pediatr., 90:169, 1977.
Miller, M.E.: Pathology of chemotaxis and random mobility. Semin. Hematol., 12:59, 1975.
Schur, P.H., et al.: Gamma-G-globulin deficiencies in patients with recurrent pyogenic infections. N. Engl. J. Med., 283:631, 1970.
Stiehm, E.R., and Fudenbergh, H.H.: Serum levels of immune globulins in health and disease. A survey. Pediatrics, 37:715, 1966.
Stossel, T.P.: Phagocytosis. N. Engl. J. Med., 290:717, 774, 833, 1974.

Infection in Neutropenic Patients

Anderson, E.T., Young, L.S., and Hewitt, W.L.: Antimicrobial synergism in the therapy of gram-negative bacteremia. Chemotherapy, 24:45, 1978.
Bodey, G.P., Buckley, M., Sathe, Y.S., and Freireich, E.J.: Quantitative relationships between circulating leukocytes and infection in patients with acute leukemia. Ann. Intern. Med., 64:328, 1966.
EORTC Antimicrobial Therapy Project Group: Three antibiotic regimens in the treatment of infection in febrile granulocytopenic patients with cancer. J. Infect. Dis., 137:14, 1978.
Hughes, W.T.: Fatal infections in childhood leukemia. Am. J. Dis. Child., 122:283, 1971.
Klastersky, J.: Combinations of antibiotics for therapy of severe infections in cancer patients. Eur. J. Cancer, 15(Suppl.):3, 1979.
Klastersky, J.: Granulocyte transfusions as a therapy and a prophylaxis of infections in neutropenic patients. Eur. J. Cancer, 15(Suppl.):15, 1979.
Klastersky, J., Cappel, R., and Daneau, D.: Clinical significance of in vitro synergism between antibiotics in gram-negative infections. Antimicrob. Agents Chemother., 2:470, 1972.
Klastersky, J., Meunier-Carpentier, F., and Prevost, J.M.: Significance of antimicrobial synergism for the outcome of gram-negative sepsis. Am. J. Med. Sci., 273:157, 1977.

Levine, A.S., Schimpff, S.C., Graw, R.G., Jr., and Young, R.C.: Hematologic malignancies and other marrow failure states: progress in the management of complicating infections. Semin. Hematol., 11:141, 1974.

Love, L.J., Schimpff, S.C., Schiffer, C.A., and Wiernik, P.H.: Improved prognosis for granulocytopenic patients with gram-negative bacteremia. Am. J. Med., 68:643, 1980.

Pizzo, P.A., Robichaud, K.J., Gill, F.A., and Witebsky, F.G.: Empiric antibiotic and antifungal therapy for cancer patients with prolonged fever and granulocytopenia. Am. J. Med., 72:101, 1982.

Pizzo, P.A., et al.: Duration of empiric antibiotic therapy in granulocytopenic patients with cancer. Am. J. Med., 67:194, 1979.

Quie, P.G.: Infections due to neutrophil malfunction. Medicine, 52:411, 1973.

Schimpff, S.C., Satterlee, W., Young, V.M., and Serpick, A.: Empiric therapy with carbenicillin and gentamicin for febrile patients with cancer and granulocytopenia. N. Engl. J. Med., 284:1061, 1971.

Schimpff, S.C., et al.: Origins of infection in acute nonlymphocytic leukemia. Significance of hospital acquisition of potential pathogens. Ann. Intern. Med., 77:707, 1972.

Sen, P., et al.: Superinfection: another look. Am. J. Med., 73:706, 1982.

Specific Infections

Bennett, J.E., et al.: A comparison of amphotericin B alone and combined with flucytosine in the treatment of cryptococcal meningitis. N. Engl. J. Med., 301:126, 1979.

Bishop, J.F., Schimpff, S.C., Diggs, C.H., and Wiernik, P.H.: Infections during intensive chemotherapy for non-Hodgkin's lymphoma. Ann. Intern. Med., 95:555, 1981.

Fisher, B.D., Armstrong, D., Yu, B., and Gold, J.W.M.: Invasive aspergillosis. Progress in early diagnosis and treatment. Am. J. Med., 71:571, 1981.

Hughes, W.T., et al.: Successful chemoprophylaxis for *Pneumocystis carinii* pneumonitis. N. Engl. J. Med., 297:1419, 1977.

Kaplan, M.H., Rosen, P.P., and Armstrong, D.: Cryptococcosis in a cancer hospital: clinical and pathologic correlates in 46 patients. Cancer, 39:2265, 1977.

Medoff, G., and Kobayashi, G.S.: Strategies in the treatment of systemic fungal infections. N. Engl. J. Med., 302:145, 1980.

Medoff, G., Kunz, L.J., and Weinberg, A.N.: Listeriosis in humans: an evaluation. J. Infect. Dis., 123:247, 1971.

Meltzer, R.S., et al.: Antemortem diagnosis of central nervous system strongyloidiasis. Am. J. Med. Sci., 277:91, 1979.

Meyer, R.D., Rosen, P., and Armstrong, D.: Phycomycosis complicating leukemia and lymphoma. Ann. Intern. Med., 77:871, 1972.

Meyer, R.D., et al.: Aspergillosis complicating neoplastic disease. Am. J. Med., 54:6, 1973.

Ruskin, J., and Remington, J.S.: Toxoplasmosis in the compromised host. Ann. Intern. Med., 84:193, 1976.

Schimpff, S., et al.: Varicella-zoster infection in patients with cancer. Ann. Intern. Med., 76:241, 1972.

Walzer, P.D., et al.: *Pneumocystis carinii* pneumonia in the United States. Epidemiologic, diagnostic and clinical features. Ann. Intern. Med., 80:83, 1974.

Young, D.S., Armstrong, D., Blevins, A., and Lieberman, P.: Nocardia asteroides infection complicating neoplastic disease. Am. J. Med., 50:356, 1971.

Prevention of Infection

Dekker, A.W., Rozenberg-Arska, M., Sixma, J.J., and Verhef, J.: Prevention of infection with trimethoprim-sulfamethoxazole plus amphotericin B in patients with acute nonlymphocytic leukemia. Ann. Intern. Med., 95:555, 1981.

Gurwith, M.J., et al.: A prospective controlled investigation of prophylactic trimethoprim/sulfamethoxazole in hospitalized granulocytopenic patients. Am. J. Med., 66:248, 1979.

Levine, A.S., et al.: Protected environments and prophylactic antibiotics. A prospective controlled study of their utility in the therapy of acute leukemia. N. Engl. J. Med., 288:477, 1973.

Schimpff, S.C.: Infection prevention during granulocytopenia. *In* Current Clinical Topics in Infectious Diseases—1980. Edited by J.S. Remington and M.N. Swartz. New York, McGraw-Hill, 1980.

Schimpff, S.C.: Infection prevention during profound granulocytopenia. New approaches to alimentary canal microbial suppression. Ann. Intern. Med., 93:358, 1980.

Wade, J.C., et al.: A comparison of trimethoprim-sulfamethoxazole plus nystatin with gentamicin in the prevention of infections in acute leukemia. N. Engl. J. Med., 304:1057, 1981.

Wilson, J.M., and Guiney, D.G.: Failure of oral trimethoprim-sulfamethoxazole prophylaxis in acute leukemia. N. Engl. J. Med., 306:16, 1982.

CHAPTER 34

Nosocomial Infections

J.E. McGowan, Jr., and J.A. Acar

Objective 34–1. Recognize a nosocomial infection and evaluate risk of its occurrence in specific patients.

DEFINITION AND INCIDENCE

Some patients develop an infection during the course of their hospitalization. When an infection is not likely to have been acquired before, or incubating during, the time of hospital admission, it is classified as hospital-associated or nosocomial. The term does not identify a site of infection in the patient. Instead, it identifies the hospital as the geographic location in which the individual is thought to have developed the infection. Note that the definition does not require that the infectious agent itself be acquired within the hospital. The word nosocomial is derived from the Greek and means "within the house." Infections of this type are sometimes referred to as "cross-infections."

Recent studies in the United States show that 3.5% of hospitalized patients develop nosocomial infections. These infections have considerable consequences both for patients and for the community.

Nosocomial infection is most likely to develop in the urinary tract, and bacteriuria accounts for about 40% of all hospital infections (Table 34–1). Infection is also frequent in surgical wounds and in the lower respiratory tract. The most costly infections to treat are lower respiratory tract infections and septicemias; the latter have the highest case-to-fatality ratio.

RISK FACTORS

As for most other infectious diseases, the occurrence of nosocomial infection depends upon the interaction of two factors: (1) the virulence and spread of the infecting microorganism; and (2) the potential victim, whether patient or hospital employee. Patients with compromised host defenses are at high risk of nosocomial infection. The impaired defenses may be physical, as in burns or traumatic wounds, chemical, as in pernicious anemia or gastrectomy, which can impair production of gastric acid and remove this defense mechanism, or immunologic, as in Hodgkin's disease or cancer chemotherapy.

In addition to the patient and the organism, the major determinant of nosocomial infection is the hospital environment in which organism and host interact. Included are the procedures, prescriptions, and other medical regimens employed during the patient's hospital stay. These factors also are partly responsible for determining which patients are most likely to become infected and which organisms are likely to cause the infection. Pa-

> **CONSEQUENCES OF NOSOCOMIAL (HOSPITAL) INFECTION**
>
> Nosocomial (hospital) infection can produce severe illness and even death. Studies in the United States suggest that approximately 3.5% of hospitalized patients develop such infections, and about 1 in 1000 hospitalized patients die of such an illness. These reported figures probably underestimate the incidence because they do not include infections that occur after discharge from the hospital. In addition, these infections can have major consequences for the hospital, the community, and hospital workers. The economic cost of caring for patients who develop nosocomial infections is considerable, as is the lost productivity of patients who require an additional hospital stay. The occurrence of such infections may have legal consequences in some countries. The organisms responsible for nosocomial infections are often more resistant to antimicrobial agents than those encountered in infections outside the hospital. When patients infected with these organisms during hospitalization return home, the resistant organisms may persist in their endogenous flora and may be disseminated in the community. Hospital workers, as well as hospital patients, are susceptible to a number of microorganisms encountered in the hospital. Some organisms are more likely to cause symptomatic illness in employees than in patients; for example, hepatitis B virus in hemodialysis unit personnel often causes illness, whereas infected patients in the same area usually remain asymptomatic.

tients at higher risk of acquiring these infections are those receiving immunosuppressive therapy, such as with corticosteroids, and those who must undergo numerous diagnostic and therapeutic procedures. The escalation in invasive diagnostic procedures and devices, such as catheters for blood pressure monitoring, has increased the likelihood of nosocomial infection.

Patients especially predisposed to nosocomial infection are likely to be located in specific hospital areas. For this reason, the following hospital departments are high-risk areas: the intensive care and burn units, the newborn nursery, and the oncology service. In addition, procedures that increase risk of infection are often performed in designated locations; examples are the hemodialysis area, where infection with hepatitis B virus may occur, the operating room, and the delivery suite, where fetal monitoring is frequently employed. The risk of nosocomial infection to hospital employees is also increased in the clinical laboratory, where large volumes of blood must be handled, blood that may be positive for hepatitis viruses or other infecting agents, and in medical wards where large numbers of patients with contagious diseases, such as tuberculosis and whooping cough, are treated.

NOSOCOMIAL PATHOGENS

Nosocomial infection occurs most often in patients who have impaired resistance to microorganisms. Thus, although patients with normal host defenses against infection can become infected during hospitalization, nosocomial infection is more often due to organisms that present little threat to the normal host. The bacteria that frequently cause nosocomial infection (Table 34–2) include both

Table 34–1. Occurrence of Nosocomial Infection* by Site and Hospital Service

Hospital Service	Urinary Tract	Surgical Wounds	Lower Respiratory Tract	Blood	Other	TOTAL
Medicine	1.9	0.1	0.8	0.2	0.6	3.6
Surgery	1.9	1.6	0.8	0.2	0.3	3.8
Gynecology	1.6	1.1	0.1	0.1	0.1	3.0
Obstetrics	0.5	0.9	—	—	0.6	2.0
Pediatrics	0.2	0.1	0.2	0.1	0.5	1.1
Neonatology	0.1	0.1	0.2	0.1	1.0	1.5
All Patients (average)	1.3	0.7	0.4	0.1	0.5	2.1

*Expressed as the number of infections per 100 patients discharged from 1975 to 1978. (Data from 80 hospitals throughout the United States participating in the National Nosocomial Infections Study, Centers for Disease Control, United States Public Health Service.)

Table 34–2. Major Bacterial Pathogens of Nosocomial Infection by Relative Frequency of Occurrence, Sites Usually Affected, Usual Hospital Reservoir, and Major Routes of Transmission to the Patient

Organism	Relative Occurrence*	Sites Affected	Hospital Reservoirs	Transmission Routes
Escherichia coli	19.2%	Urinary tract and blood	Gastrointestinal tract of patients and staff	Touch contact and urine catheters
Staphylococcus aureus	10.2%	Surgical wounds, skin, and blood	Skin and nares of patients and personnel	Touch contact, air, intravenous catheters
Enterococcus and other group D streptococci	9.5%	Urine and surgical wounds	Gastrointestinal tract of patients and staff	Touch contact and urine catheters
Pseudomonas aeruginosa	9.0%	Urine, burns, respiratory tract, and blood	Liquids (respiratory therapy equipment, handwashing lotion) and moist areas of the body and the environment	Touch contact and contaminated liquids
Proteus	7.7%	Urine, respiratory tract, surgical wounds, and blood	Gastrointestinal tract of patients and staff; environmental objects	Touch contact and contaminated liquids
Klebsiella	7.7%			
Enterobacter	4.3%			
Serratia	2.0%			

*Relative frequency of all organisms isolated from nosocomial infection. (Data from the National Nosocomial Infections Study, Centers for Disease Control, United States Public Health Service, 1975 to 1978.)

Table 34–3. Natural Resistance in Bacterial Species and Antibiotics that may Act as Selectors

Bacterial Species	Antibiotics
Klebsiella	Ampicillin and carbenicillin
Enterobacter	Ampicillin and cephalothin
Serratia	Ampicillin, cephalothin, and colistin
Pseudomonas aeruginosa	Ampicillin, cephalothin, trimethoprim, and nalidixic acid
Proteus morganii	Ampicillin, cephalothin, and colistin
Proteus inconstans	Ampicillin, cephalothin, gentamicin, and colistin
Enterococci	Cephalosporins and low-level resistance to all aminoglycosides

microbial agents, such as streptococci and staphylococci, that can readily infect persons with intact host defenses and agents such as klebsiella and proteus, which are often present in normal bowel flora or other endogenous sites and become pathogenic only when host resistance is impaired. Many of these organisms owe their prominence in nosocomial infection to their ability to persist on materials and equipment used in the hospital or to their transmittal by hospital personnel or equipment from one patient to another. Thus, organisms found in the hospital environment vary from those present in the community. In part, this difference results from the extensive use of antimicrobial agents in certain areas of a hospital. Such usage permits organisms resistant to the antimicrobial drugs to survive and eliminates organisms that are susceptible (Table 34–3). Specific nosocomial pathogens vary from hospital to hospital, and from time to time in the same hospital. Today, the most frequent of these nosocomial pathogens are gram-negative aerobic bacilli, staphylococci, and fungi.

Staphylococcus aureus, a gram-positive coccus and the major pathogen of hospital infection throughout the 1950s and early 1960s, still causes a number of infections in hospitals today (see Table 34–2). Infections with this organism most frequently involve surgical wounds, burns, and intravenous catheters. The organism persists in hospitals today because of its widespread presence in the skin, the hair, and the nasopharynx of patients and employees, as well as on the hands of personnel and on instruments, chairs, tubs, and other objects in hospitals. The staphylococcus joins the pneumococcus and many of the streptococci as bacteria that cause infection in patients with intact host defenses.

In contrast, illness due to gram-negative aerobic bacilli, such as *Escherichia coli* and klebsiella, most frequently occurs in patients with compromised host defenses. The importance of host defenses is shown by the increasing frequency of infections caused by these organisms, which are now the most common nosocomial pathogens. This group includes the usual aerobic organisms of the bowel, the Enterobacteriaceae or gut bacteria. Some of the organisms in the group, such as klebsiella, enterobacter, and serratia, have a unique ability to survive and thrive in the fluids commonly used for intravenous therapy, such as 5% dextrose in water and normal saline solution. During the past decade, we have also come to appreciate the pathogenicity of anaerobic organisms that inhabit the normal bowel, such as *Bacteroides fragilis*.

Distinct from the Enterobacteriaceae is another group of organisms that withstand most antimicrobial agents, either through natural resistance to penetration of their cell wall by the drug or by their ability to inactivate the drug itself (Table 34–4). Members of this group include pseudomonas, acinetobacter, and flavobacterium. The importance of these organisms as causes of nosocomial infection has increased in the past decade.

In recent years, nonbacterial organisms have become more important causes of hospital infection. These organisms include fungi, such as *Candida albicans*, aspergillus, and torulopsis; protozoan parasites, such as toxoplasma; viruses, such as cytomegalovirus, varicella-zoster virus, and rotaviruses; and other parasites and organisms not clearly classified, such as *Pneumocystis carinii*.

> **Objective 34–2.** Describe the individual measures that reduce the risk of nosocomial infection.

Some patients have such severely impaired host defenses that it is difficult to prevent or to minimize the occurrence of infection in them. Some infections clearly can be prevented, however, by steps that all physicians and hospital workers should follow. The infections primarily susceptible to control are those that occur as a result of an invasive diagnostic or therapeutic procedure, and those caused by organisms whose proliferation is controllable. Infections due to these factors often involve patients whose host defenses are intact. Thus, it is particularly important to minimize the risk of infection related to a procedure, to environmental factors, and to exposure to an organism whose spread can be contained by isolation precautions.

Nosocomial infection spreads within the hospital in a number of ways, most commonly by transmission on the hands of hospital personnel. The machinery and equipment used

Table 34–4. Acquired Resistance to Antibiotics

Mechanism of Resistance	Mutation	R. Plasmid
Alteration of target site for drug	Streptomycin (30 S ribosome) Rifampicin (RNA polymerase)	Macrolides
Impermeability of cell to antimicrobial agent (transport-defective)	Aminoglycosides Sulfonamides	Tetracycline
Detoxification and inactivation of drug	Beta-lactam compounds (overproduction of cephalosporinase)	Penicillins (beta-lactamases) Aminoglycosides (enzymes) Chloramphenicol (acetyl transferase)
Cellular bypass of blocked reaction	Trimethoprim (thymine-less bacteria)	Trimethoprim Sulfonamides

> **PSEUDOMONAS**
>
> *Pseudomonas aeruginosa* is a gram-negative aerobic bacillus that belongs to the subgroup called "nonfermenters" because they do not ferment certain sugars commonly used for testing. This bacterium characteristically produces a blue-green pigment and often can be recognized by its grape-like odor when grown on routine culture media.
>
> Pseudomonas is a frequent pathogen in nosocomial infection, in large measure because it is naturally resistant to many antimicrobial agents. Thus, in hospitals, where antibiotics are administered frequently, pseudomonas organisms have a selective advantage that allows them to overgrow other normal inhabitants of the bowel. In addition, the organism survives well in liquids, such as nebulizer wells of respiratory therapy equipment and handwashing lotions, as well as in moist areas of the human body and the environment. As a result, pseudomonas is often able to grow in areas of hospitals unsuitable for other bacteria.
>
> Pseudomonas infection is especially prominent in patients who have impaired host defenses. The predisposing defect may be physical, as in patients with burns, physiologic, as in patients with cystic fibrosis, or hematologic, as in granulocytopenic patients, those with leukemia and other hematologic malignant diseases, or those receiving immunosuppressive drugs.
>
> Other pseudomonas species beside *Pseudomonas aeruginosa* have become more important causes of nosocomial infection in the past decade. *P. cepacia* and *P. maltophilia* have been incriminated in a number of outbreaks of nosocomial infection. Because these bacteria are also frequently resistant to many commonly employed antimicrobial agents, it is difficult to manage patients with these infections.

in the hospital may also be vectors, but it is much less common today for infection to spread from walls, floors, or other environmental surfaces. Most important vehicles of infection are amenable to measures that can decrease the likelihood of spread.

ASEPTIC TECHNIQUE AND HYGIENE

The most likely mechanism of spread of nosocomial infection is from patient to patient by the hands of hospital personnel. Proper attention to handwashing can minimize the spread of virulent microorganisms by this route. This infection control procedure, probably the most important, may have the greatest impact on infection rates of any control procedure yet devised.

Once microorganisms have been removed from an object or an area, certain procedures can minimize the likelihood of the reintroduction of these potential pathogens. Taken as a whole, these procedures are known as aseptic technique and are the mainstay of surgery and many other hospital procedures.

STERILIZATION AND DISINFECTION TECHNIQUES

Microorganisms can be removed from objects in the hospital environment, to varying degrees, by different techniques. When an item is processed in a way that kills all microorganisms, including bacterial spores, it is defined as "sterile." Sterility can be achieved by a variety of techniques; exposure to steam in an autoclave, exposure to ethylene oxide gas, or immersion in glutaraldehyde solution are the procedures employed most frequently. Some objects need not be sterile and require a less-complete removal of microorganisms. For this purpose, disinfectant solutions, antiseptics, or other cleansing solutions can be used.

ISOLATION PRECAUTIONS

When the mode by which an organism is spread in the hospital is known, one can devise ways to eliminate or reduce the microbe's transmission. These precautions, known as isolation techniques, are necessary for approximately 2% of patients admitted to general hospitals at any given time. In most hospitals today, categoric isolation is employed. In this system, diseases are classified as to their likely mode of spread. For all agents likely to spread by the same route(s), a common group of isolation procedures is defined (Table 34–5). Thus, in a categoric isolation system, the procedure to control tuberculosis, which is spread by airborne transmission of droplet nuclei from the respiratory tract of a patient, varies from that used to isolate a patient infected with hepatitis A virus, which is spread from person to person by a fecal-oral route. The advantages of such a system are the ease of implementing a limited number of procedures and the effective use of

Table 34-5. Categories of Isolation Precautions and Selected Features of Procedures

Category	Purpose	Indication (Disease)	Private room	Masks, gowns, gloves	Handwashing
Strict isolation	To contain contagious disease spread by contact and by airborne transmission	Plague, smallpox, rabies, Ebola or Lassa arboviral infections, Marburg viral infection, congenital rubella	Essential, with negative-pressure ventilation	Required	After contact with patient
Respiratory isolation	To contain diseases spread by airborne transmission (droplets or droplet nuclei coughed, sneezed, or breathed into environment)	Measles, meningococcal disease, pulmonary tuberculosis, pertussis, rubella	Essential, with negative-pressure ventilation	Masks required, but not gowns or gloves	After contact with patient
Wound and skin precautions	To control diseases spread by direct contact of hands or instruments with wounds, skin lesions, or heavily contaminated articles	Burns, staphylococcal or streptococcal skin infections, extensive surgical infection, skin involved by herpes zoster	Helpful, but not essential	Masks not required, but gowns and gloves worn when handling contaminated area	After contact with patient
Enteric precautions	To control diseases spread in feces	Salmonellosis, shigellosis, campylobacter infection, cholera, poliomyelitis, hepatitis A, other diarrheal diseases of suspected infectious origin	Helpful, but not essential	Masks not required, but gowns and gloves worn when handling feces or fecally contaminated objects	After contact with patient
Secretion precautions	To control diseases spread by direct contact with contaminated secretions, body fluids, or articles contaminated by these fluids	Minor burns, syphilis, gonorrhea, selected fungal and viral diseases, acute upper respiratory disease	Not required	Masks and gowns not required, but gloves worn when handling secretions	After contact with patient
Protective isolation	To protect uninfected persons with severely impaired resistance to infection from potential pathogens	Agranulocytosis, severe neutropenia, lymphoma, leukemia	Preferred	Not required	Before contact with patient

hospital facilities. The disadvantage is that not all communicable diseases fit easily into a few categories of isolation precautions. Individual sets of isolation guidelines usually specify the following: the advisability of a private room; the necessity of hospital personnel to wear gowns, masks, and gloves when near the patient; the frequency and timing of handwashing; and the care of articles brought into and taken out of the patient's room. One must remember to discontinue isolation precautions when the patient's contagious period has ended; the extra effort required to interact with a patient in isolation interferes with care.

HOSPITAL PROCEDURES

Hospital procedures often bypass the patient's normal barriers to infection and thus predispose him to infection. Many preventable nosocomial infections involve invasive medical devices. Foremost among these infections are those due to urinary catheters, intravenous or other intravascular catheters, surgical manipulations, and respiratory therapy equipment.

Care of Urinary Catheters. About 40% of nosocomial infections occur in the urinary tract, and approximately 75% of these cases of bacteriuria occur in patients who have undergone instrumentation of the urinary tract. Up to 16% of patients in general hospitals are given indwelling urinary catheters during hospitalization. Therefore, many hospitalized patients are at risk of developing nosocomial bacteriuria. Studies show that the daily risk of developing this complication is approximately 5% for each day that the catheter remains in place. Because bladder bacteriuria is the most frequent predisposing factor in gram-negative bacteremia, serious consequences can attend this usually benign nosocomial infection.

To prevent catheter-associated urinary tract infections, the following guidelines are particularly important: (1) use a bladder catheter only when absolutely necessary; consider alternatives such as intermittent catheterization or condom catheters; (2) remove urinary catheters as soon as possible; (3) allow only well-trained hospital personnel to insert catheters, and insist on adequate cleaning of the urethral meatus with an antiseptic agent, the wearing of gloves during the procedure, and immobilization of the catheter to prevent friction on the urethra; (4) be sure that the catheter is connected to a sterile, closed collection system in which urine is not exposed to the hospital environment from the time it leaves the patient's bladder until it is emptied from a collection bag at the end of the system; the collection system must be maintained so that gravity directs the flow of urine away from the bladder; this means keeping the level of the collection bag below that of the bladder; (5) obtain specimens needed from the collection system by needle aspiration rather than by disassembling the system; (6) irrigate urinary catheter drainage systems with fluids only when indicated by clot formation or other obstruction; if frequent irrigation becomes necessary, use a triple-lumen catheter to permit irrigation without frequent opening and closing of the system; and (7) note that systemic antimicrobial agents, as "prophylaxis" against bacteriuria while a urinary catheter is in place, are ineffective, except in patients whose catheter is in place for short periods (1 or 2 days).

Care of Intravenous and Other Intravascular Catheters. Bacteremia accounts for about 5% of all nosocomial infections, but the associated case-to-fatality ratio is much higher than for most other infections of this type (between 30 and 40% in recent series). About 80% of these infections are produced by seeding of the blood from infection at some other site; many of the remaining cases are due to infection of intravenous catheters and other intrasvascular devices. These infections can arise from contamination of intravenous and arterial catheters, infusion solutions, transducers in monitoring systems, cardiopulmonary bypass machinery, and dialysis equipment. Although the rate of sepsis associated with intravenous catheters is under 1%, the use of this equipment in up to 40% of hospitalized patients, or about 16 million persons per year in the United States, makes possible a large number of such infections.

Nosocomial infections from contaminated catheters can be minimized by attention to the following: (1) restriction of the use of intravascular therapy to patients who absolutely require such treatment and the discontinuance of this therapy as soon as possible; (2) use of small-bore plastic catheters and steel needles whenever possible because infection rates are lower with this equipment; (3) replacement of intravenous cannulas at least every 48 to 72 hours; (4) careful attention to hygiene during any manipulation of the catheter system; included are a thorough cleaning of the skin site with an antiseptic at the time of catheter insertion, secure anchoring of the catheter to the skin, and covering of the cath-

Table 34–6. Methods to Strengthen Host Defenses of Patients and Hospital Personnel Against Nosocomial Infection

IMMUNIZATION
    Cytomegalovirus (patients—experimental)
    Diphtheria-tetanus (patients and personnel)
    Hepatitis B (patients and personnel)
    Influenza (patients and personnel)
    Measles (patients and personnel)
    Meningococcus (patients—experimental)
    Mumps (patients and personnel)
    Pseudomonas (patients—experimental)
    Rubella (patients and personnel)
    Shigella (patients—experimental)
    Varicella-zoster (patients—experimental)

ADMINISTRATION OF PREPARATIONS CONTAINING ANTIBODIES
    Hepatitis B immune globulin (patients and personnel)
    Immune serum globulin, which contains different antibodies in varying concentrations according to pool of donors (patients and personnel)
    Measles immune globulin (patients)
    Varicella-zoster immune globulin (patients)

ADMINISTRATION OF WHITE BLOOD CELLS (patients—experimental)

ADMINISTRATION OF ANTIMICROBIAL AGENTS TO PREVENT OR ELIMINATE COLONIZATION WITH SPECIFIC PATHOGENS
    Erythromycin: pertussis (patients and personnel)
    Mafenide and other antimicrobial ointments (burn patients)
    Penicillin: group A streptococcus (burn patients)
    Rifampin: *Haemophilus influenzae* (patients)
    Rifampin: meningococcus (patients and personnel)
    Trimethoprim-sulfamethoxazole: *Pneumocystis carinii* (patients)

WHAT IS AN EPIDEMIC?

Hospital personnel can establish the usual or baseline frequency of hospital infection by measuring either the incidence or the prevalence of occurrence. Determining how frequently nosocomial infection occurs in patients during a given time interval measures the incidence of nosocomial infection. Determining how many patients hospitalized at any one time are afflicted with such infections measures the prevalence. An epidemic or outbreak of nosocomial infection is defined as the occurrence of more than the usual number of cases. Thus, in an area where a disease is rare, a single case may be considered an epidemic. By contrast, the occurrence in 1 week of 276 cases of a disease usually encountered 200 to 300 times per week does not represent an outbreak.

For each of these measurements, then, it is necessary to know not only how many cases of infection occur, but also how many individuals are at risk of developing the infection. For example, the number of patients at risk of surgical wound infection is the subgroup that have had operations, and not the entire hospital population. A ratio in which the number of cases is the numerator and the number of persons at risk is the denominator is known as the attack rate of nosocomial infection and is the standard unit of reference in hospital epidemiology.

The epidemiologic criteria to trace a microorganism include the following: biotyping (all species), phage typing (*Staphylococcus aureus, Pseudomonas aeruginosa,* and salmonella), bacteriocin typing (*Pseudomonas aeruginosa*), serotyping (klebsiella, *Escherichia coli,* salmonella, shigella, streptococci, pneumococci, and haemophilus), and antibiotic resistance pattern (all species). In the last case, the natural resistance that involves all strains within a given species (see Table 34–3) is to be distinguished from acquired resistance, in which a single strain is affected. Acquired resistance can be chromosomally or plasmid-mediated (Tables 34–4 and 34–7).

---

eter site with a dry, sterile dressing; and (5) inspection of the catheter site every 24 hours, with immediate removal of the catheter if evidence of inflammation is found at the site and culture of the tip of the removed catheter.

Because the risk of sepsis in association with arterial catheters, central venous lines, and blood pressure monitors is even greater than that for "routine" intravenous therapy, special protocols have been developed that detail specific procedures and steps for care of these systems.

Handling of Respiratory Therapy Equipment and Suctioning. Nosocomial pneumonia is less frequent than hospital-associated bac-

Table 34-7. Frequency of Plasmid-mediated Bacterial Resistance

Antibiotics	Species	Frequency
Penicillin	*Staphylococcus aureus*	Extremely high
Ampicillin and carbenicillin	Salmonella, shigella, *Escherichia coli*, enterobacter, *Pseudomonas aeruginosa*, *Staphylococcus aureus*, proteus, haemophilus, gonococci	Extremely high
Cephalosporins	Partially inactivated by some transferable beta-lactamases	—
Tetracycline	*Escherichia coli*, klebsiella, serratia, enterobacter, *Proteus morganii*, *Pseudomonas aeruginosa*, *Staphylococcus aureus*, enterococci, *Listeria monocytogenes*, haemophilus	Extremely high
Chloramphenicol	*Escherichia coli*, klebsiella, serratia, enterobacter, *Proteus morganii*, *Pseudomonas aeruginosa*, *Staphylococcus aureus*, salmonella, groups A, B, and D streptococci	High
Kanamycin	*Escherichia coli*, klebsiella, serratia, enterobacter, proteus, *Pseudomonas aeruginosa*, *Staphylococcus aureus*, enterococci, haemophilus	High
Gentamicin	*Escherichia coli*, klebsiella, serratia, enterobacter, proteus, *Pseudomonas aeruginosa*, *Staphylococcus aureus*, enterococci	Moderate
Tobramycin	*Escherichia coli*, klebsiella, serratia, enterobacter, proteus, *Pseudomonas aeruginosa*, *Staphylococcus aureus*	Moderate
Amikacin	*Escherichia coli*, enterobacter, *Pseudomonas aeruginosa*, klebsiella, serratia	Low
Trimethoprim	Proteus, salmonella, shigella, *Vibrio cholerae*, *Escherichia coli*, klebsiella, serratia, enterobacter	Moderate
Sulfonamides	*Escherichia coli*, klebsiella, serratia, enterobacter, shigella, salmonella, proteus	High

teriuria or surgical wound infection. It remains a major problem, however, because the incidence has remained constant over the past decade, and the case-to-fatality ratio approaches 40% in many series of cases. Gram-negative aerobic bacilli are the most common pathogens, but *Staphylococcus aureus* is also encountered. In patients with compromised host defenses, less-virulent pathogens such as candida, pneumocystis, legionella, and cytomegalovirus are frequently involved.

Many cases of nosocomial pneumonia result from aspiration of oropharyngeal organisms into the lungs. Thus, efforts are directed at minimizing colonization of the oropharynx with other than endogenous flora, which pulmonary defenses handle well. Colonization of the oropharynx with potential pathogens, especially gram-negative aerobic bacilli, occurs infrequently in healthy persons, but these organisms often colonize the respiratory tree in persons with systemic illness. Procedures that predispose patients to bacterial colonization include improper decontamination of respiratory therapy equipment and faulty suctioning technique. Respiratory therapy equipment implicated in nosocomial pneumonia includes nebulizers, anesthesia apparatus, intermittent positive-pressure respirators, and humidifiers. During the past decade, procedures for proper cleaning of these implements have been developed, and the risk of infection from this equipment seems to be decreasing. One must still follow strict aseptic technique for suctioning secretions (new gloves, new catheter, and uncontaminated irrigant fluids for each episode) and for care of tracheostomies (gloves and new equipment for each episode), however. In addition, one must prevent aspiration episodes by proper positioning of patients, that is, by not placing them on their backs, and by not attempting to feed patients whose gag reflex is depressed.

ATTEMPTS TO STRENGTHEN HOST DEFENSES

Many hospital infections occur in patients whose resistance to infection is impaired. In recent years, a number of attempts have been made to restore normal defense mechanisms. These procedures include immunization against specific organisms, administration of preparations containing antibody against one or a variety of microorganisms, administration of white blood cells, and prescription of antimicrobial agents to prevent or eliminate colonization with specific pathogens (Table 34–6). The approaches that have been successful generally have had specific pathogens or specific time periods as their target; attempts to protect patients against multiple or unknown organisms for an indefinite period have usually failed.

> **Objective 34–3. Describe the measures taken in hospitals to reduce the risk of nosocomial infection.**

The preceding section discusses measures to reduce the risk of nosocomial infection in an individual patient. Because of the problem that such infections present as a group, however, many hospitals have established infection control committees. The activities of such a group usually focus on four areas: (1) identifying specific problems in the individual hospital; (2) developing steps to control the epidemic spread of infection; (3) developing steps to control day-to-day, baseline occurrences of infection; and (4) implementing and monitoring those steps to control outbreaks and the procedures to decrease the risk of infection in individual patients.

Different methods are employed from hospital to hospital and from country to country, but such efforts are the keystone of our attempts to minimize the risk of nosocomial infection.

SUGGESTED READINGS

Bennett, J.V., and Brachman, P.S.: Hospital Infection. Boston, Little, Brown, 1979.
Dixon, R.E. (ed.): Symposium on nosocomial infections. Part I. Second international conference. Am. J. Med., 70:379, 1981.
LaForce, F.M.: Hospital-acquired gram-negative rod pneumonias: an overview. Am. J. Med., 70:664, 1981.
Maki, D.G.: Nosocomial bacteremia: an epidemiologic overview. Am. J. Med., 70:719, 1981.
Sacks, T.C., and McGowan, J.E., Jr. (eds.): International symposium on control of nosocomial infection. Rev. Infect. Dis., 3:635, 1981.
Wenzel, R.P. (ed.): Handbook of Hospital-Acquired Infections. Boca Raton, FL, CRC Press, 1981.

CHAPTER 35

Travel to Tropical Countries

M. Rey

> **Objective 35–1. Advise a traveler before departure regarding precautions to take against major infectious problems.**

The high risk of acquiring an infection in a tropical country is linked to the multiplicity of pathogens and to the lack of immunologic defenses of travelers encountering these pathogens for the first time. The risk of transmission arises from (1) a natural environment favorable to the proliferation of insects that act as vectors or intermediate hosts and (2) an unclean water supply, inadequate disposal of wastes, and improper purification of drinking water.

First, the physician should find out where the traveler is going. Some infections can be contracted anywhere, such as hepatitis A, poliomyelitis, amebiasis, salmonellosis, and shigellosis. Others are specific for certain areas, as shown in Figures 35–1 to 35–3 and Table 35–1. Figure 35–4 shows the main arthropod vectors and the corresponding tropical diseases.

Pamphlets published each year by the World Health Organization (WHO) and the United States Center for Disease Control (CDC) describe the principal risks in each country. One should also determine the actual conditions on the trip. An organized tour in an air-conditioned bus between airports and deluxe hotels carries a much lower risk of infection than a prolonged stay in a village in the bush or the adventurous wanderings of a globe-trotter bent on experiencing everything. Although it may not be necessary to review every risk of infection, one must emphasize, for example, the seriousness of an attack of malignant falciparum malaria or the frequency of food poisoning.

Advice to travelers mostly concerns vaccination, malaria prophylaxis, and general hygienic measures. Table 35–2 presents some general principles, and Tables 35–3 to 35–5 review the available practical measures.

VACCINATION

Several vaccinations are in current use. Some of them, such as variola, yellow fever, and cholera vaccinations, are under international regulation. A certificate of vaccination is required to cross some borders; each country determines its own regulations, which may change from year to year. One should ask for information at a vaccination center or a travel agency. Proof of vaccination is written on a special form or booklet and should be

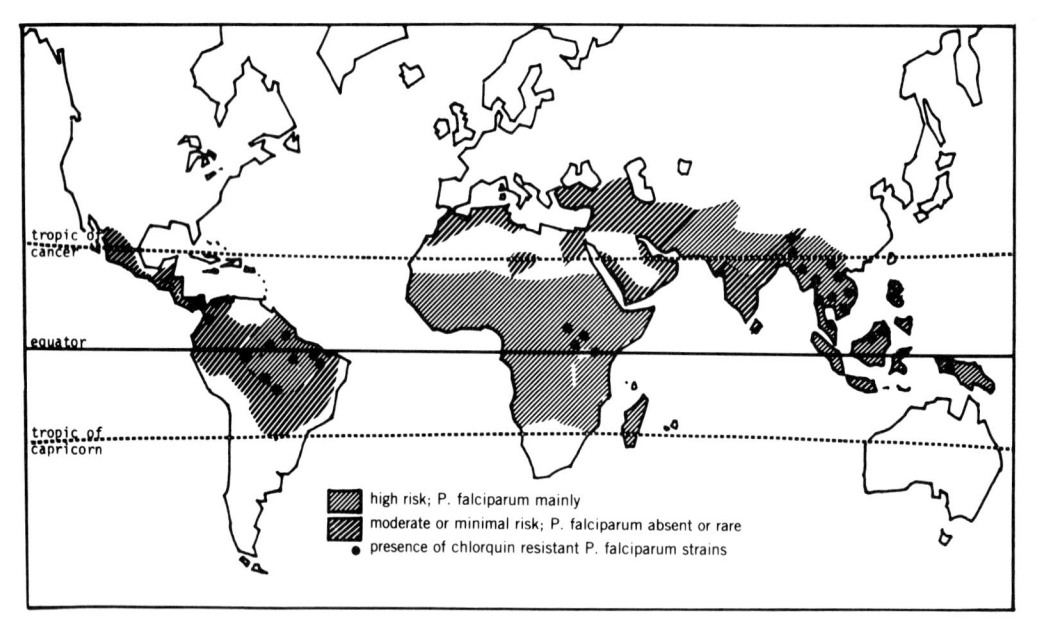

Fig. 35–1. Geographic distribution of malaria. (From data from the World Health Organization.)

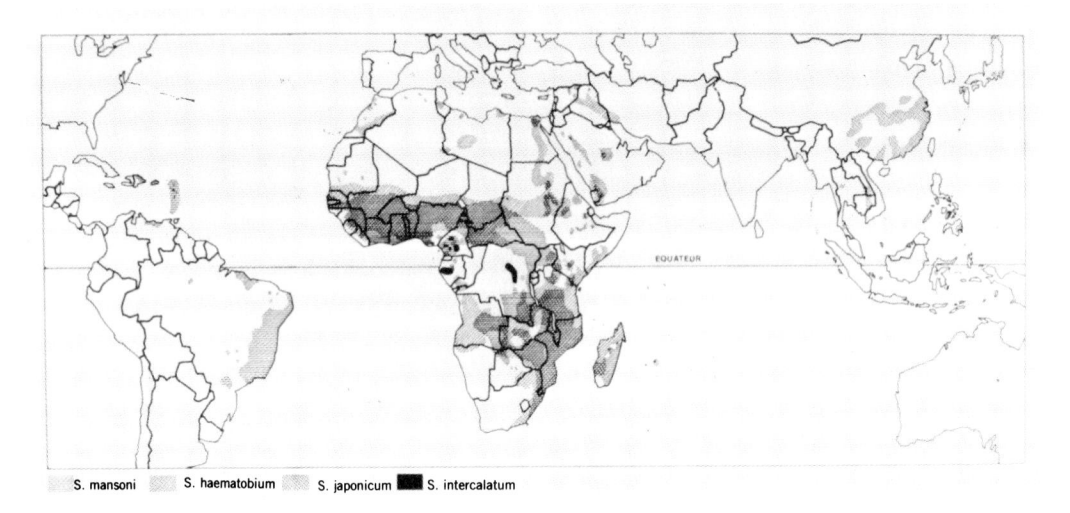

Fig. 35–2. Geographic distribution of the four forms of schistosomiasis. (From Gentilini, M., and Duflo, B.: Médecine tropicale. 3rd Ed. Paris, Flammarion, 1982.)

stamped by an appropriate public health authority. If a vaccination is contraindicated, a detailed certificate should specify the reasons.

Smallpox (Variola). Smallpox vaccination is no longer recommended by the WHO; the last endemic case was seen in Somalia in 1977. Several countries still insist on this vaccination, however. The certificate is valid for 3 years, starting 10 days after primary vaccination and from the first day after revaccination.

Because of the risk of complications, such as generalized vaccinia, necrotizing vaccinia, and encephalitis, contraindications should be sought carefully. These include eczema or other overt dermatitis, pregnancy, immunosuppressive disease or treatment, cancer

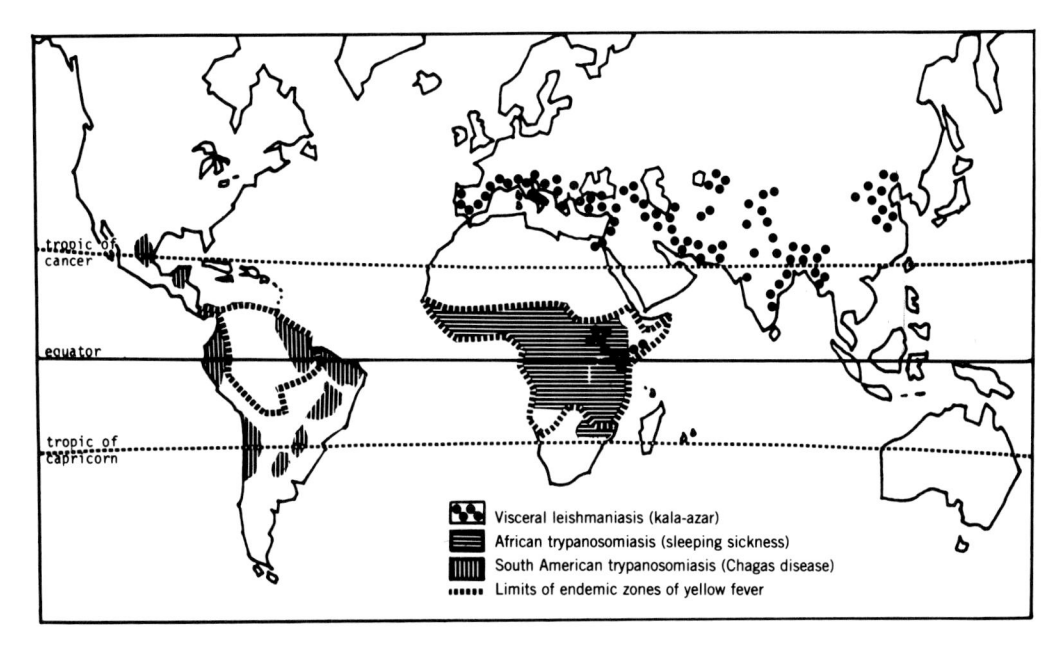

Fig. 35–3. Geographic distribution of visceral leishmaniasis, African and South American trypanosomiasis, and yellow fever.

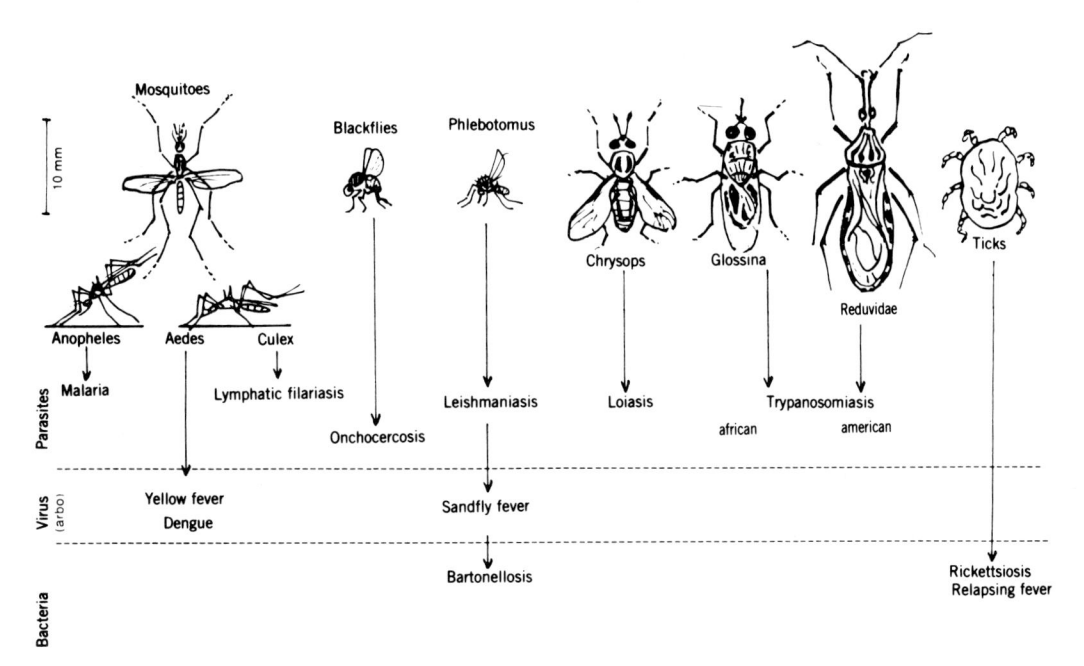

Fig. 35–4. Main arthropod vectors and corresponding tropical diseases.

Table 35–1. World Distribution of Major Endemic Tropical Diseases Likely to Infect Travelers

	America		Africa		Europe	Asia	
	Caribbean	Central and South	North	Tropical	Mediterranean	Middle East and India	Southeast
Malaria	(−)	+ +	+	+ + +	(−)	+	+ +
Trypanosomiasis							
American	−	+	−	−	−	−	−
African	−	−	−	+ +	−	−	−
Leishmaniasis							
cutaneous	−	+ +	−	+	+	+ +	−
visceral	−	−	−	+	+	+ +	−
Schistosomiasis							
urinary	−	−	+	+ + +	−	+	−
intestinal	−	+ +	+	+ + +	−	−	−
arteriovenous	−	−	−	−	−	−	+ +
Filariasis							
lymphatic	+	+ +	−	+ + +	−	+ +	+
loiasis	−	−	−	+ +	−	−	−
onchocerciasis	−	+	−	+ + +	−	−	−
Paragonimiasis and opisthorchiasis	−	+	+	+	−	−	+
Amebiasis	+ +	+	+ +	+ +	+	+ + +	+ + +
Salmonellosis and shigellosis	+ +	+ +	+ +	+ +	+	+ + +	+ + +
Cholera	−	−	+	+ +	+	+ +	+ +
Bartonellosis	−	+ +	−	−	−	−	−
Arboviral infection							
dengue and related syndromes	+ +	+	+	+	+	+ +	+ +
hemorrhagic fever	−	−	−	−	−	−	+ +
yellow fever	−	+	−	+	−	−	−
Smallpox*	−	−	−	*	−	−	−

*Last endemic case seen in Somalia in 1977.
(−), Minimal risk; −, no risk; +, low risk; + +, moderate risk; + + +, high risk.

chemotherapy, or corticosteroid therapy. Minimal proteinuria and controlled diabetes are not contraindications.

The primary smallpox vaccination of most travelers today is far outdated or nonexistent. These people develop a pustular vaccinal reaction of the primary or accelerated type if given viable vaccine, and they should be warned that they might experience general symptoms such as fever and myalgias from the fourth to the tenth day after vaccination. Primary vaccination of an adult is not considered as dangerous as that of a young child, however. The inoculation should be made with care. The multiple-pressure technique, with a needle applied obliquely or transversely, or the method of multiple pricking with a needle, stylet, or ring is now preferred to the older, scratch technique. Pustules should be protected with a dry dressing.

Yellow Fever. This vaccination differs from others in that it is only given at certain accepted facilities. Even though yellow fever vaccination is required only by a certain number of western and central African countries, it is recommended for all persons going to endemic zones: tropical Africa and several areas of Central and South America (Fig. 35–3).

Administered by a single subcutaneous injection, this well-tolerated live virus vaccine sometimes produces a minor febrile reaction with aching, around the fifth day after vaccination. The few contraindications to yellow fever vaccination are pregnancy, renal or progressive hepatic disease, and immunosuppression. Required from 1 year of age, the certificate is valid for 10 years, starting from the tenth day after initial vaccination and from the first day after revaccination.

Table 35–2. Mode of Transmission and Prevention of Principal Tropical Infections

Mode of Transmission	Infections Transmitted	Preventive Measures Nonspecific	Preventive Measures Specific
Mosquito bites	Malaria, yellow fever, dengue	Avoidance of insect bites	Chemoprophylaxis (malaria), vaccination (yellow fever)
Other insect bites	Trypanosomiasis, onchocerciasis, leishmaniasis, rickettsiosis, borrelliosis	Avoidance of insect bites	Chemoprophylaxis in hyperendemic zones; specific immunization
Skin contact	Schistosomiasis, ankylostomiasis (hookworm infection), anguilluliasis* (strongyloidiasis)	Avoidance of bathing in contaminated water; wearing of shoes	No specific measures
Contamination of food or water	Amebiasis, salmonellosis, shigellosis, cholera, poliomyelitis, hepatitis A	Drinking of boiled or disinfected water; avoidance of eating raw foods	Vaccination (typhoid, cholera, poliomyelitis), standard immunoglobulin (hepatitis)
Animal bites	Rabies	Wound disinfection	Vaccination when infection is suspected
Wounds	Tetanus	Wound disinfection	Immunization, careful cleansing of wounds

*The term "anguilluliasis" has been largely replaced by "strongyloidiasis"

Table 35–3. Immunization Calendar

Required Immunization	Suggested Schedule, with Tetanus and Polio Boosters (TP)	Interval Between First Inoculation and Departure Minimum Number of Days	Interval Between First Inoculation and Departure Maximum Number of Days
Smallpox†	Day 0: smallpox and TP	10	15
Cholera*	Day 0: TP Day 10: cholera	20	25
Smallpox and cholera*	Day 0: TP Day 10: smallpox and cholera	16	16
Yellow fever	Day 0: yellow fever and TP	10	10
Yellow fever and smallpox	Day 0: Yellow fever and TP Day 15: Smallpox (and TP if not done on day 0); or Day 0: yellow fever and TP and smallpox	25 10	30 15
Yellow fever and cholera	Day 0: yellow fever and TP Day 15, or better, Day 30: cholera	21	36
Yellow fever, smallpox, and cholera	Day 0: yellow fever and TP Day 15, or better Day 30: smallpox and cholera	25	45

*If 2 injections of cholera vaccine are used, the first is administered by itself on day 10 and the second, along with smallpox vaccine, is given 7 to 10 days later.

Note: If typhoid immunization is added, it can be limited to 2 injections, 10 to 15 days apart, and can be inserted between yellow fever vaccination (at least 15 days before the 1st typhoid) and smallpox or cholera vaccination (10 days after the second typhoid).

†A vestige of the past, we all hope.

Table 35–4. Malaria Chemoprophylaxis According to Patient's Age

| Medication | Frequency of Dose | Individual dose (mg) by age (years) |||||
		1	1–3	3–6	1–12	over 12
Chloroquine* (Nivaquine, Aralen, Avloclor)	Daily Weekly	12–25 50–100	25 100	50 150	75 200	100 300–400
Amodiaquine† (Flavoquine, Camoquin)	Weekly	50–100	100	200	300	400
Chlorguanide‡ (Paludrine, Proquanil)	Daily	25	50	75	100	100
Pyrimethamine§ (Daraprim, Malocide)	Weekly	12.5	12.5	25	25	25–50

*Tablet dosage varies according to brand: Nivaquine: 100 and 300 mg; others: 150 mg. Syrup suspension gives a dose of 25 mg/tsp. Infants under 6 kg are given ½ tsp/day or 1 tsp every other day.
†Flavoquine: 1 tablet = 200 mg.
‡Paludrine: 1 tablet = 100 mg.
§Verify tablet dosage: Daraprim: 25 mg; Malocide: 50 mg.

Table 35–5. General Precautions for Travelers to Tropical Countries

1. Aside from certain centers with a regulated water supply, beware of drinking tap water. Preliminary boiling is the only certain means of disinfection, although chemical disinfectants are more practical: javelle water (1 to 4 drops/L), hydrochlorazone (1 tablet/L), tincture of iodine (10 drops/L).
2. Avoid raw foods such as vegetables, fruits, or shellfish, as well as raw or rare meats and ice creams of local preparation.
3. Avoid bathing in stagnant or slow-moving freshwater outside of properly disinfected swimming pools.
4. Do not walk about on bare feet, above all on moist soil. Be careful at river crossings.
5. Disinfect all wounds carefully.
6. Avoid insect bites by using insect repellants or by spraying insecticides.

Cholera. Despite its mediocre efficacy, anticholera immunization is still required by certain countries and is sometimes demanded by anxious travelers. These patients should be informed that they will have little exposure to cholera and that immunization provides only 50 to 60% protection for a few months. Anticholera immunization may be given by intradermal or subcutaneous inoculation. Certain countries, such as France, do not accept intradermal immunizations. Two injections, 1 or 2 weeks apart, give the best protection, but a single injection is often accepted, especially for travelers native to endemic areas. A local reaction may be observed in the first 48 hours. The certificate is valid for 6 months starting from the sixth day after the first immunization and immediately after reimmunization.

Other Diseases. Other immunizations are just as important as those previously mentioned, even though they have escaped international regulation.

Poliomyelitis immunization should be strongly recommended. In practice, a simple booster, preferably with the killed virus (Salk) vaccine is adequate for the majority of travelers. Persons under 30 years of age who have never been vaccinated, however, should undergo a complete series, that is, at least 2 doses of live or killed vaccine, 1 month apart.

Travelers should have a current tetanus immunization, as should everyone (see Table 1–5). In infants, it is also necessary to determine the status of diphtheria and pertussis immunization. Measles vaccination in young children over 1 year of age can be recommended. If a patient plans to stay in areas where tuberculosis is prevalent, or in crowded conditions, it is advisable to know the result of the patient's pretravel purified protein derivative (PPD) test, and possibly prescribe a bacille Calmette Guérin (BCG) test or repeated tuberculin testing.

Typhoid immunization is advised only when persons are traveling to hyperendemic zones, such as North Africa, Egypt, and India, and where the risk of typhoid infection is increased by the hygienic conditions of the journey. Two injections at 2-week intervals are considered adequate, but a third injection raises antibody levels even higher. Nasal or oral typhoid vaccine may soon be available if its promises are confirmed.

Antimeningococcal immunization can be suggested to travelers to regions subject to epidemics of cerebrospinal meningitis, such as Sahel in subsaharan Africa, particularly during an epidemic. Children and adults under age 30 benefit most from immunization. Only 1 subcutaneous injection is needed, except in young infants, who should receive a subsequent booster injection. Monovalent vaccine (polysaccharide A) is appropriate for travel to Africa, where group A disease is prevalent. Bivalent (A and C) vaccine is useful under other circumstances.

Immunization against plague, which consists of 2 injections of killed bacterial vaccine, 5 days apart, or against typhus, comprising 3 injections at weekly intervals, can be added to the list under special circumstances. Examples are persons studying rodents in India, China, or the southwest of the United States and persons involved in relief efforts for refugees.

The immunization schedule should take into consideration possible combinations and the intervals between injections.

Combined Immunizations. Smallpox vaccination can be given with any other immunization, including yellow fever vaccine. Cholera and typhoid vaccines, which are killed bacterial vaccines, are capable of altering the response to viral vaccines, except smallpox, and should not be given at the same time as yellow fever or poliomyelitis vaccine. Tetanus toxoid and killed poliovirus vaccine (Salk) can be given in the same injection.

The interval between live virus vaccinations is, in principle, about 2 weeks, or 3 weeks after a primary reaction to smallpox vaccine. The vaccination schedule usually begins with yellow fever vaccine and ends, at least 10 days before departure, with smallpox vaccine. The schedules can be simplified and shortened according to the scheme developed in Table 35–3.

CHEMOPROPHYLAXIS

Malaria Prophylaxis. This is the most important of all preventive measures. Its goal is to avoid an episode of "malignant" or "pernicious" falciparum malaria. It is imperative for all ages and for every trip to tropical countries. Indeed, even if traveling to an area considered noninfected, one could still be bitten by an infected mosquito during a brief stopover, anticipated or unforeseen, in an endemic area.

Chemoprophylaxis should be started the day of departure or the day before, followed for the entire journey, and continued for at least 6 weeks after returning. It only suppresses the clinical manifestations without preventing infection or the development of the preliminary parasitic stages in the host.

Several preparations are available, as discussed in the following paragraphs:

The 4-aminoquinolines (chloroquine and amodiaquine) are the major prophylactic and therapeutic antimalarial agents. Their effectiveness is excellent, except in areas where resistant *Plasmodium falciparum* have been described (see the discussion later in this objective), where these drugs cannot be recommended. The slow elimination of these agents permits a variety of dosage schedules. Tolerance is excellent with the doses employed, although some individuals may complain of side effects such as nausea, vertigo, pruritus, and rarely, urticaria.

Proguanil, largely used in English-speaking tropical countries, has the advantage of being nontoxic and easy to use, although it must be taken daily and has produced malarial resistance in many areas. Pyrimethamine, another folic acid antagonist, has also produced some resistance, but its slow excretion permits a weekly dose.

In practice, the drug of choice for chemoprophylaxis of all plasmodia, except chloroquine-resistant *Plasmodium falciparum*, is chloroquine phosphate, in a 300 mg base dose (500 mg total) once weekly, continued for 6 weeks after the last exposure in endemic areas.

When chloroquine is not completely tolerated, it can be replaced by weekly doses of amodiaquine, daily doses of proguanil, or weekly doses of pyrimethamine.

In infants and children, acceptability and safety are important considerations. The bitter taste of most antimalarial agents is attenuated but not eliminated by flavored syrups; children may refuse it or may throw it up. This effect has the advantage of reducing the risk of accidental poisoning. The 4-aminoquinolines are dangerous drugs that must not be left within the reach of children. The only tasteless prophylactic antimalarial drug is pyrimethamine.

In the pregnant woman, the 4-aminoquinolines are not considered dangerous to the fetus. On the other hand, the antifolates (proguanil and pyrimethamine) are contraindicated.

Chloroquine-resistant strains of *Plasmodium falciparum* may be encountered in the Amazon basin, in northwestern Brazil, Guyana, Surinam, Venezuela, Colombia, Ecuador, and Panama, in Bangladesh, Burma, Thailand, Laos, Campuchea, Vietnam, Malaysia, Indonesia, and the Philippines, and in central Africa. Chloroquine resistance is increasing and may reach 60 to 80% of *P. falciparum* strains in these areas. One of the following alternatives is advised:

1. Replace the 4-aminoquinolines with an antifolate agent such as proguanil or pyrimethamine.
2. Preferably, add an antifolate drug to the chloroquine or amodiaquine regimen. Several combinations have been marked outside the United States: Draclor (chloroquine and pyrimethamine, at a dose of 1 or 2 tablets weekly), or Lapaquin (chloroquine and chlorproguanil, to be taken once a week.
3. Prescribe a pyrimethamine-sulfone combination such as Maloprim, at a dose of 1 tablet weekly (not available in the United States).
4. Prescribe a pyrimethamine-sulfonamide combination such as Fansidar, to be taken once weekly (available in the United States). If taken separately, the dose is 50 mg (2 tablets) pyrimethamine and 1000 mg sulfadoxine every other week. *Plasmodium falciparum* resistant to Fansidar has been reported on the Thai-Kampuchean border, in Indonesia, in Papua-New Guinea, and in the Amazon region of Brazil.

A new and promising product currently under study is mefloquine, to be taken in doses of 5 mg/kg/week.

Other Diseases. Chemoprophylaxis for other diseases is much less important and, for the most part, is optional. Intestinal prophylaxis against enteropathogenic *Escherichia coli* with doxycycline, 1 tablet/day may be recommended for a short trip of less than 2 to 3 weeks' duration. This regimen is ineffective against amebiasis.

Other precautions are summarized in Table 35–5.

These measures do not cover every possible infection, yet it is better to recommend those measures that are essential and realistic, to ensure compliance.

Objective 35–2. Determine which tests are necessary in an asymptomatic individual just returned from a trip to a tropical country.

No particular tests are mandatory. When pressed by a persistent individual, or in children, one can obtain a complete blood count to check for eosinophils or malaria parasites, and one may look for parasites in the patient's stool.

Objective 35–3. Distinguish malaria and hepatic amebiasis from the other possible causes of fever in a returning traveler.

The appearance of symptoms after foreign travel requires an unusual diagnostic workup. Indeed, the illness may not be related to the recent travel; however, several diseases unique to the returning traveler should be considered. Two of these diseases, malaria and amebiasis, stand out by their frequency and their severity.

MALARIA

Clinical Manifestations. A continuous or irregular fever, progressively increasing, starting 1 to 3 weeks after exposure and accompanied by headaches, myalgias, and malaise, and gastrointestinal problems such as vomiting and occasional diarrhea, should suggest a primary infection with *Plasmodium falciparum* or *P. vivax*. A pulse-fever deficit may be noted; splenomegaly is most often absent. This clinical picture also suggests typhoid fever.

Malignant falciparum malaria may follow the fever of a primary infection or may begin without prodrome. The clinical picture is that of hyperacute encephalopathy. The most typical form of falciparum malaria is associated with a fever of 104° F (40° C), with deep coma preceded or accompanied by general convulsions without meningeal or localizing signs, and with hypotonia and loss of reflexes. Fever may be absent or variable however, and coma may be replaced by severe prostration or variable alterations of consciousness. The spleen is not generally palpable. Signs of hemolysis, such as anemia or jaundice, are variable. The cerebrospinal fluid is normal or minimally disturbed (lymphocytosis of less than 50/ml). Total vascular collapse may supervene rapidly. In the absence of treatment, the course of the disease is nearly always fatal in under 3 days.

Simple intermittent paroxysmal fevers are more typical of malaria and are less dangerous than the continuous, progressive fevers. In this form of the disease, the classic malarial paroxysms of chills, then fever, then sweats, which unfold over several hours, may be accompanied by splenomegaly. The periodicity of the attack depends on the plasmodial species: daily (often *Plasmodium falciparum*), tertian or every other day (*P. falciparum*, *P. vivax*, or *P. ovale*), and quartan or every third day (*P. malariae*).

Diagnosis. The physician's practical approach can be summarized as follows:

1. The diagnosis of malaria is considered routine in a traveler who develops symptoms after returning from a country where the disease is endemic, even if the visit has been of short duration (a stopover is sufficient), even if another diagnosis appears more likely, and even if the correct chemoprophylaxis seems to have been taken. Prophylaxis does not always prevent secondary episodes or relapses; these episodes are rare with *Plasmodium falciparum* malaria and generally fade out in 3 to 6 months, but they are more common with *P. malariae* infection and may last up to 20 years.

2. The diagnosis is confirmed by the demonstration of malarial parasites by microscopic examination of a simple blood smear or thick smear on a slide stained with Giemsa stain. Often, no one capable of reading the smear is immediately available. Several slides should still be made; they can be read later, to allow a retrospective diagnosis.

3. Recognition of the specific causative species depends on the morphologic features of the parasite and is important because it establishes the duration of the risk of relapse and the need for a radical cure. Only one species, *Plasmodium falciparum*, produces malignant cerebral malaria and has chloro-

---

PREPARING A SLIDE TO LOOK FOR BLOOD-BORNE PARASITES IN A DROP OF BLOOD (PLASMODIUM, FILARIA, AND BORRELIA)

Sample at the bedside or in the laboratory.

1. *Thick smear.* Obtain a drop of blood directly from the patient's finger (or from a vein) without anticoagulant and place it on a slide. Slow the clot formation by rotating the point of the needle or stylus in the drop until it is dry (8 to 12 minutes). Lake the red blood cells with a drop of distilled water and stain with Giemsa.

2. *Thin smear.* Spread a thin layer, if necessary, on the same slide as the thick drop, using the same finger stick. The blood should be drawn with heparin as an anticoagulant. Stain with May-Grünwald-Giemsa. The reading should be done with meticulous care. At least 20 to 30 minutes should be given to the microscopic examination before concluding that the specimen is negative for parasitic infection.

quine-resistant strains. In contrast to nonfalciparum malaria, one can detect (1) high-grade parasitemia (> 2 to 3%), (2) the presence of mostly young ring trophozoites, and (3) crescent- or banana-shaped gametocytes.

4. It is often preferable to undertake treatment on clinical suspicion, without waiting for confirmation, since antimalarial therapy does not obscure other possible diagnoses and since untreated malignant malaria can be rapidly fatal.

Treatment. The treatment of nonmalignant malaria begins with oral chloroquine. In adults, a total dose of 2 to 3 g is given over 2 to 3 days: 1 g (600 mg chloroquine base) initially, then 500 (total) mg in 6 hours, and 500 mg at 24 and 48 hours. In the child, the dose should be carefully correlated with the patient's weight: a first dose of 10 mg chloroquine base per kg, then 5 mg/kg/day for 2 days.

To prevent relapses due to *Plasmodium vivax*, *P. ovale*, or *P. malariae* infection, the hepatic parasite must be eliminated. For this purpose, an 8-aminoquinoline such as primaquine, 15 mg/day for 2 weeks, should be used as the last phase of treatment of a clinical case of malaria due to these species or prophylactically on return from a hyperendemic zone.

In malignant falciparum malaria, one should administer intravenous quinine, 1.5 mg/day or 25 mg/kg for children, or intramuscular chloroquine, 250 mg every 6 hours. It is usually necessary to place the patient in an intensive care or specialized (cardiovascular, renal, or respiratory) unit, depending on the case. After 2 or 3 days of quinine administration, treatment is completed with oral chloroquine.

When the patient has just returned from an area where chloroquine-resistant *P. falciparum* are endemic, chloroquine can be replaced by or combined with Fansidar, 1.5 to 2 g as a single dose in the adult or 50 mg/kg in the child, or by trimethoprim-sulfamethoxazole, 2 tablets twice daily for 5 days, or one can use quinine, 650 mg 3 times daily for 10 to 14 days, in combination with pyrimethamine, 25 mg twice daily for 3 days, and sulfadiazine, 500 mg 4 times daily for 5 days.

HEPATIC AMEBIASIS

Clinical Manifestations. This disease can occur weeks, months, or even years after returning from an endemic area. It may be preceded by episodes of suspicious dysentery or diarrhea. A fever of 39 to 40° C (104° F) develops rapidly and is accompanied by right-upper-quadrant abdominal pain radiating to the right scapula and hepatomegaly tender to pressure or percussion. Roentgenograms show restricted movement of the right diaphragm, with elevation and obliteration of the

Table 35–6. Evocative Signs in a Febrile Patient Just Returned from a Tropical Country

In the Presence of	Think of
Diarrhea or dysentery	Salmonellosis, shigellosis, amebiasis
Tender hepatomegaly	Hepatic amebiasis
Jaundice	Viral hepatitis, malaria, yellow fever and other arboviral infections, leptospirosis, borreliosis
Encephalitic signs	Malaria (cerebral), typhoid fever, arboviral infections, trypanosomiasis
Myocardial signs	Trypanosomiasis (South American), typhoid fever
Conjunctivitis and myalgias	Arboviral infection, leptospirosis
Facial edema	Trichinosis, trypanosomiasis, schistosomiasis
Hemorrhagic syndrome	Arboviral infection (Lassa or other arenaviruses, Ebola virus)
Anemia	Malaria, bartonellosis, kala-azar
Elevated sedimentation rate	Hepatic amebiasis, kala-azar, trypanosomiasis
Hypereosinophilia	Schistosomiasis, trichinosis, tissue parasite infection such as paragonimiasis (distomiasis)

Table 35–7. Diagnostic Approaches in Acute Diarrhea or Dysentery in Travelers

Appearance of Stools	Fever	Probable Cause	Polymorphonuclear Leukocytes in Stools	Confirmation of Diagnosis
Diarrhea (sometimes cholera-like) without blood or mucus	Absent	Enterotoxin-producing *Escherichia coli*	Absent	Usually only clinical (turista)
		Vibrio cholerae	Absent	Specific culture for *V. cholerae* in stool
	Present	Salmonella	Absent	Routine culture of stool
Dysentery blood or mucus	Absent	Amoeba	Absent	Microscopic examination of fresh stool
	Present	Shigella / Salmonella	Present / Absent (relative)	Routine culture of stool

costophrenic angle, occasionally with a significant pleural effusion.

The sedimentation rate is often elevated (100 mm/hr or more). The white blood count is elevated, and neutrophilia is present. Demonstration of amebas in the stool is inconstant. Serologic tests, such as immunofluorescence, precipitation, and agglutination, confirm the diagnosis; in infected patients test results are nearly always positive at high titer.

Treatment. Hospitalization is the rule. Treatment must be started rapidly without waiting for confirmation of the diagnosis. Metronidazole, the drug of choice, is effective against amebic liver abscess in over 90% of patients. The usual recommended dose in this indication is 500 to 750 mg 3 times daily in an adult, or 25 mg/kg in a child, either orally or intravenously. The duration of therapy is still debatable. Five days have been proposed, but most authorities recommend at least 10 days, and some up to 3 weeks. Emetine dihydrochloride is used less nowadays because it requires monitoring for cardiotoxicity. Doses are 1 to 1.5 mg/kg/day (maximum 90 mg/day), intramuscularly or by deep subcutaneous injection, for 6 to 8 days.

Another alternative is chloroquine, administered at 1 g/day intramuscularly or by deep subcutaneous injection, for 6 to 8 days or alternatively administered at 1 g/day orally for 2 days, then at 500 mg/day for 2 to 3 weeks. Because emetine dihydrochloride and chloroquine are ineffective against intestinal parasites, an intraluminal amebicide must be combined: iodoquinol (diiodohydroxyquin), 650 mg 3 times a day, orally for 20 days, is often recommended. Some combine the prescription with metronidazole.

One should look for abscess formation on echograms or hepatic scans, and treat such abscesses with closed or open evacuation if rupture into the pleural or abdominal spaces seems imminent. The pus, described as chocolate, coffee-and-milk, or anchovy paste in color, is bacteriologically sterile and is usually devoid of amebas.

OTHER INFECTIONS

Many other infections have a similar clinical presentation, but in contrast to falciparum malaria and hepatic amebiasis, they generally do not require urgent action. Diagnosis can be difficult and may require consultation and special studies. Table 35–6 lists the clinical and microbiologic associations likely to aid the diagnosis of such infections. Examples of other systemic parasitic infections that require specific treatment are visceral leishmaniasis or kala-azar, African trypanosomiasis or sleeping sickness, American trypanosomiasis or Chagas' disease, and schistosomiasis in its initial invasive phase. Viral infections may also give a similar picture, especially those due to an arbovirus, such as dengue or a related syndrome. *Salmonella typhi* infec-

MAJOR TROPICAL INFECTIONS IN TRAVELERS

AMEBIASIS

This cosmopolitan, widely distributed disease most often involves the large intestine and causes rectocolitis in the form of acute or chronic amebic dysentery. This illness is occasionally extraintestinal and is manifested by abscesses of the liver, lung, or other organs. Transmitted by fecal-oral route, by food contaminated by parasitic cysts, amebiasis is due to a pathogenic ameba, *Entamoeba histolytica,* not to be confused with saprophytic amebas such as *Entamoeba coli.*

ARBOVIRAL INFECTION

These acute viral infections are transmitted by arthropod vectors, generally mosquitoes. One of the most serious is yellow fever, which often causes fatal hepatic or renal failure or a fatal hemorrhagic syndrome.

BARTONELLOSIS

This South American (Andean) bacterial infection is transmitted by sandflies and produces a febrile hemolytic anemia.

CHOLERA

This acute diarrheal disorder is due to *Vibrio cholerae* and is transmitted by the fecal-oral route from water or food. Travelers are rarely infected.

DISTOMIASIS

Pulmonary paragonimiasis and hepatobiliary opisthorchiasis are chronic systemic helminthic infections acquired by eating raw contaminated foods such as salads, fish, and crustaceans.

FILARIASIS

This systemic roundworm infection is transmitted by various flying insects. Loiasis, a subcutaneous helminthic infection with *Loa loa,* is generally benign, is restricted to central Africa, is most easily contracted by the traveler. The lymphatic filariae (wuchereria) that can produce elephantiasis and the onchocerca that can cause blindness are, on the other hand, of little risk to the traveler.

LEISHMANIASIS

This disease is due to intracellular protozoans and is transmitted by sandflies. It exists in several forms: benign cutaneous ulcerations (tropical ulcer) (Plate 14C); localized mucocutaneous ulcerations, possibly severe; and generalized visceral leishmaniasis with prolonged fever, splenomegaly, anemia, and granulocytopenia. This last form is eventually fatal if untreated.

Weeks or months after a sandfly bite, enlarging papules appear, to become a superficial ulceration covered by a crust and bordered by rolled undermined, indurated edges. After treatment with parenteral neostibosan, or after several months if no effective therapy is given, healing occurs by granulation. Caused by *Leishmania tropica,* this disease is prevalent in many tropical and subtropical regions (Asia, Mediterranean coast, Africa). Oriental sore must be distinguished from mucocutaneous leishmaniasis (espundia), which is more severe and produces large ulcerations with widespread tissue destruction. This disease is contracted throughout Central and South America and is due to *L. brasiliensis.* A Mexican cutaneous leishmaniasis, produced by *L. mexicana,* is also known. The definitive diagnosis of cutaneous leishmaniasis depends upon the demonstration of leishmania in scrapings or histologic sections of the margin of the lesion.

MALARIA

This sporozoan infection is transmitted by anopheles mosquitoes. Among the four plasmodium species capable of infecting man (*Plasmodium falciparum, P. malariae, P. vivax,* and *P. ovale*), *P. falciparum* is the most dangerous. This species causes malignant tertian malaria and represents the major risk to travelers in tropical areas.

SCHISTOSOMIASIS

Also known as bilharziasis, this chronic systemic helminthic infection is acquired by contact with contaminated water while bathing. Genitourinary infestation due to *Schistosoma haematobium* gives rise initially to hematuria and cystitis, but can produce secondary renal complications. Intestinal schistosomiasis due to *S. mansoni* can produce cirrhosis with portal hypertension. *S. japonicum,* which is limited to the Far East, produces infections (arteriovenosis) high in the portal vein and is the most serious form of schistosomiasis because of its much greater output of parasitic eggs.

TRYPANOSOMIASIS

This protozoan infection has a subacute or chronic course. The African form of the disease is transmitted by glossina (tsetse flies) and leads to a progressive, fatal meningoencephalitis, also known as sleeping sickness. The American form of trypanosomiasis, also called Chagas' disease, is transmitted by reduviid bugs and produces, among other disorders, myocardiopathy.

tion is similar in presentation, but is usually recognized. Few of these infections are actually contagious in the temperate zones, except certain rare but alarming African viral diseases such as Lassa, Marburg, and Ebola fevers, for which special isolation precautions are mandatory.

> **Objective 35–4. Determine whether diarrhea or dysentery is due to cholera or to amebic colitis.**

Most acute diarrheas or dysenteries of travelers, with or without fever, are bacterial "food poisonings." Stool cultures permit identification of the causative agent when it is an invasive microbe such as salmonella, shigella, or campylobacter. The culture results are not as clear when the disorder is due to toxigenic enteropathogens such as staphylococcus, clostridium, noncholera vibrio, or enteropathogenic *Escherichia coli*. Without waiting for culture results, one should initiate antibiotic therapy, with tetracycline or trimethoprim-sulfamethoxazole, as well as rehydration in severe cases. It is important not to miss two different infections that demand entirely different therapy: cholera and amebiasis. See Table 35–7 for diagnostic approaches to these disorders.

CHOLERA

Cholera, now widely endemic in various tropical areas of Asia and Africa, and perhaps in Louisiana, rarely infects the traveler. The disease should be suspected, however, if (1) fewer than 5 days have elapsed between the stay in the suspected area and the onset of the illness and (2) the patient is afebrile.

The typical cholera stools, which are frequent, copious, and watery ("rice water"), are not always present, nor is intense dehydration accompanied by vascular collapse. Diagnosis rests on the isolation of *Vibrio cholerae* from the stool. This procedure must be especially requested from the laboratory in addition to the routine stool culture.

Cholera falls under international regulation. The patient in question should therefore be hospitalized and isolated immediately, even though the risk of transmission in industrialized countries is slight. Treatment, which is essentially symptomatic, includes intensive rehydration suited to the seriousness of the case. Public health authorities should be informed immediately.

AMEBIC COLITIS

Amebic colitis is suggested by an acute or subacute dysentery with bloody mucoid stools and a syndrome of abdominal and pelvic pain characterized by colic, urgency, and tenesmus. Fever is not always present. The diagnosis is made by demonstrating amebas laden with red blood cells in the stool by direct examination within 10 minutes of passage. Protoscopy reveals characteristic ulcerations and permits sampling of the mucus in which one has the best chance of finding the amebas. The usual initial therapy is with metronidazole, 750 mg 3 times daily for a week (see Objective 17–3).

SUGGESTED READINGS

Bruce-Chwatt, L.J.: Essential Malariology. London, W. Heinemann, p. 354, 1980.

Center for Disease Control: Health Information for International Travel. Center for Disease Control Publication No. 78:8280. Atlanta, United States Department of Health, Education and Welfare, 1978.

Gentilini, M., Duflo, B. Lagardère, B., and Danis, M.: Médecine tropicale. 2nd Ed. Paris, Flammarion, 1977.

Hunter, G.W., Swartzwelder, J.C., and Clyde, D.F.: Tropical Medicine. 5th Ed. Philadelphia, W.B. Saunders, 1976.

Nash, T.E., Cheever, A.W., Ottesen, E.A., and Cook, J.A.: Schistosome infections in humans: perspectives and recent findings. Ann. Intern. Med., 97:740, 1982.

Weniger, B., et al.: High-level chloroquine resistance of Plasmodium falciparum malaria acquired in Kenya. N. Engl. J. Med., 307:1560, 1982.

CHAPTER 36

Principles of Antimicrobial Treatment

R.C. Moellering, Jr.

Three areas deserve special consideration when treating patients with antimicrobial agents: (1) the choice of an appropriate agent, (2) the determination of the optimal dose and route of administration; and (3) the effective monitoring of therapeutic response. Although all three factors are important, I place special emphasis on the initial choice of the therapeutic agent because it is a key determinant of therapeutic success.

> **Objective 36–1. Choose an appropriate therapeutic agent for a patient likely to have an infection.**

To make a rational choice among the many currently available antimicrobial agents, clinicians must know or must be able to estimate the infecting organism. They must ascertain the antimicrobial susceptibility of the organism, and they must consider a number of important host factors.

INFECTING ORGANISM

Drug Therapy Based on Culture Results. It is easy to choose an antibiotic if one has the luxury of waiting for the results of cultures. Such is often the case in chronic or subacute infections, such as recurrent urinary tract infections. In such infections, sufficient information is provided by the clinical microbiology laboratory as long as one has obtained adequate cultures. Unfortunately, this procedure is not always as straightforward as it might seem. It is important to obtain cultures of all potentially infected sites prior to the initiation of antimicrobial therapy. The presence of antimicrobial agents is a major factor in "negative" or unsatisfactory cultures. When antibiotics are given before cultures are taken, the clinical microbiology laboratory has several techniques for removing or inactivating these substances, including the addition of beta-lactamase to inactivate penicillin and related agents, the use of sodium polyanetholesulfonate (Liquoid or SPS) to inactivate aminoglycosides and polymyxins in blood cultures, the use of culture media with a high salt content to inactivate aminoglycosides, and the treatment of liquid specimens with exchange resins such as the antimicrobial removal device (ARD). The physician must therefore alert the clinical laboratory to the presence of antibiotics in clinical specimens.

Rapid Identification of Pathogens. In most cases, therapy must be started before the de-

---

CASE REPORT

A 53-year-old female patient was admitted to the Massachusetts General Hospital with a 2-day history of recurrent fevers and rigors. She had a long history of postprandial right-upper-quadrant discomfort and fatty food intolerance. An oral cholecystogram had revealed cholelithiasis 5 years earlier. On admission, the patient was noted to be a moderately obese female in no obvious distress. Her temperature was 37.5° C; her sclerae were slightly icteric, and she had moderate right-upper-quadrant tenderness. Two hours after hospital admission, the patient had a rigor, and her temperature rose to 40° C. Blood cultures were obtained, and intramuscular tobramycin, 1.7 mg/kg every 8 hours, was initiated.

The following day, 3 of 4 blood cultures were growing gram-negative bacilli. The patient's serum creatinine level was 1.0 mg/100 ml, her bilirubin level was 3.6 mg/100 ml, alkaline phosphatase was 120 IU (normal is 13 to 39 IU), serum glutamic-oxaloacetic transaminase (SGOT) was 42 U (normal is 10 to 40 U), and amylase was 10 U (normal is 4 to 25 U). A diagnosis of ascending cholangitis with gram-negative bacteremia was made, and further blood cultures were obtained.

Twenty-four hours later, these blood cultures were also positive, and the original blood isolate was identified as *Klebsiella pneumoniae,* susceptible to cephalothin, tetracycline, chloramphenicol, tobramycin, gentamicin, and amikacin, but resistant to ampicillin and carbenicillin. Because the patient continued to have intermittent fevers and chills, cephalothin, 1.5 g every 4 hours intravenously, was added to the drug regimen. Despite therapy with cephalothin and tobramycin, the patient remained febrile, and blood cultures remained positive.

Because of this situation, the cephalothin and tobramycin were discontinued, and doxycycline, 100 mg intravenously every 12 hours, was administered. Within 24 hours, the patient was afebrile and blood cultures were negative. She was taken to the operating room for cholecystectomy and common duct exploration with removal of a common duct stone. Doxycycline was continued for a week postoperatively. The patient's postoperative course was unremarkable, and she was discharged from the hospital in good condition 2 weeks later.

The case is particularly instructive because it illustrates several factors important in the choice of appropriate antimicrobial therapy. Even though the infecting organism was known and even though the patient was treated with two bactericidal antibiotics to which her infecting organism was susceptible in vitro, and against which these agents in combination often produce synergistic activity, the patient's fever and bacteremia persisted. How could this be? The answer is related to two important factors that often determine the balance between the success or failure of antimicrobial therapy: (1) the concentration of the antibiotic at the site of infection; and (2) the presence of an anatomic abnormality that serves as a nidus of infection.

Neither cephalothin nor tobramycin is effectively concentrated in the biliary tract, especially in obstruction. Thus, these drugs could not control the patient's cholangitis. Switching to an agent that effectively concentrates in the biliary tree led to control of the cholangitis and permitted the surgical procedure to be performed in the absence of bacteremia. Without surgical removal of the patient's common duct stone, however, it is unlikely that she could have been cured, even with an antibiotic that provides high biliary levels of drug because she would probably have had recurrent cholangitis as soon as the doxycycline was stopped. In this case, the common duct stone served as a foreign body and as a nidus of continued infection.

Thus, we have already seen several factors to consider in the effective use of antimicrobial agents. In this chapter, we consider these and other factors that determine the success or failure of antimicrobial therapy.

---

finitive results of cultures are available. In such instances, the clinician may employ one of several rapid diagnostic methods to determine the major infecting pathogen(s). Of all current techniques, none is more useful or more widely applicable than Gram's stain. Gram's staining may be performed on virtually any infected body fluid or tissue. It is especially useful for identifying organisms in body fluids that are normally sterile, such as urine, pleural fluid, cerebrospinal fluid (CSF), middle ear fluid, synovial fluid, or peritoneal exudate. Gram's staining of sputum obtained in such a way as to avoid oropharyngeal contamination, especially by nasotracheal suction or transtracheal aspiration, usually reveals the infecting pathogen in patients with bacterial bronchitis or pneumonia.

The presence of polymorphonuclear leukocytes on Gram's stain or methylene blue preparations of stool in patients with diarrhea alerts the clinician to the possible diagnosis of inflammatory bowel disease or bowel wall infection with organisms such as staphylococci, salmonella, shigella, or invasive *Escherichia coli*. Polymorphonuclear leukocytes are absent in normal stools, in the stools of patients with food poisoning, and in those of patients with diarrhea caused by viruses or toxin-producing organisms such as *Vibrio cholerae* and noninvasive *E. coli*.

Immunologic techniques may be employed in certain specialized instances to aid in the rapid identification of infecting organisms, but the availability of these techniques outside major hospitals often limits their widespread applicability. Fluorescent antibody techniques are useful in identifying organisms such as *Legionella pneumophila* in pleural fluid, lung tissue, and appropriately obtained sputum. Such techniques are also employed with varying success to identify pathogenic streptococci. The presence of specific bacterial antigens in various body fluids, especially blood, urine, and cerebrospinal fluid, may be determined by counterimmunoelectrophoresis, enzyme-linked immunoabsorbent assay (ELISA), or latex agglutination tests. These sensitive techniques can be helpful, but at present are not widely available.

Drug Therapy in Infections of Unknown Origin. Despite the applicability of the principles previously described, antimicrobial therapy must often be initiated without benefit of the exact knowledge of the infecting organism. In such instances, the clinician must make use of "bacteriologic statistics": an awareness of those organisms most likely to cause infection in a given clinical setting. Examples of such bacteriologic statistics are given in Table 36–1. This information can be used to guide initial therapy. For instance, when faced with an otherwise normal patient with cellulitis of the arm, one would logically begin therapy with a semisynthetic penicillinase-resistant penicillin or a cephalosporin to cover the likely pathogens, which are *Staphylococcus aureus* and group A streptococci. For the neonate with acute meningitis, a combination of ampicillin with gentamicin or a related aminoglycoside would be reasonable to cover the possibility of infection with coliform gram-negative bacilli, as well as group B streptococci.

ANTIMICROBIAL SUSCEPTIBILITY

Once one has determined the actual or most likely pathogen, it is necessary to obtain information concerning the antimicrobial susceptibility of the infecting organism. In chronic infections, such information may be available prior to the start of therapy. In most infections, however, one does not have this luxury, and presumptive therapy is based on the likelihood that the suspected pathogen is susceptible or resistant to commonly used antimicrobial agents. Because the drug susceptibilities of the same organism may vary from one geographic area to another, the physician must have access to information on the susceptibility patterns in his community or hospital. An example of such information is given in Table 36–2, which presents the susceptibility data on currently isolated pathogenic bacteria at the Massachusetts General Hospital in Boston. The geographic differences in prevalence of antibiotic-resistant organisms may often be traced to regional differences in patterns of antibiotic prescription. Heavy or excessive clinical use of antimicrobials can provide the selective pressure that leads to the emergence of resistant organisms.

Universally Susceptible Organisms. A few organisms are universally susceptible to antimicrobial agents. For instance, it is not currently necessary to test the penicillin susceptibility of group A streptococci (*Streptococcus pyogenes*), *Neisseria meningitidis*, and anaerobes other than *Bacteroides fragilis* because these organisms are universally susceptible to antibiotics. Even statements such as the preceding, however, may be subject to future revision, as evidenced by the recent development of penicillin resistance among *Streptococcus pneumoniae*, *Neisseria gonorrhoeae*, and *Bacteroides melaninogenicus*.

Susceptibility Testing Techniques. At present, two major types of "standard" susceptibility tests are available: disc-diffusion and dilution. Recently, however, a number of "rapid" automated methods, many of which are based on turbidimetric monitoring devices, have been developed.

Disc-diffusion methods are probably the most widely employed susceptibility testing techniques in routine clinical laboratories throughout the world. These methods are based on the principle that antimicrobial agents diffuse out of a paper disc, which is

Table 36–1. Most Frequent Bacterial Pathogens by Anatomic Site

Skin and Subcutaneous Tissues (cellulitis, pyoderma)
  Staphylococcus aureus
  Streptococcus pyogenes (group A)
  Gram-negative bacilli (traumatic and surgical wounds and in immunocompromised hosts)
  Clostridium and anaerobic streptococci (traumatic and surgical wounds)

Sinuses (sinusitis)
  Streptococcus pneumoniae
  Streptococcus pyogenes (group A)
  Haemophilus influenzae
  Staphylococcus aureus (rare)

Middle Ear (otitis media)
  Streptococcus pneumoniae
  Streptococcus pyogenes (group A)
  Haemophilus influenzae (children)
  Pseudomonas aeruginosa (diabetics, chronic otitis media)
  Proteus (chronic otitis media)

Pharynx (pharyngitis, epiglottitis)
  Streptococcus pyogenes (group A)
  Group B, C, G beta-hemolytic streptococci (rare)
  Corynebacterium diphtheriae
  Haemophilus influenzae (epiglottitis only)

Lungs (pneumonia)
  Streptococcus pneumoniae
  (Mycoplasma pneumoniae)
  Haemophilus influenzae
  Streptococcus pyogenes (group A)
  Legionella pneumophila
  Staphylococcus aureus (following influenza)
  Klebsiella (alcoholics, hospitalized patients)
  Group B streptococcus (newborns)

Lungs (abscess)
  Bacteroides (usually penicillin-susceptible)
  Other "mouth anaerobes," including fusospirochetes and anaerobic streptococci
  Klebsiella and other gram-negative bacilli (alcoholics, hospitalized patients)
  Staphylococcus aureus (may also produce pneumatocele)

Liver and Biliary Tract (cholangitis, cholecystitis)
  Escherichia coli
  Klebsiella and Enterobacter
  Proteus
  Bacteroides
  Salmonella (usually asymptomatic carriage only)

Peritoneal Cavity (peritonitis, abscess)
  Bacteroides
  Escherichia coli
  Proteus
  Other facultative gram-negative bacilli
  Clostridia and anaerobic streptococci
  Enterococci
  Streptococcus pneumoniae (nephrotic syndrome, postnecrotic cirrhosis)

Urinary Tract (cystitis, pyelonephritis, prostatitis)
  Escherichia coli
  Proteus mirabilis
  Klebsiella and Enterobacter
  Enterococci
  Other gram-negative bacilli (other Proteus species, Pseudomonas aeruginosa, and Citrobacter)
  Group B streptococci
  Staphylococcus epidermidis (cystitis, urethritis)

Table 36-1. Continued

Meninges (meningitis)
  Streptococcus pneumoniae
  Neisseria meningitidis
  Haemophilus influenzae (children)
  Staphylococcus aureus (neonates and after trauma or neurosurgery)
  Coliform bacilli (neonates)
  Group B streptococci (neonates)
  Listeria moncytogenes (rare)
  Streptococcus pyogenes and other streptococci (rare)

Endocardium (endocarditis)
  Nongroupable streptococci (alpha-hemolytic)
  Enterococci and Streptococcus bovis
  Other groupable streptococci
  Staphylococcus aureus
  Staphylococcus epidermidis (prosthetic valve endocarditis (PVE))
  Diphtheroids (PVE)
  Gram-negative bacilli (PVE)

Bones (acute osteomyelitis)
  Staphylococcus aureus
  Streptococci (all groups)
  Salmonella especially in sickle cell anemia
  Other gram-negative bacilli especially following trauma or surgery

placed on the surface of an agar plate to produce a concentration gradient of antimicrobial activity in the agar. This concentration gradient, in turn, can inhibit the growth of susceptible organisms that are seeded on the surface of the plate. The diameter of the zone of inhibition is proportional to the activity of the antimicrobial agent. If carefully done, this test, which is inexpensive and is easy to perform, provides clinically useful information. It does not, however, enable one to determine the actual capacity of antimicrobials to kill bacteria because it is based on growth inhibition and not on killing, and it cannot readily be employed for testing slow-growing, fastidious organisms or anaerobes.

Quantitative data are provided by serial dilutions of antimicrobial agents in broth- or agar-based culture media. The lowest concentration that inhibits visible growth after 18 to 24 hours of incubation is known as the minimal inhibitory concentration (MIC). In broth dilution tests, it is possible to subculture samples without visible growth to determine the minimal bactericidal concentration (MBC) or the minimal lethal concentration (MLC), which is usually based on 99.9% killing after 18 to 24 hours of incubation.

HOST FACTORS IN DRUG THERAPY

Even though the likely infecting pathogen and its probable or actual antimicrobial susceptibility have been determined, one must still consider the individual host factors before prescribing an antibiotic. These factors must be given close scrutiny because they are important determinants of both the efficacy and the potential toxicity of antibiotics in a given patient (Table 36-3).

Before administering antibiotics or, for that matter, any drug, the physician must ascertain that the patient has not had a prior adverse reaction to that agent or to related drugs. Failure to follow this simple guideline can have disastrous consequences.

Age of the Patient. The patient's age must be carefully considered both in making the initial choice of an antimicrobial agent and in determining the appropriate dose. The activity and efficiency of a number of physiologic processes vary at different ages. For instance, gastric acidity is reduced in young children and in the elderly; indeed, more than one-third of patients over age 60 are achlorhydric. These differences can affect the absorption of antibiotics administered orally, especially those that are subject to acid hydrolysis. The absorption of orally administered penicillin G

Table 36–2. Susceptibility of Commonly Isolated Bacteria to Antimicrobial Agents (Massachusetts General Hospital, Boston, 1979)*

Organism	No. of Strains†	% Susceptible to:							
		Pen	Meth	Tetr	Chlr	Eryt	Ceph	Tetr	Chlr	Clin	Nitr‡

Organism	No. of Strains†	Pen	Meth	Tetr	Chlr	Eryt	Ceph	Tetr	Chlr	Clin	Nitr‡
Staphylococcus aureus	2628	11	99	51	2	85	99	91	91	90	100
Staphylococcus epidermidis	2012	21	50	81	56	47	94	61	77	56	99
Streptococcus pneumoniae	41	100	97	59	50	100	100	97	100	100	—
Alpha-hemolytic streptococci	393	98	91	92	100	94	99	72	99	95	85
Beta-hemolytic streptococci	700	99	98	77	86	95	100	38	99	98	99
Nonhemolytic streptococci	381	99	96	90	95	97	99	51	100	98	98
Enterococci	1883	32	0	84	83	49	27	22	78	2	95
Streptococcus bovis	25	100	92	82	88	100	100	28	100	100	90

Organism	No. of Strains	% Susceptible to:								
		Ceph	Tetr	Chlr	Amp	Carb	Kana	Gent	Coli	Tobr	Amik	Nitr‡

Organism	No. of Strains	Ceph	Tetr	Chlr	Amp	Carb	Kana	Gent	Coli	Tobr	Amik	Nitr‡
Acinetobacter calcoaceticus (anitratum)	407	0	51	2	2	76	89	71	97	87	77	0
Acinetobacter calcoaceticus (lwoffi)	32	28	81	56	78	75	87	96	96	90	90	23
Alcaligenes sp.	22	59	59	50	54	76	18	54	90	54	54	42
Aeromonas sp.	13	30	92	100	7	7	100	100	76	100	100	—
Citrobacter freundii	231	19	77	86	29	59	80	87	93	87	93	95
Citrobacter diversus	65	96	90	95	0	0	93	98	98	98	100	96
Enterobacter aerogenes	294	15	84	83	13	78	90	92	98	92	96	73
Enterobacter cloacae	537	6	82	88	14	77	88	91	96	91	99	83
Escherichia coli	5557	89	68	94	77	78	85	99	99	98	98	98
Flavobacterium sp.	28	0	7	14	0	0	4	11	0	4	7	—
Klebsiella pneumoniae	1939	85	76	81	8	3	84	88	99	89	98	85
Proteus inconstans	17	5	0	41	64	84	88	70	0	88	100	0
Proteus mirabilis	1101	97	0	93	93	94	91	97	1	98	98	6
Proteus morganii	251	0	74	86	7	91	92	98	0	99	99	32
Proteus rettgeri	79	17	8	40	37	67	69	75	1	82	96	18
Proteus vulgaris	107	9	35	78	11	68	89	92	2	93	98	36
Pseudomonas aeruginosa	1566	0	2	0	0	84	4	78	99	94	81	0
Pseudomonas maltophilia	150	0	22	74	3	47	34	56	52	55	42	3
Salmonella sp.	57	100	71	98	87	88	91	100	100	100	100	—
Serratia liquefaciens	17	29	64	82	29	73	94	94	76	94	100	—
Serratia marcescens	361	0	5	77	9	64	77	85	8	81	94	10
Shigella sp.	35	94	25	91	80	82	94	100	100	100	100	—

Abbreviations: Amik, amikacin; Amp, ampicillin; Carb, carbenicillin; Ceph, cephalothin; Chlr, chloramphenicol; Clin, clindamycin; Coli, colistin; Eryt, erythromycin; Gent, gentamicin; Kana, kanamycin; Meth, methicillin; Nitr, nitrofurantoin; Pen, penicillin; Tetr, tetracycline; Tobr, tobramycin
*Susceptibilities determined by disc-diffusion (Bauer-Kirby) method.
†Unique isolates, i.e., duplicate isolates from the same patient have been excluded.
‡Urine isolates only.

Table 36–3. Host Factors that Determine Antimicrobial Efficacy and Safety

1. History of previous adverse effect
2. Age
3. Presence of genetic or metabolic abnormalities
4. Pregnancy or breast feeding
5. Renal and hepatic function
6. Site of infection

is thus more efficient in young children and in achlorhydric adults, including those with pernicious anemia.

Renal function, which also varies with age, is diminished in premature and newborn infants and reaches adult levels only after 2 months of age. This physiologic feature requires that the dosage of certain agents, such as the penicillins, the aminoglycosides, and vancomycin, which are excreted primarily by the kidney, must be altered in the neonate. Renal function diminishes physiologically in older patients. Such patients may have as much as a 50% reduction in renal function despite normal serum creatinine levels. Indeed, serum creatinine levels may be spuriously low because of the diminished muscle mass in the elderly. In such patients, the dosages of certain drugs, such as the penicillins, cephalosporins, and especially the aminoglycosides, the polymyxins, and vancomycin, must be reduced to avoid toxicity associated with excessively high serum concentrations.

That hepatic function is not fully developed in the neonate is clinically significant when such patients are given chloramphenicol, which is normally detoxified in the liver by conjugation. The presence of excessive levels of free chloramphenicol in the serum results from failure to conjugate chloramphenicol and may be associated with cardiovascular collapse and death (the so-called "gray syndrome") in the neonate if doses of the drug are not appropriately modified.

The administration of either sulfonamides, which displace bilirubin from albumin binding sites, or novobiocin, which inhibits hepatic conjugation and excretion of bilirubin, may cause hyperbilirubinemia and kernicterus in the neonate.

Tetracyclines avidly bind to developing bones and teeth. Because these agents readily cross the placenta, they can affect the development of deciduous teeth in the fetus if given to pregnant patients. When given to children up to 6 to 8 years of age, tetracyclines may also cause discoloration or enamel hyperplasia of the permanent teeth.

Adverse effects of antimicrobial agents are more frequent in the elderly than in younger patients. This incidence is related to prior exposures that predispose patients to hypersensitivity reactions, to nonspecific susceptibilities to such adverse reactions as hepatotoxicity from isoniazid and nephrotoxicity from cephaloridine and the polymyxins, and to cumulative toxic effects due to repeated exposure to drugs. These cumulative effects are exemplified by aminoglycoside ototoxicity, which may be cumulative on repeated exposure because cochlear hair cells damaged by prior exposure do not regenerate.

Genetic or Metabolic Abnormalities. The presence of genetic or metabolic abnormalities may also determine the efficacy or toxicity of antimicrobial agents. The rate at which certain drugs are inactivated by acetylation in the liver is genetically determined. The acetylation of isoniazid may produce metabolites that are associated with an increased incidence of hepatotoxicity in patients who are rapid acetylators. On the other hand, hepatotoxicity due to rifampin seems to be less frequent in rapid than in slow acetylators.

Patients who have glucose-6-phosphate dehydrogenase (G6PD) deficiency may develop significant hemolysis when exposed to various agents, including nalidixic acid, the sulfonamides, nitrofurantoin, furazolidine, dapsone (diaminodiphenylsulfone), and chloramphenicol. The sulfonamides also produce hemolytic reactions in patients with certain hemoglobinopathies such as hemoglobin H and hemoglobin Zurich.

Patients with diabetes mellitus pose unique problems for the physician contemplating antimicrobial therapy. The activity of sulfonylurea oral hypoglycemic agents, such as tolbutamide and chlorpropamide, may be potentiated by sulfonamides, which are structurally related to the hypoglycemic agents, and by chloramphenicol, which can inhibit the hepatic metabolism of these drugs and can thus prolong their activity. Many antimicrobial agents that concentrate in the urine, including cephalosporins, chloramphenicol, isoniazid, nalidixic acid, nitrofurantoin, penicillin, streptomycin, sulfanilamide, and tetracycline, can produce false-positive results for urine glucose levels if one uses tests, such as Benedict's test and Clinitest, that measure reducing substances in the urine. Antimicrobials in the urine do not interfere with glucose oxidase, which is the basis for measuring urine glucose levels by Dextrostix, Labstix, and similar products.

The microvascular disease of diabetes mellitus may impair the absorption of intramuscularly administered antibiotics. Thus, the intravenous route is preferred over the intramuscular, at least for initiating antimicrobial therapy for severe, life-threatening infections such as bacteremia or endocarditis in the diabetic.

In patients with iron-deficiency or pernicious anemia, chloramphenicol may temporarily impair the reticulocyte response to appropriate replacement therapy, but this fact is of more academic than practical interest.

Pregnancy and Lactation. The use of antimicrobial agents during pregnancy demands special considerations because of the potentiality for adverse effects on both mother and fetus and because of physiologic alterations that affect the pharmacokinetics of various drugs. All antimicrobials cross the placenta in varying degrees. Although none of these agents has proved to be teratogenic in man, studies in animals and bacteria suggest that metronidazole, in particular, should be avoided, especially during the first trimester of pregnancy. The penicillins, cephalosporins, and erythromycin have been used extensively in pregnant women and appear free of teratogenic potential in man. The safety of rifampin and trimethoprim is not known.

A number of antimicrobials are potentially toxic to the fetus or the pregnant patient. Tetracycline exhibits both possibilities. Because it crosses the placenta, this drug can interfere with fetal bone formation and dentition, as already noted. In addition, pregnant women appear to be uniquely susceptible to hepatotoxicity from the tetracyclines. This effect is dose-related. Some pregnant women given large doses of intravenous tetracycline (more than 1 to 2 g/day) have developed severe and occasionally fatal hepatitis with steatosis. Less frequently, pancreatitis and possibly renal damage have resulted from the administration of tetracycline to pregnant patients. Some have suggested that it is safe to administer tetracyclines orally in doses not exceeding 1 g/day; nevertheless, it is preferable to avoid these agents entirely during pregnancy.

A few authors have suggested that antimicrobials produce toxic effects on children exposed to these agents in utero. Mild eighth nerve damage has been documented in children whose mothers received streptomycin for treatment of tuberculosis during pregnancy. Less well documented is a claim that isoniazid can produce neurologic damage in children exposed to this drug in utero.

Because pregnant women have an increased plasma volume, the volume of distribution of various drugs is augmented. This change results in lower serum levels for some antibiotics, such as ampicillin, but the clinical significance of this observation remains to be proved.

Virtually all antibiotics are secreted, with varying degrees of efficiency, in breast milk. The drug concentrations are generally low, but under certain circumstances, these agents can have adverse effects on the nursing infant. The presence of nalidixic acid and sulfonamides in breast milk has caused hemolysis in infants with G6PD deficiency. Sulfonamides in breast milk may also be dangerous to premature babies because of the ability of this drug to displace bilirubin from albumin binding sites, as noted earlier. Recent evidence suggests, however, that for sulfisoxazole at least, the concentrations in breast milk are so low that they are unlikely to cause kernicterus.

Renal and Hepatic Abnormalities. The liver and the kidneys serve as the major routes of metabolism and excretion of most antimicrobials. Hence it is important to consider renal and hepatic function, both in choosing an agent and in determining its appropriate dose. Failure to do so may permit an accumulation of drugs, which in turn can have significant adverse effects.

Excessive levels of the penicillins may cause central nervous system abnormalities, such as myoclonus, seizures, or coma; such levels may also prolong the patient's bleeding time by interfering with platelet function. El-

Table 36–4. Antimicrobial Agents in Impaired Hepatic or Renal Function

Antimicrobial Agent	To be used with caution or in decreased doses in liver disease	Contraindicated in renal failure	Dosages to be modified in renal impairment	Dosages to be modified only in severe renal failure	Dosage not affected by renal function
Amikacin			X		
Amoxicillin				X	
Ampicillin				X	
Carbenicillin			X		
Cefaclor				X	
Cefamandole			X		
Cefazolin			X		
Cefoxitin			X		
Cefuroxime			X		
Cephalexin				X	
Cephaloridine		X			
Cephalothin				X	
Chloramphenicol	X				X
Clindamycin	X				X
Cloxacillin					X
Colistin			X		
Dicloxacillin					X
Doxycycline					X
Erythromycin	X				X
Ethambutal				X	
Gentamicin			X		
Isoniazid	X			X	
Kanamycin			X		
Lincomycin	X			X	
Methenamine		X			
Methicillin				X	
Minocycline					X
Nafcillin					X
Nalidixic acid					X
Nitrofurantoin		X			
Oxacillin					X
Para-aminosalicylic acid		X			
Penicillin G				X	
Polymyxin B			X		
Rifampin	X				X
Sisomicin			X		
Streptomycin			X		
Sulfadimidine					X
Sulfonamides (long-acting)		X			
Tetracyclines	X				
Tetracyclines (except doxycycline and minocycline)		X			
Ticarcillin			X		
Tobramycin			X		
Trimethoprim-sulfamethoxazole				X	
Vancomycin			X		

evated serum concentrations of the aminoglycosides are associated with the development of eighth nerve damage, both auditory and vestibular, and can cause neuromuscular blockade, as can the polymyxins. The tetracyclines, excluding minocycline and doxycycline, are contraindicated in patients with renal insufficiency because excessive serum concentrations are associated with a marked antianabolic effect that leads to rapid increases in azotemia and acidosis. Elevated serum levels of the tetracyclines can also produce toxic hepatitis. The reversible type of bone marrow toxicity from chloramphenicol occurs at lower doses in patients with impaired hepatic function. Table 36–4 lists antibiotics for which doses should be modified in patients with abnormal hepatic or renal function.

Site of Infection. Of all the host factors important in determining the success or failure of antimicrobial therapy, none deserves stronger consideration than the site of the infection. It is easy to measure serum concentrations of most antimicrobial agents, and such determinations are useful in monitoring therapy. Except in bacteremia, however, such concentrations may be different from the concentrations of drug present at the actual site of infection. One must provide adequate concentrations of the antimicrobial agent at the site of infection. In general, the clinician strives to achieve concentrations of antimicrobials at the site of infection that are at least equal to the MIC of the drug for the infecting microorganism. Ideally, concentrations should exceed the MIC several times, but even subinhibitory concentrations of antibiotics may have beneficial effects. Recent studies suggest that subinhibitory concentrations of various antibiotics may enhance phagocytosis of organisms, such as *Staphylococcus aureus*, and may diminish the capacity of certain bacteria to adhere to potential sites of infection. Despite such observations, most clinicians prefer to ensure highest achievable concentrations of antibiotics at the site of infection.

Antimicrobial agents vary in their binding affinities for serum proteins. Some, such as the aminoglycosides, exhibit little binding under physiologic conditions, whereas others, such as the semisynthetic penicillins, exhibit up to 96% protein binding. Antibiotics with low degrees of protein binding penetrate more easily to extravascular sites, such as interstitial and ascitic fluid. Only unbound antimicrobials are able to exhibit antibacterial activity. Binding to serum proteins is reversible, however, and thus even highly bound agents are clinically efficacious. Interestingly, raising a given drug's serum binding from 0 to 90% reduces the concentration of free drug in serum and tissues by only half. This phenomenon probably explains the difficulty of ascertaining the influence of protein binding on the clinical outcome.

Certain areas of the body present special difficulties in achieving adequate antibiotic concentrations, even after parenteral drug administration. These areas include the CSF, biliary tract, and vitreous humor of the eye.

The blood-brain barrier inhibits passage of a number of antimicrobials. Liquid-soluble agents, such as chloramphenicol, rifampin, isoniazid, and trimethoprim, produce higher CSF levels than the more highly ionized compounds such as the first- and second-generation cephalosporins and the aminoglycosides. Table 36–5 summarizes the ability of various agents to enter the CSF. Biliary penetration by antimicrobials also varies. Some agents, such as ampicillin, cefamandole, cefoxitin, third-generation cephalosporins, and doxycycline, are concentrated in the bile, whereas others, such as cephalothin and the aminoglycosides, are not concentrated there to any significant degree (Table 36–5). In the presence of complete biliary obstruction, no agents are effectively concentrated in the bile.

Antibiotic combinations may also be inadequate because of poor penetration of the vegetations of bacterial endocarditis and avascular areas such as bones and devitalized tissues. For this reason, high doses of parenteral antimicrobial agents are usually necessary in the therapy of endocarditis and acute osteomyelitis.

Table 36–5. Cerebrospinal Fluid and Bile Concentrations of Antimicrobials following Parenteral Administration

Antimicrobial Agent	Cerebrospinal Fluid Concentration				Bile Concentration		
	Adequate	Poor	Extremely poor	Inadequate data	Adequate	Poor	Inadequate data
Aminoglycosides			X			X	
Ampicillin		X			X		
Cephalosporins			X*		X†		
Chloramphenicol	X					X	
Clindamycin		X			X		
Doxycycline and minocycline				X	X		
Erythromycin		X			X		
Methicillin		X					
Nafcillin§		X			X		
Oxacillin§		X					
Penicillin§		X			X‡		
Polymyxins			X			X	
Rifampin		X					
Sulfonamides		X				X	
Tetracyclines		X			X		
Trimethoprim		X					X
Vancomycin§		X§			X		

*Cephalothin almost nil; cefoxitin and cefamandole penetrate better. The third-generation cephalosporins (cefotaxime, cefoperazone, moxalactam, ceftriaxone, and ceftazidime) penetrate well into cerebrospinal fluid.
†Cefamandole, cefazolin, cefoxitin, and third-generation cephalosporins, but not cephalothin.
‡Especially ampicillin and nafcillin.
§Adequate when given in high doses.

Even if one is able to achieve therapeutic concentrations of antibiotics at the site of infection, a number of local factors may vitiate the effectiveness of such agents. Abscess cavities provide a particularly difficult milieu for antimicrobial agents. The purulent material therein binds and inactivates polymyxins and aminoglycosides. The aminoglycosides are specifically inhibited by binding to DNA from lysed polymorphonuclear leukocytes. High concentrations of extracellular beta-lactamase produced by bacteria in abscess cavities may inactivate a number of the penicillins and cephalosporins. The acidic pH of abscess cavities antagonizes the effectiveness of the aminoglycosides and other agents, such as erythromycin, which are more effective at normal or alkaline pH. In addition, the low oxidation-reduction (redox) potential of most intra-abdominal abscesses renders aminoglycosides ineffective against facultative organisms because oxygen is required for bacterial uptake of the aminoglycosides. For all these reasons, surgical drainage of abscesses is almost always necessary for antibiotics to become effective.

Other Considerations. Other factors may also influence the effectiveness of antimicrobial drugs. Some agents such as the aminoglycosides are ineffective against intracellular organisms; this property likely explains the lack of clinical efficacy of antibiotics such as gentamicin and the cephalosporins in treating typhoid fever, despite the excellent in vitro activity of these drugs against *Salmonella typhi*. Antibiotics are often ineffective against infections in which foreign bodies are present. Thus, it is frequently necessary to remove or to replace prosthetic heart valves, joints, and vascular grafts to cure a contiguous infection. The mechanism by which foreign bodies potentiate infection is not clear, but they probably impair local host defense mechanisms that are required for optimal antibiotic efficiency.

> **Objective 36–2.** Determine the optimal dose and route of administration of antimicrobial agents.

With only a few exceptions, parenteral doses of antimicrobial agents produce higher serum levels than orally administered drugs. As a result, the oral route of administration is usually reserved for treating mild, benign infections. Oral agents vary in their absorption. Benzyl penicillin (penicillin G) is not acid stable and thus produces poor serum levels when taken with food. Equivalent doses of phenoxylmethyl penicillin (penicillin V) result in higher serum levels because the drug is acid stable. In patients with achlorhydria, the two antibiotics produce equivalent serum levels. Amoxicillin and, especially, bacampicillin and pivampicillin produce higher serum levels than ampicillin and are preferred when this class of drugs is administered orally to treat systemic extraurinary and extraintestinal infections.

The concomitant administration of milk, antacids, or iron-containing preparations impairs the oral absorption of the tetracyclines because these drugs form insoluble chelates with divalent cations such as Mg^{++}, Ca^{++}, or Fe^{++}. The aminoglycosides, polymyxins, and vancomycin are so poorly absorbed from the gastrointestinal tract that they must be given exclusively by the parenteral route. One exception is the use of oral vancomycin to treat pseudomembranous colitis due to *Clostridium difficile*, a pathologic process in which it is not necessary to achieve measurable serum drug concentrations to produce an adequate clinical response.

The parenteral route of administration is usually reserved for those agents for which oral absorption is insufficient to produce adequate serum levels or for infections in which it is necessary to achieve high serum and tissue concentrations of the drug. The intramuscular route is usually indicated for colistin (polymyxin E) and the aminoglycosides. In most instances, this route ensures adequate serum levels. In severely ill patients, however, especially those in shock or with diabetes mellitus, it is preferable to begin parenteral therapy intravenously because of unpredictable drug absorption under such circumstances. Chloramphenicol is not reliably absorbed when given intramuscularly and thus must be given intravenously when the parenteral route is indicated.

Intravenous administration permits the delivery of high concentrations of drugs with a minimum of discomfort to the patient and is preferred when treating serious infections such as endocarditis, meningitis, and acute osteomyelitis. Despite much investigation, no consensus exists as to whether continuous infusion or bolus administration is preferable. Continuous infusion is often easier to maintain, especially with modern infusion equipment. One possible advantage of bolus infusion is that the higher peak serum levels thus attained favor diffusion of drugs into avascular areas, such as vegetations and possibly abscess cavities. Whether this ability confers significant clinical advantages remains to be determined.

In treating meningitis with agents such as the aminoglycosides, polymyxins, and first- and second-generation cephalosporins, all of which cross the blood-brain barrier with difficulty, it is necessary to employ intrathecal or intraventricular therapy. Direct instillation of antibiotics into the eye, usually by subtenon injection, may be required in endophthalmitis because of the poor penetration of most agents into the vitreous humor. Direct instillation of antibiotics into peritoneal, pericardial, or synovial fluid is usually unnecessary because all parenterally administered antibiotics penetrate into these body fluids well.

Objective 36–3. Describe an effective way to monitor therapeutic response.

In many patients, it is possible to monitor therapeutic response on clinical grounds alone. Thus the subsidence of fever, the disappearance of local signs of infection, and the return of a sense of well-being in the patient all signify an appropriate response. When such changes are documented, more formal monitoring is not usually necessary. An apparent failure to respond clinically may not be due to the ineffectiveness of the antimicrobial agents themselves. For example, a persistent fever may be due to the presence of a localized collection of infectious material that requires surgical drainage, or it may be the result of a hypersensitivity reaction to one of the drugs administered. Other explanations for real or apparent failure to respond to antimicrobial therapy may be found among the various host factors discussed earlier. The physician should always review these factors when a patient fails to respond to treatment.

Measuring serum concentrations of antibiotics may be useful to avoid excessive levels of certain drugs, such as the aminoglycosides, chloramphenicol, and vancomycin, which are associated with toxicity. In addition, such measurements may be used to ascertain that serum concentrations are adequate, especially in patients who have unusually rapid clearance rates of drugs, such as burn patients, or in whom the dose has been modified for hepatic or renal failure. The serum bactericidal titer or the serum antimicrobial dilution titer may also determine the efficacy of antibiotic therapy. In this test, serial dilutions of the patient's serum after antibiotic administration are incubated with an inoculum of the infecting organism, and the highest dilution that inhibits or kills the organism is determined. This test has been used to monitor therapy in bacterial endocarditis, septicemia, infections in cancer and neutropenic patients, osteomyelitis, septic arthritis, and empyema. An inhibitory or bactericidal titer of 1:8 or greater signifies a high likelihood of success. Not all agree on the techniques used to perform and to interpret this test, however, and this controversy has hindered the widespread application of this method.

At all times during a course of antimicrobial therapy, the physician must keep in mind the myriad adverse effects of antimicrobial agents, be they due to hypersensitivity, direct toxicity, or interaction with concomitantly administered drugs. Such reactions occur in up to 30% of patients, depending upon the drug and length of therapy. Proper monitoring of laboratory studies, that is, following serum creatinine concentrations in patients receiving aminoglycosides, polymyxins, and vancomycin and watching hematologic parameters in patients taking chloramphenicol, and paying careful attention to minor complaints such as tinnitus and vertigo, which may represent early warning signs of eighth nerve damage due to aminoglycosides, are necessary to detect such adverse reactions as early as possible. By so doing, serious damage can often be averted.

In conclusion, although antimicrobial agents are invaluable, their effective use requires more than simply administering a drug to which a microorganism has been shown to be effective in vitro. Careful attention to host factors, thoughtful consideration of appropriate dose and route of administration, and close monitoring of therapeutic response are all important prerequisites for success.

SUGGESTED READINGS

Bennett, W.M., et al.: Drug therapy in renal failure: dosing guidelines for adults. Ann. Intern. Med., 93:62, 1980.

Calderwood, S.B., and Moellering R.C., Jr.: Common adverse effects of antibacterial agents on major organ systems. Surg. Clin. North Am., 60:65, 1980.

Eliopoulos, G.E., and Moellering, R.C., Jr.: Principles of antibiotic therapy. Med. Clin. North Am., 66:3, 1982.

McCracken, G.H., Jr.: Pharmacological basis for antimicrobial therapy in newborn infants. Am. J. Dis. Child., 128:407, 1974.

Moellering, R.C., Jr.: Special consideration of the use of antimicrobial agents during pregnancy, post partum and in the newborn. Clin. Obstet. Gynecol., 22:373, 1979.

Moellering, R.C., Jr.: Factors influencing the clinical use of antimicrobial agents in elderly patients. Geriatrics, 33:83, 1978.

Murray, B.E., and Moellering, R.C., Jr.: Patterns and mechanisms of antibiotic resistance. Med. Clin. North Am., 62:899, 1978.

Peterson, L.R., and Gerding, D.N.: Influence of protein binding of antibiotics on serum pharmacokinetics and extravascular penetration: clinically useful concepts. Rev. Infect. Dis., 2:340, 1980.

Pessayre, D., Allemand, H., and Benhamou, J.P.: Effets des maladies du foie et des voies biliaires sur le métabolisme des médicaments. Nouv. Presse Med., 6:3209, 1977.

Reller, L.B., and Stratton, C.W.: Serum dilution test for bactericidal activity. II. Standardization and correlation with antimicrobial assays and susceptibility tests. J. Infect. Dis., 136:196, 1977.

Weinstein, L.: Common sense (clinical judgment) in the diagnosis and antibiotic therapy of etiologically undefined infections. Pediatr. Clin. North Am., 15:141, 1968.

Weinstein, L., and Dalton, A.C.: Host determinants of response to antimicrobial agent. N. Engl. J. Med., 279:467, 524, 580, 1968.

Index

Page numbers in *italics* refer to figures; page numbers followed by "t" refer to tables; page numbers followed by "b" refer to boxes.

Abdominal infections, 249–266
   antibiotic therapy for, 262
   bacteria most often associated with, 259t
Abdominal surgical procedures, prophylaxis in, 264t–265t
Abscess(es),
   brain. See *Brain abscess(es)*
   Brodie's, 43b
      tomogram of, *433*
   dental, 61
   epidural, 461–462
   fever in drug addicts and, 163
   hepatic, *252*, 252–253
   intra-abdominal, 254–256, 255t
      microbial ecology of, 258b
   lateral pharyngeal, *57*, 57–58
   obstruction of left colon, *256*
   periapical, 61
   periodontal, 61–62
   perirectal, 253
   peritonsillar, 55–56
      repeated, 58
      treatment of, 56
   renal, 285
   retropharyngeal, 31, *56*, 56–57
      treatment of, 56
   subhepatic, 253
Acne, 387–388, *388*
   folliculitis, furunculosis, and hidradenitis, differences among, 387t
Acquired immune deficiency syndrome (AIDS), 382, 533b
   fever in drug addicts and, 169
Actinomyces israelii, 375
Actinomycosis in lymph node, *377*

Acuminate condylomas, *332*
   intraurethral, *332*
Acute paralysis of limbs, 489
Adenitis, 7
   pyogenic organisms and, 370–372
   suppurative cervical, streptococcal pharyngitis and, 44
Adenopathy, infectious, 369–383
   causes of, axillary, 369–370
      bovine tuberculous, 372
      cervical, 369–370
      miscellaneous, 375–377
      viral infections, 375
   inguinal. See *Infectious inguinal adenopathy*
   isolated inguinal, diagnostic procedure, 377–378
   superficial, caused by atypical mycobacteria, 372–373
      caused by mycobacteria, 372–373
      causes of, animal origin, and treatment of, 376t
      differential diagnosis of, 370t
   transmitted by animals, 374t
   zoonotic, 373
      cat-scratch disease, 374
      pasteurellosis, 375
      plague, 375
      toxoplasmosis, 373
      tularemia, 373–374
Adenovirus(es), 503b
Aeromonas hydrophila, cellulitis and, 15
Amebiasis, 572b
   drugs active against, 233t
   hepatic, 570–571
      clinical manifestations of, 570–571
      treatment of, 571
   intestinal, 231–232

Amebiasis, intestinal *(Continued)*
    clinical features of, 232
    diagnosis of, 232
    pathogenesis of, 231–232
    treatment of, 232
Aminoglycosides, pregnancy and, 365
Anaerobes, antibiotics effective against, 262t
Anaerobic bacilli, gram-negative, features of, 262t
Anaerobic bacteria, identification of, 258–261
    nontoxigenic anaerobes, 258
    toxigenic anaerobes, 258
Anaerobic infections, clues for recognizing, 260t
Anemia, helminthiasis and, 239
Angina, Ludwig's, 62
Angiography, contrast, infective endocarditis and, 197
Animal bites, preventing infection of, 11–15
Anthrax, 16
    cutaneous, treatment of, 17
Antibiotic(s), acquired resistance to, 554t
    beta-lactum, 365
    coryza and, 22
    disc susceptibility test (Kirby-Bauer), 261
    human breast milk excretion and, 366t
    pregnancy and, 365–366
        general, 365
        specific, 365–366
    urinary, requirements for optimal, 299b
Antibody function testing, 535
Antimicrobial agents, in impaired hepatic or renal function, 583t
    optimal dose and route of administration, 585–586
Antimicrobial susceptibility, 577–579
    testing techniques, 577–579
    universally susceptible organisms, 577
Antimicrobial treatment, principles of, 575–587
Antimycotic drugs, major characteristics of, 140t–141t
Antinuclear antibody test, 160
Antistreptolysin O (ASLO), 160
Antituberculosis chemoprophylaxis, indications for, 120
Antituberculous agents, dosages, side effects, and activity of major, 119t
    pregnancy and, 365
Appendicitis, 250–251
Arboviral infections, 572b
Arbovirus(es), 456
Arenavirus(es), 456–457
Argyll-Robertson pupil, 340
Arthritis, bacterial, 442–445
    joint aspiration, 443
    rheumatoid, 147
    septic. See *Septic arthritis*
Arthropod vectors, 563
Ascariasis, treatment of, 246
Ascaris lumbricoides, 242
Aspergillosis, 138–142
    lung tissue biopsy in, *137*
Aspergillus, 134–136
Aspergillus fumigatus fungal ball, *136*
Aspiration pneumonia, 96
    antimicrobial therapy for, 98
    diagnosis of, 97–98
    treatment of, 98
Atelectasis, 79
Athlete's foot, *396*
Automated reagin test (ART), 342

Autonomic urogenital syndrome, 325

Bacille Calmette Guerin (BCG) adenitis, 373
Bacille Calmette Guerin (BCG) test, 566
Bacille Calmette Guerin (BCG) vaccination, 122
    tuberculin skin test and, 117
Bacillus anthracis, 16
Bacteremia, blood cultures and, 171
    number of, 172
    timing of, 172–173
    enterococcal, 178
    gram-negative, 175–177
    negative blood cultures and, 184
    organism responsible for, 174–175
    positive blood cultures and, 184
    septicemia and, 171–187
    staphylococcal, 177–178
Bacteria, pyogenic, 369
    susceptibility of, to antimicrobial agents, 580t
Bacterial pathogens by anatomic site, most frequent, 578t–579t
Bacteriuria, asymptomatic, 349
Bacteroides fragilis, 8, 20, 97
    polymorphic aspect of, *261*
Bacteroides melaninogenicus, pneumonia due to, 97
Balloon catheter, 79
Baronellosis, 572b
Behçet's disease, 66
Biopsy, lung, 86
    cystlike structures in, *540*
    needle, of tuberculous kidney, 294
    of skin lesions, 160
    transbronchoscopic, 539
Blastomyces dermatitidis, 134
Blastomycosis, *135*, 138
    North American, *400*
Blood collection, aseptic precautions for, 173
Blood count, 535
Blood culture(s), bacteremia and, 171–173
    indications for, 172t
    infective endocarditis and, 199–200
    procedure, acceleration of, 173
Bone and joint infections, 431–449
    bone scans, 433
    depth of, 431
    fever in drug addicts and, 165–166
    roentgenograms, 432–433
    signs of, 431
Bone or joint prosthetic material, infection adjacent to, 439–440
    diagnostic problems, 439–440
    therapeutic problems, 440
Bone scans, 433
Bone versus joint lesions, 431–432
Bordetella pertussis, 107, 109b
Borreliosis, 404–405
Botulism, 233, 489–491
    clinical evidence of, 489–490
        gastrointestinal signs as, 489–490
        paralysis as, 490
    epidemiologic evidence of, 490
    in Canada, France, and United States, 491t
    infant, 490
    laboratory confirmation of diagnosis of, 490
    pathogenesis of, 491t
    treatment of, 490–491
Bovine tuberculous adenopathy, 372

Index

Brain abscess(es), 458–461
  causes of, 460
  clinical features of, 460
  treatment of, 460
Branhamella catarrhalis, 26
Brodie's abscess, 436
  tomogram of, *433*
Bronchiolitis, acute, causes of, 103
  cardiorespiratory decompensation in, 104
  diagnosis of, 103–104
  duration of, 105
  prognosis of, 104–105
  treatment of, 105
Bronchitis, chronic, 78
Bronchopneumonia, 80, *83*
  measles and, 419
Bronchopulmonary infection, causes of, 108
  neonatal, 108
Bronchoscopy, fiberoptic, 539
  fiberscopic, 86
Brucellosis, 179–180
  meningitis due to, 477
Burns, 7
  third degree, 8

CAMP test, *364*
Campylobacter fetus, 228b
Candida, 138
Candida albicans, 68, *310*
  cellulitis and, 15
  urethritis and, 321
  vaginitis and, 313–316
Candida onychomycosis, 397
Candidemia, diagnostic management of, 176b
  manifestations of, 176b
  risk factors of, 176b
  treatment of, 176b
Candidiasis, 143. See also *Moniliasis*
  chronic hyperplastic, 60
Canker sores, 65
Cardiac tamponade, 208
  pericardiocentesis in, 208
  treatment of, 208
Cardiorespiratory decompensation, signs of incipient, 104
Catheter(s), balloon, 79
  maintenance, guidelines for, 300–301
  Swan-Ganz, 79
Catheter-associated urinary tract infections, 557
Cat-scratch disease, 374
Cellophane tape test, *243*
Cellulitis, *Aeromonas hydrophila* and, 15
  air in retropharyngeal space and, *58*
  anaerobic, 163–164
  deep, 18–20, 257t
    indications of, 18
  extensive necrotizing, *58*
  fever in drug addicts and, 163
  gangrenous, 18
  Haemophilus influenzae and, 15
  orbital, differential diagnosis of, 16t
    treatment of, 17
  Pasteurella multocida, 16
    treatment of, 17
  periorbital, 15
  Proteus species and, 15
    differential diagnosis of, 16t
  Staphylococcus aureus and, 15
  Streptococcus pneumoniae and, 15
  Streptococcus pyogenes and, 15
  superficial, 14–17
  synergistic necrotizing, 20
  treatment of, 17–18
Center for Disease Control (CDC), United States, 561
Central nervous system (CNS) infections, initial diagnostic studies, 452–454
  cerebrospinal fluid examination, 452–454
  lumbar puncture technique, 452
  localized symptoms of, 458–463
  medical history, 451
  physical examination, 451–452
  processing of cerebrospinal fluid specimens in, 453t
Cephalosporin(s), 8
  third-generation, 185t
Cerebrospinal fluid (CSF), bile concentrations of antimicrobials following parenteral administration and, 585t
  examination of, 452–454, 466–468
    central nervous system infections and, 452–454
Cervicitis, causes of, 311
  chlamydial, 312–313
  treatment of, 313
Chagas' disease, 571
Chalazion, *508*
Chancre, 336
Chancroid (soft chancre), 326
  diagnosis of, 326–327
Chemoprophylaxis, 567
  antituberculosis, indications for, 120
  defined, 263
  malaria, 566t, 567
  other diseases, 568
Chemotaxis, 5–6
Chest roentgenogram(s), abnormal, 114–115
  indications for, 77
  infective endocarditis and, 199
  other indications for, 78
  staphylococcal pleuropulmonary infection and, 110
Chickenpox. See *Varicella*
Chlamydia trachomatis, 108–109, *320*, *323*, *380*
  neonatal infection, determination of, 108
Chlamydiae, 504b
  classification of according to serotypes and disorders, 321t
  infections caused by, pregnancy and, 361
Chloramphenicol, pregnancy and, 366
Cholecystectomy, typhoid fever and, 219
Cholecystitis, acute, 251–252
Cholera, 229, 572b, 373
  immunization, 566
  pathophysiology and epidemiology of, 229b
  treatment of, 229
Choleric toxin and colibacillary enterotoxin, activity of, *230*
Chorioretinitis, acute, *524*
  cicatricial, *524*
Citrobacter, 286b
Clostridia, 234b

Clostridia (Continued)
  infection caused by, 7
  myonecrosis caused by, 18
Clostridium perfringens, 18, 307, 308
  gas gangrene, 19t
Clostridium tetani, 8, 9
Clue cell, 311
Coagulation, disseminated intravascular, 182
Coccidioidal, 546
Coccidioides immitis, 132–134
Coccidioidin skin test, 130
Coccidioidomycosis, 133, 138
Cold sores, 65
Colitis, amebic, 573
Complement activity, measurement of, 535
Computerized axial tomographic (CT) scanning, 453, 458
  and infective endocarditis, 197
Condyloma latum, 341
  syphilis and, 339
Congestive heart failure, 104
Conjunctival flora, 502t
Conjunctivitis, 363, 505–511, 512t–513t
  chlamydial, 363
  follicular, 510
Contrast angiography, and infective endocarditis, 197
Coombs' test, 160
Cornea (keratitis), infections of, 514t–515t
Corneal ulcer, staphylococcal, 516
Corynebacterium diphtheriae, 45, 48
Coryza, simple, 21
Cough, rhinorrhea and, 23
Countercurrent immunoelectrophoresis (CIE), 217, 540
  Cryptococcus neoformans and, 138
Coxsackievirus A, and viral pericarditis, 208
Coxsackievirus B, and viral myocarditis, 210
  and viral pericarditis, 208
Cranial meninges, 459
Croup, 24, 32. See also Laryngotracheobronchitis, viral
Cryptococcosis, 142
Cryptococcus neoformans, 137–138, 484, 484b, 544–545
  diagnosis of, 544–545
  signs and symptoms of, 544
  treatment of, 545
Cutaneous flora, normal, 4t
Cutaneous hemorrhagic eruption, 403–405
  borreliosis, 404
  endocarditis, 404
  meningococcemia, 403
  pneumococcal and gram-negative septicemias, 403–404
  viral infections, 405
Cutaneous manifestations of serious infectious disease, 404t
Cyanosis, 31
Cystitis, "honeymoon," 288
  in young women, 296–298
  relapsing, 288
  simple, 288
  viral, 286
Cytomegalovirus (CMV), 267, 359, 359b, 455–456
  fever in drug addicts and, 168–169

infections with, 357–358
  diagnosis of, 358
  incidence of, 357–358
  prevention of, 358
  viral transmission of, 358

Dacryoadenitis, 505
Dacryocystitis, purulent, 508
Dane particle, 271, 275
  diagram of, 271
"Daughter" cells, 134
Dengue, 571
Dermatitis, exfoliative, 408–411
Dermatophytosis, 393
Diarrhea, acute, with gastroenteritis, 226
  acute infectious, 221–236
    determining cause of, 222–223
    neonate, 235–236
    principal causes of, 223t
  antibiotic therapy and, 233
  campylobacter, caused by, 228–229
  cholera-like, 223
  clinical features of, 223
  diagnostic tests for, 224
    stool culture, 224
  dysenteric, 223
  enteropathogenic viruses, caused by, 230–231
  Escherichia coli, caused by, 227–228
    pathogenesis of, 227–228
    treatment of, 228
  infant with, fluid/electrolyte replacement in, 222t
  other bacterial, 229–230
  traveler's, 227
  viral, 224
  volume depletion, evaluation of, 221–222
  water and electrolyte depletion caused by severe, 222t
Diarrhea or dysentery in travelers, acute, diagnostic approaches in, 571t
Dicloxacillin, 17
Digestive tract below diaphragm, normal flora of, 259t
Diphtheria, 31, 45
  alimentary disorders in infants and, 489
  antibiotic therapy in, 49
  diagnosis of, 46–48
  immunization, 47, 50
  immunofluoresence tests, 48
    pertussis, 566
    polyvalent preparations, 50
  laryngeal, 31, 32
  malignant, 46
  other therapeutic measures in, 49–50
  paralysis and, 498
  pharyngitis and, 37
  serosanguineous discharge and, 23
  serotherapy and, 48
  specific therapy in, 48–49
  throat culture in, 48
Diphtheria antitoxin, hypersensitivity reactions and, 49
Diphtheria toxin, 46b
Diphtheroids, 48
Disseminated gonococcal infection (DGI), 179
Distomiasis, 572b
Diverticulitis, 251
Dressler's syndrome, 147, 157

Drug(s), antimycotic, 140t–141t
  overdose, and fever, 165
  therapy, host factors in. See *Host factors in drug therapy*
Dyspnea, 24
  inspiratory, of rapid onset, 33
  mononucleosis and, 53
  progressive onset of, 32–33

Earache, rhinorrhea and, 23–24
Early antigen (EA), 52
Echocardiogram, infective endocarditis and, 200
Ecthyma gangrenosum, 411
Edema,
  of the uvula, 56
  pulmonary, 79
Electrocardiogram, infective endocarditis and, 199
Electrophoresis, protein, 160
Elek test, 48
Embolism, major artery, and infective endocarditis, 198
Embolization, catastrophic, 167
  septic pulmonary, 167
Emphysema, 78
  in infants, 106
Empyema, antibiotic therapy for, 151
  organisms responsible for, 150t
  sterile, 150
  subdural, 461
    associated with meningitis, 461
    clinical features of, 361
    diagnosis of, 461
    treatment of, 461
  surgical treatment of, 151
Encephalitis, 65
  agents associated with postinfectious and postvaccination, 458t
  arboviral, 457t
  disturbances of consciousness in, 452
  infectious nonviral causes of acute, 455t
  treatable causes of, 454
Encephalomyelitis, following infection and vaccination, 457
Endocarditis, candidal, 166, 167
  characteristics of left- and right-sided, 166t
  chest roentgenograms and, 199
  cutaneous hemorrhagic eruption and, 404
  in drug addicts, fever and, 166–167
    therapy for, 168t
  infective. See *Infective endocarditis*
  native-valve, definitive therapy of, 202t
  staphylococcal tricuspid, 165
Endometritis, 316–317
Endophthalmitis, 511, 517t
  immediate treatment of, 511–518
  principles of evaluation, 511
Enterobacter, 186b
Enterococci, group D, 286b
Enterocolitis, 223
  necrotizing, 364
    acute, 236
  pseudomembranous. See *Pseudomembranous enterocolitis*
Enterotoxins, 228

Enteroviruses, 456, 480
Enzyme-linked immunosorbent assay (ELISA), 160, 231, 350
  Chagas myocarditis and, 212
  rotavirus and, 224
Eosinophilia, helminthiasis and, 239
  tropical, 81
Epidemic, definition of, 558b
Epidemic parotitis. See *Mumps*
Epididymo-orchitis, 318, 329–330
  diagnosis of, 330
  treatment of, 330
Epidural abscess, 461–462
  in spine, 462
Epiglottitis, 32
  acute, 31, 33, 34
    antibiotic treatment of, 33
Epstein-Barr nuclear antigen (EBNA), 52–53
Epstein-Barr virus (EBV), 51, 52, 54b, 267, 456
  cancer and, 54b
  diagnosis confirmation of, 53
  epidemiology of, 54b
  pathology of, 54b
  viral myocarditis and, 210
  viral pericarditis and, 208
Erysipelas, 15
Erysipelothrix infections, 17
Erysipelothrix rhusiopathiae, 17
  treatment of, 17
Erythema, 408–411
  infectiosum, 422
  multiforme, 66
Erythromycin, 17
Escherichia coli, 285b
  cellulitis and, 15
  enterotoxins from, 228b
Ewing's sarcoma, 436
Exanthem(s), diagnosis of, 413
  epidemiologic features of, 412t
  infectious, 411
  maculopapular, 414t
  with vesicular rashes, 416t
Exanthema subitum, 422
Exposure, occupational, fever and, 157
Eye infections, 501–528
  clinical evaluation of, 501–502
    nervous tissue, 502
    nonvascularized tissue, 502
    tissue fluid, 502
    vascularized tissue, 501–502
  microbiologic diagnosis of, 503–505
    smears, 504
    special cases, 504–505
    specimen collection, 503–504
  principal bacteria in, 502t
  types of, 502
Eyebrows and eyelids, infections of, 505, 506t

Fasciitis, necrotizing, 19–20
  in drug users, 163–164
Favus, 397–398
Felon (whitlow), 389
Fetal defenses against infection, 353
Fever(s), 153–161

Fever(s) *(Continued)*
  as sign of serious illness, 154–156
  blisters. See *Cold sores*
  drug users and, 162–169, 164t
    bone and joint infections, 431–449
    tetanus, 167
  drug-associated, 157
  factitious, 157
  in infants, 153
  in pregnancy, 360–361
    other disorders, 361
    urinary tract infection, 361
    viral infection, 361
  isolated, 157–158
    clinical features of, 157–158
    laboratroy and radiologic findings of, 158
  mechanisms of, 154b
  or unknown origin, 158–159
    chief metabolic causes of, 159t
    classification of, 158–159, 159t
  paratyphoid, 215–219, 405
  patients, returned from tropical country, 570
  polypnea and, 153
  Pontiac, 94
  pulmonary embolism and, 156
  rat-bite, 12
  rheumatic. See *Rheumatic fever*
  rhinorrhea and, 23
  Rocky Mountain spotted, 405, 407, 479
  scarlet, 423–425
  severity of, 153–156
  sore throat and, 37–59
  thrombophlebitis, 156
  tobia, 407
  tropical diseases and, 157
  typhoid. See *Typhoid fever*
  viral hemorrhagic, 157, 406t
  with localized signs and symptoms, 156
  without localized signs and symptoms, 156–157
Fifth disease, 422
Filariasis, 572b
Fistula(s), orodermal, 58
FitzHugh-Curtis syndrome, 312
Flu syndrome. See *Influenza*
Fluorescent treponemal antibody absorption, 326, 340, 343, 344
Folliculitis, 388, 389
  treatment of, 389–390
Food poisoning, bacterial, 573
  main causes of, 232–233
  origin of, 234t
Foreign body ingestion, 33
Fournier's gangrene, 19
Francisella tularensis, 5
FTA-ABS. See *Fluorescent treponemal antibody absorption*
Fungal infections. See also *specific infections*
  acute primary, 125–143
  of skin and various tissues, 391t
Fungus, description of, 143b
Furunculosis, 388–389
  treatment of, 389–390
Fusobacterium, 16

Gallbladder and biliary tract, infections of, 269

Gangrene, 182
Gardnerella vaginalis, 308
  vaginitis and, 316
Gas gangrene, spontaneous, 18
Genital herpes, 327, 328. See also *Genital infections*
  diagnosis of, 327
  primary infection, 327
  recurrences, 327
  treatment of, 327
Genital infections, 303–334
  culture, 308–311
  female, 305–306
    causes of, 307t
    clinical diagnostic clues to, 306t
    site of infection and microbial causes of, 308t
  gynecologic examination, 305–306
  infected patients, contacts of, 304–305
    follow-up of, 303–304
  male, epididymo-orchitis, 318
    genital ulcerations, 318
    prostatitis, 318
    urethritis, 318
    venereal warts, 318
  microscopic examinations, 307–308
  patient and physician relationship, 303
  pregnancy and, 361
    risk factors, 362–363
  reports to health authorities, 305
    medical history of patients, 305
  specimen collection methods, 306–307
Giardiasis, 231
Gingivectomy, 63
Gingivitis, 63
  acute necrotizing ulcerative, 63
    treatment of, 63–64
Glabrous skin, 392–395
  dermatophytosis of, 393
  tinea versicolor, 393–395
Glomerulonephritis, erysipelas and, 15
Gonococcal infection(s), treatment for, 314t–315t
  disseminated, 179
Gonococcemia, 179, 447
Gonorrhea, 179, 311–312
  pregnancy and, 361
Gooseberry jelly sputum, 90
Gram stain of bacterial pus, *260*
Gram-negative bacilli meningitis, 472
Granuloma inguinale, 327–329
  diagnosis of, 327–329
  treatment of, 329
  tuberculous, *121*
Gray syndrome, 581
Grippe. See *Influenza*
Guillain-Barré syndrome, causes of, 495
  infectious causes of, 493t
  influenza immunization and, 75
Gummas, 340
Gynecologic examinations, 305–306
Gynecologic infection, causes of, 306–311

Haemophilus influenzae, 16, 17, 33, 74
  bacterial meningitis and, 470–471
  cellulitis and, 15
  mortality rate in, 90

otitis and, 29–30
plasmid-mediated resistance of, 27b
pneumonias due to, 90
satellite phenomenon of, *471*
septic arthritis and, 446
sinusitis and, 26
transtracheal aspirate of, *87*
type B vaccine, 486
Hair follicle, *387*
Hand-foot-mouth disease, 428–429
Headache, rhinorrhea and, 24
Helminthiasis, causes of, 238t
  symptoms of, anemia, 239
    cutaneous larva migrans (creeping eruption), 239
    eosinophilia, 239
    gastrointestinal, 239
    intestinal, 238–239
    pneumonia in immunocompromised host, 239
    pneumonitis, 239
    pruritus ani and vulvae, 238
  treatment of intestinal, 247t
Helminthic infections, intestinal, 237–248
  treatment of, 246–248, 247t
Helminths, characteristics of, 240b
  eggs of intestinal, *242*
  in humans, cestodes, 240
    nematodes, 240
    trematodes, 240
  intestinal, biologic cycles of, 241t
  patterns of biologic cycle, *241*
Hematogenous bone infection, age and microbiologic findings in, 435t
Hematogenous osteomyelitis,
  acute, *439*
  adults for, treatment of, 437t
  roentgenograms and bone scan of, *434*
Hemianopia, left, *460*
Hemorrhages, measles and, 419
Heparin therapy, in thrombophlebitis and embolism, 156
Hepatitis, acute and chronic, distinction between, 274–275
  B Virus, acute viral, 272
    Guillain-Barré syndrome and, 495
    homosexual activity and, 272
    pregnancy and, 365
  chronic, biochemical features of, 275
    clinical features of, 275
    treatment of, 275
  clinical and biochemical surveillance of, 273–274
  fever in drug addicts and, 169
  granulomatous, causes of and diagnostic tests for, 276t
    sarcoidosis and, 277
    tuberculosis and, 277
  immunization and preventive measures, 274
  non-healing, 275
  prognostic factors in, hepatocellular insufficiency, 273–274
    infection itself, 273
    previous liver condition, 273
  treatment of acute, 273
  viral, 270–273
    Reye's syndrome and, 273
  viruses,
    non-A and non-B, 272
    possible protection against, 274t
    three principal, 271t
Hepatosplenomegaly, 116
Herpangina, 38
  vesicles, *39*
Herpes genitalis, 336
Herpes labialis. See *Cold sores*
Herpes simplex virus (HSV), 64–65, 454–455
  meningitis and, 481
  oral ulceration and, 541
  primary infection, 65
  recurrent infection, 65
  type 1 (HSV-1), 64, 427
    type 2 (HSV-2) and, distinction between, 64t
  type 2 (HSV-2), 64, 327, 358, 427
    type 1 (HSV-1) and, distinction between, 64t
Herpes varicella-zoster virus, 359–360, 455
Herpesvirus(es), Guillain-Barré syndrome and, 495
Heterophile antibody, serologic tests for, 52
Hidradenitis, 389
  treatment of, 389–390
Histocytes, *129*
Histoplasma, 546
Histoplasma capsulatum, 129, 130–132
Histoplasmosis, *128*, 138
  ocular, 526
Hodgkin's disease, 100, 544–546
  cryptococcosis and, 127
  stage IV-B, 546
    causes of infection, 546
    prevention of, 546
    treatment of, 546
Hookworm infection, treatment of, 247
Host defense mechanisms, defects in, 531t
  infections not requiring investigation of, 534–535
  infections requiring investigation of, 535–536
    further tests, 536
    screening studies, 535
    treatment of, 536
Host factors in drug therapy, 579–586
  age of patient, 579–581
  antimicrobial efficacy and safety, 581t
  genetic or metabolic abnormalities, 581–582
  other considerations, 585
  pregnancy and lactation, 582
  renal and hepatic abnormalities, 583–584
  site of infection, 584–585
Host infections, immunocompromised, 529–549
  cellular defense mechanisms, 529–530
    lymphocytes, 530
    macrophages, 530
    neutrophilic polymorphonuclear leukocytes, 529–530
  humoral defense mechanisms, 530
    complement system, 530
  infections that frequently cause, 534t
  opportunistic pathogens in,
    Nocardia asteroides, 541b
    Pneumocystis carinii, 541b
    Strongyloides stercoralis, 541b
  oral gut decontamination and, 547
  prevention of, 546–548
    catheter maintenance, 547
    general measures, 547

Host infections, prevention of *(Continued)*
   laminar air flow isolation, 547
   miscellaneous techniques, 548
  structural and functional defense mechanisms, 530–531
Hutchinson's triad, 341
Hypercapnia, 104
Hyperthermia, malignant, 153
Hypovolemia, 181
Hypoxemia, 78, 104

Immune effusions, 147
Immune system, defects in, 531–534
Immunity, schematic representation of, 371
Immunization(s), antimeningococcal, 567
  antityphoid, 219
  calendar, 565t
  cholera, 566
  combined, 567
  diphtheria, 47, 50
  influenza, 74t
  plague, 567
  pneumococcal, 100
  poliomyelitis, 566
  schedule, 567
  tetanus, 10t, 13t, 566
Immunofluoresence tests, in diphtheria, 48
Immunoglobulin levels, quantitation of, 535
Impetigo, 385–387, 386
Indirect fluorescent antibody (IFA) test, 350
Indirect hemagglutination (IHA) test, 350
Infarction, myocardial, fever and, 156–157
Infecting organism, 575–577
  drug therapy based on culture results, 575
  drug therapy in infections of unknown origin, 577
  rapid identification of pathogens, 575–577
Infection(s). See also specific infections
  abdominal, 249–266
  capable of transplacental transmission, 358–360
    herpes simplex virus 2, 358–359
    listeria bacteremia, 360
    syphilis, 360
    varicella-zoster, 359–360
  defense agents against, 529–531
  fetal defenses against, 353b
  fever and, 160
  intestinal helminthic, 237–248
  intra-abdominal, therapy for, 261–263
  intravenous catheter, 542
  oral, 541–542
  other types of recurrent, 534–535
  pelvic, 253–254
  pinworm, 238
  pregnancy and, 349–368
  with rashes, 403–429
  wound, 256–258
Infectious inguinal adenopathy(ies), 378t
  nonvenereal causes of, 378–379
    common bacterial infections, 378–379
    plague, 379
    tick-borne infections, 379
  venereal causes of, 379
    chancroid, 379–380
    chlamydial infection, 380
    granuloma inguinale, 380
    lymphogranuloma venereum, 380
Infectious lesions, open and closed, 386t
Infective endocarditis (IE), 189–204
  alcoholism and, 191
  antibiotic prophylaxis, 191–193
  bacteremia and, 191
  blood culture and, 199–200
  cardiac lesions, predisposing, 189–191
  chest roentgenograms and, 199
  clinical manifestations of, 193–196
  computerized axial tomographic (CT) scanning and, 197
  definition and epidemiology of, 190b
  dental procedures and, 193
  diagnosis of, blood and other cultures, 199–200
    chest roentgenogram, 199
    echocardiogram, 200
    electrocardiogram, 199
    laboratory tests, 198–199
  drug abusers and, 190
  negative blood cultures and, 203
  neurologic signs of, 196–197
  pathophysiology of, 191b
  peripheral signs of, 197–198
  prophylaxis of, 194t–195t
  rheumatic heart disease and, 189
  Roth's spots and, 197
  staphylococcemia and, 178t
  treatment of, 200–202
    antimicrobial therapy, indications for, 201
    surgical treatment, indications for, 201–202
Inflammation(s), fever and, 160
Influenza, causes of, 71
  complications of, 74
  deaths by pneumonia as complication of, 73
  diseases which mimic, 71
  prophylaxis, 75
  treatment of, 74–75
Influenza A, 75
Influenza B, 75
Influenza immunization, indications for, 74t
Influenza syndrome, 71–76
Influenza viruses, 72b
Inguinal adenopathy. See *Infectious inguinal adenopathy(ies)*
Inguinal intertrigo, 390–392
  causes of, 390
  dermatophytic, 392
  diagnosis of, 390–392
  treatment of, 392
Interstitial pneumonia, 80
Intertrigo, due to *Candida albicans*, 396
  inguinal. See *Inguinal intertrigo*
  of interdigital spaces, 395
Intestinal flukes, 245–246
  Fasciolopsis buski, 245–246
  Heterophyes heterophyes, 246
  Metagonimus yokogawai, 246
Intraorbital infections, 505, 507t
Intrathecal therapy, 486
Intrauterine infections, consequences of, 351t
Intravenous catheter infections, 542
Invader, 1–5
Isolation precautions, categories of, 556t

Jaffe-Lichtenstein tumor, 436
Janeway lesions, 166
　infective endocarditis and, 197
Jarisch-Herxheimer reaction, 346–347

Kala-azar, 571
Kawasaki's syndrome, 428b
　scarlet fever and, 424
Keratitis, 511, 514t–515t
Keratoconjunctivitis, adenovirus, *510*
Kidney, putty, 294
Klebsiella, 285b
Klebsiella pneumoniae, 90–91, 92
　transtracheal aspirate of, *87*
Koplik's spots, 417

Lacrimal apparatus infections, 505, 509t
Lactose dehydrogenase activity (LDH), pleural effusion and, 146
Laminar air flow isolation, 547
Laryngeal, obstruction, 31
　tuberculosis, 31
Laryngitis, 31–35
　diphtheritic, 31, 32
　in adults, 31
　in children, 31–35
　spasmodic, 32, 34–35
　　rhinorrhea and, 24
Laryngotracheobronchitis, necrotizing, 32
　organisms identified in, 32t
　rhinorrhea and, 24
　viral, 32
　treatment of, 32
Lassa fever, 407b
Legionella, 100b
Legionella pneumophila, 94–95, *95*
　clinical features of, 94
　diagnosis of, 95
　treatment of, 95
Legionnaire's disease, 94
Leishmaniasis, 572b
　visceral, 571
Leprosy, *497*
　cardinal neurologic manifestations, 496–497
　diagnosis of, 496
　other clinical manifestations, 497–498
　treatment of, 498
　types of, lepromatous, 496
　　tuberculoid, 496
Leptospira, 478b
Leptospirosis, meningitis due to, 477
Lesions, infectious, open and closed, 386t
Leukemia, myelocytic, acute, 536–538
　clinical examination of, 536–537
　other investigations of, 537
Lincoln Highway of the neck, 55
Lipopolysaccharides (LPS), 183
Listeria bacteremia, 360
Listeria monocytogenes, 361b, 471–472, 545
　diagnosis of, 545
　signs and symptoms of, 545
　treatment of, 545

Liver, abscess and tumor of, difference between, 277–279
　amebic abscess of, 278
　infiltrative lesions of, 275–277
　treatment of abscesses in, 278–279
Liver infections, 267–279
　clinical manifestations of, 267–268
　　fever, 267–268
　　flank pain, 268
　　hepatomegaly, 268
　　jaundice, 268
　diagnostic procedures, 269
　hepatic involvement, types of, 268–269
　treatment, principles of, 269–270
Liver scan, normal, 252
Lobular pneumonia, 80
Ludwig's angina, 62
Lumbar puncture, 452
　clinical indications for, 465
　considerations prior to, 452t
　in diagnosis of *Cryptococcus neoformans*, 544
　Listeria monocytogenes and, 545
　technique for, 465–466
Lung abscess, 88
Lung scan, 79
Lyell's syndrome, 410
Lyme disease, 449b
Lymph node(s), swelling of, 369
Lymph node puncture, 369, 370b
Lymphadenopathy, infectious mononucleosis and, 50
　syphilis and, 339
Lymphangitis, 7
Lymphedema, erysipelas and, 15
Lymphocyte disorders, 532–634
　B-cell immune deficiency, 532–533
　combined B- and T-cell immune deficiency, 533–534
　T-cell immune deficiency, 533
Lymphocytes, atypical, 54b
Lymphocytic choriomeningitis virus, 480–481
Lymphogranuloma venereum (LGV), 326, 329, 380
　diagnosis of, 329
　treatment of, 329

McCoy cells, *322*
Maculopapular rash, 405–408
　rickettsioses, 405–408
　typhoid or paratyphoid fever, 405
Malaria, 154, 560–570, 572b
　chemoprophylaxis and, 566t
　clinical manifestations of, 569
　diagnosis of, 569
　fever in drug addicts and, 168–169
　geographic distribution of, *562*
　prophylaxis and, 567
　treatment of, 570
Malformation(s), anatomic, in young children, 298
Malignant disease, fever and, 160
Mammal bite(s), 11
　infections transmitted by, 14t
Marfan's syndrome, 190, 192
Mastoiditis, 28
　streptococcal pharyngitis and, 44

Maternal, fetal, and neonatal infections, prevalence of, 350t
Measles, 413–420
  circumstances that worsen prognosis, 418
  clinical features of, 417
  complications of, 419
    bronchopneumonias, 419
    hemorrhages, 419
    neurologic complications, 419
    otitis media, 419
    tracheolaryngitis, 419
  differential diagnosis of, 417–418
  epidemics in United States, causes of, 420
  treatment of, 418
  vaccination, 419–420, 566
  vaccine, 419–420
    contraindications, 420
    Edmondston B, 419
    epidemiologic changes associated with, 420
    indications for, 420
    Schwartz type, 419–420
    side effects of, 420
  virus, 417b
Meig's syndrome, 147
Mendelson's syndrome, 96
Meninges, cranial, *459*
Meningitis, acute infectious, 465–487
  aseptic, 67
  bacterial,
    Haemophilus influenzae and, 470–471
    pneumococci and, 468–470
    prophylactic measures in, 486–487
  brucellosis, due to, 477
  candidal, 546
  clear fluid, bacterial cause of, 476–478
    diagnostic guidelines, 476–477
  comparative cerebrospinal fluid findings in, 467t
  differential diagnosis of, 473b
  due to brucellosis, 477
  due to leptospirosis, 477–478
  fungi and, 483
  gram-negative bacilli, 472
  immediate treatment of, 472–476
  level of consciousness in, 473
  meningococcal, 468
    cerebrospinal fluid in, *469*
  nonpurulent or "aseptic," 479–483
  other causes of, 472, 483
    Campylobacter fetus, 472
    Staphylococcus aureus, 472
    Staphylococcus epidermidis, 472
  other forms of, 485–486
  parasites and, 482–483
    amebas, 482–483
  pneumococcal, groups at risk for, 470b
  purulent, 483–485
    antibiotic therapy for, 474t–475t
    first 24 hours of treatment, 483–484
    second to fourth day of treatment, 484–485
    tenth to fourteenth day and after, 485
  tuberculous, 114, 546
    clinical features of, 478
    laboratory and diagnostic tests for, 478–479
    treatment of, 479
  viruses, 479–482
    enteroviruses, 480
    herpes simplex, 481
    lymphocytic choriomeningitis, 480–481
    mumps, 480
    mycoplasma, 481
Meningococcemia, 182
  cutaneous hemorrhagic eruption and, 404
Meningococci, 469b
Meningoencephalitis, 67, 479
  viral, 546
Mesothelioma, neoplastic effusions and, 147
Metapneumonic effusions, 149
Microbe, 1–5
Microbiology laboratory, indications for use of, 24
Moniliasis, 68
  oral, 68–69
    acute, 68–69
    chronic, 68–69
    chronic hyperplastic candidiasis, 69
    severe, 68
Monoarthritis, cause of low-grade, 445
Mononucleosis, infectious, 47, 50–53
  diagnosis of, 52
  pharyngitis and, *51*
  polyadenopathy and, 381
  serological tests in, 55
  treatment of, 53
  without heterophile antibody, 52–53
Monospot, 51
Monosticon, 51
Monotest, 47, 51
Moraxella, 503b
Mucocutaneous lymph node syndrome. See *Kawasaki's syndrome*
Mucormycosis, 142
Mucoviscidosis, 27
Mumps, 67–68, 480
  treatment of, 67
Mumps orchitis, 67
Murphy's sign, 268, 269
Mycobacteria of medical importance, 114t
Mycobacterial disease, disseminated, 542–543
Mycobacterium tuberculosis, biologic properties of, 123b
  characteristic appearance of, *121*
Mycoplasma, 481
Mycoplasma hominis, 324
Mycoplasma pneumoniae, 85, 92–94
  Guillain-Barré syndrome and, 495
  presumptive diagnosis of, 93
Mycoplasma T. See *Ureaplasma urealyticum*
Mycosis, pulmonary. See *Pulmonary mycosis*
Myeloma, multiple, 543–544
  causes of infection, 543–544
  treatment of fever and sepsis, 544
Myocarditis, Chagas, 211–212
  treatment of, 212
  diphtheria and, 49, 212–213
    treatment of, 212–213
  pericarditis and, 205–213
  viral, 210–211
    clinical manifestations of, 210–211
    treatment of, 211
Mycosis, pulmonary. See *Pulmonary mycosis*
Myositis, 18–19
Myringitis, bullous, 29

antibiotic treatment of, 30
Myringotomy, 31
Myxovirus influenzae, 71
   kinds of type A, 72t
   schematic diagram of type A, 73

Nafcillin, 17
Nails, infections of, 395–397
Necrosis, hepatocellular, diagnosis of, 270
Neisseria gonorrhoeae, 4, 308, 311, *312*, 331b
   pelvic inflammatory disease and, 317
   penicillinase-producing (PPNG), 312
Neisseria meningitidis, serogroup A, 468
Neonatal disease and vaginal flora, 362t
Neonatal eye infections, 363t
Neoplasms, 147
Nephrostomy, 300
Nephrotic syndrome, erysipelas and, 15
Nephrotomography during intravenous urogram, *290*
Nervous system, peripheral, infections affecting, 489–499
Neuritis, optic, 518
Neuropathy, alimentary disorders in infants and, 489
Neurosyphilis, 346
   asymptomatic, 345
Neutropenia, 531–532
   bacteria-killing defects, 532
   causes of fever in, 537–538
   chemotactic defects in, 531–532
   diagnosis of, 538–541
      endoscopic study and biopsy in, 539
      laboratory techniques in, 539
      noninfectious disorders, 541
      problems in, 539
      serologic studies in, 540–541
   empiric treatment of fever in, 538t
   fever and, causes of, 537–538
      treatment of, 537–538
   impaired opsonization, 532
Neutrophil function testing, 536
Node(s), Osler's, 166
   infective endocarditis and, 197
Nonbacterial thrombotic endocarditis (NBTE), 191
Nosocomial infections, 551–560
   bacterial pathogens of, 553t
   consequences of, 552b
   definition and incidence of, 551
   methods to strengthen host defenses against, 558t
   natural resistance in bacterial species and antibiotics that act as selectors, 553t
   nosocomial pathogens and, 552–554
   occurrence of, by site and hospital service, 552t
   reducing risk of, 554–560
      aseptic technique and hygiene, 555
      care of intravenous and intravascular catheters, 557
      care of urinary catheters, 557
      handling of respiratory therapy equipment, 558–560
      hospital procedures in, 557–560
      isolation precautions, 555–557
      sterilization and disinfection technique, 555
   risk factors, 551–552
   Staphylococcus aureus and, 553

strengthening host defenses, 560
Nursing, restrictions on antibiotics during, 365–366

Onychomycosis, 395–397
   candida, 397
   dermatophytic, *397*
Ophthalmitis, 363
Opsonization, 5–6
   impaired, 532
Optic nerve, infections of, 518t
Oral bacterial flora, predominant, 62t
Oral infections, 61–69
Organisms found in nose and oropharynx, 24t
Osteitis, 28
Osteomyelitis, 165
   chronic, 441–442
   hematogenous. See *Hematogenous osteomyelitis*
   vertebral, 440–441, *442*
      bacteriologic and surgical diagnosis of, 441
      clinical and radiologic signs of, 441
Osteomyelitis, acute, 434–436
   criteria for cure, 438
      therapeutic failure, 438–439
   diagnosis of, 435–436
   diagnostic principles, 434–435
   monitoring of therapeutic efficacy, 437–438
   treatment of, 436–439
Otitis, 28–30
   clinical signs of, 29–30
   pathogenesis of, 28–29
Otitis media, acute, 28
   antibiotic treatment of, 30
   treatment of, 30
   measles and, 419
   right-sided, *460*
   streptococcal pharyngitis and, 44

Palsy(ies), ocular, 489
   peripheral facial, 489
Paracoccidioides brasiliensis, 134
Paralysis, diphtheritic, 498
Parameningeal infections, 451–463
Parasite(s), blood-borne, slide of, 569b
   facultative intracellular, biologic properties and their meaning, 371t
Paresis, 340
Paronychia, 389
Parotitis, 67
   purulent, 67
Pasteurella multocida, 12
Pasteurella multocida cellulitis, treatment of, 17
Pasteurellosis, 375
Pediculosis pubis, 331–333
   diagnosis of, 333
   treatment of, 333
Pelvic infections, 253–254
Pelvic inflammatory disease (PID), 313, 317–318
Penicillin, cellulitis and, 17
   mammal bites and, 12
Peptostreptococcus, 16
Perianal infections, 543
Pericardial constriction, pericardectomy in, 208
Pericardial effusion, 205–208

Pericardial effusion (Continued)
  bidimensional echocardiogram showing, 206, 207
  subcostal view of, 207
Pericarditis, acute, treatment of, 205
  bacterial, 209
  dry, 205
  fibrinous, 205, 208
  fibrous, 205, 208
    treatment of, 208
  myocarditis and, 205–213
  other types of infectious, 210
  tuberculous, 209–210
    treatment of, 210
  viral, 208–209
    coxsackievirus A and, 208
    treatment of, 209
Pericoronitis, 61
Periodontitis, 62, 64
  advanced, 63
    treatment of, 63
  chronic, 63
  rapidly advancing, 63
Peritonitis, secondary, 249–250
  spontaneous, 16, 250
Pertussis, 105–108
  clinical features of, 105
  diagnosis of, 107
  neurologic complications in, 106–107
  paroxysmal respiratory insufficiency in, 106
  pulmonary complications in, 106
  serious, indications of, 106
  treatment of, 107
  vaccination for, 108
  vaccine, complications from, 108
Petechiae, subconjunctival, 197
Phagocytosis, 5–7
Pharyngitis, 37
  antibiotic therapy in, 37
  causes of, 38t
  diagnosis of, 44
  diphtheritic, 47
  in course of infectious mononucleosis, 51
  scarlet fever and, 38
  streptococcal,
    indications for throat culture and, 40
    otitis media and, 44
    use of penicillin in, 44–45
  uncertainty of clinical diagnosis of, 38–40
  viral origin of, 38
Pharyngotonsillitis, streptococcal, treatment of, 44–45
Phthirus pubis, 331
Pinta, 407
Pinworm, 243
  infection, 238
  treatment of, 246–247
Placoid epithelial disorder, 525
Plague, 375
  immunization, 567
Plasmid-mediated bacterial resistance, frequency of, 559t
Plasmodium vivax, 168
Pleural effusion, 145–151
  clinical features of, 146
  culture media for, 149
  laboratory values in, 146–147

  major types of, 148t
  metapneumonic, 151
  microorganisms responsible for, 149–150
  pulmonary infections and, 149
  radiographic features of, 146
  tuberculous, 147–149, 150–151
Pleurisy, tuberculous, 114, 117
Pneumatocele and pyopneumothorax typical of pleuropulmonary infection, 111
Pneumococci, and bacterial meningitis, 468–470
Pneumonia(s), 78
  acute, in adults, 77–101
    in children, 103–111
  aspiration, 96–98
    diphtheria and, 49
  atypical, defined, 92
    diagnosis and treatment of, 92–96
    useful features in diagnosis of, 93t
  bacterial, failure of therapy in, 99
    influenza and, 74
  Bacteroides melaninogenicus, due to, 97
  causes of therapeutic failures during, 99t
  community-acquired, etiologic diagnosis of, 86
  clinical findings in, 79
  due to *Bacteroides melaninogenicus*, 97
  due to *Pneumocystis carinii*, 540
  etiologic diagnosis of, 79
  exposure to cold and, 78
  fever in drug addicts and, 165
  hospital-acquired, etiologic diagnosis of, 91
    treatment of, 92
  in aged, 78
  in immunocompromised host, 239
  in immunosuppressed patients, treatment of, 541t, 542
  indications for chest roentgenogram, 77
  interstitial, 80
  invasive investigations, 86
  laboratory tests for, 81–86
    blood count, 81–83
    blood culture, 83
    pleural fluid examination, 83, 86
    sputum examination and culture, 83
  lobar (alveolar), 80
  lobular (bronchopneumonia), 80
  major causes of, 80t
  necrotizing, principal bacteria responsible for, 85t
  other causes of, 91
  parasitic infections and, 81
  pneumococcal, 82, 88
    mortality rates in, 89t
  possible responsible organisms in, 81t
  radiologic findings in, 79–80
  risk factors in, 77–78
  staphylococcal, 84, 91
  viral, causes of, 96t
    influenza and, 74
Pneumonitis, helminthiasis and, 239
Poliomyelitis, acute anterior (AAP), alimentary disorders in infants and, 489
  clinical manifestations of, 491–492
  differential diagnosis of, 492t
  epidemiologic considerations, 492–493
  Guillain-Barré syndrome and, difference between, 491
  immunization, 566

laboratory findings, 493
preventive measures when identified, 494–495
  primary vaccination, 494–495
  revaccination, 495
vaccination, 493
  attenuated live vaccine, 494
  inactivated vaccine, 493–494
viral, 95–96
Polyadenopathy, infectious, causes of, 380–382
  mononucleosis and, 381
  other infections and, 382
  skin eruptions and, 380–381
  toxoplasmosis and, 381
noninfectious and non-neoplastic inflammatory, 382
superficial, 381t
Polyarthritis, 447–449
Polypnea, fever and, 153
Postcardiotomy syndrome, 147
Postoperative infections, 317
Pregnancy, aminoglycosides and, 365
  antituberculous agents and, 365
  chlamydiae and, infections caused by, 361
  chloramphenicol and, 366
  genital infections in, 361
  infection and, 349–368
  rash in, 361
  recommended antibiotics during, 366–367
  restrictions on antibiotics during, 365–366
  sulfonamides and, 366
  tetracycline and, 365–366
  Trichomonas vaginalis and, 307–308, *310*
  use of antimicrobial agents during, 582
Prenatal and neonatal infections, clinical manifestations of, 352t
Prophylaxis, abdominal surgical procedures and, 264t–265t
  malaria and, 567
  rabies and, 12
  wound infections and, 7
Prostatitis, 288–289, 298, 318
  acute bacterial, 288, 324
    treatment of, 325
  causes of, 324
  chronic bacterial, 288, 324
    treatment of, 325–326
  clinical manifestations of, 289
  diagnosis of, 325
  diagnostic tests for, 289
  nonbacterial, 288–289
  prostatodynia, 325
    treatment of, 326
Prostatodynia, 289, 325
Prosthetics, bone or joint, infection adjacent to, 439–440
  valve endocarditis and, 202–203
Protein electrophoresis, 160
Proteus, 286b
Proteus species, cellulitis and, 15
Pseudomembranous enterocolitis (PMEC), 233–235
  clinical features of, 234–235
  clostridial versus staphylococcal enterocolitis, 235
  diagnosis of, 235
  treatment of, 235
Pseudomonas, 555b
Pseudomonas aeruginosa, 92

ecthyma gangrenosum and, 411
Pseudomonas cepacia, 92
Pseudomonas species, 26
  cellulitis and, 15
Pulmonary edema, 79
Pulmonary embolism, 78–79
  fever and, 156
Pulmonary infections, pleural effusions and, 149
Pulmonary infiltrate-eosinophilia syndrome, causes of, 81
Pulmonary infiltrates, evidence of, 78
Pulmonary mycosis, 125–143
  acute, 126
  bat droppings and, 125
  bird droppings and, 125
  chronic, 126–127
  diagnosis of, 125
  disseminated, 127
  specific, diagnosis of, 127–130
    selected features of, 131t
  therapy of, 139t
Pulpitis, 61
Punch biopsy, 15
Pupil, Argyll-Robertson, 340
Purified protein derivative (PPD), 113
Purified protein derivative (PPD) test, 566
Pus, 1, 26, 28
  dishwater, 20
  in sinusitis, 25
Pyelography, 293
Pyelonephritis, *291*
  acute, 289–292, 299–300
  chronic, 292
  diagnosis of, 292–294
Pyoderma gangrenosum and chronic cutaneous ulcers, 400
Pyorrhea. See *Periodontitis*

Rabies, 12, 13b
  measures in suspected, 14t
  prophylaxis, 12
  vaccines for, 13–14
    duck embryo vaccine (DEV), 13
    human diploid cell culture (HDCV), 13
Rapid Plasma Reagin (RPR), 326, 342
Rash(es), infections with, 403–429
  in pregnancy, 361
  lesions, types of, 411–413
    macules, 411–413
    papules, 413
    petechiae, 413
    vesicles, 413
  maculopapular, infectious diseases producing, 415t
Rectal infections, 543
Red eardrums, 29
Reiter's syndrome, 447
Respiratory infections, principal viruses implicated in, 22t
Respiratory syncytial virus (RSV), 103, 104b
Respiratory tract, viral infections of, 22t
Reye's syndrome, 458
  viral hepatitis and, 273
Rhagades, 341
Rheumatic fever (RF), 43

Rheumatic fever (RF) *(Continued)*
  acute, 447–448
  severe pharyngitis and, 40
  streptococcal pharyngitis and, 45
Rheumatic heart disease, infective endocarditis and, 189
Rheumatoid arthritis (RA), immune effusions and, 147
Rhinitis, 21–25
Rhinorrhea, 21–25
  as sign of coryza, 21
  cough and, 23
  earache and, 23–24
  fever and, 23
  headache and, 24
  laryngitis and, 31
  laryngotracheobronchitis and, 24
  persistent or bloody, 22–23
  respiratory difficulty and, 24
  sore throat and, 23
Rickettsia, 407b, 479
  infections caused by, 409t
Ringworm of scalp, 398
Ritter's disease, 408
Rocky Mountain spotted fever, 405, 407, 479
Roentgenogram(s), abdominal, 236, 252, 255
  bone and joint infections and, 432–433
  chest. See *Chest roentgenogram(s)*
Roseola infantum, 422
Rotavirus(es), 224, 230–231
Roth's spots, infective endocarditis and, 197
Roundworms, intestinal, 240–244
  Ascaris lumbricoides, 243–244
  hookworms, 244
  pinworms, 240–241
  Strongyloides stercoralis, 244
  whipworms, 241
Rubella, 421–422
  congenital, 354
    diagnosis of, 356, 357b
    prevention of, 356
    risk of infection, 356
  diagnosis of, 421
  transmission of, 421
Rubella immunization, 422–423
  indications for, 423
  nasal instillation, 423
  subcutaneous injection, 422–423
  side effects of, 423
Rubella virus, 356b

Sabin-Feldman dye test, 350
Salmonella, 226
Salmonella typhi carrier, 215
  management of, 219
Salmonellosis, 226–227
  clinical features of, 226–227
  epidemiology of, 226b
  treatment of, 227
Sao Paulo fever, 407
Sarcoidosis, hepatitis and, 277
Sarcoma, Ewing's, 436
Scalded skin syndrome, toxic epidermal necrolysis versus, 410t
Scalp infections, 397–398
  diagnosis of, 397–398
  treatment of, 398
Scarlet fever, 423–425
  clinical features of, 424
  differential diagnosis of, 424
  Kawasaki's syndrome and, 424
  pharyngitis and, 38
  toxic shock syndrome and, 424
  treatment of, 424–425
Schick test, 50, 51b
Schistosoma haematobium, 5
Schistosomiasis, 277, 571, 572b
  geographic distribution of, 562
  urinary tract, 285–286
Sclera and episclera, infections of, 518
Septic arthritis, 445–447
  antibiotic therapy for, 445–446
  frequency of infecting organisms in, by age, 444t
  haemophilus influenzae and, 446
  mobilization, 447
  other therapeutic measures, 446–447
  treatment of, in adults, 446t
Septic shock, 177
  consequences of, 181–182
  disseminated intravascular coagulation and, 182
  endotoxin and, 183b
Septicemia, 7, 78
  antibiotic treatment for, 182
  bacteremia and, 171–187
  blood cultures and, 171
    number of, 172
    timing of, 172–173
  cause of shock in, 181t
  cutaneous signs of, 175t
  due to gram-negative bacilli, 184–186
  etiologic probabilities according to portal of entry of, 174t
  infection, drainage of, 184
  initial treatment for, 182–184
  localization and complications of, 175t
  pneumococcal and gram-negative, 403–404
  shock and, 180–182
  Staphylococcus aureus and, 186
    treatment of, 186
  treatment of, 184–186
Serotherapy, in diphtheria, 48
Serratia, 286b
Serratia marcescens, 92, 286
Serum haptoglobins test, 160
Serum iron test, 160
Sexually transmitted diseases, 304t
Shigella, 225b
  group A, 225
  group B, 225
Shigellosis, 224–226
  clinical features of, 225
  diagnosis of, 225
  treatment of, 225
Ship's wheel cell, 134
Shock, cold, 181
  identifying cause of, 180–181
  measures against, 182–184
  recognizing, 180
  septic. See *Septic shock*
  septicemia and, 180–182, 181t
  warm, 181

Shock lung, 181–182
Sinusitis, 25–28
  bilateral maxillary, 26
  clinical signs of, 25
  common acute, 26–27
  ethmoid, 25
  maxillary, dental infections and, 27
  microbiologic diagnosis of, 25–26
  nasal discharge in, purulent, 25
  relapsing, 27–28
  severe, 28
  sphenoid, 25
  streptococcal pharyngitis and, 44
Skin infections, primary, 385–401
Skin lesions, syphilis and, 338
  types of, 411–413
Skin testing, 535–536
Sleeping sickness, 571
Smallpox vaccination, 562–564
Sore throat, fever and, 37–59
  rhinorrhea and, 23
Spanish flu, 74
Sporothrix schenckii, 134
Sporotrichosis, 138
Stamey test, 330
Staphylococcal infections, predisposing causes for, 6t
Staphylococcal pleuropulmonary infections (SPPI),
  clinical features and diagnosis of, 110
  treatment and care of, 110–111
Staphylococcemia, 177
  infective endocarditis and, 178t
Staphylococcus aureus, 1–5, 16, 26, 74, 177
  cellulitis and, 15
  distinctive characteristics of, 6
  nosocomial infection and, 553
  osteomyelitis and, 437
  pathogenicity of, 4–5
    factors linked to, 5t
  purulent parotitis and, 67
  pus from abscess due to, 2
  septicemia and, 186
  spinal epidural abscess and, 462
Staphylococcus epidermidis, 5
  distinctive characteristics of, 6t
Staphylococcus infection, malignant (facial), 16
Stomatitis, aphthous, 65
Stools, microscopic examination of, 224b
  normal, bacteria found in, 225t
Stools of infant, normal or diarrheal, value and mean composition of fecal losses of water and electrolytes in, 222t
Streptococcal infection(s), 363–364
  early neonatal, 363–364
  group A, 42t
  late neonatal, 364
Streptococcus, group A, enzymes and toxins secreted by, 43t
  erysipelas and, 15
  impetigo and, 23
  laboratory diagnosis of, 43
  laboratory procedures in, 41–43
  necrotizing fasciitis and, 19
  pharyngitis and, 37
  possible sequelae and, relationship between, 42t
  throat culture, technique for, 41

  two key antigens in, 42t
  group B, neonatal sepsis and meningitis and, 471
  group D, 286b
Streptococcus pneumoniae, 16, 74, 86–90, 89b
  cellulitis and, 15
  sinusitis and, 26
Streptococcus pyogenes, 16, 26, *40*, 41b
  cellulitis and, 15
  group B, chains of, 39
Strongyloides stercoralis, 543
  larva in feces, *242*
Strongyloidiasis, 543
  treatment of, 247–248
Sulfonamides, pregnancy and, 366
Swan-Ganz catheter, 79
Syndrome(s). See *specific syndromes*
Synergy, microbial, mechanisms of, 259b
Synovial fluid, chemical analysis and cell count of, 443
  composition of, in articular disorders, 444t
  microbiologic examination of, 443–445
    other microbiologic tests, 444–445
Syphilis, 335–348, 360
  chronic cutaneous ulcers and, 400
  congenital, 341
    serosanguineous discharge and, 23
  dark-field microscopic examination, 341–342
  diagnosis of latent, 344–345
  epidemiology of, 347b
  generalized rash, 338–340
    acute lymphocytic meningitis, 339
    alopecia, 339
    cerebrovascular accident in young person, 339–340
    Condyloma latum, 339
    course of, 339
    lymphadenopathy, generalized, 339
    mucous membrane lesions, 338–339
  pathogenesis and stages of, 337b
  primary, course of, 337
    extragenital lesions, 336
    genital lesions, 335–336
    regional adenopathy, 337
  secondary, 337–340
  serologic response to therapy, 347
  serologic tests, 342–344
    congenital syphilis, 344
    incubating syphilis, 343
    late syphilis, 343
    latent syphilis, 343
    primary syphilis, 343
    secondary syphilis, 343
    syphilis in pregnancy, 344
  sexual partners of patients with, 335
  tertiary, dementia (general paralysis), 340
    destructive skin and bone lesions, 340
    peripheral neuropathy, 340
    posterior column disease, 340
    proximal aortic and aortic valvular disease, 340–341
  treatment of, 345–347
Syphilitic chancre, *326*, *336*
  diagnosis of, 326
Syphilitic mucous plaques, *339*
Syphilitic papule, 338

Systemic lupus erythematosus (SLE), immune effusions and, 147

Taenia proglottids, 243
Taenia saginata, 245
Tampons. See Toxic shock syndrome
Tapeworm infections, treatment of, 248
Tapeworms, intestinal, 244–245
  beef and pork, 245
  dwarf, 245
  fish, 244–245
Tetanus, 8–11
  fever in drug addicts and, 167
  muscle spasms in, 9, 10
  prevention of, 11
  recognizing at outset, 11
  smiling and surprised look in, 12
Tetanus antitoxins, 9–11
  heterologous (horse), 10
  homologous (human), 10
Tetanus immunization, 566
  practical program of, 13t
  primary series, 10t
    comparison of, 10
Tetanus infections, 7
Tetracycline, pregnancy and, 365–366
Therapeutic response, ways to monitor, 586–587
Throat culture, in diphtheria, 48
  indications for, 40
  interpretation of results of, 43–44
  technique for, 41
Thrombophlebitis, 167
  fever and, 156
  heparin therapy in, 156
  in drug users, 163
  intracranial, 462–463
    clinical features of, 462
    diagnosis of, 462–463
    treatment of, 463
Thrush, 68
Tick, brush, 405–408
  dog, 405–408
  paralysis, diagnosis of, 495–496
Tick-borne infections, 379
Tinea capitis, 397–398
Tinea circinata, 393
Tinea versicolor, 393–395, 394
Tobia fever, 407
Tonsillitis, 37
  causes of, 38t
  due to group A streptococci, diagnosis of, 44
TORCH groups, 350
Toxic shock syndrome, 410–411
  scarlet fever and, 424
Toxocara canis infection, 527
Toxoplasma gondii, 354b, 545–546
  diagnosis of, 545–546
  signs and symptoms of, 545
  transmission of, 355
  treatment of, 546
Toxoplasmosis, 373
  congenital, 350–354
    diagnosis of, 350–351
    incidence of, 353t

prevalence and prevention of, 351–354
  therapy for, 351
polyadenopathy and, 381
Tracheolaryngitis, measles and, 419
Tracheostomy, in laryngotracheobronchitis, 32
  in spasmodic laryngitis, 35
Transtracheal aspiration, 86
Transudates and exudates, distinction between, 146–147
Travelers to tropical countries, precautions for, 566t
Trench mouth, 63
Treponema pallidum, 308, 342b
  hemagglutinating antibodies (TPHA) test, 326
  microhemagglutination test for (MHATP), 343
Treponematoses, nonvenereal, 346b
Trichinosis, 212, 213b
Trichomonas vaginalis, 307, 308, 310
  pregnancy and, 361
  urethritis and, 321
  vaginitis and, 316
Trismus, 11b, 55
  absence of, 56, 57
Tropical countries, travel to, 561–573
  vaccinations for, 561–567
Tropical diseases, fever and, 157
  likely to infect travelers, 564t
Tropical infections, in travelers, 572b
  mode of transmission and prevention of, 565t
Trypanosoma cruzi, 210, 211
Trypanosomiasis, 572b
  African, 571
  American, 571
Tubercle, 122
Tuberculosis, annual risk of development of, 120t
  bilateral ulcerocaseous, 116
  diagnostic examinations in, 118t
  hepatitis and, 277
  laryngeal, 31
  miliary, 114, 115–117, 116
  prevention of, 120–124
  reducing incidence of infection, 120
  renal, 295
  testing for, 566
  urinary, 294
Tuberculosis, primary, 113–114
  adenopathy and pneumatelectasis during, 115
  infiltration of medial lobe in, 114
Tuberculosis, pulmonary, 113–124
  diagnosis of, 117–118
    bacteriologic studies, 118
    tuberculin skin test, 117–118
  reactivated, 117
  treatment of, 118–120
    drug therapy in, 119–120
  urinary. See Urinary tuberculosis
Tuberculous granuloma, 121
  pericarditis, 209–210
Tuberculous infection, tuberculous disease and, 124
Tularemia, 373–374
Tumors caused by viruses, benign, 330–331
  diagnosis of, 330–331
  treatment of, 331
Turista, 227
Tympanometry, 29
Typhoid fever, 215–219, 226, 405

clinical features of, 216, 217t
complications, treatment of, 218
cross-infection, prevention of, 218–219
epidemiology, 215–216
laboratory methods, direct, 216
  indirect, 216–217
psychiatric symptoms and, 216
specific treatment, 218
supportive treatment, 218
treatment of, 217–219
typhoid carrier state and, chemotherapy of, 218t
Typhoid immunization, 566
Typhus, epidemic, 405, 408
  scrub, 405, 408
Tzanck test, 327

Ulcer(s), aphthous, 66, 66t
  chronic cutaneous, 398–401, 399t
    clinical features of, 398
    diagnosis of, 398–401
    self-inflicted injuries and, 400
    treatment of, 400–401
  corneal, 516
  dendritic, *516*
  genital, 309t
  herpetic, 66, 66t
  male genital, 318
  malignant, 401
  oral, HSV and, 541
  pyoderma gangrenosum and chronic cutaneous, 400
  staphylococcal corneal, *516*
  tertiary syphilis of, *400*
  vascular, 401
    treatment of, 401
Urethral and arthritic syndromes, differential diagnosis of, 448t
Urethral syndrome, 313
Urethritis, 300, 318
  cause of, 318–319
  gonococcal, clinical manifestations of, 319
    microbiologic features, 319
    treatment of, 319–320
  male, causes of in, 319t
  nongonococcal, 322
    Candida albicans, 321
    Chlamydia trachomatis, 320–321
    herpesvirus hominis, 322
    miscellaneous bacterial causes, 321–322
    Reiter's syndrome, 322
    treatment of, 322–324
    Trichomonas vaginalis, 321
    Ureaplasma urealyticum, 321
  treatment of, 319
Urethritis syndrome, postgonococcal, 320
Urinalysis, 283b
  interpretation of culture, 283–284
Urinary tract infections, 281–301
  antimicrobial agents in treatment of, 297t–298t
  catheter-associated, 557
  factors precluding short-term treatment of, 298t
  follow up treatment of, 300
  frequency of bacteria responsible for, 289t
  general measures, 296–300
  in different groups of patients, 281–282

    aged individuals, 282
    children, 281–282
    diabetics, 282
    individuals who have had invasive examinations, 282
    older men, 282
    women, 282
  in elderly patients, 299
  organisms that cause, 286b
  recurrent, in women, 299
  schistosomiasis and, 277, 571, 572b
  signs and symptoms of, 281
  symptomatic, disorders in young women, 286–288
    genitourinary tuberculosis, 284
    obstruction, 284–285
    other causes of, without bacteriuria, 288
    renal abscesses, 285
    suppressed infections, 284
    urethral syndrome, 284
    urinary tract schistosomiasis, 285–286
    viral cystitis, 286
  treatment of, 296
    duration of, 296
  with *Proteus mirabilis*, 287
Urinary tuberculosis, 294
  diagnostic tests, 294
    culture, 294
    needle biopsy, 294–296
    radiography, 294
Urine collection,
  clean-catch method of, 282–283
    in infants, 282
    suprapubic puncture, 282
  in patients with urinary catheters, 282–283
Urine sample, delivery of to laboratory, 283
Uveal tract and retina, infections of, 519t–523t, 528
Uveitis, anterior, *524*

Vaccination(s),
  smallpox, 562–564
  travel to tropical countries and, 561–567
Vaginitis, 313–316
  Candida albicans, 313–316
  causes of, 311
  Gardnerella vaginalis, 316
  general considerations, 316
  Trichomonas vaginalis, 316
Varicella (chickenpox), 425–427
  clinical features of, 425
  differential diagnosis of, 425
  other measures, 427
  preventive measures, 426–427
  treatment and complications of, 425–426
Varicella syndrome, severe, 426–427
Varicella-zoster infections, 359–360, 455
Vector(s), arthropod, 563
Venereal Disease Research Laboratory (VDRL), 326, 339, 342
Venereal infections, epidemiologic control of, 303–305
Venereal warts, 318
Vibrio parahaemolyticus, cellulitis and, 15
Vibro fetus, 472
Viral capsid antigen (VCA), 52–53
Viral hemorrhagic fevers, 406t

Viral infections, recurrent, 534
Viral myocarditis, 210–211
Viral pericarditis, 210–211
Viral pneumonias, 95–96
    causes of, 96
    influenza, 72b
    norwalk-like, 231
    rubella, 356b
    tumors caused by, 330–331
Visceral leishmaniasis, geographic distribution of, 563

Waterhouse-Friderichsen syndrome, 182
Weil-Felix reaction, 408
Weil's disease, 477
Widal reaction, 217
World Health Organization (WHO), 561, 562
Worms, passing of, 237–238

Wound infection prophylaxis, purpose of, 7
Wound infections, 1–20, 256–258. See also *Infection(s)*
    factors contributing to, 7
    patient, 5–7
    prevention of, 7–11
Wright's technique, 180

Yeasts and molds with dimorphic fungi, comparison of, 142t
Yellow fever, viral hepatitis and, 273
Yellow fever vaccination, 564
Yersinia, infections with, 448–449

Ziehl-Neelsen sputum stain, 118
Zoster infection and relapsing herpes infection, difference between, 427–428
Zygomycetes, 137